Springer Series in Statistics

Springer Series in Statistics

(continued after index)

Frank E. Harrell, Jr.

Regression Modeling Strategies

With Applications to Linear Models, Logistic Regression, and Survival Analysis

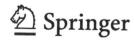 Springer

Frank E. Harrell, Jr.
Department of Biostatistics
Vanderbilt University School of Medicine
S-2323 MCN 2158
Nashville, TN 37232-2637
f.harrell@vanderbilt.edu

Library of Congress Cataloging-in-Publication Data
Harrell, Jr., Frank E.
    Regression modeling strategies : with applications to linear models, logistic regression,
and survival analysis / Frank E. Harrell, Jr.
        p.   cm. — (Springer series in statistics)
    Includes bibliographical references and index.
    ISBN 0-387-95232-2 (alk. paper)
    1. Regression analysis.   2. Linear models (Statistics).   3. Logistic regression.   4. Survival
analysis.   I. Title.   II. Series.
    QA278.2 .H387 2001
    519.5′36—dc21   2001020045

SAS is a registered trademark of SAS Institute Inc.
S-Plus is registered trademark of Insightful Corporation.

ISBN-10: 0-387-95232-2
ISBN-13: 978-0387-95232-1

Printed on acid-free paper.

Printed in the United States of America.   (EB)

9 8 7

springer.com

To the memories of Frank E. Harrell, Sr., Richard Jackson, L. Richard Smith, and John Burdeshaw, and with appreciation to Lea Anne and Charlotte Harrell and to two high school math teachers: Ms. Gaston and Mr. Christian.

Preface

There are many books that are excellent sources of knowledge about individual statistical tools (survival models, general linear models, etc.), but the art of data analysis is about choosing and using multiple tools. In the words of Chatfield [69, p. 420] "...students typically know the technical details of regression for example, but not necessarily when and how to apply it. This argues the need for a better balance in the literature and in statistical teaching between *techniques* and problem solving *strategies.*" Whether analyzing risk factors, adjusting for biases in observational studies, or developing predictive models, there are common problems that few regression texts address. For example, there are missing data in the majority of datasets one is likely to encounter (other than those used in textbooks!) but most regression texts do not include methods for dealing with such data effectively, and most texts on missing data do not cover regression modeling.

This book links standard regression modeling approaches with

- methods for relaxing linearity assumptions that still allow one to easily obtain predictions and confidence limits for future observations, and to do formal hypothesis tests,

- nonadditive modeling approaches not requiring the assumption that interactions are always linear × linear,

- methods for imputing missing data and for penalizing variances for incomplete data,

- methods for handling large numbers of predictors without resorting to problematic stepwise variable selection techniques,

- data reduction methods (some of which are based on multivariate psychometric techniques too seldom used in statistics) that help with the problem of "too many variables to analyze and not enough observations" as well as making the model more interpretable when there are predictor variables containing overlapping information,

- methods for quantifying predictive accuracy of a fitted model,

- powerful model validation techniques based on the bootstrap, that allow the analyst to estimate predictive accuracy nearly unbiasedly without holding back data from the model development process, and

- graphical methods for understanding complex models.

On the last point, this text has special emphasis on what could be called "presentation graphics for fitted models" to help make regression analyses more palatable to nonstatisticians. For example, nomograms have long been used to make equations portable, but they are not drawn routinely because doing so is very labor intensive. An S language (S-Plus or R) function called `nomogram` in the library described below draws nomograms from a regression fit, and these diagrams can be used to communicate modeling results as well as to obtain predicted values manually even in the presence of complex variable transformations.

Most of the methods in this text apply to all regression models, but special emphasis is given to some of the most popular ones: multiple regression using least squares, the binary logistic model, two logistic models for ordinal responses, parametric survival regression models, and the Cox semiparametric survival model. There is also a chapter on nonparametric transform-both-sides regression. Emphasis is given to detailed case studies for these methods as well as for data reduction, imputation, model simplification, and other tasks. The majority of examples are from biomedical research. However, the methods presented here have broad application to other areas including economics, epidemiology, sociology, psychology, engineering, and predicting consumer behavior and other business outcomes.

This text is intended for Masters or PhD level graduate students who have had a general introductory probability and statistics course and who are well versed in ordinary multiple regression and intermediate algebra. The book is also intended to serve as a reference for data analysts and statistical methodologists. Readers without a strong background in applied statistics may wish to first study one of the many introductory applied statistics and regression texts that are available; Katz' small book on multivariable analysis[232] is especially helpful to clinicians and epidemiologists. The paper by Nick and Hardin[325] also provides a good introduction to multivariable modeling and interpretation.

The overall philosophy of this book is summarized by the following statements.

- Satisfaction of model assumptions improves precision and increases statistical power.

- It is more productive to make a model fit step by step (e.g., transformation estimation) than to postulate a simple model and find out what went wrong.

- Graphical methods should be married to formal inference.

- Overfitting occurs frequently, so data reduction and model validation are important.

- In most research projects the cost of data collection far outweighs the cost of data analysis, so it is important to use the most efficient and accurate modeling techniques, to avoid categorizing continuous variables, and to not remove data from the estimation sample just to be able to validate the model.

- The bootstrap is a breakthrough for statistical modeling, and the analyst should use it for many steps of the modeling strategy, including derivation of distribution-free confidence intervals and estimation of optimism in model fit that takes into account variations caused by the modeling strategy.

- Imputation of missing data is better than discarding incomplete observations.

- Variance often dominates bias, so biased methods such as penalized maximum likelihood estimation yield models that have a greater chance of accurately predicting future observations.

- Carefully fitting an improper model is better than badly fitting (and overfitting) a well-chosen one.

- Methods that work for all types of regression models are the most valuable.

- Using the data to guide the data analysis is almost as dangerous as not doing so.

- There are benefits to modeling by deciding how many degrees of freedom (i.e., number of regression parameters) can be "spent," deciding where they should be spent, and then spending them.

On the last point, the author believes that significance tests and P-values are problematic, especially when making modeling decisions. Judging by the increased emphasis on confidence intervals in scientific journals there is reason to believe that hypothesis testing is gradually being deemphasized. Yet the reader will notice that this text contains many P-values. How does that make sense when, for example, the text recommends against simplifying a model when a test of linearity is not significant? First, some readers may wish to emphasize hypothesis testing in general, and some hypotheses have special interest, such as in pharmacology where one may be interested in whether the effect of a drug is linear in log dose. Second, many of the more interesting hypothesis tests in the text are tests of complexity (nonlinearity, interaction) of the overall model. Null hypotheses of linearity of effects in particular are frequently rejected, providing formal evidence that the analyst's investment of time to use more than simple statistical models was warranted.

The text emphasizes predictive modeling, but as discussed in Chapter 1, developing good predictions goes hand in hand with accurate estimation of effects and with hypothesis testing (when appropriate). Besides emphasis on multivariable modeling, the text includes a chapter (16) introducing survival analysis and methods for analyzing various types of single and multiple events. This book does not provide examples of analyses of one common type of response variable, namely, cost and related measures of resource consumption. However, least squares modeling presented in Chapter 7, the robust rank-based methods presented in Chapters 13 and 19, and the transform-both-sides regression models discussed in Chapter 15 are very applicable and robust for modeling economic outcomes. See [120] and [177] for example analyses of such dependent variables using, respectively, the Cox model and nonparametric additive regression. The central Web site for this book (see the Appendix) has much more material on the use of the Cox model for analyzing costs.

Heavy use is made of the S-Plus statistical software environment from Insightful Corporation (Seattle, Washington). A few small examples using SAS (SAS Institute, Inc., Cary, North Carolina) are also described. S-Plus is the focus because it is an elegant object-oriented system in which it is easy to implement new statistical ideas. Many S-Plus users around the world have done so, and their work has benefitted many of the procedures described here. S-Plus also has a uniform syntax for specifying statistical models (with respect to categorical predictors, interactions, etc.), no matter which type of model is being fitted.[65]

A free, open-source statistical software system called R has become available in the past few years. The R language is similar to the S language on which S-Plus is based. Most of the functions used in this text are expected to be adapted to the R system. See the book's Web site for updated information about software availability.

Readers who don't use S-Plus, R, or any other statistical software environment will still find the statistical methods and case studies in this text useful, and it is hoped that the code that is presented will make the statistical methods more concrete. At the very least, the code demonstrates that all of the methods presented in the text are feasible.

This text does not teach analysts how to use S-Plus or R. For that, the reader may wish to consult Venables and Ripley[434] (which is an excellent companion to this text) as well as texts by Spector,[395] Krause and Olson,[250] and others, along with S-Plus manuals.[308] A free resource is a book by Alzola and Harrell[15] available on this text's Web site. That document teaches general S-Plus concepts as well as how to use add-on libraries described below. The document is also useful for SAS users who are new to S-Plus. See the Appendix for more information.

In addition to powerful features that are built into S-PLUS, this text uses a library of freely available S-PLUS functions called `Design` written by the author. `Design`, so named because of its tracking of modeling details related to the expanded X or design matrix, is a series of over 200 functions for model fitting, testing, estimation, validation, graphics, prediction, and typesetting by storing enhanced model design attributes in the fit. `Design` includes functions for least squares and penalized least squares multiple regression modeling in addition to functions for binary and ordinal logistic regression and survival analysis that are emphasized in this text. Other freely available miscellaneous S-PLUS functions used in the text are found in the `Hmisc` library also written by the author. Functions in `Hmisc` include facilities for data reduction, imputation, power and sample size calculation, advanced table making, recoding variables, importing and inspecting data, and general graphics. Consult the Appendix for information on obtaining `Hmisc` and `Design`.

The author and his colleagues have written SAS macros for fitting restricted cubic splines and for other basic operations. See the Appendix for more information as well as notes on using SAS procedures for many of the models discussed in this text. It is unfair not to mention some excellent capabilities of other statistical packages such as Stata and SYSTAT, but the extendibility and graphics of S-PLUS and R make them especially attractive for all aspects of the comprehensive modeling strategy presented in this book.

Portions of Chapters 4 and 19 were published as reference [185]. Some of Chapter 13 was published as reference [188].

The author may be contacted by electronic mail at `f.harrell@vanderbilt.edu` and would appreciate being informed of unclear points, errors, and omissions in this book. Suggestions for improvements and for future topics are also welcome. As described in the Web site, instructors may contact the author to obtain copies of quizzes and extra assignments (both with answers) related to much of the material in the earlier chapters, and to obtain full solutions (with graphical output) to the majority of assignments in the text.

Acknowledgements

A good deal of the writing of this book was done during my 17 years on the faculty of Duke University. I wish to thank my close colleague Kerry Lee for providing many valuable ideas, fruitful collaborations, and well-organized lecture notes from which I have greatly benefited over the past years. Terry Therneau of Mayo Clinic has given me many of his wonderful ideas for many years, and has written state-of-the-art S-PLUS software for survival analysis that forms the core of survival analysis software in my `Design` library. Michael Symons of the Department of Biostatistics of the University of North Carolina at Chapel Hill and Timothy Morgan of the Biometry Department at Wake Forest University School of Medicine also provided course materials, some of which motivated portions of this text. My former clinical colleagues in the Cardiology Division at Duke University, Robert Califf, Phillip Harris, Mark Hlatky, Dan Mark, David Pryor, and Robert Rosati for many years provided valuable motivation, feedback, and ideas through our interaction on clinical problems. Besides Kerry Lee, statistical colleagues L. Richard Smith, Lawrence Muhlbaier, and Elizabeth DeLong clarified my thinking and gave me new ideas on numerous occasions. Charlotte Nelson and Carlos Alzola have frequently helped me debug S-PLUS routines when they thought they were just analyzing data.

Former students Bercedis Peterson, James Herndon, Robert McMahon, and Yuan-Li Shen have provided many insights into logistic and survival modeling. Associations with Doug Wagner and William Knaus of the University of Virginia, Ken Offord of Mayo Clinic, David Naftel of the University of Alabama in Birmingham, Phil Miller of Washington University, and Phil Goodman of the University of Nevada Reno have provided many valuable ideas and motivations for this work, as have Michael Schemper of Vienna University, Janez Stare of Ljubljana University, Slovenia, and Ewout Steyerberg of Erasmus University, Rotterdam. Richard Goldstein of Qualitas, Inc., along with several anonymous reviewers, provided many helpful criticisms of a previous version of this manuscript that resulted in significant improvements, and critical reading by Bob Edson (VA Cooperative Studies Program, Palo Alto) resulted in many error corrections. Thanks to Brian Ripley of the University of Oxford for providing many helpful software tools and statistical insights that greatly aided in the production of this book, and to Bill Venables of CSIRO Australia for wisdom, both statistical and otherwise. Thanks also to John Kimmel of Springer-Verlag whose ideas and encouragement have been invaluable. This work would also not have been possible without the S environment developed by Rick Becker, John Chambers, Allan Wilks, and many other researchers at Lucent Technologies and several universities, or without the S-PLUS environment developed by many programmers and researchers at Insightful Corporation.

This work was supported by grants and contracts from the following U.S. agencies: Agency for Healthcare Research and Quality; National Library of Medicine; National Heart, Lung and Blood Institute and the National Center for Research Resources of the National Institutes of Health; National Cancer Institute; Robert Wood Johnson Foundation; National Center for Health Statistics; Roche Pharmaceuticals; the Biometry Training Program, Duke University; and the Department of Health Evaluation Sciences, University of Virginia School of Medicine.

Frank E. Harrell, Jr.
Vanderbilt University
November 2005

Contents

Typographical Conventions

Boxed numbers in the margins such as ① correspond to numbers at the end of chapters in sections named "Further Reading." Bracketed numbers and numeric superscripts in the text refer to the bibliography while alphabetic superscripts indicate footnotes.

S-PLUS language commands and names of S-PLUS functions and libraries are set in `typewriter font`, as are most variable names. When S-PLUS commands are interspersed with output printed by those commands, the > indicates a prompt for an S-PLUS command, and a + at the left indicates a prompt for a continuation line. Neither of these prompts is entered by users.

In the S language upon which S-PLUS is based, $x \leftarrow y$ is read "x gets the value of y." The assignment operator $\leftarrow$, used in the text for esthetic reasons, is entered by the user as `<-`. Comments begin with #, subscripts use brackets ([ ]), and the missing value is denoted by `NA` (not available).

Chapter 1

Introduction

1.1 Hypothesis Testing, Estimation, and Prediction

Statistics comprises among other areas study design, hypothesis testing, estimation, and prediction. This text aims at the last area, by presenting methods that enable an analyst to develop models that will make accurate predictions of responses for *future* observations. Prediction could be considered a superset of hypothesis testing and estimation, so the methods presented here will also assist the analyst in those areas. It is worth pausing to explain how this is so.

In traditional hypothesis testing one often chooses a *null hypothesis* defined as the absence of some effect. For example, in testing whether a variable such as cholesterol is a risk factor for sudden death, one might test the null hypothesis that an increase in cholesterol does not increase the risk of death. Hypothesis testing can easily be done within the context of a statistical model, but a model is not required. When one only wishes to assess whether an effect is zero, P-values may be computed using permutation or rank (nonparametric) tests while making only minimal assumptions. But there are still reasons for preferring a model-based approach over techniques that only yield P-values.

1. Permutation and rank tests do not easily give rise to estimates of *magnitudes* of effects.

2. These tests cannot be readily extended to incorporate complexities such as cluster sampling or repeated measurements within subjects.

3. Once the analyst is familiar with a model, that model may be used to carry out many different statistical tests; there is no need to learn specific formulas

to handle the special cases. The two-sample t-test is a special case of the ordinary multiple regression model having as its sole X variable a dummy variable indicating group membership. The Wilcoxon-Mann-Whitney test is a special case of the proportional odds ordinal logistic model.[452] The analysis of variance (multiple group) test and the Kruskal–Wallis test can easily be obtained from these two regression models by using more than one dummy predictor variable.

Even without complexities such as repeated measurements, problems can arise when many hypotheses are to be tested. Testing too many hypotheses is related to fitting too many predictors in a regression model. One commonly hears the statement that "the dataset was too small to allow modeling, so we just did hypothesis tests." It is unlikely that the resulting inferences would be reliable. If the sample size is insufficient for modeling it is often insufficient for tests or estimation. This is especially true when one desires to publish an estimate of the effect corresponding to the hypothesis yielding the smallest P-value. Ordinary point estimates are known to be badly biased when the quantity to be estimated was determined by "data dredging." This can be remedied by the same kind of shrinkage used in multivariable modeling (Section 9.10).

Statistical estimation is usually model-based. For example, one might use a survival regression model to estimate the relative effect of increasing cholesterol from 200 to 250 mg/dl on the hazard of death. Variables other than cholesterol may also be in the regression model, to allow estimation of the effect of increasing cholesterol, holding other risk factors constant. But accurate estimation of the cholesterol effect will depend on how cholesterol as well as each of the adjustment variables is assumed to relate to the hazard of death. If linear relationships are incorrectly assumed, estimates will be inaccurate. Accurate estimation also depends on avoiding overfitting the adjustment variables. If the dataset contains 200 subjects, 30 of whom died, and if one adjusted for 15 "confounding" variables, the estimates would be "overadjusted" for the effects of the 15 variables, as some of their apparent effects would actually result from spurious associations with the response variable (time until death). The overadjustment would reduce the cholesterol effect. The resulting unreliability of estimates equals the degree to which the overall model fails to validate on an independent sample.

It is often useful to think of effect estimates as differences between two predicted values from a model. This way, one can account for nonlinearities and interactions. For example, if cholesterol is represented nonlinearly in a logistic regression model, predicted values on the "linear combination of X's scale" are predicted log odds of an event. The increase in log odds from raising cholesterol from 200 to 250 mg/dl is the difference in predicted values, where cholesterol is set to 250 and then to 200, and all other variables are held constant. The point estimate of the 250:200mg/dl odds ratio is the antilog of this difference. If cholesterol is represented nonlinearly in the model, it does not matter how many terms in the model involve cholesterol as long as the correct predicted values are obtained.

Thus when one develops a reliable multivariable prediction model, hypothesis testing and estimation of effects are byproducts of the fitted model. So predictive modeling is often desirable even when prediction is not the main goal.

1.2   Examples of Uses of Predictive Multivariable Modeling

There is an endless variety of uses for multivariable models. Predictive models have long been used in business to forecast financial performance and to model consumer purchasing and loan pay-back behavior. In ecology, regression models are used to predict the probability that a fish species will disappear from a lake. Survival models have been used to predict product life (e.g., time to burn-out of an mechanical part, time until saturation of a disposable diaper). Models are commonly used in discrimination litigation in an attempt to determine whether race or sex is used as the basis for hiring or promotion, after taking other personnel characteristics into account.

Multivariable models are used extensively in medicine, epidemiology, biostatistics, health services research, pharmaceutical research, and related fields. The author has worked primarily in these fields, so most of the examples in this text come from those areas. In medicine, two of the major areas of application are diagnosis and prognosis. There models are used to predict the probability that a certain type of patient will be shown to have a specific disease, or to predict the time course of an already diagnosed disease.

In observational studies in which one desires to compare patient outcomes between two or more treatments, multivariable modeling is very important because of the biases caused by nonrandom treatment assignment. Here the simultaneous effects of several uncontrolled variables must be controlled (held constant mathematically if using a regression model) so that the effect of the factor of interest can be more purely estimated. A newer technique for more aggressively adjusting for nonrandom treatment assignment, the *propensity score*,[81, 357] provides yet another opportunity for multivariable modeling (see Section 10.1.4). The propensity score is merely the predicted value from a multivariable model where the response variable is the exposure or the treatment actually used. The estimated propensity score is then used in a second step as an adjustment variable in the model for the response of interest.

It is not widely recognized that multivariable modeling is extremely valuable even in well-designed randomized experiments. Such studies are often designed to make *relative* comparisons of two or more treatments, using odds ratios, hazard ratios, and other measures of relative effects. But to be able to estimate *absolute* effects one must develop a multivariable model of the response variable. This model can predict, for example, the probability that a patient on treatment A with characteristics X will survive five years, or it can predict the life expectancy for this patient. By making the same prediction for a patient on treatment B with the same characteristics, one can estimate the absolute difference in probabilities or life expectancies. This approach recognizes that low-risk patients must have less absolute benefit of treatment (lower change in outcome probability) than high-risk patients,[240] a fact that has been ignored in many clinical trials. Another reason for multivariable modeling in randomized clinical trials is that when the basic response model is nonlinear (e.g., logistic, Cox, parametric survival models), the unadjusted estimate of the treatment effect is not correct if there is moderate heterogeneity of subjects, even with perfect balance of baseline characteristics across the treatment groups.[a,17, 142] So even when investigators are interested in simple comparisons of two groups' responses, multivariable modeling can be advantageous and sometimes mandatory.

Cost-effectiveness analysis is becoming increasingly used in health care research, and the "effectiveness" (denominator of the cost-effectiveness ratio) is always a measure of absolute effectiveness. As absolute effectiveness varies dramatically with the risk profiles of subjects, it must be estimated for individual subjects using a multivariable model.

1.3   Planning for Modeling

When undertaking the development of a model to predict a response, one of the first questions the researcher must ask is "will this model actually be used?" Many models are never used, for several reasons including: (1) it was not deemed relevant to make predictions in the setting envisioned by the authors; (2) potential users of the model did not trust the relationships, weights, or variables used to make the predictions; and (3) the variables necessary to make the predictions were not routinely available.

Once the researcher convinces herself that a predictive model is worth developing, there are many study design issues to be addressed.[13, 260] Models are often developed using a "convenience sample," that is, a dataset that was not collected with such predictions in mind. The resulting models are often fraught with difficulties such as the following.

---

[a]For example, unadjusted odds ratios from 2×2 tables are different from adjusted odds ratios when there is variation in subjects' risk factors within each treatment group, even when the distribution of the risk factors is identical between the two groups.

1. The most important predictor or response variables may not have been collected, tempting the researchers to make do with variables that do not capture the real underlying processes.

2. The subjects appearing in the dataset are ill-defined, or they are not representative of the population for which inferences are to be drawn; similarly, the data collection sites may not represent the kind of variation in the population of sites.

3. Key variables are missing in large numbers of subjects.

4. Data are not missing at random; for example, data may not have been collected on subjects who dropped out of a study early, or on patients who were too sick to be interviewed.

5. Operational definitions of some of the key variables were never made.

6. Observer variability studies may not have been done, so that the reliability of measurements is unknown.

A predictive model will be more accurate, as well as useful, when data collection is planned prospectively. That way one can design data collection instruments containing the necessary variables, and all terms can be given standard definitions (for both descriptive and response variables) for use at all data collection sites. Also, steps can be taken to minimize the amount of missing data.

In the context of describing and modeling health outcomes, Iezzoni[218] has an excellent discussion of the dimensions of risk that should be captured by variables included in the model. She lists these general areas that should be quantified by predictor variables:

1. age,

2. sex,

3. acute clinical stability,

4. principal diagnosis,

5. severity of principal diagnosis,

6. extent and severity of comorbidities,

7. physical functional status,

8. psychological, cognitive, and psychosocial functioning,

9. cultural, ethnic, and socioeconomic attributes and behaviors,

10. health status and quality of life, and

11. patient attitudes and preferences for outcomes.

1.3.1 Emphasizing Continuous Variables

When designing the data collection it is important to emphasize the use of continuous variables over categorical ones. Some categorical variables are subjective and hard to standardize, and on the average they do not contain the same amount of statistical information as continuous variables. Above all, it is unwise to categorize naturally continuous variables during data collection,[b] as the original values can then not be recovered, and if another researcher feels that the (arbitrary) cutoff values were incorrect, other cutoffs cannot be substituted. Many researchers make the mistake of assuming that categorizing a continuous variable will result in less measurement error. This is a false assumption, for if a subject is placed in the wrong interval this will be as much as a 100% error. Thus the magnitude of the error multiplied by the probability of an error is no better with categorization.   ⊡1

1.4 Choice of the Model

The actual method by which an underlying statistical model should be chosen by the analyst is not well developed. A. P. Dawid is quoted in Lehmann[277] as saying the following.

> Where do probability models come from? To judge by the resounding silence over this question on the part of most statisticians, it seems highly embarrassing. In general, the theoretician is happy to accept that his abstract probability triple (Ω, A, P) was found under a gooseberry bush, while the applied statistician's model "just growed".

⊡2

In biostatistics, epidemiology, economics, psychology, sociology, and many other fields it is seldom the case that subject matter knowledge exists that would allow the analyst to prespecify a model (e.g., Weibull or log-normal survival model), a transformation for the response variable, and a structure for how predictors appear in the model (e.g., transformations, addition of nonlinear terms, interaction terms). Indeed, some authors question whether the notion of a model even exists in many cases.[69] We are for better or worse forced to develop models empirically in the majority of cases. Fortunately, careful and objective validation of the accuracy of model predictions against observable responses can lend credence to a model, if a good validation is not merely the result of overfitting (see Section 5.2).

There are a few general guidelines that can help in choosing the basic form of the statistical model.

---

[b]An exception may be sensitive variables such as income level. Subjects may be more willing to check a box corresponding to a wide interval containing their income. It is unlikely that a reduction in the probability that a subject will inflate her income will offset the loss of precision due to categorization of income, but there will be a decrease in the number of refusals. This reduction in missing data can more than offset the lack of precision.

1. The model must use the data efficiently. If, for example, one were interested in predicting the probability that a patient with a specific set of characteristics would live five years from diagnosis, an inefficient model would be a binary logistic model. A more efficient method, and one that would also allow for losses to follow-up before five years, would be a semiparametric (rank based) or parametric survival model. Such a model uses individual times of events in estimating coefficients, but it can easily be used to estimate the probability of surviving five years. As another example, if one were interested in predicting patients' quality of life on a scale of excellent, very good, good, fair, and poor, a polytomous (multinomial) categorical response model would not be efficient as it would not make use of the ordering of responses.

2. Choose a model that fits overall structures likely to be present in the data. In modeling survival time in chronic disease one might feel that the importance of most of the risk factors is constant over time. In that case, a proportional hazards model such as the Cox or Weibull model would be a good initial choice. If on the other hand one were studying acutely ill patients whose risk factors wane in importance as the patients survive longer, a model such as the log-normal or log-logistic regression model would be more appropriate.

3. Choose a model that is robust to problems in the data that are difficult to check. For example, the Cox proportional hazards model and ordinal logistic models are not affected by monotonic transformations of the response variable.

4. Choose a model whose mathematical form is appropriate for the response being modeled. This often has to do with minimizing the need for interaction terms that are included only to address a basic lack of fit. For example, many researchers have used ordinary linear regression models for binary responses, because of their simplicity. But such models allow predicted probabilities to be outside the interval $[0, 1]$, and strange interactions among the predictor variables are needed to make predictions remain in the legal range.

5. Choose a model that is readily extendible. The Cox model, by its use of stratification, easily allows a few of the predictors, especially if they are categorical, to violate the assumption of equal regression coefficients over time (proportional hazards assumption). The continuation ratio ordinal logistic model can also be generalized easily to allow for varying coefficients of some of the predictors as one proceeds across categories of the response.

R. A. Fisher as quoted in Lehmann[277] had these suggestions about model building: "(a) We must confine ourselves to those forms which we know how to handle," and (b) "More or less elaborate forms will be suitable according to the volume of the data." Ameen [69, p. 453] stated that a good model is "(a) satisfactory in performance relative to the stated objective, (b) logically sound, (c) representative, (d) questionable and subject to on-line interrogation, (e) able to accommodate external or expert information and (f) able to convey information."

It is very typical to use the data to make decisions about the form of the model as well as about how predictors are represented in the model. Then, once a model is developed, the entire modeling process is routinely forgotten, and statistical quantities such as standard errors, confidence limits, P-values, and R^2 are computed as if the resulting model were entirely prespecified. However, Faraway,[134] Draper,[117] Chatfield,[69] Buckland et al.[55] and others have written about the severe problems that result from treating an empirically derived model as if it were prespecified and as if it were the correct model. As Chatfield states [69, p. 426]: "It is indeed strange that we often admit model uncertainty by searching for a best model but then ignore this uncertainty by making inferences and predictions as if certain that the best fitting model is actually true."

Stepwise variable selection is one of the most widely used and abused of all data analysis techniques. Much is said about this technique later (see Section 4.3), but there are many other elements of model development that will need to be accounted for when making statistical inferences, and unfortunately it is difficult to derive quantities such as confidence limits that are properly adjusted for uncertainties such as the data-based choice between a Weibull and a log-normal regression model.   ③

Ye[458] developed a general method for estimating the "generalized degrees of freedom" (GDF) for any "data mining" or model selection procedure based on least squares. The GDF is an extremely useful index of the amount of "data dredging" or overfitting that has been done in a modeling process. It is also useful for estimating the residual variance with less bias. In one example, Ye developed a regression tree using recursive partitioning involving 10 candidate predictor variables on 100 observations. The resulting tree had 19 nodes and GDF of 76. The usual way of estimating the residual variance involves dividing the pooled within-node sum of squares by $100 - 19$, but Ye showed that dividing by $100 - 76$ instead yielded a much less biased (and much higher) estimate of σ^2. In another example, Ye considered stepwise variable selection using 20 candidate predictors and 22 observations. When there is no true association between any of the predictors and the response, Ye found that GDF = 14.1 for a strategy that selected the best five-variable model.   ④

Given that the choice of the model has been made (e.g., a log-normal model), penalized maximum likelihood estimation has major advantages in the battle between making the model fit adequately and avoiding overfitting (Sections 9.10 and 13.4.7). Penalization lessens the need for model selection.

1.5   Further Reading

[1]   More problems caused by dichotomizing continuous variables are discussed in [9, 12, 31, 57, 133, 202, 261, 349, 405].

[2]   See the excellent editorial by Mallows[300] for more about model choice.

3   See [10, 55, 69, 117, 134, 286] for information about accounting for model selection in making final inferences. Faraway[134] demonstrated that the bootstrap has good potential in related although somewhat simpler settings, and Buckland et al.[55] developed a promising bootstrap weighting method for accounting for model uncertainty.

4   Tibshirani and Knight[418] developed another approach to estimating the generalized degrees of freedom.

Chapter 2

General Aspects of Fitting Regression Models

2.1   Notation for Multivariable Regression Models

The ordinary multiple linear regression model is frequently used and has parameters that are easily interpreted. In this chapter we study a general class of regression models, those stated in terms of a weighted sum of a set of independent or predictor variables. It is shown that after linearizing the model with respect to the predictor variables, the parameters in such regression models are also readily interpreted. Also, all the designs used in ordinary linear regression can be used in this general setting. These designs include analysis of variance (ANOVA) setups, interaction effects, and nonlinear effects. Besides describing and interpreting general regression models, this chapter also describes, in general terms, how the three types of assumptions of regression models can be examined.

First we introduce notation for regression models. Let Y denote the response (dependent) variable, and let $X = X_1, X_2, \ldots, X_p$ denote a list or vector of predictor variables (also called covariables or independent, descriptor, or concomitant variables). These predictor variables are assumed to be constants for a given individual or subject from the population of interest. Let $\beta = \beta_0, \beta_1, \ldots, \beta_p$ denote the list of regression coefficients (parameters). β_0 is an optional intercept parameter, and $\beta_1, \ldots, \beta_p$ are weights or regression coefficients corresponding to $X_1, \ldots, X_p$. We use matrix or vector notation to describe a weighted sum of the Xs:

$$X\beta = \beta_0 + \beta_1 X_1 + \ldots + \beta_p X_p, \tag{2.1}$$

where there is an implied $X_0 = 1$.

A regression model is stated in terms of a connection between the predictors X and the response Y. Let $C(Y|X)$ denote a property of the distribution of Y given X (as a function of X). For example, $C(Y|X)$ could be $E(Y|X)$, the expected value or average of Y given X, or $C(Y|X)$ could be the probability that $Y = 1$ given X (where $Y = 0$ or 1).

2.2   Model Formulations

We define a regression function as a function that describes interesting properties of Y that may vary across individuals in the population. X describes the list of factors determining these properties. Stated mathematically, a general regression model is given by

$$C(Y|X) = g(X). \tag{2.2}$$

We restrict our attention to models that, after a certain transformation, are linear in the unknown parameters, that is, models that involve X only through a weighted sum of all the Xs. The *general linear regression model* is given by

$$C(Y|X) = g(X\beta). \tag{2.3}$$

For example, the ordinary linear regression model is

$$C(Y|X) = E(Y|X) = X\beta, \tag{2.4}$$

and given X, Y has a normal distribution with mean $X\beta$ and constant variance σ^2. The binary logistic regression model[89, 440] is

$$C(Y|X) = \text{Prob}\{Y = 1|X\} = (1 + \exp(-X\beta))^{-1}, \tag{2.5}$$

where Y can take on the values 0 and 1. In general the model, when stated in terms of the property $C(Y|X)$, may not be linear in $X\beta$; that is $C(Y|X) = g(X\beta)$, where $g(u)$ is nonlinear in u. For example, a regression model could be $E(Y|X) = (X\beta)^{.5}$. The model may be made linear in the unknown parameters by a transformation in the property $C(Y|X)$:

$$h(C(Y|X)) = X\beta, \tag{2.6}$$

where $h(u) = g^{-1}(u)$, the inverse function of g. As an example consider the binary logistic regression model given by

$$C(Y|X) = \text{Prob}\{Y = 1|X\} = (1 + \exp(-X\beta))^{-1}. \tag{2.7}$$

If $h(u) = \text{logit}(u) = \log(u/(1-u))$, the transformed model becomes

$$h(\text{Prob}(Y = 1|X)) = \log(\exp(X\beta)) = X\beta. \tag{2.8}$$

The transformation $h(C(Y|X))$ is sometimes called a *link function*. Let $h(C(Y|X))$ be denoted by $C'(Y|X)$. The general linear regression model then becomes

$$C'(Y|X) = X\beta. \tag{2.9}$$

In other words, the model states that some property C' of Y, given X, is a weighted sum of the Xs ($X\beta$). In the ordinary linear regression model, $C'(Y|X) = E(Y|X)$. In the logistic regression case, $C'(Y|X)$ is the logit of the probability that $Y = 1$, $\log \text{Prob}\{Y = 1\}/[1 - \text{Prob}\{Y = 1\}]$. This is the log of the odds that $Y = 1$ versus $Y = 0$.

It is important to note that the general linear regression model has two major components: $C'(Y|X)$ and $X\beta$. The first part has to do with a property or transformation of Y. The second, $X\beta$, is the *linear regression* or *linear predictor* part. The method of least squares can sometimes be used to fit the model if $C'(Y|X) = E(Y|X)$. Other cases must be handled using other methods such as maximum likelihood estimation or nonlinear least squares.

2.3   Interpreting Model Parameters

In the original model, $C(Y|X)$ specifies the way in which X affects a property of Y. Except in the ordinary linear regression model, it is difficult to interpret the individual parameters if the model is stated in terms of $C(Y|X)$. In the model $C'(Y|X) = X\beta = \beta_0 + \beta_1 X_1 + \ldots + \beta_p X_p$, the regression parameter β_j is interpreted as the change in the property C' of Y per unit change in the descriptor variable X_j, all other descriptors remaining constant:

$$\beta_j = C'(Y|X_1, X_2, \ldots, X_j + 1, \ldots, X_p) - C'(Y|X_1, X_2, \ldots, X_j, \ldots, X_p). \tag{2.10}$$

In the ordinary linear regression model, for example, β_j is the change in expected value of Y per unit change in X_j. In the logistic regression model β_j is the change in log odds that $Y = 1$ per unit change in X_j. When a noninteracting X_j is a dichotomous variable or a continuous one that is linearly related to C', X_j is represented by a single term in the model and its contribution is described fully by β_j.

In all that follows, we drop the ′ from C' and assume that $C(Y|X)$ is the property of Y that is linearly related to the weighted sum of the Xs.

2.3.1   Nominal Predictors

Suppose that we wish to model the effect of two or more treatments and be able to test for differences between the treatments in some property of Y. A nominal or polytomous factor such as treatment group having k levels, in which there is no definite ordering of categories, is fully described by a series of $k-1$ binary dummy descriptor variables. Suppose that there are four treatments, J, K, L, and M, and the treatment factor is denoted by T. The model can be written as

$$
\begin{aligned}
C(Y|T = J) &= \beta_0 \\
C(Y|T = K) &= \beta_0 + \beta_1 \\
C(Y|T = L) &= \beta_0 + \beta_2 \\
C(Y|T = M) &= \beta_0 + \beta_3.
\end{aligned}
\tag{2.11}
$$

The four treatments are thus completely specified by three regression parameters and one intercept that we are using to denote treatment J, the reference treatment. This model can be written in the previous notation as

$$
C(Y|T) = X\beta = \beta_0 + \beta_1 X_1 + \beta_2 X_2 + \beta_3 X_3,
\tag{2.12}
$$

where

$$
\begin{aligned}
X_1 &= 1 \quad \text{if } T = K, \quad 0 \text{ otherwise} \\
X_2 &= 1 \quad \text{if } T = L, \quad 0 \text{ otherwise} \\
X_3 &= 1 \quad \text{if } T = M, \quad 0 \text{ otherwise.}
\end{aligned}
\tag{2.13}
$$

For treatment J $(T = J)$, all three Xs are zero and $C(Y|T = J) = \beta_0$. The test for any differences in the property $C(Y)$ between treatments is $H_0 : \beta_1 = \beta_2 = \beta_3 = 0$.

This model is an *analysis of variance* or *k-sample*-type model. If there are other descriptor covariables in the model, it becomes an *analysis of covariance*-type model.

2.3.2   Interactions

Suppose that a model has descriptor variables X_1 and X_2 and that the effect of the two Xs cannot be separated; that is the effect of X_1 on Y depends on the level of X_2 and vice versa. One simple way to describe this *interaction* is to add the constructed variable $X_3 = X_1 X_2$ to the model:

$$
C(Y|X) = \beta_0 + \beta_1 X_1 + \beta_2 X_2 + \beta_3 X_1 X_2.
\tag{2.14}
$$

It is now difficult to interpret β_1 and β_2 in isolation. However, we may quantify the effect of a one-unit increase in X_1 if X_2 is held constant as

$$
\begin{aligned}
C(Y|X_1 + 1, X_2) \quad - \quad & C(Y|X_1, X_2) \\
= \quad & \beta_0 + \beta_1(X_1 + 1) + \beta_2 X_2 \\
+ \quad & \beta_3(X_1 + 1)X_2 \\
- \quad & [\beta_0 + \beta_1 X_1 + \beta_2 X_2 + \beta_3 X_1 X_2] \\
= \quad & \beta_1 + \beta_3 X_2.
\end{aligned}
\tag{2.15}
$$

Likewise, the effect of a one-unit increase in X_2 on C if X_1 is held constant is $\beta_2 + \beta_3 X_1$. Interactions can be much more complex than can be modeled with a product of two terms. If X_1 is binary, the interaction may take the form of a difference in shape (and/or distribution) of X_2 versus $C(Y)$ depending on whether $X_1 = 0$ or $X_1 = 1$ (e.g., logarithm vs. square root). When both variables are continuous, the possibilities are much greater (this case is discussed later). Interactions among more than two variables can be exceedingly complex.

2.3.3 Example: Inference for a Simple Model

Suppose we postulated the model

$$
C(Y|age, sex) = \beta_0 + \beta_1 age + \beta_2(sex = f) + \beta_3 age(sex = f),
$$

where $sex = f$ is a dummy indicator variable for sex = female; that is the reference cell is sex = male. This is a model that assumes

1. age is linearly related to $C(Y)$ for males,

2. age is linearly related to $C(Y)$ for females, and

3. whatever distribution, variance, and independence assumptions are appropriate for the model being considered.

We are thus assuming that the interaction between age and sex is simple; that is it only alters the slope of the age effect. The parameters in the model have interpretations shown in Table 2.1. β_3 is the difference in slopes (female – male).

There are many useful hypotheses that can be tested for this model. First let's consider two hypotheses that are seldom appropriate although they are routinely tested.

1. $H_0 : \beta_1 = 0$: This tests whether age is associated with Y for males.

2. $H_0 : \beta_2 = 0$: This tests whether sex is associated with Y for zero-year olds.

TABLE 2.1

Parameter	Meaning
β_0	$C(Y|age = 0, sex = m)$
β_1	$C(Y|age = x + 1, sex = m) - C(Y|age = x, sex = m)$
β_2	$C(Y|age = 0, sex = f) - C(Y|age = 0, sex = m)$
β_3	$C(Y|age = x + 1, sex = f) - C(Y|age = x, sex = f) -$
	$[C(Y|age = x + 1, sex = m) - C(Y|age = x, sex = m)]$

Now consider more useful hypotheses. For each hypothesis we should write what is being tested, translate this to tests in terms of parameters, write the alternative hypothesis, and describe what the test has maximum power to detect. The latter component of a hypothesis test needs to be emphasized, as almost every statistical test is focused on one specific pattern to detect. For example, a test of association against an alternative hypothesis that a slope is nonzero will have maximum power when the true association is linear. If the true regression model is exponential in X, a linear regression test will have some power to detect "nonflatness" but it will not be as powerful as the test from a well-specified exponential regression effect. If the true effect is U-shaped, a test of association based on a linear model will have almost no power to detect association. If one tests for association against a quadratic (parabolic) alternative, the test will have some power to detect a logarithmic shape but it will have very little power to detect a cyclical trend having multiple "humps." In a quadratic regression model, a test of linearity against a quadratic alternative hypothesis will have reasonable power to detect a quadratic nonlinear effect but very limited power to detect a multiphase cyclical trend. Therefore in the tests in Table 2.2 keep in mind that power is maximal when linearity of the age relationship holds for both sexes. In fact it may be useful to write alternative hypotheses as, for example, "H_a : age is associated with $C(Y)$, powered to detect a *linear* relationship." Note that if there is an interaction effect, we know that there is both an age and a sex effect. However, there can also be age or sex effects when the lines are parallel. That's why the tests of total association have 2 d.f.

2.4   Relaxing Linearity Assumption for Continuous Predictors

2.4.1   Simple Nonlinear Terms

If a continuous predictor is represented, say, as X_1 in the model, the model is assumed to be linear in X_1. Often, however, the property of Y of interest does not behave linearly in all the predictors. The simplest way to describe a nonlinear effect

TABLE 2.2: Most Useful Tests for Linear *Age* × *Sex* Model

Null or Alternative Hypothesis	Mathematical Statement
Effect of age is independent of sex or Effect of sex is independent of age or Age and sex are additive Age effects are parallel	$H_0 : \beta_3 = 0$
Age interacts with sex Age modifies effect of sex Sex modifies effect of age Sex and age are nonadditive (synergistic)	$H_a : \beta_3 \neq 0$
Age is not associated with Y Age is associated with Y Age is associated with Y for either Females or males	$H_0 : \beta_1 = \beta_3 = 0$ $H_a : \beta_1 \neq 0$ or $\beta_3 \neq 0$
Sex is not associated with Y Sex is associated with Y Sex is associated with Y for some Value of age	$H_0 : \beta_2 = \beta_3 = 0$ $H_a : \beta_2 \neq 0$ or $\beta_3 \neq 0$
Neither age nor sex is associated with Y Either age or sex is associated with Y	$H_0 : \beta_1 = \beta_2 = \beta_3 = 0$ $H_a : \beta_1 \neq 0$ or $\beta_2 \neq 0$ or $\beta_3 \neq 0$

of X_1 is to include a term for $X_2 = X_1^2$ in the model:

$$C(Y|X_1) = \beta_0 + \beta_1 X_1 + \beta_2 X_1^2. \tag{2.16}$$

If the model is truly linear in X_1, β_2 will be zero. This model formulation allows one to test H_0 : model is linear in X_1 against H_a : model is quadratic (parabolic) in X_1 by testing $H_0 : \beta_2 = 0$.

Nonlinear effects will frequently not be of a parabolic nature. If a transformation of the predictor is known to induce linearity, that transformation (e.g., $\log(X)$) may be substituted for the predictor. However, often the transformation is not known. Higher powers of X_1 may be included in the model to approximate many types of relationships, but polynomials have some undesirable properties (e.g., undesirable peaks and valleys, and the fit in one region of X can be greatly affected by data in other regions[299]) and will not adequately fit many functional forms.[112] For example, polynomials do not adequately fit logarithmic functions or "threshold" effects.

2.4.2   Splines for Estimating Shape of Regression Function and Determining Predictor Transformations

A draftman's *spline* is a flexible strip of metal or rubber used to draw curves. Spline functions are piecewise polynomials used in curve fitting. That is, they are polynomials within intervals of X that are connected across different intervals of X. Splines have been used, principally in the physical sciences, to approximate a wide variety of functions. The simplest spline function is a linear spline function, a piecewise linear function. Suppose that the x axis is divided into intervals with endpoints at a, b, and c, called *knots*. The linear spline function is given by

$$f(X) = \beta_0 + \beta_1 X + \beta_2 (X - a)_+ + \beta_3 (X - b)_+ + \beta_4 (X - c)_+, \tag{2.17}$$

where

$$\begin{aligned}(u)_+ = \quad & u, \quad u > 0, \\ & 0, \quad u \le 0. \end{aligned} \tag{2.18}$$

The number of knots can vary depending on the amount of available data for fitting the function. The linear spline function can be rewritten as

$$\begin{aligned} f(X) \quad &= \beta_0 + \beta_1 X, & X \le a \\ &= \beta_0 + \beta_1 X + \beta_2 (X - a) & a < X \le b \\ &= \beta_0 + \beta_1 X + \beta_2 (X - a) + \beta_3 (X - b) & b < X \le c \\ &= \beta_0 + \beta_1 X + \beta_2 (X - a) \\ &\quad + \beta_3 (X - b) + \beta_4 (X - c) & c < X. \end{aligned} \tag{2.19}$$

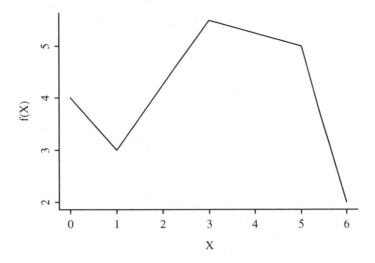

FIGURE 2.1: A linear spline function with knots at $a = 1, b = 3, c = 5$.

A linear spline is depicted in Figure 2.1. The general linear regression model can be written assuming only piecewise linearity in X by incorporating constructed variables X_2, X_3, and X_4 :

$$C(Y|X) = f(X) = X\beta, \tag{2.20}$$

where $X\beta = \beta_0 + \beta_1 X_1 + \beta_2 X_2 + \beta_3 X_3 + \beta_4 X_4$, and

$$X_1 = X \quad X_2 = (X - a)_+$$
$$X_3 = (X - b)_+ \quad X_4 = (X - c)_+. \tag{2.21}$$

By modeling a slope increment for X in an interval $(a, b]$ in terms of $(X - a)_+$, the function is constrained to join ("meet") at the knots. Overall linearity in X can be tested by testing $H_0 : \beta_2 = \beta_3 = \beta_4 = 0$.

2.4.3 Cubic Spline Functions

Although the linear spline is simple and can approximate many common relationships, it is not smooth and will not fit highly curved functions well. These problems can be overcome by using piecewise polynomials of order higher than linear. Cubic polynomials have been found to have nice properties with good ability to fit sharply curving shapes. Cubic splines can be made to be smooth at the join points (knots) by forcing the first and second derivatives of the function to agree at the knots.

Such a smooth cubic spline function with three knots (a, b, c) is given by

$$
\begin{aligned}
f(X) &= \beta_0 + \beta_1 X + \beta_2 X^2 + \beta_3 X^3 \\
&+ \beta_4 (X - a)_+^3 + \beta_5 (X - b)_+^3 + \beta_6 (X - c)_+^3 \\
&= X\beta
\end{aligned} \tag{2.22}
$$

with the following constructed variables:

$$
\begin{aligned}
X_1 &= X \qquad X_2 = X^2 \\
X_3 &= X^3 \qquad X_4 = (X - a)_+^3 \\
X_5 &= (X - b)_+^3 \qquad X_6 = (X - c)_+^3.
\end{aligned} \tag{2.23}
$$

If the cubic spline function has k knots, the function will require estimating $k + 3$ regression coefficients besides the intercept. See Section 2.4.5 for information on choosing the number and location of knots. ☐1

There are more numerically stable ways to form a design matrix for cubic spline functions that are based on B-splines instead of the truncated power basis[110, 389] used here. However, B-splines are more complex and do not allow for extrapolation beyond the outer knots, and the truncated power basis seldom presents estimation problems (see Section 4.6) when modern methods such as the Q–R decomposition are used for matrix inversion. ☐2

2.4.4   Restricted Cubic Splines

Stone and Koo[403] have found that cubic spline functions do have a drawback in that they can be poorly behaved in the tails, that is before the first knot and after the last knot. They cite advantages of constraining the function to be linear in the tails. Their restricted cubic spline function (also called *natural splines*) has the additional   ☐3 advantage that only $k - 1$ parameters must be estimated (besides the intercept) as opposed to $k + 3$ parameters with the unrestricted cubic spline. The restricted spline function with k knots $t_1, \ldots, t_k$ is given by[112]

$$
f(X) = \beta_0 + \beta_1 X_1 + \beta_2 X_2 + \ldots + \beta_{k-1} X_{k-1}, \tag{2.24}
$$

where $X_1 = X$ and for $j = 1, \ldots, k - 2$,

$$
\begin{aligned}
X_{j+1} &= (X - t_j)_+^3 - (X - t_{k-1})_+^3 (t_k - t_j)/(t_k - t_{k-1}) \\
&+ (X - t_k)_+^3 (t_{k-1} - t_j)/(t_k - t_{k-1}).
\end{aligned} \tag{2.25}
$$

It can be shown that X_j is linear in X for $X \geq t_k$. Figure 2.2 displays the spline component variables X_j for $j = 2, 3, 4$ and $k = 5$ and one set of knots. The left graph magnifies the lower portion of the curves. Figure 2.3 displays some typical

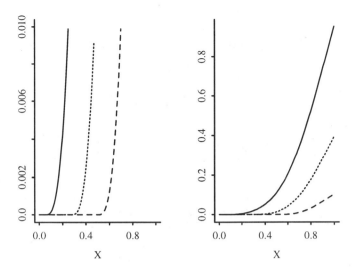

FIGURE 2.2: Restricted cubic spline component variables for $k = 5$ and knots at $X =$ .05, .275, .5, .725, and .95.

shapes of restricted cubic spline functions with $k = 3, 4, 5$, and 6. These functions were generated using random β.

   Once $\beta_0, \ldots, \beta_{k-1}$ are estimated, the restricted cubic spline can be restated in the form

$$\begin{aligned} f(X) &= \beta_0 + \beta_1 X + \beta_2 (X - t_1)^3_+ + \beta_3 (X - t_2)^3_+ \\ &\quad + \ldots + \beta_{k+1}(X - t_k)^3_+ \end{aligned} \tag{2.26}$$

by computing

$$\beta_k = [\beta_2(t_1 - t_k) + \beta_3(t_2 - t_k) + \ldots + \beta_{k-1}(t_{k-2} - t_k)]/(t_k - t_{k-1}) \tag{2.27}$$
$$\beta_{k+1} = [\beta_2(t_1 - t_{k-1}) + \beta_3(t_2 - t_{k-1}) + \ldots + \beta_{k-1}(t_{k-2} - t_{k-1})]/(t_{k-1} - t_k).$$

A test of linearity in X can be obtained by testing

$$H_0 : \beta_2 = \beta_3 = \ldots = \beta_{k-1} = 0. \tag{2.28}$$

4

   The truncated power basis for restricted cubic splines does allow for rational (i.e., linear) extrapolation beyond the outer knots. However, when the outer knots are in the tails of the data, extrapolation can still be dangerous.

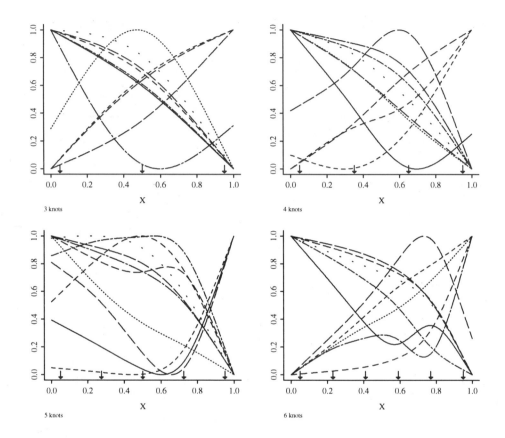

FIGURE 2.3: Some typical restricted cubic spline functions for $k = 3, 4, 5, 6$. The y-axis is $X\beta$. Arrows indicate knots.

TABLE 2.3

k				Quantiles			
3			.10	.5	.90		
4			.05	.35	.65	.95	
5		.05	.275	.5	.725	.95	
6	.05	.23	.41	.59	.77	.95	
7	.025	.1833	.3417	.5	.6583	.8167	.975

When nonlinear terms in Equation 2.25 are normalized, for example, by dividing them by the square of the difference in the outer knots to make all terms have units of X, the ordinary truncated power basis has no numerical difficulties when modern matrix algebra software is used.

2.4.5   Choosing Number and Position of Knots

We have assumed that the locations of the knots are specified in advance; that is, the knot locations are not treated as free parameters to be estimated. If knots were free parameters, the fitted function would have more flexibility but at the cost of instability of estimates, statistical inference problems, and inability to use standard regression modeling software for estimating regression parameters.

How then does the analyst preassign knot locations? If the regression relationship were described by prior experience, prespecification of knot locations would be easy. For example, if a function were known to change curvature at $X = a$, a knot could be placed at a. However, in most situations there is no way to prespecify knots. Fortunately, Stone[401] has found that the location of knots in a restricted cubic spline model is not very crucial in most situations; the fit depends much more on the choice of k, the number of knots. Placing knots at fixed quantiles (percentiles) of a predictor's marginal distribution is a good approach in most datasets. This ensures that enough points are available in each interval, and also guards against letting outliers overly influence knot placement. Recommended equally spaced quantiles are shown in Table 2.3.

⑤

The principal reason for using less extreme default quantiles for $k = 3$ and more extreme ones for $k = 7$ is that one usually uses $k = 3$ for small sample sizes and $k = 7$ for large samples. When the sample size is less than 100, the outer quantiles should be replaced by the fifth smallest and fifth largest datapoints, respectively.[403] What about the choice of k? The flexibility of possible fits must be tempered by the sample size available to estimate the unknown parameters. Stone[401] has found that more than 5 knots are seldom required in a restricted cubic spline model. The principal decision then is between $k = 3, 4$, or 5. For many datasets, $k = 4$ offers an adequate fit of the model and is a good compromise between flexibility and loss of precision caused by overfitting a small sample. When the sample size is large (e.g., $n \geq 100$ with a continuous uncensored response variable), $k = 5$ is a good choice. Small samples (< 30, say) may require the use of $k = 3$. Akaike's information criterion (AIC, Section 9.8.1) can be used for a data-based choice of k. The value of k maximizing the model likelihood ratio $\chi^2 - 2k$ would be the best "for the money" using AIC.

The analyst may wish to devote more knots to variables that are thought to be more important, and risk lack of fit for less important variables. In this way the total number of estimated parameters can be controlled (Section 4.1).

2.4.6   Nonparametric Regression

One of the most important results of an analysis is the estimation of the tendency (trend) of how X relates to Y. This trend is useful in its own right and it may be sufficient for obtaining predicted values in some situations, but trend estimates can also be used to guide formal regression modeling (by suggesting predictor variable transformations) and to check model assumptions.

Nonparametric smoothers are excellent tools for determining the shape of the relationship between a predictor and the response. The standard nonparametric smoothers work when one is interested in assessing one continuous predictor at a time and when the property of the response that *should* be linearly related to the predictor is a standard measure of central tendency. For example, when $C(Y)$ is $E(Y)$ or $\Pr[Y = 1]$, standard smoothers are useful, but when $C(Y)$ is a measure of variability or a rate (instantaneous risk), or when Y is only incompletely measured for some subjects (e.g., Y is censored for some subjects), simple smoothers will not work.

The oldest and simplest nonparametric smoother is the moving average. Suppose that the data consist of the points $X = 1, 2, 3, 5$, and 8, with the corresponding Y values $2.1, 3.8, 5.7, 11.1$, and 17.2. To smooth the relationship we could estimate $E(Y|X = 2)$ by $(2.1+3.8+5.7)/3$ and $E(Y|X = (2+3+5)/3)$ by $(3.8+5.7+11.1)/3$. Note that overlap is fine; that is one point may be contained in two sets that are averaged. You can immediately see that the simple moving average has a problem in estimating $E(Y)$ at the outer values of X. The estimates are quite sensitive to the choice of the number of points (or interval width) to use in "binning" the data.

A moving least squares linear regression smoother is far superior to a moving flat line smoother (moving average). Cleveland's[76] moving linear regression smoother *loess* has become the most popular smoother. To obtain the smoothed value of Y at $X = x$, we take all the data having X values within a suitable interval about x. Then a linear regression is fitted to all of these points, and the predicted value from this regression at $X = x$ is taken as the estimate of $E(Y|X = x)$. Actually, `loess` uses weighted least squares estimates, which is why it is called a *locally weighted least squares* method. The weights are chosen so that points near $X = x$ are given the most weight[a] in the calculation of the slope and intercept. Surprisingly, a good default choice for the interval about x is an interval containing $2/3$ of the datapoints! The weighting function is devised so that points near the extremes of this interval receive almost no weight in the calculation of the slope and intercept.

Because `loess` uses a moving straight line rather than a moving flat one, it provides much better behavior at the extremes of the Xs. For example, one can fit a straight line to the first three datapoints and then obtain the predicted value at the lowest X, which takes into account that this X is not the middle of the three Xs.

`loess` obtains smoothed values for $E(Y)$ at each observed value of X. Estimates for other Xs are obtained by linear interpolation.

The `loess` algorithm has another component. After making an initial estimate of the trend line, `loess` can look for outliers off this trend. It can then delete or downweight those apparent outliers to obtain a more robust trend estimate. Now, different points will appear to be outliers with respect to this second trend estimate. The new set of outliers is taken into account and another trend line is derived. By default, the process stops after these three iterations. `loess` works exceptionally well for binary Y as long as the iterations that look for outliers are not done, that is only one iteration is performed.

For a single X, Friedman's "super smoother"[146] is another efficient and flexible nonparametric trend estimator. For both `loess` and the super smoother the amount of smoothing can be controlled by the analyst. Hastie and Tibshirani[191] provided an excellent description of smoothing methods and developed a generalized additive model for multiple Xs, in which each continuous predictor is fitted with a nonparametric smoother (see Chapter 16). Interactions are not allowed. Cleveland et al.[65] have extended two-dimensional smoothers to multiple dimensions without assuming additivity. Their *local regression model* is feasible for up to four or so predictors. Local regression models are extremely flexible, allowing parts of the model to be parametrically specified, and allowing the analyst to choose the amount of smoothing or the effective number of degrees of freedom of the fit.

Smoothing splines are related to nonparametric smoothers. Here a knot is placed at every datapoint, but a penalized likelihood is maximized to derive the smoothed estimates. Gray[161, 162] developed a general method that is halfway between smoothing splines and regression splines. He prespecified, say, 10 fixed knots, but uses a penalized likelihood for estimation. This allows the analyst to control the effective number of degrees of freedom used.

Besides using smoothers to estimate regression relationships, smoothers are valuable for examining trends in residual plots. See Sections 14.6 and 20.2 for examples.

---

[a]This weight is not to be confused with the regression coefficient; rather the weights are $w_1, w_2, \ldots, w_n$ and the fitting criterion is $\sum_i^n w_i(Y_i - \hat{Y}_i)^2$.

2.4.7 Advantages of Regression Splines over Other Methods

There are several advantages of regression splines:[187]

1. Parametric splines are piecewise polynomials and can be fitted using any existing regression program after the constructed predictors are computed. Spline regression is equally suitable to multiple linear regression, survival models, and logistic models for discrete outcomes.

2. Regression coefficients for the spline function are estimated using standard techniques (maximum likelihood or least squares), and statistical inferences can readily be drawn. Formal tests of no overall association, linearity, and additivity can readily be constructed. Confidence limits for the estimated regression function are derived by standard theory.

3. The fitted spline function directly estimates the transformation that a predictor should receive to yield linearity in $C(Y|X)$. The fitted spline transformation often suggests a simple transformation (e.g., square root) of a predictor that can be used if one is not concerned about the proper number of degrees of freedom for testing association of the predictor with the response.

4. The spline function can be used to represent the predictor in the final model. Nonparametric methods do not yield a prediction equation.

5. Splines can be extended to nonadditive models (see below). Multidimensional nonparametric estimators often require burdensome computations.

2.5   Recursive Partitioning: Tree-Based Models

Breiman et al.[48] have developed an essentially model-free approach called *classification and regression trees* (CART), a form of recursive partitioning. For some implementations of CART, we say "essentially" model-free since a model-based statistic is sometimes chosen as a splitting criterion. The essence of recursive partitioning is as follows.

1. Find the predictor so that the best possible binary split on that predictor has a larger value of some statistical criterion than any other split on any other predictor. For ordinal and continuous predictors, the split is of the form $X < c$ versus $X \geq c$. For polytomous predictors, the split involves finding the best separation of categories, without preserving order.

2. Within each previously formed subset, find the best predictor and best split that maximizes the criterion in the subset of observations passing the previous split.

3. Proceed in like fashion until fewer than k observations remain to be split, where k is typically 20 to 100.

4. Obtain predicted values using a statistic that summarizes each terminal node (e.g., mean or proportion).

5. Prune the tree backward so that a tree with the same number of nodes developed on 0.9 of the data validates best on the remaining 0.1 of the data (average over the 10 cross-validations). Alternatively, shrink the node estimates toward the mean, using a progressively stronger shrinkage factor, until the best cross-validation results.

Tree models have the advantage of not requiring any functional form for the predictors and of not assuming additivity of predictors (i.e., recursive partitioning can identify complex interactions). Trees can deal with missing data flexibly. They have the disadvantages of not utilizing continuous variables effectively and of overfitting in three directions: searching for best predictors, for best splits, and searching multiple times. The penalty for the extreme amount of data searching required by recursive partitioning surfaces when the tree does not cross-validate optimally until it is pruned all the way back to two or three splits. Thus reliable trees are often not very discriminating.

Tree models are especially useful in messy situations or settings in which overfitting is not so problematic, such as confounder adjustment using propensity scores[82] or in missing value imputation (Section 8.4). A major advantage of tree modeling is savings of analyst time.

2.6   Multiple Degree of Freedom Tests of Association

When a factor is a linear or binary term in the regression model, the test of association for that factor with the response involves testing only a single regression parameter. Nominal factors and predictors that are represented as a quadratic or spline function require multiple regression parameters to be tested simultaneously in order to assess association with the response. For a nominal factor having k levels, the overall ANOVA-type test with $k-1$ d.f. tests whether there are any differences in responses between the k categories. It is recommended that this test be done before attempting to interpret individual parameter estimates. If the overall test is not significant, it can be dangerous to rely on individual pairwise comparisons because the type I error will be increased. Likewise, for a continuous predictor for which linearity is not assumed, all terms involving the predictor should be tested simultaneously to check whether the factor is associated with the outcome. This test should precede the test for linearity and should usually precede the attempt to eliminate nonlinear terms. For example, in the model

$$C(Y|X) = \beta_0 + \beta_1 X_1 + \beta_2 X_2 + \beta_3 X_2^2, \tag{2.29}$$

one should test $H_0 : \beta_2 = \beta_3 = 0$ with 2 d.f. to assess association between X_2 and outcome. In the five-knot restricted cubic spline model

$$C(Y|X) = \beta_0 + \beta_1 X + \beta_2 X' + \beta_3 X'' + \beta_4 X''', \tag{2.30}$$

the hypothesis $H_0 : \beta_1 = \ldots = \beta_4 = 0$ should be tested with 4 d.f. to assess whether there is any association between X and Y. If this 4 d.f. test is insignificant, it is dangerous to interpret the shape of the fitted spline function because the hypothesis that the overall function is flat has not been rejected.

A dilemma arises when an overall test of association, say one having 4 d.f., is insignificant, the 3 d.f. test for linearity is insignificant, but the 1 d.f. test for linear association, after deleting nonlinear terms, becomes significant. Had the test for linearity been borderline significant, it would not have been warranted to drop these terms in order to test for a linear association. But with the evidence for nonlinearity not very great, one could attempt to test for association with 1 d.f. This however is not fully justified, because the 1 d.f. test statistic does not have a χ^2 distribution with 1 d.f. since pretesting was done. The original 4 d.f. test statistic does have a χ^2 distribution with 4 d.f. because it was for a prespecified test.

For quadratic regression, Grambsch and O'Brien[158] showed that the 2 d.f. test of association is nearly optimal when pretesting is done, even when the true relationship is linear. They considered an ordinary regression model $E(Y|X) = \beta_0 + \beta_1 X + \beta_2 X^2$ and studied tests of association between X and Y. The strategy they studied was as follows. First, fit the quadratic model and obtain the partial test of $H_0 : \beta_2 = 0$, that is the test of linearity. If this partial F-test is significant at the $\alpha = 0.05$ level, report as the final test of association between X and Y the 2 d.f. F-test of $H_0 : \beta_1 = \beta_2 = 0$. If the test of linearity is insignificant, the model is refitted without the quadratic term and the test of association is then a 1 d.f. test, $H_0 : \beta_1 = 0|\beta_2 = 0$. Grambsch and O'Brien demonstrated that the type I error from this two-stage test is greater than the stated α, and in fact a fairly accurate P-value can be obtained if it is computed from an F distribution with 2 numerator d.f. even when testing at the second stage. This is because in the original 2 d.f. test of association, the 1 d.f. corresponding to the nonlinear effect is deleted if the nonlinear effect is very small; that is one is retaining the most significant part of the 2 d.f. F statistic.

If we use a 2 d.f. F critical value to assess the X effect even when X^2 is not in the model, it is clear that the two-stage approach can only lose power and hence it has no advantage whatsoever. That is because the sum of squares due to regression from the quadratic model is greater than the sum of squares computed from the linear model.

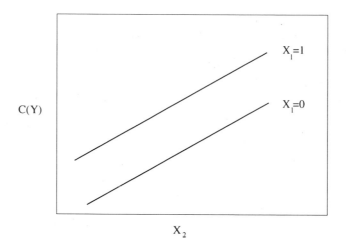

FIGURE 2.4: Regression assumptions for one binary and one continuous predictor.

2.7   Assessment of Model Fit

2.7.1   Regression Assumptions

In this section, the regression part of the model is isolated, and methods are de-scribed for validating the regression assumptions or modifying the model to meet the assumptions. The general linear regression model is

$$C(Y|X) = X\beta = \beta_0 + \beta_1 X_1 + \beta_2 X_2 + \ldots + \beta_k X_k. \tag{2.31}$$

The assumptions of linearity and additivity need to be verified. We begin with a special case of the general model,

$$C(Y|X) = \beta_0 + \beta_1 X_1 + \beta_2 X_2, \tag{2.32}$$

where X_1 is binary and X_2 is continuous. One needs to verify that the property of the response $C(Y)$ is related to X_1 and X_2 according to Figure 2.4. There are several methods for checking the fit of this model. The first method below is based on critiquing the simple model, and the other methods directly "estimate" the model.

1. Fit the simple linear additive model and critically examine residual plots for evidence of systematic patterns. For least squares fits one can compute esti-mated residuals $e = Y - X\hat{\beta}$ and box plots of e stratified by X_1 and scatterplots of e versus X_1 and $\hat{Y}$ with trend curves. If one is assuming constant conditional variance of Y, the spread of the residual distribution against each of the vari-ables can be checked at the same time. If the normality assumption is needed (i.e., if significance tests or confidence limits are used), the distribution of e

can be compared with a normal distribution with mean zero. **Advantage**: Simplicity. **Disadvantages**: Standard residuals can only be computed for continuous uncensored response variables. The judgment of nonrandomness is largely subjective, it is difficult to detect interaction, and if interaction is present it is difficult to check any of the other assumptions. Unless trend lines are added to plots, patterns may be difficult to discern if the sample size is very large. Detecting patterns in residuals does not always inform the analyst of what corrective action to take, although partial residual plots can be used to estimate the needed transformations if interaction is absent.

2. Make a scatterplot of Y versus X_2 using different symbols according to values of X_1. **Advantages**: Simplicity, and one can sometimes see all regression patterns including interaction. **Disadvantages**: Scatterplots cannot be drawn for binary, categorical, or censored Y. Patterns are difficult to see if relationships are weak or if the sample size is very large.

3. Stratify the sample by X_1 and quantile groups (e.g., deciles) of X_2. Within each $X_1 \times X_2$ stratum an estimate of $C(Y|X_1, X_2)$ is computed. If X_1 is continuous, the same method can be used after grouping X_1 into quantile groups. **Advantages**: Simplicity, ability to see interaction patterns, can handle censored Y if care is taken. **Disadvantages**: Subgrouping requires relatively large sample sizes and does not use continuous factors effectively as it does not attempt any interpolation. The ordering of quantile groups is not utilized by the procedure. Subgroup estimates have low precision (see p. 477 for an example). Each stratum must contain enough information to allow trends to be apparent above noise in the data. The method of grouping chosen (e.g., deciles vs. quintiles vs. rounding) can alter the shape of the plot.

4. Fit a nonparametric smoother separately for levels of X_1 (Section 2.4.6) relating X_2 to Y. **Advantages**: All regression aspects of the model can be summarized efficiently with minimal assumptions. **Disadvantages**: Does not easily apply to censored Y, and does not easily handle multiple predictors.

5. Fit a flexible parametric model that allows for most of the departures from the linear additive model that you wish to entertain. **Advantages**: One framework is used for examining the model assumptions, fitting the model, and drawing formal inference. Degrees of freedom are well defined and all aspects of statistical inference "work as advertised." **Disadvantages**: Complexity, and it is generally difficult to allow for interactions when assessing patterns of effects.

The first four methods each have the disadvantage that if confidence limits or formal inferences are desired it is difficult to know how many degrees of freedom were effectively used so that, for example, confidence limits will have the stated coverage probability. For method five, the restricted cubic spline function is an excellent tool for estimating the true relationship between X_2 and $C(Y)$ for continuous variables without assuming linearity. By fitting a model containing X_2 expanded into $k - 1$ terms, where k is the number of knots, one can obtain an estimate of the function of X_2 that could be used linearly in the model:

$$
\begin{aligned}
\hat{C}(Y|X) &= \hat{\beta}_0 + \hat{\beta}_1 X_1 + \hat{\beta}_2 X_2 + \hat{\beta}_3 X_2' + \hat{\beta}_4 X_2'' \\
&= \hat{\beta}_0 + \hat{\beta}_1 X_1 + \hat{f}(X_2),
\end{aligned} \tag{2.33}
$$

where

$$
\hat{f}(X_2) = \hat{\beta}_2 X_2 + \hat{\beta}_3 X_2' + \hat{\beta}_4 X_2'', \tag{2.34}
$$

and X_2' and X_2'' are constructed spline variables (when $k = 4$) as described previously. We call $\hat{f}(X_2)$ the spline-estimated transformation of X_2. Plotting the estimated spline function $\hat{f}(X_2)$ versus X_2 will generally shed light on how the effect of X_2 should be modeled. If the sample is sufficiently large, the spline function can be fitted separately for $X_1 = 0$ and $X_1 = 1$, allowing detection of even unusual interaction patterns. A formal test of linearity in X_2 is obtained by testing $H_0 : \beta_3 = \beta_4 = 0$, using a computationally efficient score test, for example (Section 9.2.3).

If the model is nonlinear in X_2, either a transformation suggested by the spline function plot (e.g., $\log(X_2)$) or the spline function itself (by placing X_2, X_2', and X_2'' simultaneously in any model fitted) may be used to describe X_2 in the model. If a tentative transformation of X_2 is specified, say $g(X_2)$, the adequacy of this transformation can be tested by expanding $g(X_2)$ in a spline function and testing for linearity. If one is concerned only with prediction and not with statistical inference, one can attempt to find a simplifying transformation for a predictor by plotting $g(X_2)$ against $\hat{f}(X_2)$ (the estimated spline transformation) for a variety of g, seeking a linearizing transformation of X_2. When there are nominal or binary predictors in the model in addition to the continuous predictors, it should be noted that there are no shape assumptions to verify for the binary/nominal predictors. One need only test for interactions between these predictors and the others.

If the model contains more than one continuous predictor, all may be expanded with spline functions in order to test linearity or to describe nonlinear relationships. If one did desire to assess simultaneously, for example, the linearity of predictors X_2 and X_3 in the presence of a linear or binary predictor X_1, the model could be specified as

$$
\begin{aligned}
C(Y|X) &= \beta_0 + \beta_1 X_1 + \beta_2 X_2 + \beta_3 X_2' + \beta_4 X_2'' \\
&+ \beta_5 X_3 + \beta_6 X_3' + \beta_7 X_3'',
\end{aligned} \tag{2.35}
$$

where X_2', X_2'', X_3', and X_3'' represent components of four knot restricted cubic spline functions.

The test of linearity for X_2 (with 2 d.f.) is $H_0 : \beta_3 = \beta_4 = 0$. The overall test of linearity for X_2 and X_3 is $H_0 : \beta_3 = \beta_4 = \beta_6 = \beta_7 = 0$, with 4 d.f. But as described further in Section 4.1 even though there are many reasons for allowing relationships to be nonlinear, there are reasons for not testing the nonlinear components for significance, as this might tempt the analyst to simplify the model.[158] Testing for linearity is usually best done to justify to nonstatisticians the need for complexity to explain or predict outcomes.

2.7.2   Modeling and Testing Complex Interactions

For testing interaction between X_1 and X_2 (after a needed transformation may have been applied), often a product term (e.g., $X_1 X_2$) can be added to the model and its coefficient tested. A more general simultaneous test of linearity and lack of interaction for a two-variable model in which one variable is binary (or is assumed linear) is obtained by fitting the model

$$
\begin{aligned}
C(Y|X) &= \beta_0 + \beta_1 X_1 + \beta_2 X_2 + \beta_3 X_2' + \beta_4 X_2'' \\
&+ \beta_5 X_1 X_2 + \beta_6 X_1 X_2' + \beta_7 X_1 X_2''
\end{aligned} \tag{2.36}
$$

and testing $H_0 : \beta_3 = \ldots = \beta_7 = 0$. This formulation allows the shape of the X_2 effect to be completely different for each level of X_1. There is virtually no departure from linearity and additivity that cannot be detected from this expanded model formulation if the number of knots is adequate and X_1 is binary. For binary logistic models, this method is equivalent to fitting two separate spline regressions in X_2.   9

Interactions can be complex when all variables are continuous. An approximate approach is to reduce the variables to two transformed variables, in which case interaction may sometimes be approximated by a single product of the two new variables. A disadvantage of this approach is that the estimates of the transformations for the two variables will be different depending on whether interaction terms are adjusted for when estimating "main effects." Another method involves fitting interactions of the form $X_1 f(X_2)$ and $X_2 g(X_1)$:

$$
\begin{aligned}
C(Y|X) &= \beta_0 + \beta_1 X_1 + \beta_2 X_1' + \beta_3 X_1'' \\
&+ \beta_4 X_2 + \beta_5 X_2' + \beta_6 X_2'' \\
&+ \beta_7 X_1 X_2 + \beta_8 X_1 X_2' + \beta_9 X_1 X_2'' \\
&+ \beta_{10} X_2 X_1' + \beta_{11} X_2 X_1''
\end{aligned} \tag{2.37}
$$

(for $k = 4$ knots for both variables). The test of additivity is $H_0 : \beta_7 = \beta_8 = \ldots = \beta_{11} = 0$ with 5 d.f. A test of lack of fit for the simple product interaction with X_1 is $H_0 : \beta_8 = \beta_9 = 0$, and a test of lack of fit for the simple product interaction with X_2 is $H_0 : \beta_{10} = \beta_{11} = 0$.

A general way to model and test interactions, although one requiring a larger number of parameters to be estimated, is based on modeling the $X_1 \times X_2 \times Y$ relationship with a smooth three-dimensional surface. A cubic spline surface can be constructed by covering the $X_1 - X_2$ plane with a grid and fitting a patchwise cubic polynomial in two variables. The grid is $(u_i, v_j), i = 1, \ldots, k, j = 1, \ldots, k$, where knots for X_1 are $(u_1, \ldots, u_k)$ and knots for X_2 are $(v_1, \ldots, v_k)$. The number of parameters can be reduced by constraining the surface to be of the form $aX_1 + bX_2 + cX_1X_2$ in the lower left and upper right corners of the plane. The resulting restricted cubic spline surface is described by a multiple regression model containing spline expansions in X_1 and X_2 and all cross-products of the restricted cubic spline components (e.g., $X_1 X_2'$). If the same number of knots k is used for both predictors, the number of interaction terms is $(k - 1)^2$. Examples of various ways of modeling interaction are given in Chapter 10. Spline functions made up of cross-products of all terms of individual spline functions are called *tensor splines*.[190] $\boxed{10}$

The presence of more than two predictors increases the complexity of tests for interactions because of the number of two-way interactions and because of the possibility of interaction effects of order higher than two. For example, in a model containing age, sex, and diabetes, the important interaction could be that older male diabetics have an exaggerated risk. However, higher-order interactions are often ignored unless specified a priori based on knowledge of the subject matter. Indeed, the number of two-way interactions alone is often too large to allow testing them all with reasonable power while controlling multiple comparison problems. Often, the only two-way interactions we can afford to test are those that were thought to be important before examining the data. A good approach is to test for all such prespecified interaction effects with a single global (pooled) test. Then, unless interactions involving only one of the predictors is of special interest, one can either drop all interactions or retain all of them.

For some problems a reasonable approach is, for each predictor separately, to test simultaneously the joint importance of all interactions involving that predictor. For p predictors this results in p tests each with $p - 1$ degrees of freedom. The multiple comparison problem would then be reduced from $p(p - 1)/2$ tests (if all two-way interactions were tested individually) to p tests.

In the fields of biostatistics and epidemiology, some types of interactions that have consistently been found to be important in predicting outcomes and thus may be prespecified are the following.

1. Interactions between treatment and the severity of disease being treated. Patients with little disease can receive little benefit.

2. Interactions involving age and risk factors. Older subjects are generally less affected by risk factors. They had to have been robust to survive to their current age with risk factors present.

3. Interactions involving age and type of disease. Some diseases are incurable and have the same prognosis regardless of age. Others are treatable or have less effect on younger patients.

4. Interactions between a measurement and the state of a subject during a measurement. Respiration rate measured during sleep may have greater predictive value and thus have a steeper slope versus outcome than respiration rate measured during activity.

5. Interaction between menopausal status and treatment or risk factors.

6. Interactions between race and disease.

7. Interactions between calendar time and treatment. Some treatments have learning curves causing secular trends in the associations.

8. Interactions between month of the year and other predictors, due to seasonal effects.

9. Interaction between the quality and quantity of a symptom, for example, daily frequency of chest pain × severity of a typical pain episode.

10. Interactions between study center and treatment.   11

2.7.3 Fitting Ordinal Predictors

For the case of an ordinal predictor, spline functions are not useful unless there are so many categories that in essence the variable is continuous. When the number of categories k is small (three to five, say), the variable is usually modeled as a polytomous factor using dummy variables or equivalently as one linear term and $k-2$ dummies. The latter coding facilitates testing for linearity. For more categories, it may be reasonable to stratify the data by levels of the variable and to compute summary statistics (e.g., logit proportions for a logistic model) or to examine regression coefficients associated with dummy variables over categories. Then one can attempt to summarize the pattern with a linear or some other simple trend. Later hypothesis tests must take into account this data-driven scoring (by using > 1 d.f., for example), but the scoring can save degrees of freedom when testing for interaction with other factors. In one dataset, the number of comorbid diseases was used to summarize the risk of a set of diseases that was too large to model. By plotting the logit of the proportion of deaths versus the number of diseases, it was clear that the square of the number of diseases would properly score the variables.

Sometimes it is useful to code an ordinal predictor with $k-1$ dummy variables of the form $I(X \geq v_j)$, where $j = 2, \ldots, k$ and $I(h) = 1$ if h is true, 0 otherwise.[441] Although a test of linearity does not arise immediately from this coding, the regression coefficients are interpreted as amounts of change from the previous category.

A test of whether the last m categories can be combined with the category $k - m$ does follow easily from this coding.

2.7.4   Distributional Assumptions

The general linear regression model is stated as $C(Y|X) = X\beta$ to highlight its regression assumptions. For logistic regression models for binary or nominal responses, there is no distributional assumption if simple random sampling is used and subjects' responses are independent. That is, the binary logistic model and all of its assumptions are contained in the expression logit$\{Y = 1|X\} = X\beta$. For ordinary multiple regression with constant variance σ^2, we usually assume that $Y - X\beta$ is normally distributed with mean 0 and variance σ^2. This assumption can be checked by estimating β with $\hat{\beta}$ and plotting the overall distribution of the residuals $Y - X\hat{\beta}$, the residuals against $\hat{Y}$, and the residuals against each X. For the latter two, the residuals should be normally distributed within each neighborhood of $\hat{Y}$ or X. A weaker requirement is that the overall distribution of residuals is normal; this will be satisfied if all of the stratified residual distributions are normal. Note a hidden assumption in both models, namely, that there are no omitted predictors. Other models, such as the Weibull survival model or the Cox[92] proportional hazards model, also have distributional assumptions that are not fully specified by $C(Y|X) = X\beta$. However, regression and distributional assumptions of some of these models are encapsulated by

$$C(Y|X) = C(Y = y|X) = d(y) + X\beta \qquad (2.38)$$

for some choice of C. Here $C(Y = y|X)$ is a property of the response Y evaluated at $Y = y$, given the predictor values X, and $d(y)$ is a component of the distribution of Y. For the Cox proportional hazards model, $C(Y = y|X)$ can be written as the log of the hazard of the event at time y, or equivalently as the log of the $-$ log of the survival probability at time y, and $d(y)$ can be thought of as a log hazard function for a "standard" subject.

If we evaluated the property $C(Y = y|X)$ at predictor values X^1 and X^2, the difference in properties is

$$
\begin{aligned}
C(Y = y|X^1) - C(Y = y|X^2) &= d(y) + X^1\beta \qquad (2.39)\\
&\quad - [d(y) + X^2\beta]\\
&= (X^1 - X^2)\beta,
\end{aligned}
$$

which is independent of y. One way to verify part of the distributional assumption is to estimate $C(Y = y|X^1)$ and $C(Y = y|X^2)$ for set values of X^1 and X^2 using a method that does not make the assumption, and to plot $C(Y = y|X^1) - C(Y = y|X^2)$ versus y. This function should be flat if the distributional assumption holds. The assumption can be tested formally if $d(y)$ can be generalized to be a function of X as well as y. A test of whether $d(y|X)$ depends on X is a test of one part of the distributional assumption. For example, writing $d(y|X) = d(y) + X\Gamma \log(y)$ where

$$X\Gamma = \Gamma_1 X_1 + \Gamma_2 X_2 + \ldots + \Gamma_k X_k \qquad (2.40)$$

and testing $H_0 : \Gamma_1 = \ldots = \Gamma_k = 0$ is one way to test whether $d(y|X)$ depends on X. For semiparametric models such as the Cox proportional hazards model, the only distributional assumption is the one stated above, namely, that the difference in properties between two subjects depends only on the difference in the predictors between the two subjects. Other, parametric, models assume in addition that the property $C(Y = y|X)$ has a specific shape as a function of y, that is that $d(y)$ has a specific functional form. For example, the Weibull survival model has a specific assumption regarding the shape of the hazard or survival distribution as a function of y.

Assessments of distributional assumptions are best understood by applying these methods to individual models is demonstrated in later chapters.

2.8   Further Reading

1 References [110, 389, 392] have more information about cubic splines.

2 See Smith[392] for a good overview of spline functions.

3 More material about natural splines may be found in [110, pp. 55, 236, 273]. Mc-Neil et al.[310] discuss the overall smoothness of natural splines in terms of the integral of the square of the second derivative of the regression function, over the range of the data.

4 A tutorial on restricted cubic splines is in [187].

5 Durrleman and Simon[121] provide examples in which knots are allowed to be estimated as free parameters, jointly with the regression coefficients. They found that even though the "optimal" knots were often far from a priori knot locations, the model fits were virtually identical.

6 Contrast Hastie and Tibshirani's generalized nonparametric additive models[191] with Stone and Koo's[403] additive model in which each continuous predictor is represented with a restricted cubic spline function.

7 Gray[161, 162] provided some comparisons with ordinary regression splines, but he compared penalized regression splines to nonrestricted splines with only two knots. Two knots were chosen so as to limit the degrees of freedom needed by the regression spline method to a reasonable number. Gray argued that regression splines are sensitive to knot locations, and he is correct when only two knots are allowed and no linear tail restrictions are imposed. Two knots also prevent the (ordinary maximum likelihood) fit from utilizing some local behavior of the regression relationship. For penalized likelihood estimation using B-splines, Gray[162] provided extensive simulation studies of type I and II error for testing association in which the true regression

function, number of knots, and amount of likelihood penalization were varied. He studied both normal regression and Cox regression.

[8] Breiman et al.'s original CART method[48] used the Gini criterion for splitting. Later work has used log-likelihoods.[75] Segal,[381] LeBlanc and Crowley,[270] and Ciampi et al.[73, 74] have extended recursive partitioning to censored survival data using the log-rank statistic as the criterion. Zhang[461] extended tree models to handle multivariate binary responses. Schmoor et al.[376] used a more general splitting criterion that is useful in therapeutic trials, namely, a Cox test for main and interacting effects. Davis and Anderson[107] used an exponential survival model as the basis for tree construction. Ahn and Loh[6] developed a Cox proportional hazards model adaptation of recursive partitioning along with bootstrap and cross-validation-based methods to protect against "over-splitting." The Cox-based regression tree methods of Ciampi et al.[73] have a unique feature that allows for construction of "treatment interaction trees" with hierarchical adjustment for baseline variables. Zhang et al.[462] provided a new method for handling missing predictor values that is simpler than using surrogate splits. See [100, 186] for examples using recursive partitioning for binary responses in which the prediction trees did not validate well.

[9] For ordinary linear models, the regression estimates are the same as obtained with separate fits, but standard errors are different (since a pooled standard error is used for the combined fit). For Cox[92] regression, separate fits can be slightly different since each subset would use a separate ranking of Y.

[10] Gray's penalized fixed-knot regression splines can be useful for estimating joint effects of two continuous variables while allowing the analyst to control the effective number of degrees of freedom in the fit [161, 162, Section 3.2]. When Y is a non-censored variable, the local regression model of Cleveland et al.,[65] a multidimensional scatterplot smoother mentioned in Section 2.4.6, provides a good graphical assessment of the joint effects of several predictors so that the forms of interactions can be chosen. See Wang et al.[445] and Gustafson[169] for several other flexible approaches to analyzing interactions among continuous variables.

[11] Study site by treatment interaction is often the interaction that is worried about the most in multicenter randomized clinical trials, because regulatory agencies are concerned with consistency of treatment effects over study centers. However, this type of interaction is usually the weakest and is difficult to assess when there are many centers due to the number of interaction parameters to estimate. Schemper[367] discusses various types of interactions and a general nonparametric test for interaction.

2.9   Problems

For problems 1 to 3, state each model statistically, identifying each predictor with one or more component variables. Identify and interpret each regression parameter except for coefficients of nonlinear terms in spline functions. State each hypothesis below as a formal statistical hypothesis involving the proper parameters, and give the (numerator) degrees of freedom of the test. State alternative hypotheses carefully with respect to unions or intersections of conditions and list the type of alternatives to the null hypothesis that the test is designed to detect.[b]

1. A property of Y such as the mean is linear in age and blood pressure and there may be an interaction between the two predictors. Test H_0 : there is no interaction between age and blood pressure. Also test H_0 : blood pressure is not associated with Y (in any fashion). State the effect of blood pressure as a function of age, and the effect of age as a function of blood pressure.

2. Consider a linear additive model involving three treatments (control, drug Z, and drug Q) and one continuous adjustment variable, age. Test H_0 : treatment group is not associated with response, adjusted for age. Also test H_0 : response for drug Z has the same property as the response for drug Q, adjusted for age.

3. Consider models each with two predictors, temperature and white blood count (WBC), for which temperature is always assumed to be linearly related to the appropriate property of the response, and WBC may or may not be linear (depending on the particular model you formulate for each question). Test:

   (a) H_0 : WBC is not associated with the response versus H_a : WBC is linearly associated with the property of the response.

   (b) H_0 : WBC is not associated with Y versus H_a : WBC is quadratically associated with Y. Also write down the formal test of linearity against this quadratic alternative.

   (c) H_0 : WBC is not associated with Y versus H_a : WBC related to the property of the response through a smooth spline function; for example, for WBC the model requires the variables WBC, WBC′, and WBC″ where WBC′ and WBC″ represent nonlinear components (if there are four knots in a restricted cubic spline function). Also write down the formal test of linearity against this spline function alternative.

   (d) Test for a lack of fit (combined nonlinearity or nonadditivity) in an overall model that takes the form of an interaction between temperature and WBC, allowing WBC to be modeled with a smooth spline function.

4. For a fitted model $Y = a + bX + cX^2$ derive the estimate of the effect on Y of changing X from x_1 to x_2.

5. In "The Class of 1988: A Statistical Portrait," the College Board reported mean SAT scores for each state. Use an ordinary least squares multiple regression model to study the mean verbal SAT score as a function of the percentage of students taking the test in each state. Provide plots of fitted functions and defend your choice of the "best" fit. Make sure the shape of the chosen fit

---

[b]In other words, under what assumptions does the test have maximum power.

agrees with what you know about the variables. Add the raw data points to any plots, showing fitted equations (e.g., `points(x,y)` in S-PLUS).

(a) Fit a linear spline function with a knot at X = 50%. Plot the data and the fitted function and do a formal test for linearity and a test for association between X and Y. Give a detailed interpretation of the estimated coefficients in the linear spline model, and use the partial t-test to test linearity in this model.

(b) Fit a restricted cubic spline function with knots at X = 6, 12, 58, and 68% (not percentile).[c] Plot the fitted function and do a formal test of association between X and Y. Do two tests of linearity that test the same hypothesis:

    i. by using a *contrast* to simultaneously test the correct set of coefficients against zero (done by the `anova` function in `Design`);[d]

    ii. by comparing the R^2 from the complex model with that from a simple linear model using a partial F-test.

Explain why the tests of linearity have the d.f. they have.

(c) Using subject matter knowledge, pick a final model (from among the previous models or using another one) that makes sense.

The data are found in Table 2.4.

---

[c]Note: To prespecify knots for restricted cubic spline functions, use something like `rcs(predictor, c(t1,t2,t3,t4))`, where the knot locations are `t1, t2, t3, t4`.

[d]Note that `anova` in `Design` computes all needed test statistics from a single model fit object.

TABLE 2.4

% Taking SAT (X)	Mean Verbal Score (Y)	% Taking SAT (X)	Mean Verbal Score (Y)
4	482	24	440
5	498	29	460
5	513	37	448
6	498	43	441
6	511	44	424
7	479	45	417
9	480	49	422
9	483	50	441
10	475	52	408
10	476	55	412
10	487	57	400
10	494	58	401
12	474	59	430
12	478	60	433
13	457	62	433
13	485	63	404
14	451	63	424
14	471	63	430
14	473	64	431
16	467	64	437
17	470	68	446
18	464	69	424
20	471	72	420
22	455	73	432
23	452	81	436

Chapter 3

Missing Data

3.1 Types of Missing Data

There are missing data in the majority of datasets one is likely to encounter. Before discussing some of the problems of analyzing data in which some variables are missing for some subjects, we define some nomenclature.

Missing completely at random (MCAR)

Data elements are missing for reasons that are unrelated to any characteristics or responses for the subject, including the value of the missing value, were it to be known. Examples include missing laboratory measurements because of a dropped test tube (if it was not dropped because of knowledge of any measurements), a study that ran out of funds before some subjects could return for follow-up visits, and a survey in which a subject omitted her response to a question for reasons unrelated to the response she would have made or to any other of her characteristics.

Missing at random (MAR)

Data elements are not missing at random, but the probability that a value is missing depends on values of variables that were actually measured. As an example, consider a survey in which females are less likely to provide their personal income in general (but the likelihood of responding is independent of her actual income). If we know the sex of every subject and have income levels for some of the females, unbiased sex-specific income estimates can be made. That is because the incomes we do have for some of the females are a random sample of all females' incomes. Another way of saying that a variable is MAR is that given the values of other available variables, subjects having missing values are only randomly different from other subjects.[360] Or to paraphrase Greenland and Finkle,[165] for MAR the missingness of a covariable cannot depend on unobserved covariable values; for example whether a predictor is observed cannot depend on another predictor when the latter is missing but it can depend on the latter when it is observed. MAR and MCAR data are also called *ignorable* nonresponses.

Informative missing (IM)

Elements are more likely to be missing if their true values of the variable in question are systematically higher or lower. An example is when subjects with lower income levels or very high incomes are less likely to provide their personal income in an interview. IM is also called nonignorable nonresponse.

IM is the most difficult type of missing data to handle. In many cases, there is no fix for IM nor is there a way to use the data to test for the existence of IM. External considerations must dictate the choice of missing data models, and there are few clues for specifying a model under IM. MCAR is the easiest case to handle. Our ability to correctly analyze MAR data depends on the availability of auxiliary variables (the sex of the subject in the example above). Most of the methods available for dealing with missing data assume the data are MAR.

3.2   Prelude to Modeling

No matter whether one deletes incomplete cases, carefully imputes (estimates) missing data, or uses a full maximum likelihood technique to incorporate partial data, it is beneficial to characterize patterns of missingness using exploratory data analysis techniques. These techniques include binary logistic models and recursive partitioning for predicting the probability that a given variable is missing. Patterns of missingness should be reported to help readers understand the limitations of incomplete data. If you do decide to use imputation, it is also important to describe how variables are simultaneously missing. A cluster analysis of missing value status of all the variables is useful here. This can uncover cases where imputation is not as effective. For example, if the only variable moderately related to diastolic blood pressure is systolic pressure, but both pressures are missing on the same subject, systolic pressure cannot be used to estimate diastolic blood pressure. S-PLUS functions `naclus` and `naplot` in the `Hmisc` library (see p. 120) can help detect how variables are simultaneously missing. Recursive partitioning (regression tree) algorithms (see Section 2.5) are invaluable for describing which kinds of subjects are missing on a variable. Logistic regression is also an excellent tool for this purpose. A later example (p. 312) demonstrates these procedures.

3.3   Missing Values for Different Types of Response Variables

When the response variable Y is collected serially but some subjects drop out of the study before completion, there is a variety of ways of dealing with partial information such as multiple imputation in phases.[263] When Y is the time until an event, there are actually no missing values of Y but follow-up will be curtailed for some subjects. That leaves the case where the response is once, so that when it is not measured it is completely missing.

It is common practice to discard subjects having missing Y. Before doing so, at minimum an analysis should be done to characterize the tendency for Y to be missing, as just described. For example, logistic regression or recursive partitioning can be used to predict whether Y is missing and to test for systematic tendencies as opposed to Y being missing completely at random. In many models, though, more efficient estimates of regression coefficients can be made by also utilizing observations missing on Y that are nonmissing on X. Hence there is a definite place for imputation of Y.

[1]

3.4   Problems with Simple Alternatives to Imputation

Incomplete predictor information is a very common missing data problem. Statistical software packages use casewise deletion in handling missing predictors; that is, any subject having *any* predictor or Y missing will be excluded from a regression analysis. Casewise deletion results in regression coefficient estimates that can be terribly biased, imprecise, or both. First consider an example where bias is the problem. Suppose that the response is death and the predictors are age, sex, and blood pressure, and that age and sex were recorded for every subject. Suppose that blood pressure was not measured for a fraction of 0.10 of the subjects, and the most common reason for not obtaining a blood pressure was that the subject was about to die. Deletion of these very sick patients will cause a major bias (downward) in the model's intercept parameter. In general, casewise deletion will bias the estimate of the model's intercept parameter when missingness is dependent on Y in a way that is not explained by the nonmissing Xs.

[2]

Now consider an example in which casewise deletion of incomplete records is inefficient. The inefficiency comes from the reduction of sample size, which causes standard errors to increase,[116] confidence intervals to widen, and power of tests of association and tests of lack of fit to decrease. Suppose that the response is the presence of coronary artery disease and the predictors are age, sex, LDL cholesterol, HDL cholesterol, blood pressure, triglyceride, and smoking status. Suppose that age, sex, and smoking are recorded for all subjects, but that LDL is missing in 0.18 of the subjects, HDL is missing in 0.20, and triglyceride is missing in 0.21. Assume that all missing data are MCAR and that all of the subjects missing LDL are also missing HDL and that overall 0.28 of the subjects have one or more predictors missing and hence would be excluded from the analysis. If total cholesterol were known on every subject, even though it does not appear in the model, it (along perhaps with age and sex) can be used to estimate (*impute*) LDL and HDL cholesterol and triglyceride, perhaps using regression equations from other studies. Doing the analysis on a "filled in" dataset will result in more precise estimates because the sample size would then include the other 0.28 of the subjects.

In general, observations should only be discarded if there is a rarely missing predictor of overriding importance that cannot be reliably imputed from other information, or if the fraction of observations excluded is very small and the original sample size is large. Even then, there is no advantage of such deletion other than saving analyst time.

The first blood pressure example points out why it can be dangerous to handle missing values by adding a dummy variable to the model. Many analysts would set missing blood pressures to a constant (it doesn't matter which constant) and add a variable to the model such as `is.na(blood.pressure)` in S-PLUS notation. The coefficient for the latter dummy variable will be quite large in this example, and the model will appear to have great ability to predict death. This is because some of the left-hand side of the model contaminates the right-hand side; that is, `is.na(blood.pressure)` is correlated with death.

There are rare occasions when it is permissible to add a new category to a polytomous predictor to indicate missingness. This is the case when missing is a meaningful response or when missingness is independent of Y.

3.5   Strategies for Developing Imputation Algorithms

Except in special circumstances that usually involve only very simple models, the primary alternative to deleting incomplete observations is imputation of the missing values. Many nonstatisticians find the notion of estimating data distasteful, but the way to think about imputation of missing values is that "making up" data is better than discarding valuable data. It is especially distressing to have to delete subjects who are missing on an adjustment variable when a major variable of interest is not missing. So one goal of imputation is to use as much information as possible for examining any one predictor's adjusted association with Y. However, when single conditional mean imputation is used (see below) it may be beneficial to temporarily exclude subjects that are missing on a predictor of major interest, for the purpose of estimating that predictor's strength in predicting Y.

At this point the analyst must make some decisions about which information to use in computing predicted values for missing values.

1. Imputation of missing values for one of the variables can ignore all other information. Missing values can be filled in by sampling nonmissing values of the variable, or by using a constant such as the median or mean nonmissing value.

2. Imputation algorithms can be based only on external information not otherwise used in the model for Y in addition to variables included in later modeling. For example, family income can be imputed on the basis of location of residence when such information is to remain confidential for other aspects of the analysis or when such information would require too many degrees of freedom to be spent in the ultimate response model.

3. Imputations can be derived by only analyzing interrelationships among the Xs.

4. Imputations can use relationships among the Xs and between X and Y.

5. Imputations can take into account the reason for nonresponse if known.

When a variable, say X_j, is to be included as a predictor of Y, and X_j is sometimes missing, ignoring the relationship between X_j and Y for those observations for which both are known will bias regression coefficients for X_j toward zero.[291] On the other hand, using Y to singly impute X_j using a conditional mean will cause a large inflation in the apparent importance of X_j in the final model. In other words, when the missing X_j are replaced with a mean that is conditional on Y without a random component, this will result in a falsely strong relationship between the imputed X_j values and Y.

At first glance it might seem that using Y to impute one or more of the Xs, even with allowance for the correct amount of random variation, would result in a circular analysis in which the importance of the Xs will be exaggerated. But the relationship between X and Y in the subset of imputed observations will only be as strong as the associations between X and Y that are evidenced by the nonmissing data. In other words, regression coefficients estimated from a dataset that is completed by imputation will not in general be biased high as long as the imputed values have similar variation as nonmissing data values.

The next important decision about developing imputation algorithms is the choice of how missing values are estimated.

1. Missings can be estimated using single "best guesses" (e.g., predicted conditional expected values or means) based on relationships between nonmissing values. This is called single imputation of conditional means.

2. Missing X_j (or Y) can be estimated using single individual predicted values, where by predicted value we mean a random variable value from the whole conditional distribution of X_j. If one uses ordinary multiple regression to estimate X_j from Y and the other Xs, a random residual would be added to

the predicted mean value. If assuming a normal distribution for X_j conditional on the other data, such a residual could be computed by a Gaussian random number generator given an estimate of the residual standard deviation. If normality is not assumed, the residual could be a randomly chosen residual from the actual computed residuals. When m missing values need imputation for X_j, the residuals could be sampled with replacement from the entire vector of residuals as in the bootstrap. Better still according to Rubin and Schenker[360] would be to use the "approximate Bayesian bootstrap" which involves sampling n residuals with replacement from the original n estimated residuals (from observations not missing on X_j), then sampling m residuals with replacement from the first sampled set.

3. More than one random predicted value (as just defined) can be generated for each missing value. This process is called *multiple imputation* and it has many advantages over the other methods in general. This is discussed in Section 3.7.

4. Matching methods can be used to obtain random draws of other subject's values to replace missing values. Nearest neighbor matching can be used to select a subject that is "close" to the subject in need of imputation, on the basis of a series of variables. This method requires the analyst to make decisions about what constitutes "closeness." To simplify the matching process into a single dimension, Little[290] proposed the *predictive mean matching* method where matching is done on the basis of predicted values from a regression model for predicting the sometimes-missing variable. According to Little, in large samples predictive mean matching may be more robust to model misspecification than the method of adding a random residual to the subject's predicted value, but because of difficulties in finding matches the random residual method may be better in smaller samples. The random residual method is also easier to use when multiple imputations are needed.   5

What if X_j needs to be imputed for some subjects based on other variables that themselves may be missing on the same subjects missing on X_j? This is a place where recursive partitioning with "surrogate splits" in case of missing predictors may be a good method for developing imputations (see Section 2.5 and p. 119). If using regression to estimate missing values, an algorithm to cycle through all sometimes-missing variables for multiple iterations may perform well. This algorithm is used by the S-PLUS `transcan` function described in Section 4.7. First, all missing values are initialized to medians (modes for categorical variables). Then every time missing values are estimated for a certain variable, those estimates are inserted the next time the variable is used to predict other sometimes-missing variables.

If you want to assess the importance of a specific predictor that is frequently missing, it is a good idea to perform a sensitivity analysis in which all observations containing imputed values for that predictor are temporarily deleted. The test based on a model that included the imputed values may be diluted by the imputation or it may test the wrong hypothesis, especially if Y is not used in imputing X.

Little argues for down-weighting observations containing imputations, to obtain a more accurate variance–covariance matrix. For the ordinary linear model, the weights have been worked out for some cases [291, p. 1231].

3.6   Single Conditional Mean Imputation

For a continuous or binary X that is unrelated to all other Xs, the mean or median may be substituted for missing values without much loss of efficiency,[116] although regression coefficients will be biased low since Y was not utilized in the imputation. When the variable of interest is related to the other Xs it is far more efficient to use an individual predictive model for each X based on the other variables.[54, 352, 419] The "best guess" imputation method fills in missings with predicted expected values from using the multivariable imputation model based on nonmissing data. It is true that conditional means are the best estimates of unknown values, but except perhaps for binary logistic regression[425, 427] their use will result in biased estimates and very biased (low) variance estimates. The latter problem arises from the reduced variability of imputed values [126, p. 464].

Tree-based models (Section 2.5) may be very useful for imputation since they do not require linearity or additivity assumptions, although such models often have poor discrimination when they don't overfit. When a continuous X being imputed needs to be nonmonotonically transformed to best relate it to the other Xs (e.g., blood pressure vs. heart rate), trees and ordinary regression are inadequate. Here a general transformation modeling procedure (Section 4.7) may be needed.

Schemper et al.[372, 374] proposed imputing missing binary covariables by predicted probabilities. For categorical sometimes-missing variables, imputation models can be derived using polytomous logistic regression or a classification tree method. For missing values, the most likely value for each subject (from the series of predicted probabilities from the logistic or recursive partitioning model) can be substituted to avoid creating a new category that is falsely highly correlated with Y. For an ordinal X, the predicted mean value (possibly rounded to the nearest actual data value) or median value from an ordinal logistic model is sometimes useful.

3.7   Multiple Imputation

Imputing missing values and then doing an ordinary analysis as if the imputed values were real measurements is usually better than excluding subjects with incomplete data. However, ordinary formulas for standard errors and other statistics are invalid unless imputation is taken into account.[443] Methods for properly accounting for having incomplete data can be complex. The bootstrap (described later) is an easy method to implement, but the computations can be slow. To use the bootstrap to correctly estimate variances of regression coefficients one must repeat the imputation process and the model fitting perhaps 100 times using a resampling procedure[126, 383] (see Section 5.1). Still, the bootstrap can estimate the right variance for the wrong parameter estimates if the imputations are not done correctly.

Multiple imputation uses random draws from the conditional distribution of the target variable given the other variables (and any additional information that is relevant)[288, 291, 361] (but see [313]). The additional information used to predict the missing values can contain any variables that are potentially predictive, including variables measured in the future; the causal chain is not relevant.[291] When a regression model is used for imputation, the process involves adding a random residual to the "best guess" for missing values, to yield the same conditional variance as the original variable. Methods for estimating residuals were listed in Section 3.5. To properly account for variability due to unknown values, the imputation is repeated M times, where $M \geq 3$. Each repetition results in a "completed" dataset that is analyzed using the standard method. Parameter estimates are averaged over these multiple imputations to obtain better estimates than those from single imputation. The variance–covariance matrix of the averaged parameter estimates, adjusted for variability due to imputation, is estimated using

$$V = M^{-1} \sum_i^M V_i + \frac{M+1}{M} B, \qquad (3.1)$$

where V_i is the ordinary complete data estimate of the variance–covariance matrix for the model parameters from the ith imputation, and B is the between-imputation sample variance–covariance matrix, the diagonal entries of which are the ordinary sample variances of the M parameter estimates.

⑥

Section 4.7.3 discusses the S-Plus `transcan` function for single and multiple imputation and the associated `fit.mult.impute` function for averaging regression coefficients over multiple imputations and computing V in Equation 3.1.

3.8   Summary and Rough Guidelines

Table 3.1 summarizes the advantages and disadvantages of three methods of dealing with missing data. Here "Single" refers to single conditional mean imputation (which cannot utilize Y) and "Multiple" refers to multiple random-draw imputation (which can incorporate Y).

The following contains very crude guidelines. Simulation studies are needed to refine the recommendations. Here "proportion" refers to the proportion of observations having *any* variables missing.

TABLE 3.1: Summary of Methods for Dealing with Missing Values

Method	Deletion	Single	Multiple
Allows nonrandom missing	–	x	x
Reduces sample size	x	–	–
Apparent S.E. of $\hat{\beta}$ too low	–	x	–
Increases real S.E. of $\hat{\beta}$	x	–	–
$\hat{\beta}$ biased	if not MCAR	x	–

Proportion of missings ≤ 0.05: It doesn't matter very much how you impute missings or whether you adjust variance of regression coefficient estimates for having imputed data in this case. For continuous variables imputing missings with the median nonmissing value is adequate; for categorical predictors the most frequent category can be used. Complete case analysis is an option here.

Proportion of missings 0.05 **to** 0.15: If a predictor is unrelated to all of the other predictors, imputations can be done the same as the above (i.e., impute a reasonable constant value). If the predictor is correlated with other predictors, develop a customized model (or have the `transcan` function do it for you) to predict the predictor from all of the other predictors. Then impute missings with predicted values. For categorical variables, classification trees are good methods for developing customized imputation models. For continuous variables, ordinary regression can be used if the variable in question does not require a nonmonotonic transformation to be predicted from the other variables. For either the related or unrelated predictor case, variances may need to be adjusted for imputation. Single imputation is probably OK here, but multiple imputation doesn't hurt.

Proportion of missings > 0.15: This situation requires the same considerations as in the previous case, and adjusting variances for imputation is even more important. To estimate the strength of the effect of a predictor that is frequently missing, it may be necessary to refit the model on the subset of observations for which that predictor is not missing, if Y is not used for imputation. Multiple imputation is preferred for most models.

Multiple predictors frequently missing: Here we have the same considerations as the previous case but effects of imputations are more pronounced.

It should be emphasized that the only way to know that one of these rules of thumb is adequate for a given dataset is to actually take missing values fully into account and to see if the results change! It is also important to note that the reasons for missing data are more important determinants of how missing values should be handled than is the quantity of missing values.

If the main interest is prediction and not interpretation or inference about individual effects, it is worth trying a simple imputation (e.g., median or normal value substitution) to see if the resulting model predicts the response almost as well as one developed after using customized imputation.   [7]

3.9   Further Reading

[1]   Crawford et al.[98] give an example where responses are not MCAR for which deleting subjects with missing responses resulted in a biased estimate of the response distribution. They found that multiple imputation of the response resulted in much improved estimates.

[2]   See van Buuren et al.[430] for an example in which subjects having missing baseline blood pressure had shorter survival time.

[3]   Another problem with the missingness indicator approach arises when more than one predictor is missing and these predictors are missing on almost the same subjects. The missingness indicator variables will be collinear, that is impossible to disentangle.[223]

[4]   But see [427, pp. 2645–2646] for several problems with the "missing category" approach. D'Agostino and Rubin[105] developed methods for propensity score modeling that allow for missing data. They mentioned that extra categories may be added to allow for missing data in propensity models and that adding indicator variables describing patterns of missingness will also allow the analyst to match on missingness patterns when comparing nonrandomly assigned treatments.

[5]   Kalton and Kasprzyk[227] proposed a hybrid approach to imputation in which missing values are imputed with the predicted value for the subject plus the residual from the subject having the closest predicted value to the subject being imputed.

[6]   van Buuren et al.[430] presented an excellent case study in multiple imputation in the context of survival analysis. Barnard and Rubin[29] derived an estimate of the d.f. associated with the imputation-adjusted variance matrix for use in a t-distribution approximation for hypothesis tests about imputation-averaged coefficient estimates. When d.f. is not very large, the t approximation will result in more accurate P-values than using a normal approximation that we use with Wald statistics after inserting Equation 3.1 as the variance matrix.

[7]   A good general reference on missing data is Little and Rubin,[292] and Volume 16, Nos. 1 to 3 of *Statistics in Medicine*, a large issue devoted to incomplete covariable data. Vach[424] is an excellent text describing properties of various methods of dealing with missing data in binary logistic regression (see also [425, 426, 428]). The last six references show how to use maximum likelihood to explicitly model the missing data process. Little and Rubin show how imputation can be avoided if the analyst is willing to assume a multivariate distribution for the joint distribution of X and Y. Since X usually contains a strange mixture of binary, polytomous, and continuous but highly skewed predictors, it is unlikely that this approach will work optimally in many problems. That's the reason the imputation approach is emphasized. See Rubin[361] for a comprehensive source on multiple imputation. See Little,[289] Vach and Blettner,[427]

Rubin and Schenker,[360] Greenland and Finkle,[165] and Hunsberger et al.[214] for excellent reviews of missing data problems and approaches to solving them. Reilly and Pepe have a nice comparison of the "hot-deck" imputation method and a maximum likelihood-based method.[350]

3.10   Problems

The SUPPORT Study (Study to Understand Prognoses Preferences Outcomes and Risks of Treatments) was a five-hospital study of 10,000 critically ill hospitalized adults.[241] Patients were followed for in-hospital outcomes and for long-term survival. We analyze 35 variables and a random sample of 1000 patients from this extensive dataset. This random sample is available on the Web page.

1. Explore the variables and patterns of missing data in the SUPPORT dataset.

   (a) Print univariable summaries of all variables. Make a plot (showing all variables on one page) that describes especially the continuous variables.

   (b) Make a plot showing the extent of missing data and tendencies for some variables to be missing on the same patients. Functions in the `Hmisc` library may be useful.

   (c) Total hospital costs (variable `totcst`) were estimated from hospital-specific Medicare cost-to-charge ratios. Characterize what kind of patients have missing `totcst`. For this characterization use the following patient descriptors: `age, sex, dzgroup, num.co, edu, income, scoma, meanbp, hrt, resp, temp`.

2. Prepare for later development of a model to predict costs by developing reliable imputations for missing costs. Remove the observation having zero `totcst`.[a]

   (a) The cost estimates are not available on 105 patients. Total hospital charges (bills) are available on all but 25 patients. Relate these two variables to each other with an eye toward using `charges` to predict `totcst` when `totcst` is missing. Make graphs that will tell whether linear regression or linear regression after taking logs of both variables is better.

   (b) Impute missing total hospital costs in SUPPORT based on a regression model relating charges to costs, when charges are available. You may want to use a statement like the following in S-PLUS:

---

[a]You can use the S-PLUS command `attach(support[is.na(support $ totcst) | support $ totcst > 0,])`. The `is.na` condition tells S-PLUS that it is permissible to include observations having missing `totcst` without setting all columns of such observations to `NA`.

```
totcst ← ifelse(is.na(totcst),
                (expression in charges), totcst)
```

If in the previous problem you felt that the relationship between costs and charges should be based on taking logs of both variables, the "expression in charges" above may look something like `exp(intercept + slope * log(charges))`, where constants are inserted for `intercept` and `slope`.

(c) Compute the likely error in approximating total cost using charges by computing the median absolute difference between predicted and observed total costs in the patients having both variables available. If you used a log transformation, also compute the median absolute percent error in imputing total costs by antilogging the absolute difference in predicted logs.

Chapter 4

Multivariable Modeling Strategies

Chapter 2 dealt with aspects of modeling such as transformations of predictors, relaxing linearity assumptions, modeling interactions, and examining lack of fit. Chapter 3 dealt with missing data, focusing on utilization of incomplete predictor information. All of these areas are important in the overall scheme of model development, and they cannot be separated from what is to follow. In this chapter we concern ourselves with issues related to the whole model, with emphasis on deciding on the amount of complexity to allow in the model and on dealing with large numbers of predictors. The chapter concludes with three default modeling strategies depending on whether the goal is prediction, estimation, or hypothesis testing. ☐

4.1   Prespecification of Predictor Complexity Without Later Simplification

There are rare occasions in which one actually expects a relationship to be linear. For example, one might predict mean arterial blood pressure at two months after beginning drug administration using as baseline variables the pretreatment mean blood pressure and other variables. In this case one expects the pretreatment blood pressure to linearly relate to follow-up blood pressure, and modeling is simple. In the vast majority of studies, however, there is every reason to suppose that all relationships involving nonbinary predictors are nonlinear. In these cases, the only reason to represent predictors linearly in the model is that there is insufficient information in the sample to allow us to reliably fit nonlinear relationships.[a]

Supposing that nonlinearities are entertained, analysts often use scatter diagrams or descriptive statistics to decide how to represent variables in a model. The result will often be an adequately fitting model, but confidence limits will be too narrow, P-values too small, R^2 too large, and calibration too good to be true. The reason is that the "phantom d.f." that represented potential complexities in the model that were dismissed during the subjective assessments are forgotten in computing standard errors, P-values, and R^2_{adj}. The same problem is created when one entertains several transformations (log, $\sqrt{\ }$, etc.) and uses the data to see which one fits best, or when one tries to simplify a spline fit to a simple transformation.

An approach that solves this problem is to prespecify the complexity with which each predictor is represented in the model, without later simplification of the model. The amount of complexity (e.g., number of knots in spline functions or order of ordinary polynomials) one can afford to fit is roughly related to the "effective sample size." It is also very reasonable to allow for greater complexity for predictors that are thought to be more powerfully related to Y. For example, errors in estimating the curvature of a regression function are consequential in predicting Y only when the regression is somewhere steep. Once the analyst decides to include a predictor in every model, it is fair to use general measures of association to quantify the predictive potential for a variable. If a predictor has a low rank correlation with the response, it will not "pay" to devote many degrees of freedom to that predictor in a spline function having many knots. On the other hand, a potent predictor (with a high rank correlation) not known to act linearly might be assigned five knots if the sample size allows.

This approach does not require the analyst to really prespecify predictor complexity, so how is it unbiased? There are two reasons: the analyst has already agreed to retain the variable in the model even if the rank correlation is low, and the rank correlation coefficient does not reveal the degree of nonlinearity of the predictor to allow the analyst to "tweak" the number of knots. Any predictive ability a variable might have may be concentrated in its nonlinear effects, so using the rank correlation to decide to save degrees of freedom by restricting the variable to be linear may result in no predictive ability. Likewise, a low Spearman multiple correlation between a categorical variable and Y might lead the analyst to collapse some of the categories based on their frequencies. This often helps, but sometimes the categories that are so combined are the ones that are most different from one another. So if using rank correlation to reduce degrees of freedom can harm the model, one might argue that it is fair to allow this strategy to also benefit the analysis. However,

---

[a]Shrinkage (penalized estimation) is a general solution (see Section 4.5). One can always use complex models that are "penalized towards simplicity," with the amount of penalization being greater for smaller sample sizes.

the bivariable correlation method can be misleading if marginal relationships vary greatly from ones obtained after adjusting for other predictors.

2

When Y is binary or continuous (but not censored), a good general-purpose measure of association that is useful in making decisions about the number of parameters to devote to a predictor is an extension of Spearman's ρ rank correlation. This is the ordinary R^2 from predicting the rank of Y based on the rank of X and the square of the rank of X. This ρ^2 will detect not only nonlinear relationships (as will ordinary Spearman ρ) but nonmonotonic ones as well. It is important that the ordinary Spearman ρ not be computed, as this would tempt the analyst to simplify the regression function (towards monotonicity) if the generalized ρ^2 does not significantly exceed the square of the ordinary Spearman ρ. For categorical predictors, ranks are not squared but instead the predictor is represented by a series of dummy variables. The resulting ρ^2 is related to the Kruskal–Wallis test. See pp. 127 and 452 for examples.

An open question is that if the rank correlation screening procedure is unbiased or conservative, can we reduce degrees of freedom based on partial χ^2 of F tests from a full model fit when we are still careful to conceal the separation between linear and nonlinear effects? This procedure would not assume that unadjusted relationships are informative about adjusted ones. Some simulation results may be found on the text's Web site.

Once one expands a predictor into linear and nonlinear terms and estimates the coefficients, the best way to understand the relationship between predictors and response is to graph this estimated relationship. One can also perform a joint test of all parameters associated with nonlinear effects. This can be useful in demonstrating to the reader that some complexity was actually needed. If the plot appears almost linear or the test of nonlinearity is very insignificant there is a temptation to simplify the model. The Grambsch and O'Brien result described in Section 2.6 demonstrates why this is a bad idea.

From the above discussion a general principle emerges. Whenever the response variable is informally or formally linked to particular parameters that may be deleted from the model, special adjustments must be made in P-values, standard errors, test statistics, and confidence limits, in order for these statistics to have the correct interpretation. Examples of strategies that are improper without special adjustments (e.g., using the bootstrap) include examining a frequency table or scatterplot to decide that an association is too weak for the predictor to be included in the model at all or to decide that the relationship appears so linear that all nonlinear terms should be omitted. It is also valuable to consider the reverse situation; that is, one posits a simple model and then additional analysis or outside subject matter information makes the analyst want to generalize the model. Once the model is generalized (e.g., nonlinear terms are added), the test of association can be recomputed using multiple d.f. So another general principle is that when one makes the model more complex, the d.f. properly increases and the new test statistics for association have the claimed distribution. Thus moving from simple to more complex models presents no problems other than conservatism if the new complex components are truly unnecessary.

4.2   Checking Assumptions of Multiple Predictors Simultaneously

Before developing a multivariable model one must decide whether the assumptions of each continuous predictor can be verified by ignoring the effects of all other potential predictors. In some cases, the shape of the relationship between a predictor and the property of response will be different if an adjustment is made for other correlated factors when deriving regression estimates. Also, failure to adjust for an important factor can frequently alter the nature of the distribution of Y. Occasionally, however, it is unwieldy to deal simultaneously with all predictors at each stage in the analysis, and instead the regression function shapes are assessed separately for each continuous predictor.

4.3   Variable Selection

The material covered to this point dealt with a prespecified list of variables to be included in the regression model. For reasons of developing a concise model or because of a fear of collinearity or of a false belief that it is not legitimate to include "insignificant" regression coefficients when presenting results to the intended audience, stepwise variable selection is very commonly employed. Variable selection is used when the analyst is faced with a series of potential predictors but does not have (or use) the necessary subject matter knowledge to enable her to prespecify the "important" variables to include in the model. But using Y to compute P-values to decide which variables to include is similar to using Y to decide how to pool treatments in a five–treatment randomized trial, and then testing for global treatment differences using fewer than four degrees of freedom.

Stepwise variable selection has been a very popular technique for many years, but if this procedure had just been proposed as a statistical method, it would most likely be rejected because it violates every principle of statistical estimation and hypothesis testing. Here is a summary of the problems with this method.

1. It yields R^2 values that are biased high.

2. The ordinary F and χ^2 test statistics do not have the claimed distribution.[158] Variable selection is based on methods (e.g., F tests for nested models) that were intended to be used to test only prespecified hypotheses.

3. The method yields standard errors of regression coefficient estimates that are biased low and confidence intervals for effects and predicted values that are falsely narrow.[11]

4. It yields P-values that are too small (i.e., there are severe multiple comparison problems) and that do not have the proper meaning, and the proper correction for them is a very difficult problem.

5. It provides regression coefficients that are biased high in absolute value and need shrinkage. Even if only a single predictor were being analyzed and one only reported the regression coefficient for that predictor if its association with Y were "statistically significant," the estimate of the regression coefficient $\hat{\beta}$ is biased (too large in absolute value). To put this in symbols for the case where we obtain a positive association $(\hat{\beta} > 0)$, $E(\hat{\beta}|P < 0.05, \hat{\beta} > 0) > \beta$.[69]

6. Rather than solving problems caused by collinearity, variable selection is made arbitrary by collinearity.

7. It allows us to not think about the problem.

The problems of P-value-based variable selection are exacerbated when the analyst (as she so often does) interprets the final model as if it were prespecified. Copas and Long[87] stated one of the most serious problems with stepwise modeling eloquently when they said, "The choice of the variables to be included depends on estimated regression coefficients rather than their true values, and so X_j is more likely to be included if its regression coefficient is over-estimated than if its regression coefficient is underestimated." Derksen and Keselman[111] studied stepwise variable selection, backward elimination, and forward selection, with these conclusions:

1. "The degree of correlation between the predictor variables affected the frequency with which authentic predictor variables found their way into the final model.

2. The number of candidate predictor variables affected the number of noise variables that gained entry to the model.

3. The size of the sample was of little practical importance in determining the number of authentic variables contained in the final model.

4. The population multiple coefficient of determination could be faithfully estimated by adopting a statistic that is adjusted by the total number of candidate predictor variables rather than the number of variables in the final model."

They found that variables selected for the final model represented noise 0.20 to 0.74 of the time and that the final model usually contained less than half of the actual number of authentic predictors. Hence there are many reasons for using methods such as full-model fits or data reduction, instead of using any stepwise variable selection algorithm.

If stepwise selection must be used, a global test of no regression should be made before proceeding, simultaneously testing all candidate predictors and having degrees of freedom equal to the number of candidate variables (plus any nonlinear or interaction terms). If this global test is not significant, selection of individually significant predictors is usually not warranted.

The method generally used for such variable selection is forward selection of the most significant candidate or backward elimination of the least significant predictor in the model. One of the recommended stopping rules is based on the "residual χ^2" with degrees of freedom equal to the number of candidate variables remaining at the current step. The residual χ^2 can be tested for significance (if one is able to forget that because of variable selection this statistic does not have a χ^2 distribution), or the stopping rule can be based on Akaike's information criterion (AIC[26]), here residual $\chi^2 - 2 \times d.f.$[174] Of course, use of more insight from knowledge of the subject matter will generally improve the modeling process substantially. It must be remembered that no currently available stopping rule was developed for data-driven variable selection. Stopping rules such as AIC or Mallows' C_p are intended for comparing only two *prespecified* models [46, Section 1.3].   ③

If the analyst insists on basing the stopping rule on P-values, the optimum (in terms of predictive accuracy) α to use in deciding which variables to include in the model is $\alpha = 1.0$ unless there are a few powerful variables and several completely irrelevant variables. A reasonable α that does allow for deletion of *some* variables is $\alpha = 0.5$.[399] These values are far from the traditional choices of $\alpha = 0.05$ or 0.10.   ④

Even though forward stepwise variable selection is the most commonly used method, the step-down method is preferred for the following reasons.

1. It usually performs better than forward stepwise methods, especially when collinearity is present.[301]

2. It makes one examine a full model fit, which is the only fit providing accurate standard errors, error mean square, and P-values.

3. The method of Lawless and Singhal[267] allows extremely efficient step-down modeling using Wald statistics, in the context of any fit from least squares or maximum likelihood. This method requires passing through the data matrix only to get the initial full fit.

For a given dataset, bootstrapping (Efron et al.[108, 124, 129, 130]) can help decide between using full and reduced models. Bootstrapping can be done on the whole model and compared with bootstrapped estimates of predictive accuracy based on stepwise variable selection for each resample. Unless most predictors are either very significant or clearly unimportant, the full model usually outperforms the reduced model.

Full model fits have the advantage of providing meaningful confidence intervals using standard formulas. Altman and Andersen[11] gave an example in which the lengths of confidence intervals of predicted survival probabilities were 60% longer when bootstrapping was used to estimate the simultaneous effects of variability caused by variable selection and coefficient estimation, as compared with confidence intervals computed ignoring how a "final" model came to be. On the other hand, models developed on full fits after data reduction will be optimum in many cases.

⬚5

In some cases you may want to use the full model for prediction and variable selection for a "best bet" parsimonious list of independently important predictors. This could be accompanied by a list of variables selected in 50 bootstrap samples to demonstrate the imprecision in the "best bet."

Sauerbrei and Schumacher[364] present a method to use bootstrapping to actually select the set of variables. However, there are a number of potential drawbacks to this approach:

1. The choice of an α cutoff for determining whether a variable is retained in a given bootstrap sample is arbitrary.

2. The choice of a cutoff for the proportion of bootstrap samples for which a variable is retained, in order to include that variable in the final model, is somewhat arbitrary.

3. Selection from among a set of correlated predictors is arbitrary, and all highly correlated predictors may have a low bootstrap selection frequency. It may be the case that none of them will be selected for the final model even though when considered individually each of them may be highly significant.

4. By using the bootstrap to choose variables, one must use the double bootstrap to resample the entire modeling process in order to validate the model and to derive reliable confidence intervals. This may be computationally prohibitive.

For some applications the list of variables selected may be stabilized by grouping variables according to subject matter considerations or empirical correlations and testing each related group with a multiple degree of freedom test. Then the entire group may be kept or deleted and, if desired, groups that are retained can be summarized into a single variable or the most accurately measured variable within the group can replace the group. See Section 4.7 for more on this.

Kass and Raftery[231] showed that Bayes factors have several advantages in variable selection, including the selection of less complex models that may agree better with subject matter knowledge. However, as in the case with more traditional stopping rules, the final model may still have regression coefficients that are too large. This problem is solved by Tibshirani's *lasso* method,[415, 416] which is a penalized estimation technique in which the estimated regression coefficients are constrained so that the sum of their scaled absolute values falls below some constant k chosen by cross-validation. This kind of constraint forces some regression coefficient estimates to be exactly zero, thus achieving variable selection while shrinking the remaining coefficients toward zero to reflect the overfitting caused by data-based model selection. The lasso is computationally demanding.

A final problem with variable selection is illustrated by comparing this approach with the sensible way many economists develop regression models. Economists frequently use the strategy of deleting only those variables that are "insignificant" and whose regression coefficients have a nonsensible direction. Standard variable selection on the other hand yields biologically implausible findings in many cases by setting certain regression coefficients exactly to zero. In a study of survival time for patients with heart failure, for example, it would be implausible that patients having a specific symptom live exactly as long as those without the symptom just because the symptom's regression coefficient was "insignificant." The lasso method shares this difficulty with ordinary variable selection methods and with any method that in the Bayesian context places nonzero prior probability on β being *exactly* zero.   ⌐6¬

Many papers claim that there were insufficient data to allow for multivariable modeling, so they did "univariable screening" wherein only "significant" variables (i.e., those that are separately significantly associated with Y) were entered into the model.[b] This is just a forward stepwise variable selection in which insignificant variables from the first step are not reanalyzed in later steps. Univariable screening is thus even worse than stepwise modeling as it can miss important variables that are only important after adjusting for other variables.[406] Overall, neither univariable screening nor stepwise variable selection in any way solve the problem of "too many variables, too few subjects," and they cause severe biases in the resulting multivariable model fits while losing valuable predictive information from deleting marginally significant variables.   ⌐7¬

4.4   Overfitting and Limits on Number of Predictors

When a model is fitted that is too complex, that is it has too many free parameters to estimate for the amount of information in the data, the worth of the model (e.g., R^2) will be exaggerated and future observed values will not agree with predicted values. In this situation, *overfitting* is said to be present, and some of the findings of the analysis come from fitting noise or finding spurious associations between X and Y. In this section general guidelines for preventing overfitting are given. Here we concern ourselves with the *reliability* or *calibration* of a model, meaning the ability of the model to predict future observations as well as it appeared to predict the responses at hand. For now we avoid judging whether the model is adequate for the

---

[b]This is akin to doing a t-test to compare the two treatments (out of 10, say) that are apparently most different from each other.

TABLE 4.1: Limiting Sample Sizes for Various Response Variables

Type of Response Variable	Limiting Sample Size m
Continuous	n (total sample size)
Binary	$\min(n_1, n_2)$ [c]
Ordinal (k categories)	$n - \frac{1}{n^2}\sum_{i=1}^{k} n_i^3$ [d]
Failure (survival) time	number of failures [e]

task, but restrict our attention to the likelihood that the model has significantly overfitted the data.

Studies in which models are validated on independent datasets[184, 186, 391] have shown that in many situations a fitted regression model is likely to be reliable when the number of predictors (or *candidate* predictors if using variable selection) p is less than $m/10$ or $m/20$, where m is the "limiting sample size" given in Table 4.1. For example, Smith et al.[391] found in one series of simulations that the expected error in Cox model predicted five–year survival probabilities was below 0.05 when $p < m/20$ for "average" subjects and below 0.10 when $p < m/20$ for "sick" subjects, where m is the number of deaths. For "average" subjects, $m/10$ was adequate for preventing expected errors > 0.1.   Narrowly distributed predictor variables (e.g., if all subjects' ages are between 30 and 45 or only 5% of subjects are female) will require even higher sample sizes. Note that the number of candidate variables must include all variables screened for association with the response, including nonlinear terms and interactions. Instead of relying on the rules of thumb in the table, the shrinkage factor estimate presented in the next section can be used to guide the analyst in determining how many d.f. to model (see p. 73).

4.5 Shrinkage

The term *shrinkage* is used in regression modeling to denote two ideas. The first meaning relates to the slope of a *calibration plot*, which is a plot of observed responses against predicted responses. When a dataset is used to fit the model param-

---

[c]See [329]. If one considers the power of a two-sample binomial test compared with a Wilcoxon test if the response could be made continuous and the proportional odds assumption holds, the effective sample size for a binary response is $3n_1 n_2/n \approx 3\min(n_1, n_2)$ if n_1/n is near 0 or 1 [452, Eq. 10, 15]. Here n_1 and n_2 are the marginal frequencies of the two response levels.

[d]Based on the power of a proportional odds model two-sample test when the marginal cell sizes for the response are $n_1, \ldots, n_k$, compared with all cell sizes equal to unity (response is continuous) [452, Eq. 3]. If all cell sizes are equal, the relative efficiency of having k response categories compared to a continuous response is $1 - 1/k^2$ [452, Eq. 14], for example, a five-level response is almost as efficient as a continuous one if proportional odds holds across category cutoffs.

[e]This is approximate, as the effective sample size may sometimes be boosted somewhat by censored observations, especially for nonproportional hazards methods such as Wilcoxon-type tests.[34]

eters as well as to obtain the calibration plot, the usual estimation process will force the slope of observed versus predicted values to be one. When, however, parameter estimates are derived from one dataset and then applied to predict outcomes on an independent dataset, overfitting will cause the slope of the calibration plot (i.e., the *shrinkage factor*) to be less than one, a result of *regression to the mean*. Typically, low predictions will be too low and high predictions too high. Predictions near the mean predicted value will usually be quite accurate. The second meaning of *shrinkage* is a statistical estimation method that preshrinks regression coefficients towards zero so that the calibration plot for new data will not need shrinkage as its calibration slope will be one.

We turn first to shrinkage as an adverse result of traditional modeling. In ordinary linear regression, we know that all of the coefficient estimates are exactly unbiased estimates of the true effect when the model fits. Isn't the existence of shrinkage and overfitting implying that there is some kind of bias in the parameter estimates? The answer is no because each separate coefficient has the desired expectation. The problem lies in how we use the coefficients. We tend not to pick out coefficients at random for interpretation but we tend to highlight very small and very large coefficients.

A simple example may suffice. Consider a clinical trial with 10 randomly assigned treatments such that the patient responses for each treatment are normally distributed. We can do an ANOVA by fitting a multiple regression model with an intercept and nine dummy variables. The intercept is an unbiased estimate of the mean response for patients on the first treatment, and each of the other coefficients is an unbiased estimate of the difference in mean response between the treatment in question and the first treatment. $\hat{\beta}_0 + \hat{\beta}_1$ is an unbiased estimate of the mean response for patients on the second treatment. But if we plotted the predicted mean response for patients against the observed responses from new data, the slope of this calibration plot would typically be smaller than one. This is because in making this plot we are not picking coefficients at random but we are sorting the coefficients into ascending order. The treatment group having the lowest sample mean response will usually have a higher mean in the future, and the treatment group having the highest sample mean response will typically have a lower mean in the future. The sample mean of the group having the highest sample mean is *not* an unbiased estimate of its population mean.

As an illustration, let us draw 20 samples of size $n = 50$ from a uniform distribution for which the true mean is 0.5. Figure 4.1 displays the 20 means sorted into ascending order, similar to plotting Y versus $\hat{Y} = X\hat{\beta}$ based on least squares after sorting by $X\hat{\beta}$. Bias in the very lowest and highest estimates is evident.

When we want to highlight a treatment that is not chosen at random (or a priori), the data-based selection of that treatment needs to be compensated for in

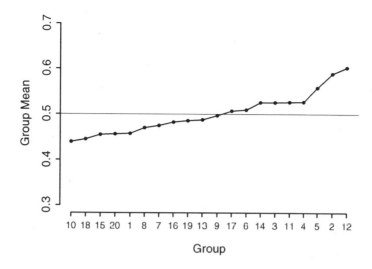

FIGURE 4.1: Sorted means from 20 samples of size 50 from a uniform $[0, 1]$ distribution. The reference line at 0.5 depicts the true population value of all of the means.

the estimation process.[f] It is well known that the use of shrinkage methods such as the James–Stein estimator to pull treatment means toward the grand mean over all treatments results in estimates of treatment-specific means that are far superior to ordinary stratified means.[128]

Turning from a cell means model to the general case where predicted values are general linear combinations $X\hat{\beta}$, the slope γ of properly transformed responses Y against $X\hat{\beta}$ (sorted into ascending order) will be less than one on new data. Estimation of the shrinkage coefficient γ allows quantification of the amount of overfitting present, and it allows one to estimate the likelihood that the model will reliably predict new observations. van Houwelingen and le Cessie [433, Eq. 77] provided a heuristic shrinkage estimate that has worked well in several examples:

$$\hat{\gamma} = \frac{\text{model } \chi^2 - p}{\text{model } \chi^2},$$ (4.1)

where p is the total degrees of freedom for the predictors and model χ^2 is the likelihood ratio χ^2 statistic for testing the joint influence of all predictors simultaneously (see Section 9.3.1). For ordinary linear models, van Houwelingen and le Cessie proposed a shrinkage factor $\hat{\gamma}$ that can be shown to equal $\frac{n-p-1}{n-1}\frac{R^2_{\text{adj}}}{R^2}$, where

⑨

---

[f]It is interesting that researchers are quite comfortable with adjusting P-values for post hoc selection of comparisons using, for example, the Bonferroni inequality, but they do not realize that post hoc selection of comparisons also biases point estimates.

the adjusted R^2 is given by

$$R^2_{\text{adj}} = 1 - (1 - R^2)\frac{n-1}{n-p-1}. \qquad (4.2)$$

For such linear models with an intercept β_0, the shrunken estimate of β is

$$
\begin{aligned}
\hat{\beta}_0^s &= (1 - \hat{\gamma})\overline{Y} + \hat{\gamma}\hat{\beta}_0 \\
\hat{\beta}_j^s &= \hat{\gamma}\hat{\beta}_j, j = 1, \ldots, p,
\end{aligned}
\qquad (4.3)
$$

where $\overline{Y}$ is the mean of the response vector. Again, when stepwise fitting is used, the p in these equations is much closer to the number of *candidate* degrees of freedom rather than the number in the "final" model. See Section 5.2 for methods of estimating γ using the bootstrap (p. 95) or cross-validation.

    Now turn to the second usage of the term *shrinkage*. Just as clothing is sometimes preshrunk so that it will not shrink further once it is purchased, better calibrated predictions result when shrinkage is built into the estimation process in the first place. The object of shrinking regression coefficient estimates is to obtain a shrinkage coefficient of $\gamma = 1$ on new data. Thus by somewhat discounting $\hat{\beta}$ we make the model underfitted on the data at hand (i.e., apparent $\gamma < 1$) so that on new data extremely low or high predictions are correct.

    Ridge regression[269, 433] is one technique for placing restrictions on the parameter estimates that results in shrinkage. A *ridge parameter* must be chosen to control the amount of shrinkage. Penalized maximum likelihood estimation,[161, 188, 269, 436] a generalization of ridge regression, is a general shrinkage procedure. A method such as cross-validation or optimization of a modified AIC must be used to choose an optimal penalty factor. An advantage of penalized estimation is that one can differentially penalize the more complex components of the model such as nonlinear or interaction effects. A drawback of ridge regression and penalized maximum likelihood is that the final model is difficult to validate unbiasedly since the optimal amount of shrinkage is usually determined by examining the entire dataset. Penalization is one of the best ways to approach the "too many variables, too little data" problem. See Section 9.10 for details.

4.6 Collinearity

When at least one of the predictors can be predicted well from the other predictors, the standard errors of the regression coefficient estimates can be inflated and corresponding tests have reduced power.[149] In stepwise variable selection, collinearity can cause predictors to compete and make the selection of "important" variables arbitrary. Collinearity makes it difficult to estimate and interpret a particular regression coefficient because the data have little information about the effect of changing one variable while holding another (highly correlated) variable constant [70, p. 173]. However, collinearity does not affect the joint influence of highly correlated variables when tested simultaneously. Therefore, once groups of highly correlated predictors are identified, the problem can be rectified by testing the contribution of an entire set with a multiple d.f. test rather than attempting to interpret the coefficient or one d.f. test for a single predictor.

Collinearity does not affect predictions made on the same dataset used to estimate the model parameters or on new data that have the same degree of collinearity as the original data [321, pp. 379–381] as long as extreme extrapolation is not attempted. Consider as two predictors the total and LDL cholesterols that are highly correlated. If predictions are made at the same combinations of total and LDL cholesterol that occurred in the training data, no problem will arise. However, if one makes a prediction at an inconsistent combination of these two variables, the predictions may be inaccurate and have high standard errors.

When the ordinary truncated power basis is used to derive component variables for fitting linear and cubic splines, as was described earlier, the component variables can be very collinear. It is very unlikely that this will result in any problems, however, as the component variables are connected algebraically. Thus it is not possible for a combination of, for example, x and $\max(x - 10, 0)$ to be inconsistent with each other. Collinearity problems are then more likely to result from partially redundant subsets of predictors as in the cholesterol example above.

One way to quantify collinearity is with *variance inflation factors* or *VIF*, which in ordinary least squares are diagonals of the inverse of the $X'X$ matrix scaled to have unit variance (except that a column of 1s is retained corresponding to the intercept). Note that some authors compute VIF from the correlation matrix form of the design matrix, omitting the intercept. VIF_i is $1/(1 - R_i^2)$ where R_i^2 is the squared multiple correlation coefficient between column i and the remaining columns of the design matrix. For models that are fitted with maximum likelihood estimation, the information matrix is scaled to correlation form, and VIF is the diagonal of the inverse of this scaled matrix.[106, 446] Then the VIF are similar to those from a weighted correlation matrix of the original columns in the design matrix. Note that indexes such as VIF are not very informative as some variables are algebraically connected to each other.

[11]

The SAS VARCLUS procedure[362] and S-PLUS varclus function can identify collinear predictors. Summarizing collinear variables using a summary score is more powerful and stable than arbitrary selection of one variable in a group of collinear variables (see the next section).

4.7 Data Reduction

The sample size need not be as large as shown in Table 4.1 if the model is validated independently and if you don't care that the model may fail to validate. However, it is likely that the model will be overfitted and will not validate if the sample size does not meet the guidelines. Use of data reduction methods before model development is strongly recommended if the conditions in Table 4.1 are not satisfied and if shrinkage is not incorporated into parameter estimation. Methods such as shrinkage and data reduction reduce the effective d.f. of the model, making it more likely for the model to validate on future data. Some available data reduction methods are given below.

1. Use the literature to eliminate unimportant variables.

2. Eliminate variables whose distributions are too narrow.

3. Eliminate candidate predictors that are missing in a large number of subjects, especially if those same predictors are likely to be missing for future applications of the model.

4. Use a statistical data reduction method such as incomplete principal components regression, nonlinear generalizations of principal components such as principal surfaces, sliced inverse regression, variable clustering, or ordinary cluster analysis on a measure of similarity between variables.

| 12 |

See Chapters 8 and 14 for detailed case studies in data reduction.

4.7.1   Variable Clustering

Although the use of subject matter knowledge is usually preferred, statistical clustering techniques can be useful in determining independent dimensions that are described by the entire list of candidate predictors. Once each dimension is scored (see below), the task of regression modeling is simplified, and one quits trying to separate the effects of factors that are measuring the same phenomenon. One type of variable clustering[362] is based on a type of oblique-rotation principal components (PC) analysis that attempts to separate variables so that the first PC of each group is representative of that group (the first PC is the linear combination of variables having maximum variance subject to normalization constraints on the coefficients[102, 104]). Another approach, that of doing a hierarchical cluster analysis on an appropriate similarity matrix (such as squared correlations) will often yield the same results. For either approach, it is often advisable to use robust (e.g., rank-based) measures for continuous variables if they are skewed, as skewed variables can greatly affect ordinary correlation coefficients. Pairwise deletion of missing values is also advisable for this procedure—casewise deletion can result in a small biased sample.

When variables are not monotonically related to each other, Pearson or Spearman squared correlations can miss important associations and thus are not always good similarity measures. A general and robust similarity measure is Hoeffding's D,[203] which for two variables X and Y is a measure of the agreement between $F(x,y)$ and $G(x)H(y)$, where G, H are marginal cumulative distribution functions and F is the joint CDF. The D statistic will detect a wide variety of dependencies between two variables.

See pp. 152, 169, 347, and 448 for examples of variable clustering.

4.7.2 Transformation and Scaling Variables Without Using Y

Scaling techniques often allow the analyst to reduce the number of parameters to fit by estimating transformations for each predictor using only information about associations with other predictors. It may be advisable to cluster variables before scaling so that patterns are derived only from variables that are related. For purely categorical predictors, methods such as correspondence analysis (see, for example, [74, 99, 163, 272, 314]) can be useful for data reduction. Often one can use these techniques to scale multiple dummy variables into a few dimensions. For mixtures of categorical and continuous predictors, qualitative principal components analysis such as the *maximum total variance* (MTV) method of Young et al.[314, 460] is useful. For the special case of representing a series of variables with one PC, the MTV method is quite easy to implement.

1. Compute PC_1, the first PC of the variables to reduce $X_1, \ldots, X_q$ using the correlation matrix of Xs.

2. Use ordinary linear regression to predict PC_1 on the basis of functions of the Xs, such as restricted cubic spline functions for continuous Xs or a series of dummy variables for polytomous Xs. The expansion of each X_j is regressed separately on PC_1.

3. These separately fitted regressions specify the working transformations of each X.

4. Recompute PC_1 by doing a PC analysis on the transformed Xs (predicted values from the fits).

5. Repeat steps 2 to 4 until the proportion of variation explained by PC_1 reaches a plateau. This typically requires three to four iterations.

A transformation procedure that is similar to MTV is the maximum generalized variance (MGV) method due to Sarle [252, pp. 1267–1268]. MGV involves predicting each variable from (the current transformations of) all the other variables. When predicting variable i, that variable is represented as a set of linear and nonlinear terms (e.g., spline components). Analysis of canonical variates[194] can be used to find the linear combination of terms for X_i (i.e., find a new transformation for X_i) and the linear combination of the current transformations of all other variables (representing each variable as a single, transformed, variable) such that these two linear combinations have maximum correlation. (For example, if there are only two variables X_1 and X_2 represented as quadratic polynomials, solve for a, b, c, d such that $aX_1 + bX_1^2$ has maximum correlation with $cX_2 + dX_2^2$.) The process is repeated until the transformations converge. The goal of MGV is to transform each variable so that it is most similar to predictions from the other transformed variables. MGV does not use PCs (so one need not precede the analysis by variable clustering), but once all variables have been transformed, you may want to summarize them with the first PC.

The SAS PRINQUAL procedure of Kuhfeld[252] implements the MTV and MGV methods, and allows for very flexible transformations of the predictors, including monotonic splines and ordinary cubic splines.

A very flexible automatic procedure for transforming each predictor in turn, based on all remaining predictors, is the ACE (alternating conditional expectation) procedure of Breiman and Friedman.[47] Like SAS PROC PRINQUAL, ACE handles monotonically restricted transformations and categorical variables. It fits transformations by maximizing R^2 between one variable and a set of variables. It automatically transforms all variables, using the "super smoother"[146] for continuous variables. Unfortunately, ACE does not handle missing values. See Chapter 15 for more about ACE.

It must be noted that at best these automatic transformation procedures generally find only *marginal* transformations, not transformations of each predictor adjusted for the effects of all other predictors. When adjusted transformations differ markedly from marginal transformations, only joint modeling of all predictors (and the response) will find the correct transformations.

Once transformations are estimated using only predictor information, the adequacy of each predictor's transformation can be checked by graphical methods, nonparametric smooths of transformed X_j versus Y, or by expanding the transformed X_j using a spline function. This approach of checking that transformations are optimal with respect to Y uses the response data, but it accepts the initial transformations unless they are significantly inadequate. If the sample size is low, or if PC_1 for the group of variables used in deriving the transformations is deemed an adequate summary of those variables, that PC_1 can be used in modeling. In that way, data reduction is accomplished two ways: by not using Y to estimate multiple coefficients for a single predictor, and by reducing related variables into a single score, after transforming them. See Chapter 8 for a detailed example of these scaling techniques.

4.7.3 Simultaneous Transformation and Imputation

As mentioned in Chapter 3 (p. 47) if transformations are complex or nonmonotonic, ordinary imputation models may not work. SAS PROC `PRINQUAL` implemented a method for simultaneously imputing missing values while solving for transformations. Unfortunately, the imputation procedure frequently converges to imputed values that are outside the allowable range of the data. This problem is more likely when multiple variables are missing on the same subjects, since the transformation algorithm may simply separate missings and nonmissings into clusters.

A simple modification of the MGV algorithm of `PRINQUAL` that simultaneously imputes missing values without these problems is implemented in the S-PLUS function `transcan`. Imputed values are initialized to medians of continuous variables and the most frequent category of categorical variables. For continuous variables, transformations are initialized to linear functions. For categorical ones, transformations may be initialized to the identify function, to dummy variables indicating whether the observation has the most prevalent categorical value, or to random numbers. Then when using canonical variates to transform each variable in turn, observations that are missing on the current "dependent" variable are excluded from consideration, although missing values for the current set of "predictors" are imputed. Transformed variables are normalized to have mean 0 and standard deviation 1. Although categorical variables are scored using the first canonical variate, `transcan` has an option to use the S-PLUS `tree` function to obtain imputed values on the original scale using recursive partitioning (Section 2.5) for these variables. It defaults to imputing categorical variables using the category whose predicted canonical score is closest to the predicted score.

`transcan` uses restricted cubic splines to model continuous variables. It does not implement monotonicity constraints. `transcan` automatically constrains imputed values (both on the transformed and original scales) to be in the same range as nonimputed ones. This adds much stability to the resulting estimates although it can result in a boundary effect. Also, imputed values can optionally be shrunken using Eq. 4.3 to avoid overfitting when developing the imputation models. Optionally, missing values can be set to specified constants rather than estimating them. These constants are ignored during the transformation-estimation phase[g]. This technique has proved to be helpful when, for example, a laboratory test is not ordered because a physician thinks the patient has returned to normal with respect to the lab parameter measured by the test. In that case, it's better to use a normal lab value for missings.

The `transcan` function can also generate multiple imputations, by sampling with replacement from the residuals for the transformed variables, and then back-trans-

---

[g]If one were to estimate transformations without removing observations that had these constants inserted for the current Y-variable, the resulting transformations would likely have a spike at Y = imputation constant.

forming so that imputations are on the original scale. The two "bootstrap" approaches implemented by transcan[h] do away with the need for a normality assumption for the residuals. After running transcan you can run the Hmisc library's fit.mult.impute function to fit the chosen model separately for each artificially completed dataset corresponding to each imputation. After fit.mult.impute fits all of the models, it averages the sets of regression coefficients and computes variance and covariance estimates that are adjusted for imputation (using Eq. 3.1). transcan makes one short cut: for each sample from the residuals it does not refit the imputation models to add the uncertainty in those models to the sources of variation accounted for by multiple imputation. If the sample size is reasonably large this will not matter, as variation in residuals from observation to observation is typically much greater than variation in predicted values due to having estimated the regression coefficients.

The transformation and imputation information created by transcan may be used to transform/impute variables in datasets not used to develop the transformation and imputation formulas. There is also an S-PLUS function to create S-PLUS functions that compute the final transformed values of each predictor given input values on the original scale.

As an example of nonmonotonic transformation and imputation, consider a sample of 415 acutely ill hospitalized patients from the SUPPORT[i] study.[241] All patients had heart rate measured and 413 had mean arterial blood pressure measured. Somers' D_{xy} rank correlation[393] between the 413 pairs of heart rate and blood pressure was 0.02, because these variables each require U-shaped transformations. Using restricted cubic splines with five knots placed at default quantiles, transcan provided the transformations shown in Figure 4.2. The correlation between transformed variables is $D_{xy} = 0.14$. The two imputed values for blood pressure are nearly normal. The fitted transformations are similar to those obtained from relating these two variables to time until death.

4.7.4   Simple Scoring of Variable Clusters

If a subset of the predictors is a series of related dichotomous variables, a simpler data reduction strategy is sometimes employed. First, construct two new predictors representing whether any of the factors is positive and a count of the number of positive factors. For the ordinal count of the number of positive factors, score the summary variable to satisfy linearity assumptions as discussed previously. For the more powerful predictor of the two summary measures, test for adequacy of scoring by using all dichotomous variables as candidate predictors after adjusting for the new summary variable. A residual χ^2 statistic can be used to test whether the

---

[h]The default is Rubin's approximate Bayesian bootstrap (double sampling with replacement of residuals); single sampling with replacement can also be specified.

[i]Study to Understand Prognoses Preferences Outcomes and Risks of Treatments

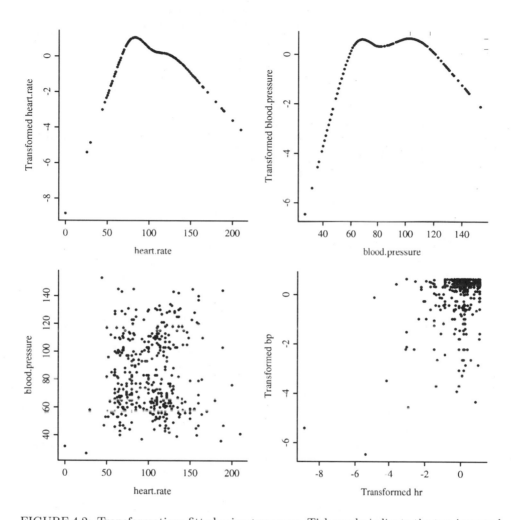

FIGURE 4.2: Transformations fitted using `transcan`. Tick marks indicate the two imputed values for blood pressure. The lower left plot contains raw data ($D_{xy} = 0.02$); the lower right is a scatterplot of the corresponding transformed values ($D_{xy} = 0.14$). Data courtesy of the SUPPORT study.[241]

summary variable adequately captures the predictive information of the series of binary predictors.[j] This statistic will have degrees of freedom equal to one less than the number of binary predictors when testing for adequacy of the summary count (and hence will have low power when there are many predictors). Stratification by the summary score and examination of responses over cells can be used to suggest a transformation on the score.

Another approach to scoring a series of related dichotomous predictors is to have "experts" assign severity points to each condition and then to either sum these points or use a hierarchical rule that scores according to the condition with the highest points (see Section 14.3 for an example). The latter has the advantage of being easy to implement for field use. The adequacy of either type of scoring can be checked using tests of linearity in a regression model. The S-PLUS function `score.binary` in the `Hmisc` library (see Section 6.2) assists in computing a summary variable from the series of binary conditions.

4.7.5   Simplifying Cluster Scores

If a variable cluster contains many individual predictors, parsimony may sometimes   13
be achieved by predicting the cluster score from a subset of its components (using linear regression or CART (Section 2.5), for example). Then a new cluster score is created and the response model is rerun with the new score in the place of the original one. If one constituent variable has a very high R^2 in predicting the original cluster score, the single variable may sometimes be substituted for the cluster score in refitting the model without loss of predictive discrimination.

Sometimes it may be desired to simplify a variable cluster by asking the question "which variables in the cluster are really the predictive ones?," even though this approach will usually cause true predictive discrimination to suffer. For clusters that are retained after limited step-down modeling, the entire list of variables can be used as candidate predictors and the step-down process repeated. All variables contained in clusters that were not selected initially are ignored. A fair way to validate such two-stage models is to use a resampling method (Section 5.2) with scores for deleted clusters as candidate variables for each resample, along with all the individual variables in the clusters the analyst really wants to retain. A method called *battery reduction* can be used to delete variables from clusters by determining if a subset of the variables can explain most of the variance explained by PC_1 [102, Chapter 12]. This approach does not require examination of associations with Y.

---

[j]Whether this statistic should be used to change the model is problematic in view of model uncertainty.

4.7.6   How Much Data Reduction Is Necessary?

In addition to using the sample size to degrees of freedom ratio as a rough guide to how much data reduction to do before model fitting, the heuristic shrinkage estimate in Equation 4.1 can also be informative. First, fit a full model with all candidate variables, nonlinear terms, and hypothesized interactions. Let p denote the number of parameters in this model, aside from any intercepts. Let LR denote the log likelihood ratio χ^2 for this full model. The estimated shrinkage is $(\text{LR} - p)/\text{LR}$. If this falls below 0.9, for example, we may be concerned with the lack of calibration the model may experience on new data. Either a shrunken estimator or data reduction is needed. A reduced model may have acceptable calibration if associations with Y are not used to reduce the predictors.

A simple method, with an assumption, can be used to estimate the target number of total regression degrees of freedom q in the model. In a "best case," the variables removed to arrive at the reduced model would have no association with Y. The expected value of the χ^2 statistic for testing those variables would then be $p - q$. The shrinkage for the reduced model is then on average $[\text{LR}-(p-q)-q]/[\text{LR}-(p-q)]$. Setting this ratio to be ≥ 0.9 and solving for q gives $q \leq (\text{LR} - p)/9$. Therefore, reduction of dimensionality down to q degrees of freedom would be expected to achieve $< 10\%$ shrinkage. With these assumptions, there is no hope that a reduced model would have acceptable calibration unless $\text{LR} > p + 9$. If the information explained by the omitted variables is less than one would expect by chance (e.g., their total χ^2 is extremely small), a reduced model could still be beneficial, as long as the conservative bound $(\text{LR} - q)/\text{LR} \geq 0.9$ or $q < \text{LR}/10$ were achieved. This conservative bound assumes that no χ^2 is lost by the reduction, that is that the final model $\chi^2 \approx \text{LR}$. This is unlikely in practice. Had the $p - q$ omitted variables had a larger χ^2 of $2(p-q)$ (the break-even point for AIC), q must be $\leq (LR-2p)/8$.

As an example, suppose that a binary logistic model is being developed from a sample containing 45 events on 150 subjects. The 10:1 rule suggests we can analyze 4.5 degrees of freedom. The analyst wishes to analyze age, sex, and 10 other variables. It is not known whether interaction between age and sex exists, and whether age is linear. A restricted cubic spline is fitted with four knots, and a linear interaction is allowed between age and sex. These two variables then need $3 + 1 + 1 = 5$ degrees of freedom. The other 10 variables are assumed to be linear and to not interact with themselves or age and sex. There is a total of 15 d.f. The full model with 15 d.f. has $\text{LR} = 50$. Expected shrinkage from this model is $(50 - 15)/50 = 0.7$. Since $\text{LR} > 15 + 9 = 24$, some reduction might yield a better validating model. Reduction to $q = (50 - 15)/9 \approx 4$ d.f. would be necessary, assuming the reduced LR is about $50 - (15 - 4) = 39$. In this case the 10:1 rule yields about the same value for q. The analyst may be forced to assume that age is linear, modeling 3 d.f. for age and sex. The other 10 variables would have to be reduced to a single variable using principal components or another scaling technique. The AIC-based calculation yields a maximum of 2.5 d.f.

If the goal of the analysis is to make a series of hypothesis tests (adjusting P-values for multiple comparisons) instead of to predict future responses, the full model would have to be used.

A summary of the various data reduction methods is given in Figure 4.3.

When principal components analysis or related methods are used for data reduction, the model may be harder to describe since internal coefficients are "hidden." The S-PLUS program on p. 118 shows how an ordinary linear model fit can be used in conjunction with a logistic model fit based on principal components, to draw a nomogram with axes for all predictors.

[14]

4.8   Overly Influential Observations

Every observation should influence the fit of a regression model. It can be disheartening, however, if a significant treatment effect or the shape of a regression effect rests on one or two observations. Overly influential observations also lead to increased variance of predicted values, especially when variances are estimated by bootstrapping after taking variable selection into account. In some cases, overly influential observations can cause one to abandon a model, "change" the data, or get more data. Observations can be *overly influential* for several major reasons.

1. The most common reason is having too few observations for the complexity of the model being fitted. Remedies for this have been discussed in Sections 4.7 and 4.3.

2. Data transcription or data entry errors can ruin a model fit.

3. Extreme values of the predictor variables can have a great impact, even when these values are validated for accuracy. Sometimes the analyst may deem a subject so atypical of other subjects in the study that deletion of the case is warranted. On other occasions, it is beneficial to truncate measurements where the data density ends. In one dataset of 4000 patients and 2000 deaths, white blood count (WBC) ranged from 500 to 100,000 with .05 and .95 quantiles of 2755 and 26,700, respectively. Predictions from a linear spline function of WBC were sensitive to WBC $> 60,000$, for which there were 16 patients. There were 46 patients with WBC $> 40,000$. Predictions were found to be more stable when WBC was truncated at 40,000, that is, setting WBC to 40,000 if WBC $> 40,000$.

4. Observations containing disagreements between the predictors and the response can influence the fit. Such disagreements should not lead to discarding the observations unless the predictor or response values are erroneous as in Reason 3, or the analysis is made conditional on observations being unlike the influential ones. In one example a single extreme predictor value in a sample

FIGURE 4.3: Summary of Some Data Reduction Methods

Goals	Reasons	Methods
		Variable clustering • Subject matter knowledge • Group predictors to maximize proportion of variance explained by PC_1 of each group • Hierarchical clustering using a matrix of similarity measures between predictors
Group predictors so that each group represents a single dimension that can be summarized with a single score	• ↓ d.f. arising from multiple predictors • Make PC_1 more reasonable summary	
Transform predictors	• ↓ d.f. due to nonlinear and dummy variable components • Allows predictors to be optimally combined • Make PC_1 more reasonable summary • Use in customized model for imputing missing values on each predictor	• Maximum total variance on a group of related predictors • Canonical variates on the total set of predictors
Score a group of predictors	↓ d.f. for group to unity	• PC_1 • Simple point scores
Multiple dimensional scoring of all predictors	↓ d.f. for all predictors combined	Principal components $1, 2, \ldots, k, k < p$ computed from all transformed predictors

of size 8000 that was not on a straight line relationship with the other (X, Y) pairs caused a χ^2 of 36 for testing nonlinearity of the predictor. Remember that an imperfectly fitting model is a fact of life, and discarding the observations can inflate the model's predictive accuracy. On rare occasions, such lack of fit may lead the analyst to make changes in the model's structure, but ordinarily this is best done from the "ground up" using formal tests of lack of fit (e.g., a test of linearity or interaction).

Influential observations of the second and third kinds can often be detected by careful quality control of the data. Statistical measures can also be helpful. The most common measures that apply to a variety of regression models are *leverage*, *DFBETAS*, *DFFIT*, and *DFFITS*.

Leverage measures the capacity of an observation to be influential due to having extreme predictor values. Such an observation is not *necessarily* influential. To compute leverage in ordinary least squares, we define the *hat matrix* H given by

$$H = X(X'X)^{-1}X'. \tag{4.4}$$

H is the matrix that when multiplied by the response vector gives the predicted values, so it measures how an observation estimates its own predicted response. The diagonals h_{ii} of H are the leverage measures and they are not influenced by Y. It has been suggested[33] that $h_{ii} > 2(p+1)/n$ signal a high leverage point, where p is the number of columns in the design matrix X aside from the intercept and n is the number of observations. Some believe that the distribution of h_{ii} should be examined for values that are higher than typical.

DFBETAS is the change in the vector of regression coefficient estimates upon deletion of each observation in turn, scaled by their standard errors.[33] Since DFBETAS encompasses an effect for each predictor's coefficient, DFBETAS allows the analyst to isolate the problem better than some of the other measures. DFFIT is the change in the predicted $X\beta$ when the observation is dropped, and DFFITS is DFFIT standardized by the standard error of the estimate of $X\beta$. In both cases, the standard error used for normalization is recomputed each time an observation is omitted. Some classify an observation as overly influential when $|\text{DFFITS}| > 2\sqrt{(p+1)/(n-p-1)}$, while others prefer to examine the entire distribution of DFFITS to identify "outliers".[33]

Section 10.7 discusses influence measures for the logistic model, which requires maximum likelihood estimation. These measures require the use of special residuals and information matrices (in place of $X'X$).

If truly influential observations are identified using these indexes, careful thought is needed to decide how (or whether) to deal with them. Most important, there is no substitute for careful examination of the dataset before doing any analyses.[68] Spence and Garrison [396, p. 16] feel that

Although the identification of aberrations receives considerable attention in most modern statistical courses, the emphasis sometimes seems to be on disposing of embarrassing data by searching for sources of technical error or minimizing the influence of inconvenient data by the application of resistant methods. Working scientists often find the most interesting aspect of the analysis inheres in the lack of fit rather than the fit itself.

4.9   Comparing Two Models

Frequently one wants to choose between two competing models on the basis of a common set of observations. The methods that follow assume that the performance of the models is evaluated on a sample not used to develop either one. In this case, predicted values from the model can usually be considered as a single new variable for comparison with responses in the new dataset. These methods listed below will also work if the models are compared using the same set of data used to fit each one, as long as both models have the same effective number of (candidate or actual) parameters. This requirement prevents us from rewarding a model just because it overfits the training sample (see Section 9.8.1 for a method comparing two models of differing complexity). The methods can also be enhanced using bootstrapping or cross-validation on a single sample to get a fair comparison when the playing field is not level, for example, when one model had more opportunity for fitting or overfitting the responses.

Some of the criteria for choosing one model over the other are

1. calibration,

2. discrimination,

3. face validity,

4. measurement errors in required predictors,

5. use of continuous predictors (which are usually better defined than categorical ones),

6. omission of "insignificant" variables that nonetheless make sense as risk factors,

7. simplicity (although this is less important with the availability of computers), and

8. lack of fit for specific types of subjects.

Items 3 through 7 require subjective judgment, so we focus on the other aspects. If the purpose of the models is only to rank-order subjects, calibration is not an issue. Otherwise, a model having poor calibration can be dismissed outright. Given that the two models have similar calibration, discrimination should be examined critically. Various statistical indexes can quantify discrimination ability (e.g., R^2, model χ^2, Somers' D_{xy}, Spearman's ρ, area under ROC curve—see Section 10.8). Rank measures (D_{xy}, ρ, ROC area) only measure how well predicted values can rank-order responses. For example, predicted probabilities of 0.01 and 0.99 for a pair of subjects are no better than probabilities of 0.2 and 0.8 using rank measures, if the first subject had a lower response value than the second. Therefore, rank measures, although fine for describing a given model, may not be very sensitive in choosing between two models. This is especially true when the models are strong, as it is easier to move a rank correlation from 0.6 to 0.7 than it is to move it from 0.9 to 1.0. Measures such as R^2 and the model χ^2 statistic (calculated from the predicted and observed responses) are more sensitive. Still, one may not know how to interpret the added utility of a model that boosts the R^2 from 0.80 to 0.81.

Again given that both models are equally well calibrated, discrimination can be studied more simply by examining the distribution of predicted values $\hat{Y}$. Suppose that the predicted value is the probability that a subject dies. Then high-resolution histograms of the predicted risk distributions for the two models can be very revealing. If one model assigns 0.02 of the sample to a risk of dying above 0.9 while the other model assigns 0.08 of the sample to the high risk group, the second model is more discriminating. The worth of a model can be judged by how far it goes out on a limb while still maintaining good calibration.

Frequently, one model will have a similar discrimination index to another model, but the likelihood ratio χ^2 statistic is meaningfully greater for one. Assuming corrections have been made for complexity, the model with the higher χ^2 usually has a better fit for *some* subjects, although not necessarily for the *average* subject. A crude plot of predictions from the first model against predictions from the second can help describe the differences in the models. More specific analyses will determine the characteristics of subjects where the differences are greatest. Large differences may be caused by an omitted, underweighted, or improperly transformed predictor, among other reasons. In one example, two models for predicting hospital mortality in critically ill patients had the same discrimination index (to two decimal places). For the relatively small subset of patients with extremely low white blood counts or serum albumin, the model that treated these factors as continuous variables provided predictions that were very much different from a model that did not.

When comparing predictions for two models that may not be calibrated (from overfitting, e.g.), the two sets of predictions may be shrunk so as to not give credit for overfitting (see Equation 4.1).

Sometimes one wishes to compare two models that used the response variable differently, a much more difficult problem. For example, an investigator may want to choose between a survival model that used time as a continuous variable, and a binary logistic model for dead/alive at six months. Here, other considerations are also important (see Section 16.1). A model that predicts dead/alive at six months does not use the response variable effectively, and it provides no information on the chance of dying within three months.

4.10   Summary: Possible Modeling Strategies

As stated in the Preface, it is only a mild oversimplification to say that a good overall strategy is to decide how many degrees of can be "spent," where they should be spent, and then to spend them. If statistical tests or confidence limits are required, later reconsideration of how d.f. are spent is not usually recommended. In what follows some default strategies are elaborated. These strategies are far from failsafe, but they should allow the reader to develop a strategy that is tailored to a particular problem. At the least these default strategies are concrete enough to be criticized so that statisticians can devise better ones.

4.10.1   Developing Predictive Models

The following strategy is generic although it is aimed principally at the development of accurate predictive models.

1. Assemble as much accurate pertinent data as possible, with wide distributions for predictor values. For survival time data, follow-up must be sufficient to capture enough events as well as the clinically meaningful phases if dealing with a chronic process.

2. Formulate good hypotheses that lead to specification of relevant candidate predictors and possible interactions. Don't use Y (either informally using graphs, descriptive statistics, or tables, or formally using hypothesis tests or estimates of effects such as odds ratios) in devising the list of candidate predictors.

3. If there are missing Y values on a small fraction of the subjects but Y can be reliably substituted by a surrogate response, use the surrogate to replace the missing values. Characterize tendencies for Y to be missing using, for example, recursive partitioning or binary logistic regression. Depending on the model used, even the information on X for observations with missing Y can be used to improve precision of $\hat{\beta}$, so multiple imputation of Y can sometimes be effective. Otherwise, discard observations having missing Y.

4. Impute missing Xs if the fraction of observations with any missing Xs is not tiny. Characterize observations that had to be discarded. Special imputation models may be needed if a continuous X needs a nonmonotonic transformation

(p. 47). These models can simultaneously impute missing values while determining transformations. In most cases, multiply impute missing Xs based on other Xs and Y, and other available information about the missing data mechanism.

5. For each predictor specify the complexity or degree of nonlinearity that should be allowed (see Section 4.1). When prior knowledge does not indicate that a predictor has a linear effect on the property $C(Y|X)$ (the property of the response that *can* be linearly related to X), specify the number of degrees of freedom that should be devoted to the predictor. The d.f. (or number of knots) can be larger when the predictor is thought to be more important in predicting Y or when the sample size is large.

6. If the number of terms fitted or tested in the modeling process (counting nonlinear and cross-product terms) is too large in comparison with the number of outcomes in the sample, use data reduction (ignoring Y) until the number of remaining free variables needing regression coefficients is tolerable. Use the $m/10$ or $m/15$ rule or an estimate of likely shrinkage or overfitting (Section 4.7) as a guide. Transformations determined from the previous step may be used to reduce each predictor into 1 d.f., or the transformed variables may be clustered into highly correlated groups if more data reduction is required. Alternatively, use penalized estimation with the entire set of variables. This will also effectively reduce the total degrees of freedom.[188]

7. Use the entire sample in the model development as data are too precious to waste. If steps listed below are too difficult to repeat for each bootstrap or cross-validation sample, hold out test data from all model development steps that follow.

8. When you can test for model complexity in a very structured way, you may be able to simplify the model without a great need to penalize the final model for having made this initial look. For example, it can be advisable to test an entire group of variables (e.g., those more expensive to collect) and to either delete or retain the entire group for further modeling, based on a single P-value (especially if the P value is not between 0.05 and 0.2). Another example of structured testing to simplify the "initial" model is making *all* continuous predictors have the same number of knots k, varying k from 0 (linear), $3, 4, 5, \ldots$, and choosing the value of k that optimizes AIC.

9. Check linearity assumptions and make transformations in Xs as needed. But beware that any examination of the response that might result in simplifying the model needs to be accounted for in computing confidence limits and other statistics. It may be preferable to retain the complexity that was prespecified in Step 5 regardless of the results of assessments of nonlinearity.

10. Check additivity assumptions by testing prespecified interaction terms. If the global test for additivity is significant or equivocal, all prespecified interactions should be retained in the model. If the test is decisive (e.g., $P > 0.3$), all interaction terms can be omitted, and in all likelihood there is no need to repeat this pooled test for each resample during model validation. In other words, one can assume that had the global interaction test been carried out for each bootstrap resample it would have been insignificant at the 0.05 level more than, say, 0.9 of the time. In this large P-value case the pooled interaction test did not induce an uncertainty in model selection that needed accounting.

11. Check to see if there are overlyinfluential observations.

12. Check distributional assumptions and choose a different model if needed.

13. Do limited backwards step-down variable selection if parsimony is more important than accuracy.[397] The cost of doing any aggressive variable selection is that the variable selection algorithm must also be included in a resampling procedure to properly validate the model or to compute confidence limits and the like.

14. This is the "final" model.

15. Interpret the model graphically (Section 5.3) and by examining predicted values and using appropriate significance tests without trying to interpret some of the individual model parameters. For collinear predictors obtain pooled tests of association so that competition among variables will not give misleading impressions of their total significance.

16. Validate the final model for calibration and discrimination ability, preferably using bootstrapping (see Section 5.2). Steps 9 to 13 must be repeated for each bootstrap sample, at least approximately. For example, if age was transformed when building the final model, and the transformation was suggested by the data using a fit involving age and age^2, each bootstrap repetition should include both age variables with a possible step-down from the quadratic to the linear model based on automatic significance testing at each step.

17. Shrink parameter estimates if there is overfitting but no further data reduction is desired, if shrinkage was not built into the estimation process.

18. When missing values were imputed, adjust final variance–covariance matrix for imputation wherever possible (e.g., using bootstrap or multiple imputation). This may affect some of the other results.

19. When all steps of the modeling strategy can be automated, consider using Faraway's method[134] to penalize for the randomness inherent in the multiple steps.

20. Develop simplifications to the full model by approximating it to any desired degrees of accuracy (Section 5.4).

4.10.2   Developing Models for Effect Estimation

By effect estimation is meant point and interval estimation of differences in properties of the responses between two or more settings of some predictors, or estimating some function of these differences such as the antilog. In ordinary multiple regression with no transformation of Y such differences are absolute estimates. In regression involving $\log(Y)$ or in logistic or proportional hazards models, effect estimation is, at least initially, concerned with estimation of relative effects. As discussed on pp. 4 and 221, estimation of absolute effects for these models must involve accurate prediction of overall response values, so the strategy in the previous section applies.

When estimating differences or relative effects, the bias in the effect estimate, besides being influenced by the study design, is related to how well subject heterogeneity and confounding are taken into account. The variance of the effect estimate is related to the distribution of the variable whose levels are being compared, and, in least squares estimates, to the amount of variation "explained" by the entire set of predictors. Variance of the estimated difference can increase if there is overfitting. So for estimation, the previous strategy largely applies.

The following are differences in the modeling strategy when effect estimation is the goal.

1. There is even less gain from having a parsimonious model than when developing overall predictive models, as estimation is usually done at the time of analysis. Leaving insignificant predictors in the model increases the likelihood that the confidence interval for the effect of interest has the stated coverage. By contrast, overall predictions are conditional on the values of all predictors in the model. The variance of such predictions is increased by the presence of unimportant variables, as predictions are still conditional on the particular values of these variables (Section 5.4.1) and cancellation of terms (which occurs when differences are of interest) does not occur.

2. Careful consideration of inclusion of interactions is still a major consideration for estimation. If a predictor whose effects are of major interest is allowed to interact with one or more other predictors, effect estimates must be conditional on the values of the other predictors and hence have higher variance.

3. A major goal of imputation is to avoid lowering the sample size because of missing values in adjustment variables. If the predictor of interest is the only variable having a substantial number of missing values, multiple imputation is less worthwhile, unless it corrects for a substantial bias caused by deletion of nonrandomly missing data.

4. The analyst need not be very concerned about conserving degrees of freedom devoted to the predictor of interest. The complexity allowed for this variable is usually determined by prior beliefs, with compromises that consider the bias-variance trade-off.

5. If penalized estimation is used, the analyst may wish to not shrink parameter estimates for the predictor of interest.

6. Model validation is not necessary unless the analyst wishes to use it to quantify the degree of overfitting.

4.10.3 Developing Models for Hypothesis Testing

A default strategy for developing a multivariable model that is to be used as a basis for hypothesis testing is almost the same as the strategy used for estimation.

1. There is little concern for parsimony. A full model fit, including insignificant variables, will result in more accurate P-values for tests for the variables of interest.

2. Careful consideration of inclusion of interactions is still a major consideration for hypothesis testing. If one or more predictors interacts with a variable of interest, either separate hypothesis tests are carried out over the levels of the interacting factors, or a combined "main effect + interaction" test is performed. For example, a very well–defined test is whether treatment is effective for *any* race group.

3. If the predictor of interest is the only variable having a substantial number of missing values, multiple imputation is less worthwhile. In some cases, multiple imputation may increase power (e.g., in ordinary multiple regression one can obtain larger degrees of freedom for error) but in others there will be little net gain. However, the test can be biased due to exclusion of nonrandomly missing observations if imputation is not done.

4. As before, the analyst need not be very concerned about conserving degrees of freedom devoted to the predictor of interest. The degrees of freedom allowed for this variable is usually determined by prior beliefs, with careful consideration of the trade-off between bias and power.

5. If penalized estimation is used, the analyst should not shrink parameter estimates for the predictors being tested.

6. Model validation is not necessary unless the analyst wishes to use it to quantify the degree of overfitting. This may shed light on whether there is overadjustment for confounders.

4.11   Further Reading

[1]   Some good general references that address modeling strategies are [185, 325, 400].

[2]   Simulation studies are needed to determine the effects of modifying the model based on assessments of "predictor promise." Although it is unlikely that this strategy will result in regression coefficients that are biased high in absolute value, it may on some occasions result in somewhat optimistic standard errors and a slight elevation in type I error probability. Some simulation results my be found on the Web site. Initial promising findings for least squares models for two uncorrelated predictors indicate that the procedure is conservative in its estimation of σ^2 and in preserving type I error.

[3]   Verweij and van Houwelingen[437] and Shao[382] describe how cross-validation can be used in formulating a stopping rule.

[4]   Roecker[355] compared forward variable selection (FS) and all possible subsets selection (APS) to full model fits in ordinary least squares. APS had a greater tendency to select smaller, less accurate models than FS. Neither selection technique was as accurate as the full model fit unless more than half of the candidate variables was redundant or unnecessary.

[5]   Other results on how variable selection affects inference may be found in Hurvich and Tsai[217] and Breiman [46, Section 8.1].

[6]   Steyerberg et al.[399] have comparisons of smoothly penalized estimators with the lasso and with several stepwise variable selection algorithms.

[7]   See Weiss,[448] Faraway,[134] and Chatfield[69] for more discussions of the effect of not prespecifying models, for example, dependence of point estimates of effects on the variables used for adjustment.

[8]   See Peduzzi et al.[328, 329] for studies of the relationship between "events per variable" and types I and II error, accuracy of variance estimates, and accuracy of normal approximations for regression coefficient estimators. Their findings are consistent with those given above.

[9]   Copas [84, Eq. 8.5] adds 2 to the numerator of Equation 4.1 (see also [337, 431]).

[10]   Efron [125, Eq. 4.23] and van Houwelingen and le Cessie[433] showed that the average expected optimism in a mean logarithmic quality score for a p-predictor binary logistic model is p/n. Taylor et al.[408] showed that the ratio of variances for certain quantities is proportional to the ratio of the number of parameters in two models. Copas stated that "Shrinkage can be particularly marked when stepwise fitting is used: the shrinkage is then closer to that expected of the full regression rather than of the subset regression actually fitted."[84, 337, 431] Spiegelhalter,[397] in arguing against variable selection, states that better prediction will often be obtained by fitting all candidate variables in the final model, shrinking the vector of regression coefficient estimates towards zero.

[11]   See Belsley [32, pp. 28–30] for some reservations about using VIF.

[12]   For incomplete principal components regression see [70, 102, 104, 220, 222]. See [271] for principal surfaces. Sliced inverse regression is described in [137, 278, 279]. For

material on variable clustering see [102, 104, 184, 305, 362]. A good general reference on cluster analysis is [434, Chapter 11].

[13]   Principal components are commonly used to summarize a cluster of variables. Vines[439] developed a method to constrain the principal component coefficients to be integers without much loss of explained variability.

[14]   See D'Agostino et al.[104] for excellent examples of variable clustering (including a two-stage approach) and other data reduction techniques using both statistical methods and subject-matter expertise.

Chapter 5

Resampling, Validating, Describing, and Simplifying the Model

5.1 The Bootstrap

When one assumes that a random variable Y has a certain population distribution, one can use simulation or analytic derivations to study how a statistical estimator computed from samples from this distribution behaves. For example, when Y has a log-normal distribution, the variance of the sample median for a sample of size n from that distribution can be derived analytically. Alternatively, one can simulate 500 samples of size n from the log-normal distribution, compute the sample median for each sample, and then compute the sample variance of the 500 sample medians. Either case requires knowledge of the population distribution function.

Efron's *bootstrap*[108, 129, 130] is a general-purpose technique for obtaining estimates of the properties of statistical estimators without making assumptions about the distribution giving rise to the data. Suppose that a random variable Y comes from a cumulative distribution function $F(y) = \text{Prob}\{Y \leq y\}$ and that we have a sample of size n from this unknown distribution, $Y_1, Y_2, \ldots, Y_n$. The basic idea is to repeatedly simulate a sample of size n from F, computing the statistic of interest, and assessing how the statistic behaves over B repetitions. Not having F at our disposal, we can estimate F by the empirical cumulative distribution function

$$F_n(y) = \frac{1}{n} \sum_{i=1}^{n} I(Y_i \le y), \tag{5.1}$$

where $I(w)$ is 1 if w is true, 0 otherwise. F_n corresponds to a density function that places probability $1/n$ at each observed datapoint (k/n if that point were duplicated k times and its value listed only once). Now pretend that $F_n(y)$ is the original population distribution $F(y)$. Sampling from F_n is equivalent to sampling with replacement from the observed data $Y_1, \ldots, Y_n$. For large n, the expected fraction of original datapoints that are selected for each bootstrap sample is $1 - e^{-1} = 0.632$. Some points are selected twice, some three times, a few four times, and so on. We take B samples of size n with replacement, with B chosen so that the summary measure of the individual statistics is nearly as good as taking $B = \infty$. The bootstrap is based on the fact that the distribution of the *observed* differences between a resampled estimate of a parameter of interest and the original estimate of the parameter from the whole whole sample tells us about the distribution of *unobservable* differences between the original estimate and the unknown population value of the parameter.

As an example, consider the data $(1, 5, 6, 7, 8, 9)$ and suppose that we would like to obtain a 0.80 confidence interval for the population median, as well as an estimate of the population expected value of the sample median (the latter is only used to estimate bias in the sample median). The first 20 bootstrap samples (after sorting data values) and the corresponding sample medians are shown in Table 5.1. For a given number B of bootstrap samples, our estimates are simply the sample 0.1 and 0.9 quantiles of the sample medians, and the mean of the sample medians. Not knowing how large B should be, we could let B range from, say, 50 to 1000, stopping when we are sure the estimates have converged. In the left plot of Figure 5.1, B varies from 1 to 400 for the mean (10 to 400 for the quantiles). It can be seen that the bootstrap estimate of the population mean of the sample median can be estimated satisfactorily when $B > 50$. For the lower and upper limits of the 0.8 confidence interval for the population median Y, B must be at least 200. For more extreme confidence limits, B must be higher still. For the final set of 400 sample medians, a histogram (right plot in Figure 5.1) can be used to assess the form of the sampling distribution of the sample median. Here, the distribution is almost normal, although there is a slightly heavy left tail that comes from the data themselves having a heavy left tail. For large samples, sample medians are normally distributed for a wide variety of population distributions. Therefore we could use bootstrapping to estimate the variance of the sample median and then take ± 1.28 standard errors as a 0.80 confidence interval. In other cases (e.g., regression coefficient estimates for certain models), estimates are asymmetrically distributed, and the bootstrap quantiles are better estimates than confidence intervals that are based on a normality assumption. Note that because sample quantiles are more or

TABLE 5.1

Bootstrap Sample	Sample Median
1 6 6 6 9 9	6.0
5 5 6 7 8 8	6.5
1 1 1 5 8 9	3.0
1 1 1 5 8 9	3.0
1 6 8 8 8 9	8.0
1 6 7 8 9 9	7.5
6 6 8 8 9 9	8.0
1 1 7 8 8 9	7.5
1 5 7 8 9 9	7.5
5 6 6 6 7 7	6.0
1 6 8 8 9 9	8.0
1 5 6 6 9 9	6.0
1 6 7 8 8 9	7.5
1 6 7 7 9 9	7.0
1 5 7 8 9 9	7.5
5 6 7 9 9 9	8.0
5 5 6 7 8 8	6.5
6 6 6 7 8 8	6.5
1 1 1 1 6 9	1.0
1 5 7 7 9 9	7.0

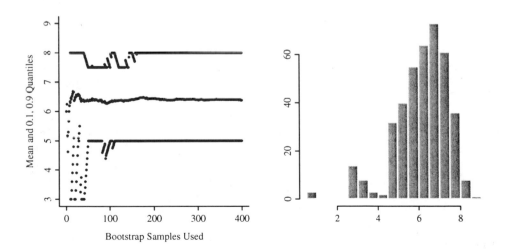

FIGURE 5.1: Estimating properties of sample median using the bootstrap.

less restricted to equal one of the values in the sample, the bootstrap distribution is discrete and can be dependent on a small number of outliers. For this reason, bootstrapping quantiles does not work particularly well for small samples [108, pp. 41–43].

The method just presented for obtaining a nonparametric confidence interval for the population median is called the *bootstrap percentile method*. It is the simplest but not necessarily the best performing bootstrap method.   ①

In this text we use the bootstrap primarily for computing statistical estimates that are much different from standard errors and confidence intervals, namely, estimates of model performance.

5.2   Model Validation

5.2.1   Introduction

The surest method to have a model fit the data at hand is to discard much of the data. A p-variable fit to $p+1$ observations will perfectly predict Y as long as no two observations have the same Y. Such a model will, however, yield predictions that appear almost random with respect to responses on a different dataset. Therefore, unbiased estimates of predictive accuracy are essential.

Model validation is done to ascertain whether predicted values from the model are likely to accurately predict responses on future subjects or subjects not used to develop our model. Three major causes of failure of the model to validate are   ②
overfitting, changes in measurement methods/changes in definition of categorical variables, and major changes in subject inclusion criteria.

There are two major modes of model validation, *external* and *internal*. The most stringent external validation involves testing a final model developed in one country on subjects in another country at another time. This validation would test whether the data collection instrument was translated into another language properly, whether cultural differences make earlier findings nonapplicable, and whether secular trends have changed associations or base rates. Testing a finished model on   ③
new subjects from the same geographic area but from a different institution as subjects used to fit the model is a less stringent form of external validation. The least stringent form of external validation involves using the first m of n observations for model training and using the remaining $n - m$ observations as a test sample. This is very similar to data-splitting (Section 5.2.3). For details about methods for external validation see the S-PLUS functions `val.prob` and `val.surv` functions in the `Design` library.

Even though external validation is frequently favored by nonstatisticians, it is often problematic. Holding back data from the model-fitting phase results in lower precision and power, and one can increase precision and learn more about geographic or time differences by fitting a unified model to the entire subject series including, for example, country or calendar time as a main effect and/or as an interacting effect.

Internal validation involves fitting and validating the model by carefully using one series of subjects. One uses the combined dataset in this way to estimate the likely performance of the final model on new subjects, which after all is often of most interest. Most of the remainder of Section 5.2 deals with internal validation.

5.2.2   Which Quantities Should Be Used in Validation?

For ordinary multiple regression models, the R^2 index is a good measure of the model's predictive ability, especially for the purpose of quantifying drop-off in predictive ability when applying the model to other datasets. R^2 is biased, however. For example, if one used nine predictors to predict outcomes of 10 subjects, $R^2 = 1.0$ but the R^2 that will be achieved on future subjects will be close to zero. In this case, dramatic overfitting has occurred. The *adjusted* R^2 (Equation 4.2) solves this problem, at least when the model has been completely prespecified and no variables or parameters have been "screened" out of the final model fit. That is, R^2_{adj} is only valid when p in its formula is honest; when it includes all parameters ever examined (formally or informally, e.g., using graphs or tables) whether these parameters are in the final model or not.

Quite often we need to validate indexes other than R^2 for which adjustments for p have not been created.[a] We also need to validate models containing "phantom degrees of freedom" that were screened out earlier, formally or informally. For these purposes, we obtain nearly unbiased estimates of R^2 or other indexes using data splitting, cross-validation, or the bootstrap. The bootstrap provides the most precise estimates.

R^2 measures only one aspect of predictive ability. In general, there are two major aspects of predictive accuracy that need to be assessed. As discussed in Section 4.5, *calibration* or *reliability* is the ability of the model to make unbiased estimates of outcome. *Discrimination* is the model's ability to separate subjects' outcomes. Validation of the model is recommended even when a data reduction technique is used. This is a way to ensure that the model was not overfitted or is otherwise inaccurate.

5.2.3   Data-Splitting

The simplest validation method is one-time *data-splitting*. Here a dataset is split into *training* (model development) and *test* (model validation) samples by a ran-

---

[a]For example, in the binary logistic model, there is a generalization of R^2 available, but no adjusted version. For logistic models we often validate other indexes such as the ROC area or rank correlation between predicted probabilities and observed outcomes. We also validate the calibration accuracy of $\hat{Y}$ in predicting Y.

dom process with or without balancing distributions of the response and predictor variables in the two samples. In some cases, a chronological split is used so that the validation is prospective. The model's calibration and discrimination are validated in the test set.

In ordinary least squares, calibration may be assessed by, for example, plotting Y against $\hat{Y}$. Discrimination here is assessed by R^2 and it is of interest in comparing R^2 in the training sample to that achieved in the test sample. A drop in R^2 indicates overfitting, and the absolute R^2 in the test sample is an unbiased estimate of predictive discrimination. Note that in extremely overfitted models, R^2 in the test set can be negative, since it is computed on "frozen" intercept and regression coefficients using the formula $1 - SSE/SST$, where SSE is the error sum of squares, SST is the total sum of squares, and SSE can be greater than SST (when predictions are worse than the constant predictor $\overline{Y}$).

[4]

To be able to validate predictions from the model over an entire test sample (without validating it separately in particular subsets such as in males and females), the test sample must be large enough to precisely fit a model containing one predictor. For a study with a continuous uncensored response variable, the test sample size should ordinarily be ≥ 100 at a bare minimum. For survival time studies, the test sample should at least be large enough to contain a minimum of 100 outcome events. For binary outcomes, the test sample should contain a bare minimum of 100 subjects in the least frequent outcome category. Once the size of the test sample is determined, the remaining portion of the original sample can be used as a training sample. Even with these test sample sizes, validation of extreme predictions is difficult.

Data-splitting has the advantage of allowing hypothesis tests to be confirmed in the test sample. However, it has the following disadvantages.

1. Data-splitting greatly reduces the sample size for both model development and model testing. Because of this, Roecker[355] found this method "appears to be a costly approach, both in terms of predictive accuracy of the fitted model and the precision of our estimate of the accuracy." Breiman [46, Section 1.3] found that bootstrap validation on the original sample was as efficient as having a separate test sample twice as large.

2. It requires a larger sample to be held out than cross-validation (see below) to be able to obtain the same precision of the estimate of predictive accuracy.

3. The split may be fortuitous; if the process were repeated with a different split, different assessments of predictive accuracy may be obtained.

4. Data-splitting does not validate the final model, but rather a model developed on only a subset of the data. The training and test sets are recombined for fitting the final model, which is not validated.

5. Data-splitting requires the split before the *first* analysis of the data. With other methods, analyses can proceed in the usual way on the complete dataset. Then, after a "final" model is specified, the modeling process is rerun on multiple resamples from the original data to mimic the process that produced the "final" model.

5.2.4 Improvements on Data-Splitting: Resampling

Bootstrapping, jackknifing, and other resampling plans can be used to obtain nearly unbiased estimates of model performance without sacrificing sample size. These methods work when either the model is completely specified except for the regression coefficients, or all important steps of the modeling process, especially variable selection, are automated. Only then can each bootstrap replication be a reflection of all sources of variability in modeling. Note that most analyses involve examination of graphs and testing for lack of model fit, with many intermediate decisions by the analyst such as simplification of interactions. These processes are difficult to automate. But variable selection alone is often the greatest source of variability because of multiple comparison problems, so the analyst must go to great lengths to bootstrap or jackknife variable selection.

The ability to study the arbitrariness of how a stepwise variable selection algorithm selects "important" factors is a major benefit of bootstrapping. A useful display is a matrix of blanks and asterisks, where an asterisk is placed in column x of row i if variable x is selected in bootstrap sample i (see p. 295 for an example). If many variables appear to be selected at random, the analyst may want to turn to a data reduction method rather than using stepwise selection (see also [364]).

Cross-validation is a generalization of data-splitting that solves some of the problems of data-splitting. *Leave-out-one cross-validation*,[382, 433] the limit of cross-validation, is similar to jackknifing.[457] Here one observation is omitted from the analytical process and the response for that observation is predicted using a model derived from the remaining $n - 1$ observations. The process is repeated n times to obtain an average accuracy. Efron[124] reports that grouped cross-validation is more accurate; here groups of k observations are omitted at a time. Suppose, for example, that 10 groups are used. The original dataset is divided into 10 equal subsets at random. The first 9 subsets are used to develop a model (transformation selection, interaction testing, stepwise variable selection, etc. are all done). The resulting model is assessed for accuracy on the remaining 1/10th of the sample. This process is repeated at least 10 times to get an average of 10 indexes such as R^2.

A drawback of cross-validation is the choice of the number of observations to hold out from each fit. Another is that the number of repetitions needed to achieve accurate estimates of accuracy often exceeds 200. For example, one may have to omit 1/10th of the sample 200 times to accurately estimate the index of interest. Thus the sample would need to be split into tenths 20 times. Another possible problem is that cross-validation may not fully represent the variability of variable selection. If

20 subjects are omitted each time from a sample of size 1000, the lists of variables selected from each training sample of size 980 are likely to be much more similar than lists obtained from fitting independent samples of 1000 subjects. Finally, as with data-splitting, cross-validation does not validate the full 1000-subject model.

An interesting way to study overfitting could be called the randomization method. Here we ask the question "How well can the response be predicted when we use our best procedure on random responses when the predictive accuracy should be near zero?" The better the fit on random Y, the worse the overfitting. The method takes a random permutation of the response variable and develops a model with optional variable selection based on the original X and permuted Y. Suppose this yields $R^2 = .2$ for the fitted sample. Apply the fit to the original data to estimate optimism. If overfitting is not a problem, R^2 would be the same for both fits and it will ordinarily be very near zero. $\boxed{7}$

5.2.5 Validation Using the Bootstrap

Efron,[124, 125] Efron and Gong,[127] Gong,[153] Efron and Tibshirani,[129, 130] Linnet,[287] and Breiman[46] describe several bootstrapping procedures for obtaining nearly unbiased estimates of future model performance without holding back data when making the final estimates of model parameters. With the "simple bootstrap" [130, p. 247], one repeatedly fits the model in a bootstrap sample and evaluates the performance of the model on the original sample. The estimate of the likely performance of the final model on future data is estimated by the average of all of the indexes computed on the original sample.

Efron showed that an enhanced bootstrap estimates future model performance more accurately than the simple bootstrap. Instead of estimating an accuracy index directly from averaging indexes computed on the original sample, the enhanced bootstrap uses a slightly more indirect approach by estimating the bias due to overfitting or the "optimism" in the final model fit. After the optimism is estimated, it can be subtracted from the index of accuracy derived from the original sample to obtain a bias-corrected or overfitting-corrected estimate of predictive accuracy. The bootstrap method is as follows. From the original X and Y in the sample of size n, draw a sample with replacement also of size n. Derive a model in the bootstrap sample and apply it without change to the original sample. The accuracy index from the bootstrap sample minus the index computed on the original sample is an estimate of optimism. This process is repeated for 100 or so bootstrap replications to obtain an average optimism, which is subtracted from the final model fit's apparent accuracy to obtain the overfitting-corrected estimate. $\boxed{8}$

Note that bootstrapping validates the *process* that was used to fit the original model. It provides an estimate of the *expected value* of the optimism, which when subtracted from the original index, provides an estimate of the *expected* bias-corrected index. $\boxed{9}$

Note that by drawing samples from X and Y, we are estimating aspects of the *unconditional* distribution of statistical quantities. One could instead draw samples from quantities such as residuals from the model to obtain a distribution that is conditional on X. However, this approach requires that the model be specified correctly, whereas the unconditional bootstrap does not. Also, the unconditional estimators are similar to conditional estimators except for very skewed or very small samples [134, p. 217].

Bootstrapping can be used to estimate the optimism in virtually any index. Besides discrimination indexes such as R^2, slope and intercept calibration factors can be estimated. When one fits the model $C(Y|X) = X\beta$, and then refits the model $C(Y|X) = \gamma_0 + \gamma_1 X \hat{\beta}$ on the same data, where $\hat{\beta}$ is an estimate of β, $\hat{\gamma}_0$ and $\hat{\gamma}_1$ will necessarily be 0 and 1, respectively. However, when $\hat{\beta}$ is used to predict responses on another dataset, $\hat{\gamma}_1$ may be < 1 if there is overfitting, and $\hat{\gamma}_0$ will be different from zero to compensate. Thus a bootstrap estimate of γ_1 will not only quantify overfitting nicely, but can also be used to shrink predicted values to make them more calibrated (similar to [397]). Efron's optimism bootstrap is used to estimate the optimism in $(0, 1)$ and then (γ_0, γ_1) are estimated by subtracting the optimism in the constant estimator $(0, 1)$. Note that in cross-validation one estimates β with $\hat{\beta}$ from the training sample and fits $C(Y|X) = \gamma X \hat{\beta}$ on the test sample directly. Then the γ estimates are averaged over all test samples. This approach does not require the choice of a parameter that determines the amount of shrinkage as does ridge regression or penalized maximum likelihood estimation; instead one estimates how to make the initial fit well calibrated.[85, 433] However, this approach is not as reliable as building shrinkage into the original estimation process. The latter allows different parameters to be shrunk by different factors. 〔10〕

Ordinary bootstrapping can sometimes yield overly optimistic estimates of optimism, that is, may underestimate the amount of overfitting. This is especially true when the ratio of the number of observations to the number of parameters estimated is not large.[145] A variation on the bootstrap that improves precision of the assessment is the ".632" method, which Efron found to be optimal in several examples.[124] This method provides a bias-corrected estimate of predictive accuracy by substituting $0.632\times$ [apparent accuracy $-\hat{\epsilon}_0$] for the estimate of optimism, where $\hat{\epsilon}_0$ is a weighted average of accuracies evaluated on observations *omitted* from bootstrap samples [130, Eq. 17.25, p. 253]. 〔11〕

For ordinary least squares, where the genuine per-observation .632 estimator can be used, several simulations revealed close agreement with the modified .632 estimator, even in small, highly overfitted samples. In these overfitted cases, the ordinary bootstrap bias-corrected accuracy estimates were significantly higher than the .632 estimates. Simulations[176] have shown, however, that for most types of indexes of accuracy of binary logistic regression models, Efron's original bootstrap has lower mean squared error than the .632 bootstrap when $n = 200, p = 30$. 〔12〕

TABLE 5.2

Method	Apparent Rank Correlation of Predicted vs. Observed	Over-Optimism	Bias-Corrected Correlation
Full Model	0.50	0.06	0.44
Stepwise Model	0.47	0.05	0.42

Bootstrap overfitting-corrected estimates of model performance can be biased in favor of the model. Although cross-validation is less biased than the bootstrap, Efron[124] showed that it has much higher variance in estimating overfitting-corrected predictive accuracy than bootstrapping. In other words, cross-validation, like data-splitting, can yield significantly different estimates when the entire validation process is repeated.

It is frequently very informative to estimate a measure of predictive accuracy forcing all candidate factors into the fit and then to separately estimate accuracy allowing stepwise variable selection, possibly with different stopping rules. Consistent with Spiegelhalter's proposal to use all factors and then to shrink the coefficients to adjust for overfitting,[397] the full model fit will outperform the stepwise model more often than not. Even though stepwise modeling has slightly less optimism in predictive discrimination, this improvement is not enough to offset the loss of information from deleting even marginally significant variables. Table 5.2 shows a typical scenario. In this example, stepwise modeling lost a possible $0.50-0.47 = 0.03$ predictive discrimination. The full model fit will especially be an improvement when

1. the stepwise selection deletes several variables that are almost significant;

2. these marginal variables have *some* real predictive value, even if it's slight; and

3. there is no small set of extremely dominant variables that would be easily found by stepwise selection.

[13]

Faraway[134] has a fascinating study showing how resampling methods can be used to estimate the distributions of predicted values and of effects of a predictor, adjusting for an automated multistep modeling process. Bootstrapping can be used, for example, to penalize the variance in predicted values for choosing a transformation for Y and for outlier and influential observation deletion, in addition to variable selection. Estimation of the transformation of Y greatly increased the variance in Faraway's examples. Brownstone [53, p. 74] states that "In spite of considerable efforts, theoretical statisticians have been unable to analyze the sampling properties of [usual multistep modeling strategies] under realistic conditions" and concludes that the modeling strategy must be completely specified and then bootstrapped to get consistent estimates of variances and other sampling properties.

[14]

5.3   Describing the Fitted Model

Before addressing issues related to describing and interpreting the model and its coefficients, one can never apply too much caution in attempting to interpret results in a causal manner. Regression models are excellent tools for estimating and inferring *associations* between an X and Y given that the "right" variables are in the model. Any ability of a model to provide *causal* inference rests entirely on the faith of the analyst in the experimental design, completeness of the set of variables that are thought to measure confounding and are used for adjustment when the experiment is not randomized, lack of important measurement error, and lastly the goodness of fit of the model.

The first line of attack in interpreting the results of a multivariable analysis is to interpret the model's parameter estimates. For simple linear, additive models, regression coefficients may be readily interpreted. If there are interactions or non-linear terms in the model, however, simple interpretations are usually impossible. Many programs ignore this problem, routinely printing such meaningless quantities as the effect of increasing age^2 by one day while holding age constant. A meaningful age change needs to be chosen, and connections between mathematically related variables must be taken into account. These problems can be solved by relying on predicted values and differences between predicted values.

Even when the model contains no nonlinear effects, it is difficult to compare regression coefficients across predictors having varying scales. Some analysts like to gauge the relative contributions of different predictors on a common scale by multiplying regression coefficients by the standard deviations of the predictors that pertain to them. This does not make sense for nonnormally distributed predictors (and regression models should not need to make assumptions about the distributions of predictors). When a predictor is binary (e.g., sex), the standard deviation makes no sense as a scaling factor as the scale would depend on the prevalence of the predictor.[b]

It is more sensible to estimate the change in Y when X_j is changed by an amount that is subject-matter relevant. For binary predictors this is a change from 0 to 1. For many continuous predictors the interquartile range is a reasonable default choice. If the 0.25 and 0.75 quantiles of X_j are g and h, linearity holds, and the estimated coefficient of X_j is b; $b \times (h - g)$ is the effect of increasing X_j by $h - g$ units, which is a span that contains half of the sample values of X_j.

---

[b]The s.d. of a binary variable is approximately $\sqrt{a(1-a)}$, where a is the proportion of ones.

For the more general case of continuous predictors that are monotonically but not linearly related to Y, a useful point summary is the change in $X\beta$ when the variable changes from its 0.25 quantile to its 0.75 quantile. For models for which $\exp(X\beta)$ is meaningful, antilogging the predicted change in $X\beta$ results in quantities such as interquartile-range odds and hazards ratios. When the variable is involved in interactions, these ratios are estimated separately for various levels of the interacting factors. For categorical predictors, ordinary effects are computed by comparing each level of the predictor to a reference level. See Section 10.10 and Chapter 11 for tabular and graphical examples of this approach.

The model can be described graphically in a straightforward fashion by plotting each X against $X\hat{\beta}$ holding other predictors constant. For an X that interacts with other factors, separate curves are drawn on the same graph, one for each level of the interacting factor.

Nomograms[28, 172, 295] provide excellent graphical depictions of all the variables in the model, in addition to enabling the user to obtain predicted values manually. Nomograms are especially good at helping the user envision interactions. See Section 10.10 and Chapter 11 for examples.

15

5.4   Simplifying the Final Model by Approximating It

5.4.1   Difficulties Using Full Models

A model that contains all prespecified terms will usually be the one that predicts the most accurately on new data. It is also a model for which confidence limits and statistical tests have the claimed properties. Often, however, this model will not be very parsimonious. The full model may require more predictors than the researchers care to collect in future samples. It also requires predicted values to be conditional on all of the predictors, which can increase the variance of the predictions.

As an example suppose that least squares has been used to fit a model containing several variables including race (with four categories). Race may be an insignificant predictor and may explain a tiny fraction of the observed variation in Y. Yet when predictions are requested, a value for race must be inserted. If the subject is of the majority race, and this race has a majority of, say 0.75, the variance of the predicted value will not be significantly greater than the variance for a predicted value from a model that excluded race for its list of predictors. If, however, the subject is of a minority race (say "other" with a prevalence of 0.01), the predicted value will have much higher variance. One approach to this problem, that does not require development of a second model, is to ignore the subject's race and to get a weighted average prediction. That is, we obtain predictions for each of the four races and weight these predictions by the relative frequencies of the four races.[c] This weighted average estimates the expected value of Y unconditional on race. It has the advantage of having exactly correct confidence limits when model assumptions are satisfied, because the correct "error term" is being used (one that deducts 3 d.f. for having ever estimated the race effect). In regression models having nonlinear link functions, this process does not yield such a simple interpretation.

When predictors are collinear, their competition results in larger P-values when predictors are (often inappropriately) tested individually. Likewise, confidence intervals for individual effects will be wide and uninterpretable (can other variables really be held constant when one is changed?).

5.4.2 Approximating the Full Model

When the full model contains several predictors that do not appreciably affect the predictions, the above process of "unconditioning" is unwieldy. In the search for a simple solution, the most commonly used procedure for making the model parsimonious is to remove variables on the basis of P-values, but this results in a variety of problems as we have seen. Our approach instead is to consider the full model fit as the "gold standard" model, especially the model from which formal inferences are made. We then proceed to approximate this full model to any desired degree of accuracy. For any approximate model we calculate the accuracy with which it approximates the best model. One goal this process accomplishes is that it provides different degrees of parsimony to different audiences, based on their needs. One investigator may be able to collect only three variables, another one seven. Each investigator will know how much she is giving up by using a subset of the predictors. In approximating the gold standard model it is very important to note that there is nothing gained in removing certain nonlinear terms; gains in parsimony come only from removing entire predictors. Another accomplishment of model approximation is that when the full model has been fitted using shrinkage (penalized estimation, Section 9.10), the approximate models will inherit the shrinkage (see Section 14.10 for an example).

Approximating complex models with simpler ones has been used to decode "black boxes" such as artificial neural networks. Recursive partitioning trees (Section 2.5) may sometimes be used in this context. One develops a regression tree to predict the predicted value $X\hat{\beta}$ on the basis of the unique variables in X, using R^2, the average absolute prediction error, or the maximum absolute prediction error as a stopping rule, for example. The user desiring simplicity may use the tree to obtain predicted values, using the first k nodes, with k just large enough to yield a low enough absolute error in predicting the more comprehensive prediction. Overfitting is not

---

[c]Using the S-PLUS Design library described in Chapter 6, such estimates and their confidence limits can easily be obtained, using for example contrast(fit, list(age=50, disease='hypertension', race=levels(race)), type='average', weights=table(race)).

a problem as it is when the tree procedure is used to predict the outcome, because (1) given the predictor values the predictions are deterministic and (2) the variable being predicted is a continuous, completely observed variable. Hence the best cross-validating tree approximation will be one with one subject per node. One advantage of the tree-approximation procedure is that data collection on an individual subject whose outcome is being predicted may be abbreviated by measuring only those Xs that are used in the top nodes, until the prediction is resolved to within a tolerable error.

When principal components regression is being used, trees can also be used to approximate the components or to make them more interpretable.

Full models may also be approximated using least squares as long as the linear predictor $X\hat{\beta}$ is the target, and not some nonlinear transformation of it such as a logistic model probability. When the original model was fitted using unpenalized least squares, submodels fitted against $\hat{Y}$ will have the same coefficients as if least squares had been used to fit the subset of predictors directly against Y. To see this, note that if X denotes the entire design matrix and T denotes a subset of the columns of X, the coefficient estimates for the full model are $(X'X)^{-1}X'Y$, $\hat{Y} = X(X'X)^{-1}X'Y$, estimates for a reduced model fitted against Y are $(T'T)^{-1}T'Y$, and coefficients fitted against $\hat{Y}$ are $(T'T)T'X(X'X)^{-1}X'Y$ which can be shown to equal $(T'T)^{-1}T'Y$.

When least squares is used for both the full and reduced models, the variance–covariance matrix of the coefficient estimates of the reduced model is $(T'T)^{-1}\sigma^2$, where the residual variance σ^2 is estimated using the *full* model. When σ^2 is estimated by the unbiased estimator using the d.f. from the full model, which provides the only unbiased estimate of σ^2, the estimated variance–covariance matrix of the reduced model will be appropriate (unlike that from stepwise variable selection) although the bootstrap may be needed to fully take into account the source of variation due to how the approximate model was selected.

So if in the least squares case the approximate model coefficients are identical to coefficients obtained upon fitting the reduced model against Y, how is model approximation any different from stepwise variable selection? There are several differences, in addition to how σ^2 is estimated.

1. When the full model is approximated by a backward step-down procedure against $\hat{Y}$, the stopping rule is less arbitrary. One stops deleting variables when deleting any further variable would make the approximation inadequate (e.g., the R^2 for predictions from the reduced model against the original $\hat{Y}$ drops below 0.95).

2. Because the stopping rule is different (i.e., is not based on P-values), the approximate model will have a different number of predictors than an ordinary stepwise model.

3. If the original model used penalization, approximate models will inherit the amount of shrinkage used in the full fit.

Typically, though, if one performed ordinary backward step-down against Y using a large cutoff for α (e.g., 0.5), the approximate model would be very similar to the step-down model. The main difference would be the use of a larger estimate of σ^2 and smaller error d.f. than are used for the ordinary step-down approach (an estimate that pretended the final reduced model was prespecified).

When the full model was not fitted using least squares, least squares can still easily be used to approximate the full model. If the coefficient estimates from the full model are $\hat{\beta}$, estimates from the approximate model are matrix contrasts of $\hat{\beta}$, namely, $W\hat{\beta}$, where $W = (T'T)^{-1}T'X$. So the variance–covariance matrix of the reduced coefficient estimates is given by

$$WVW', \tag{5.2}$$

where V is the variance matrix for $\hat{\beta}$. See Section 18.5 for an example.

5.5   Further Reading

[1]   There are many variations on the basic bootstrap for computing confidence limits.[108, 130] See Booth and Sarkar[43] for useful information about choosing the number of resamples. They report the number of resamples necessary to not appreciably change P-values, for example. Booth and Sarkar propose a more conservative number of resamples than others use (e.g., 800 resamples) for estimating variances. Carpenter and Bithell[63] have an excellent overview of bootstrap confidence intervals, with practical guidance. They also have a good discussion of the unconditional nonparametric bootstrap versus the conditional semiparametric bootstrap

[2]   Altman and Royston[13] have a good general discussion of what it means to validate a predictive model, including issues related to study design and consideration of uses to which the model will be put.

[3]   An excellent paper on external validation and generalizability is Justice et al.[224]

[4]   See Picard and Berk[338] for more about data-splitting.

[5]   In the context of variable selection where one attempts to select the set of variables with nonzero true regression coefficients in an ordinary regression model, Shao[382] demonstrated that leave-out-one cross-validation selects models that are "too large." Shao also showed that the number of observations held back for validation should often be larger than the number used to train the model. This is because in this case one is not interested in an accurate model (you fit the whole sample to do that), but an accurate estimate of prediction error is mandatory so as to know which variables to allow into the final model. Shao suggests using a cross-validation strategy in which approximately $n^{3/4}$ observations are used in each training sample and the remaining observations are used in the test sample. A repeated balanced or Monte

Carlo splitting approach is used, and accuracy estimates are averaged over $2n$ (for the Monte Carlo method) repeated splits.

[6]   Picard and Cook's Monte Carlo cross-validation procedure[339] is an improvement over ordinary cross-validation.

[7]   The randomization method is related to Kipnis' "chaotization relevancy principle"[237] in which one chooses between two models by measuring how far each is from a non-sense model. Tibshirani and Knight also use a randomization method for estimating the optimism in a model fit.[418]

[8]   This method used here is a slight change over that presented in [124], where Efron wrote predictive accuracy as a sum of per-observation components (such as 1 if the observation is classified correctly, 0 otherwise). Here we are writing $m \times$ the unitless summary index of predictive accuracy in the place of Efron's sum of m per-observation accuracies [287, p. 613].

[9]   See [433] and [46, Section 4] for insight on the meaning of expected optimism.

[10]   See Copas,[85] van Houwelingen and le Cessie [433, p. 1318], Verweij and van Houwelingen,[437] and others[431] for other methods of estimating shrinkage coefficients.

[11]   Efron[124] developed the ".632" estimator only for the case where the index being bootstrapped is estimated on a per-observation basis. A natural generalization of this method can be derived by assuming that the accuracy evaluated on observation i that is omitted from a bootstrap sample has the same expectation as the accuracy of any other observation that would be omitted from the sample. The modified estimate of ϵ_0 is then given by

$$\hat{\epsilon}_0 = \sum_{i=1}^{B} w_i T_i, \tag{5.3}$$

where T_i is the accuracy estimate derived from fitting a model on the ith bootstrap sample and evaluating it on the observations omitted from that bootstrap sample, and w_i are weights derived for the B bootstrap samples:

$$w_i = \frac{1}{n} \sum_{j=1}^{n} \frac{I(\text{bootstrap sample } i \text{ omits observation } j)}{\#\text{bootstrap samples omitting observation } j}, \tag{5.4}$$

where as before $I()$ denotes the indicator function. Note that $\hat{\epsilon}_0$ is undefined if any observation is included in every bootstrap sample. Increasing B will avoid this problem. This modified ".632" estimator is easy to compute if one assembles the bootstrap sample assignments and computes the w_i before computing the accuracy indexes T_i. For large n, the w_i approach $1/B$ and so $\hat{\epsilon}_0$ becomes equivalent to the accuracy computed on the observations not contained in the bootstrap sample and then averaged over the B repetitions.

[12]   Efron and Tibshirani[131] have reduced the bias of the ".632" estimator further with only a modest increase in its variance. Simulation has, however, shown no advantage of this ".632+" method over the basic optimism bootstrap for most accuracy indexes used in logistic models.

13 van Houwelingen and le Cessie[433] have several interesting developments in model validation. See Breiman[46] for a discussion of the choice of X for which to validate predictions.

14 Blettner and Sauerbrei also demonstrate the variability caused by data-driven analytic decisions.[41] Chatfield[69] has more results on the effects of using the data to select the model.

15 Hankins[172] is a definitive reference on nomograms and has multi-axis examples of historical significance. According to Hankins, Maurice d'Ocagne could be called the inventor of the nomogram, starting with alignment diagrams in 1884 and declaring a new science of "nomography" in 1899. d'Ocagne was at École des Ponts et Chaussées, a French civil engineering school.

Chapter 6

S-Plus Software

The methods described in this book are useful in any regression model that involves a linear combination of regression parameters. The software that is described below is useful in the same situations. S[30, 308] functions allow interaction spline functions as well as a wide variety of predictor parameterizations for any regression function, and facilitate model validation by resampling.

1

S is the most comprehensive tool for general regression models for the following reasons.

1. It is very easy to write S functions for new models, so S has implemented a wide variety of modern regression models.

2. Designs can be generated for any model. There is no need to find out whether the particular modeling function handles what SAS calls "class" variables— dummy variables are generated automatically when an S `category`, `factor`, `ordered`, or `character` variable is analyzed.

3. A single S object can contain all information needed to test hypotheses and to obtain predicted values for new data.

4. S has superior graphics.

5. *Classes* in S make possible the use of generic function names (e.g., `predict`, `summary`, `anova`) to examine fits from a large set of specific model–fitting functions.

S[30, 308, 395, 434] is a high-level object-oriented language for statistical analysis with more than 2000 functions available. S-PLUS (Insightful, Inc.[308]) on the UNIX, Linux, and Microsoft Windows/NT operating systems is the basis for S software used in this text. The R system[219] provides many of the same capabilities as S and uses the same syntax. See the Appendix and the Web site for more information about software implementations.

6.1 The S Modeling Language

S has a battery of functions that make up a statistical modeling language.[65] At the heart of the modeling functions is an *S formula* of the form

```
response  ~  terms
```

The `terms` represent additive components of a general linear model. Although variables and functions of variables make up the `terms`, the formula refers to additive combinations; for example, when `terms` is `age + blood.pressure`, it refers to $\beta_1 \times$ `age` $+\beta_2 \times$ `blood.pressure`. Some examples of formulas are below.

```
y ~ age + sex              # age + sex main effects
y ~ age + sex + age:sex    # add second-order interaction
y ~ age*sex                # second-order interaction +
                           # all main effects
y ~ (age + sex + pressure)^2
                           # age+sex+pressure+age:sex+age:pressure...
y ~ (age + sex + pressure)^2 - sex:pressure
                           # all main effects and all 2nd order
                           # interactions except sex:pressure
y ~ (age + race)*sex       # age+race+sex+age:sex+race:sex
y ~ treatment*(age*race + age*sex)
                           # no interact. with race,sex
sqrt(y) ~ sex*sqrt(age) + race
# functions, with dummy variables generated if
# race is an S factor (classification) variable
y ~ sex + poly(age,2)      # poly generates orthogonal polynomials
race.sex ← interaction(race,sex)
y ~ age + race.sex         # for when you want dummy variables for
                           # all combinations of the factors
```

The formula for a regression model is given to a modeling function; for example,

```
lrm(y ~ rcs(x,4))
```

is read "use a logistic regression model to model `y` as a function of `x`, representing `x` by a restricted cubic spline with four default knots."[a] You can use the S function `update` to refit a model with changes to the model terms or the data used to fit it:

---

[a]`lrm` and `rcs` are in the **Design** library.

```
f   ← lrm(y ∼ rcs(x,4) + x2 + x3)
f2  ← update(f, subset=sex=="male")
f3  ← update(f, .∼.-x2)            # remove x2 from model
f4  ← update(f, .∼. + rcs(x5,5))# add rcs(x5,5) to model
f5  ← update(f, y2 ∼ .)            # same terms, new response var.
```

6.2 User-Contributed Functions

In addition to the many functions that are packaged with S-Plus, a wide variety of user-contributed functions is available on the Internet (see the Appendix or Web site for addresses). Two libraries of functions used extensively in this text are Hmisc[15] and Design written by the author. The Hmisc library contains miscellaneous functions such as varclus, spearman2, transcan, hoeffd, rcspline.eval, impute, cut2, describe, sas.get, latex, and several power and sample size calculation functions. The varclus function uses the S hclust hierarchical clustering function to do variable clustering, and the S plclust function to draw dendograms depicting the clusters. varclus offers a choice of three similarity measures (Pearson r^2, Spearman ρ^2, and Hoeffding D) and uses pairwise deletion of missing values. varclus automatically generates a series of dummy variables for categorical factors. The Hmisc hoeffd function computes a matrix of Hoeffding Ds for a series of variables. The spearman2 function will do Wilcoxon, Spearman, and Kruskal–Wallis tests and generalizes Spearman's ρ to detect nonmonotonic relationships.

Hmisc's transcan function (see Section 4.7) performs a similar function to PROC PRINQUAL in SAS it uses restricted splines, dummy variables, and canonical variates to transform each of a series of variables while imputing missing values. An option to shrink regression coefficients for the imputation models avoids overfitting for small samples or a large number of predictors. transcan can also do multiple imputation and adjust variance–covariance matrices for imputation. See Chapter 8 for an example of using these functions for data reduction.

See the Web site for a list of S-Plus functions for correspondence analysis, principal components analysis, and missing data imputation available from other users. Venables and Ripley [434, Chapter 11] provide a nice description of the multivariate methods that are available in S-Plus, and they provide several new multivariate analysis functions.

A basic function in Hmisc is the rcspline.eval function, which creates a design matrix for a restricted (natural) cubic spline using the truncated power basis. Knot locations are optionally estimated using methods described in Section 2.4.5, and two types of normalizations to reduce numerical problems are supported. You can optionally obtain the design matrix for the antiderivative of the spline function. The rcspline.restate function computes the coefficients (after unnormalizing if needed) that translate the restricted cubic spline function to unrestricted

form (Equation 2.26). `rcspline.restate` also outputs LaTeX and S representations
of spline functions in simplified form.

6.3   The `Design` Library

A library of S functions called `Design` contains several functions that extend S to
make the analyses described in this book easy to do. A central function in `Design`
is `datadist`, which computes statistical summaries of predictors to automate estimation and plotting of effects. `datadist` exists as a separate function so that the
candidate predictors may be summarized once, thus saving time when fitting several
models using subsets or different transformations of predictors. If `datadist` is called
before model fitting, the distributional summaries are stored with the fit so that
the fit is self-contained with respect to later estimation. Alternatively, `datadist`
may be called after the fit to create temporary summaries to use as plot ranges
and effect intervals, or these ranges may be specified explicitly to `plot.Design` and
`summary.Design` (see below), without ever calling `datadist`. The input to `datadist`
may be a data frame, a list of individual predictors, a frame number, or a combination of the first two.

The characteristics saved by `datadist` include the overall range and certain quantiles for continuous variables, and the unique values for discrete variables (i.e., S
`factor` variables or variables with 10 or fewer unique values). The quantiles and set
of unique values facilitate estimation and plotting, as described later. When a function of a predictor is used (e.g., `pol(pmin(x,50),2)`), the limits saved apply to the
innermost variable (here, `x`). When a plot is requested for how `x` relates to the response, the plot will have `x` on the x-axis, not `pmin(x,50)`. The way that defaults are
computed can be controlled by the `q.effect` and `q.display` parameters to `datadist`.
By default, continuous variables are plotted with ranges determined by the tenth
smallest and tenth largest values occurring in the data (if $n < 200$, the 0.05 and
0.95 quantiles are used). The default range for estimating effects such as odds and
hazard ratios is the lower and upper quartiles. When a predictor is adjusted to a
constant so that the effects of changes in other predictors can be studied, the default constant used is the median for continuous predictors and the most frequent
category for factor variables. The S system option `datadist` is used to point to the
result returned by the `datadist` function. See the help files for `datadist` for more
information.

`Design` fitting functions save detailed information for later prediction, plotting,
and testing. `Design` also allows for special restricted interactions and sets the default
method of generating contrasts for categorical variables to `"contr.treatment"`, the
traditional dummy-variable approach.

`Design` has a special operator `%ia%` in the terms of a formula that allows for
restricted interactions. For example, one may specify a model that contains sex and

TABLE 6.1: **Design** Fitting Functions

Function	Purpose	Related S Functions
ols	Ordinary least squares linear model	lm
lrm	Binary and ordinal logistic regression model Has options for penalized MLE	glm
psm	Accelerated failure time parametric survival models	survreg
cph	Cox proportional hazards regression	coxph
bj	Buckley–James censored least squares model	survreg,lm
glmD	General linear models	glm

a five-knot linear spline for age, but restrict the age × sex interaction to be linear in age. To be able to connect this incomplete interaction with the main effects for later hypothesis testing and estimation, the following formula would be given:

```
y ~ sex + lsp(age,c(20,30,40,50,60)) +
    sex %ia% lsp(age,c(20,30,40,50,60))
```

The following expression would restrict the age × cholesterol interaction to be of the form $AF(B) + BG(A)$ by removing doubly nonlinear terms.

```
y ~ lsp(age,30) + rcs(cholesterol,4) +
    lsp(age,30) %ia% rcs(cholesterol,4)
```

Design has special fitting functions that facilitate many of the procedures described in this book, shown in Table 6.1. glmD is a slight modification of the built-in S glm function so that Design methods can be run on the resulting fit object. glm fits general linear models under a wide variety of distributions of Y.

You may want to specify to the fitting functions an option for how missing values (NAs) are handled. The method for handling missing data in S is to specify an na.action function. Some possible na.actions are given in Table 6.2. The default na.action is na.delete when you use Design's fitting functions. An easy way to specify a new default na.action is, for example,

```
options(na.action="na.omit")    # don't report frequency of NAs
```

before using a fitting function. If you use na.delete, you can also use the system option na.detail.response that makes model fits store information about Y stratified by whether each X is missing. The default descriptive statistics for Y are the sample size and mean. For a survival time response object, the sample size and proportion of events are used. Other summary functions can be specified using the na.fun.response option.

TABLE 6.2: Some `na.actions` Used in `Design`

Function Name	Method Used
na.fail	Stop with error message if any missing values present
na.omit	Function to remove observations with any predictors or responses missing
na.delete	Modified version of `na.omit` to also report on frequency of NAs for each variable
na.tree.replace	For categorical variables, adds a new level for NA. For continuous variables, groups into quantile groups first

```
options(na.action="na.delete", na.detail.response=T,
        na.fun.response="mystats")
# Just use na.fun.response="quantile" if don't care about n
mystats ← function(y) {
  z ← quantile(y, na.rm=T)
  n ← sum(!is.na(y))
  c(N=n, z)      # elements named N, 0%, 25%, etc.
}
```

When S deletes missing values during the model–fitting procedure, residuals, fitted values, and other quantities stored with the fit will not correspond row-for-row with observations in the original data frame (which retained NAs). This is problematic when, for example, `age` in the dataset is plotted against the residual from the fitted model. Fortunately, for many `na.actions` including `na.delete` and a modified version of `na.omit`, a class of S functions called `naresid` written by Therneau works behind the scenes to put NAs back into residuals, predicted values, and other quantities when the `predict` or `residuals` functions (see below) are used. Thus for some of the `na.actions`, predicted values and residuals will automatically be arranged to match the original data.

Any S function can be used in the terms for formulas given to the fitting function, but if the function represents a transformation that has data-dependent parameters (such as the standard S functions `poly` or `ns`), S will not in general be able to compute predicted values correctly for new observations. For example, the function `ns` that automatically selects knots for a B-spline fit will not be conducive to obtaining predicted values if the knots are kept "secret." For this reason, a set of functions that keep track of transformation parameters, exists in `Design` for use with the functions highlighted in this book. These are shown in Table 6.3. Of these functions, `asis`, `catg`, `scored`, and `matrx` are almost always called implicitly and are not mentioned

TABLE 6.3: Design Transformation Functions

Function	Purpose	Related S Functions
asis	No posttransformation (seldom used explicitly)	I
rcs	Restricted cubic splines	ns
pol	Polynomial using standard notation	poly
lsp	Linear spline	
catg	Categorical predictor (seldom)	factor
scored	Ordinal categorical variables	ordered
matrx	Keep variables as group for anova and fastbw	matrix
strat	Nonmodeled stratification factors (used for cph only)	strata

by the user. catg is usually called explicitly when the variable is a numeric variable to be used as a polytomous factor, and it has not been converted to an S categorical variable using the factor function.

These functions can be used with any function of a predictor. For example, to obtain a four-knot cubic spline expansion of the cube root of x, specify rcs(x^(1/3),4).

When the transformation functions are called, they are usually given one or two arguments, such as rcs(x,5). The first argument is the predictor variable or some function of it. The second argument is an optional vector of parameters describing a transformation, for example location or number of knots. Other arguments may be provided.

The Hmisc library's cut2 function is sometimes used to create a categorical variable from a continuous variable x. You can specify the actual interval endpoints (cuts), the number of observations to have in each interval on the average (m), or the number of quantile groups (g). Use, for example, cuts=c(0,1,2) to cut into the intervals $[0, 1), [1, 2]$.

A key concept in fitting models in S is that the fitting function returns an object that is an S list. This object contains basic information about the fit (e.g., regression coefficient estimates and covariance matrix, model χ^2) as well as information about how each parameter of the model relates to each factor in the model. Components of the fit object are addressed by, for example, fit$coef, fit$var, fit$loglik. Design causes the following information to also be retained in the fit object: the limits for plotting and estimating effects for each factor (if options(datadist="name") was in effect), the label for each factor, and a vector of values indicating which parameters associated with a factor are nonlinear (if any). Thus the "fit object" contains all the information needed to get predicted values, plots, odds or hazard ratios, and hypothesis tests, and to do "smart" variable selection that keeps parameters together when they are all associated with the same predictor.

S version 3.0 and later uses the notion of the *class* of an object. The object-oriented class idea allows one to write a few generic functions that decide which specific functions to call based on the class of the object passed to the generic function. An example is the function for printing the main results of a logistic model. The `lrm` function returns a fit object of class `"lrm"`. If you specify the S command `print(fit)` (or just `fit` if using S interactively—this invokes `print`), the `print` function invokes the `print.lrm` function to do the actual printing specific to logistic models. To find out which particular methods are implemented for a given generic function, type `methods(generic.name)`.

Generic functions that are used in this book include those in Table 6.4.

TABLE 6.4: **Design** Library and S Generic Functions

Function	Purpose	Related Functions
print	Print parameters and statistics of fit	
coef	Fitted regression coefficients	
formula	Formula used in the fit	
specs	Detailed specifications of fit	
robcov	Robust covariance matrix estimates	
bootcov	Bootstrap covariance matrix estimates and bootstrap distributions of estimates	
pentrace	Find optimum penalty factors by tracing effective AIC for a grid of penalties	
effective.df	Print effective d.f. for each type of variable in model, for penalized fit or **pentrace** result	
summary	Summary of effects of predictors	
plot.summary	Plot continuously shaded confidence bars for results of **summary**	
anova	Wald tests of most meaningful hypotheses	
plot.anova	Graphical depiction of **anova**	
contrast	General contrasts, C.L., tests	
plot	Plot effects of predictors	
gendata	Easily generate predictor combinations	
predict	Obtain predicted values or design matrix	
fastbw	Fast backward step-down variable selection	step
residuals	(or **resid**) Residuals, influence stats from fit	
sensuc	Sensitivity analysis for unmeasured confounder	
which.influence	Which observations are overly influential	residuals
latex	LaTeX representation of fitted model	Function
Dialog	Create a menu to enter predictor values	Function

continued on next page

		continued from previous page
Function	Purpose	Related Functions
	and obtain predicted values from fit	nomogram
Function	S function analytic representation of $X\hat{\beta}$ from a fitted regression model	
Hazard	S function analytic representation of a fitted hazard function (for psm)	
Survival	S function analytic representation of fitted survival function (for psm, cph)	
Quantile	S function analytic representation of fitted function for quantiles of survival time (for psm, cph)	
Mean	S function analytic representation of fitted function for mean survival time	
nomogram	Draws a nomogram for the fitted model	latex, plot
survest	Estimate survival probabilities (psm, cph)	survfit
survplot	Plot survival curves (psm, cph)	plot.survfit
validate	Validate indexes of model fit using resampling	
calibrate	Estimate calibration curve using resampling	val.prob
vif	Variance inflation factors for fitted model	
naresid	Bring elements corresponding to missing data back into predictions and residuals	
naprint	Print summary of missing values	
impute	Impute missing values	transcan
rm.impute	Impute repeated measures data with nonrandom dropout	transcan, fit.mult.impute

The first argument of the majority of functions is the object returned from the model fitting function. When used with ols, lrm, psm, cph, and glmD, these functions do the following. specs prints the design specifications, for example, number of parameters for each factor, levels of categorical factors, knot locations in splines, and so on. The robcov function computes the Huber robust covariance matrix estimate. bootcov uses the bootstrap to estimate the covariance matrix of parameter estimates. Both robcov and bootcov assume that the design matrix and response variable were stored with the fit. They have options to adjust for cluster sampling. Both replace the original variance–covariance matrix with robust estimates and return a new fit object that can be passed to any of the other functions. In that way, robust Wald tests, variable selection, confidence limits, and many other quantities may be computed automatically. The functions do save the old covariance estimates in component orig.var of the new fit object. bootcov also optionally returns the matrix of parameter estimates over the bootstrap simulations. These estimates can be used to derive bootstrap confidence intervals that don't assume normality or symmetry. Associated with bootcov are plotting functions for drawing histogram and smooth density estimates for bootstrap distributions. bootcov also has a feature for deriving approximate nonparametric simultaneous confidence sets. For example, the function can get a simultaneous 0.90 confidence region for the regression effect of age over its entire range.

The `pentrace` function assists in selection of penalty factors for fitting regression models using penalized maximum likelihood estimation (see Section 9.10). Different types of model terms can be penalized by different amounts. For example, one can penalize interaction terms more than main effects. The `effective.df` function prints details about the effective degrees of freedom devoted to each type of model term in a penalized fit.

`summary` prints a summary of the effects of each factor. When `summary` is used to estimate effects (e.g., odds or hazard ratios) for continuous variables, it allows the levels of interacting factors to be easily set, as well as allowing the user to choose the interval for the effect. This method of estimating effects allows for nonlinearity in the predictor. By default, interquartile range effects (differences in $X\hat{\beta}$, odds ratios, hazards ratios, etc.) are printed for continuous factors, and all comparisons with the reference level are made for categorical factors. See the example at the end of the `summary.Design` documentation for a method of quickly computing pairwise treatment effects and confidence intervals for a large series of values of factors that interact with the treatment variable. Saying `plot(summary(fit))` will depict the effects graphically, with bars for a list of confidence levels.

The `anova` function automatically tests most meaningful hypotheses in a design. For example, suppose that age and cholesterol are predictors, and that a general interaction is modeled using a restricted spline surface. `anova` prints Wald statistics for testing linearity of age, linearity of cholesterol, age effect (age + age × cholesterol interaction), cholesterol effect (cholesterol + age × cholesterol interaction), linearity of the age × cholesterol interaction (i.e., adequacy of the simple age × cholesterol 1 d.f. product), linearity of the interaction in age alone, and linearity of the interaction in cholesterol alone. Joint tests of all interaction terms in the model and all nonlinear terms in the model are also performed. The `text.anova.Design` function allows easy placement of the resulting statistics on plots, and the `plot.anova` function draws a dot chart showing the relative contribution (χ^2, χ^2 minus d.f., AIC, or P-value) of each factor in the model.

The `contrast` function is used to obtain general contrasts and corresponding confidence limits and test statistics. This is most useful for testing effects in the presence of interactions (e.g., type II and type III contrasts).

The `predict` function is used to obtain a variety of values or predicted values from either the data used to fit the model or from a new dataset. The `gendata` function makes it easy to obtain a data frame containing predictor combinations for obtaining selected predicted values.

The `fastbw` function performs a slightly inefficient but numerically stable version of fast backward elimination on factors, using a method based on Lawless and Singhal.[267] This method uses the fitted complete model and computes approximate Wald statistics by computing conditional (restricted) maximum likelihood estimates assuming multivariate normality of estimates. It can be used in simulations since it returns indexes of factors retained and dropped:

```
fit ← ols(y ∼ x1*x2*x3)
fastbw(fit, optional arguments)      # print results
z ← fastbw(fit, optional args)       # typically used in simulations
lm.fit(X[,z$parms.kept], Y)          # least sq. fit of reduced model
```

fastbw deletes factors, not columns of the design matrix. Factors requiring multiple d.f. will be retained or dropped as a group. The function prints the deletion statistics for each variable in turn, and prints approximate parameter estimates for the model after deleting variables. The approximation is better when the number of factors deleted is not large. For ols, the approximation is exact.

The which.influence function creates a list with a component for each factor in the model. The names of the components are the factor names. Each component contains the observation identifiers of all observations that are "overly influential" with respect to that factor, meaning that |dfbetas| > u for at least one β_i associated with that factor, for a given u. The default u is .2. You must have specified x=T, y=T in the fitting function to use which.influence. The first argument is the fit object, and the second argument is the cutoff u.

The following S program will print the set of predictor values that were very influential for each factor. It assumes that the data frame containing the data used in the fit is called df.

```
attach(df)                           # or use data=df in next line
f ← lrm(y ∼ x1 + x2 + ..., x=T, y=T)
w ← which.influence(f, .4)
nam ← names(w)
for(i in 1:length(nam)) {
    cat("Influential observations for effect of ",nam[i],"\n")
    print(df[w[[i]],])
}
```

The latex function is a generic function available in the Hmisc library. It invokes a specific latex function for ols, lrm, psm, or cph to create a LATEX representation of the fitted model for inclusion in a report or viewing on the screen. This representation documents all parameters in the model and the functional form being assumed for Y, and is especially useful for getting a simplified version of restricted cubic spline functions.

The Function function writes an S-PLUS function that you can use to evaluate $X\hat{\beta}$ analytically from a fitted regression model. The documentation for Function also shows how to use a subsidiary function sascode that will (almost) translate such an S-PLUS function into SAS code for evaluating predicted values in new subjects. Neither Function nor latex handle third-order interactions.

The nomogram function draws a partial nomogram for obtaining predictions from the fitted model manually. It constructs different scales when interactions (up to third-order) are present. The constructed nomogram is not complete, in that point scores are obtained for each predictor and the user must add the point scores manually before reading predicted values on the final axis of the nomogram. The constructed nomogram is useful for interpreting the model fit, especially for nonmonotonically transformed predictors (their scales wrap around an axis automatically).

The vif function computes variance inflation factors from the covariance matrix of a fitted model, using [106, 446].

The impute function is another generic function. It does simple imputation by default. It can also work with the transcan function to multiply or singly impute missing values using a flexible additive model.

As an example of using many of the functions, suppose that a categorical variable treat has values "a", "b", and "c", an ordinal variable num.diseases has values 0,1,2,3,4, and that there are two continuous variables, age and cholesterol. age is fitted with a restricted cubic spline, while cholesterol is transformed using the transformation log(cholesterol+10). Cholesterol is missing on three subjects, and we impute these using the overall median cholesterol. We wish to allow for interaction between treat and cholesterol. The following S program will fit a logistic model, test all effects in the design, estimate effects, and plot estimated transformations. The fit for num.diseases really considers the variable to be a five-level categorical variable. The only difference is that a 3 d.f. test of linearity is done to assess whether the variable can be remodeled "asis". Here we also show statements to attach the Design library and store predictor characteristics from datadist.

```
library(Design, T)                    # make new functions available
ddist ← datadist(cholesterol, treat, num.diseases, age)
# Could have used ddist ← datadist(data.frame.name)
options(datadist="ddist")             # defines data dist. to Design
cholesterol ← impute(cholesterol)
fit ← lrm(y ~ treat + scored(num.diseases) + rcs(age) +
                log(cholesterol+10) + treat:log(cholesterol+10))
describe(y ~ treat + scored(num.diseases) + rcs(age))
# or use describe(formula(fit)) for all variables used in fit
# describe function (in Hmisc) gets simple statistics on variables
# fit ← robcov(fit)                   # Would make all statistics that follow
                                      # use a robust covariance matrix
                                      # would need x=T, y=T in lrm()
specs(fit)                            # Describe the design characteristics
anova(fit)
anova(fit, treat, cholesterol)        # Test these 2 by themselves
plot(anova(fit))                      # Summarize anova graphically
summary(fit)                          # Estimate effects using default ranges
plot(summary(fit))                    # Graphical display of effects with C.I.
summary(fit, treat="b", age=60)       # Specify reference cell and adjustment val
summary(fit, age=c(50,70))            # Estimate effect of increasing age from
                                      # 50 to 70
```

```
summary(fit, age=c(50,60,70))        # Increase age from 50 to 70, adjust to
                                     # 60 when estimating effects of other
                                     # factors
# If had not defined datadist, would have to define ranges for all var.


# Estimate and test treatment (b-a) effect averaged over 3 cholesterols
contrast(fit, list(treat='b', cholesterol=c(150,200,250)),
              list(treat='a', cholesterol=c(150,200,250)),
         type='average')

plot(fit, age=seq(20,80,length=100), treat=NA, conf.int=F)
                                     # Plot relationship between age and log
                                     # odds, separate curve for each treat,
                                     # no C.I.
plot(fit, age=NA, cholesterol=NA)    # 3-dimensional perspective plot for age,
                                     # cholesterol, and log odds using default
                                     # ranges for both variables
plot(fit, num.diseases=NA, fun=function(x) 1/(1+exp(-x)) ,
     ylab="Prob", conf.int=.9)       # Plot estimated probabilities instead of
                                     # log odds
# Again, if no datadist were defined, would have to tell plot all limits
logit ← predict(fit, expand.grid(treat="b",num.dis=1:3,age=c(20,40,60),
                cholesterol=seq(100,300,length=10)))
# Could also obtain list of predictor settings interactively
logit ← predict(fit, gendata(fit, nobs=12))


# Since age doesn't interact with anything, we can quickly and
# interactively try various transformations of age, taking the spline
# function of age as the gold standard. We are seeking a linearizing
# transformation.


ag ← 10:80
logit ← predict(fit, expand.grid(treat="a", num.dis=0, age=ag,
                cholesterol=median(cholesterol)), type="terms")[,"age"]
# Note: if age interacted with anything, this would be the age
# "main effect" ignoring interaction terms
# Could also use logit ← plot(f, age=ag, ...)$x.xbeta[,2],
# which allows evaluation of the shape for any level of interacting
# factors. When age does not interact with anything, the result from
# predict(f, ..., type="terms") would equal the result from
# plot if all other terms were ignored


# Could also specify logit ← predict(fit, gendata(fit, age=ag, cholesterol=...))
# Unmentioned variables are set to reference values


plot(ag^.5, logit)                   # try square root vs. spline transform.
```

```
plot(ag^1.5, logit)                    # try 1.5 power

latex(fit)                             # invokes latex.lrm, creates fit.tex
# Draw a nomogram for the model fit
nomogram(fit)


# Compose S function to evaluate linear predictors analytically
g <- Function(fit)
g(treat='b', cholesterol=260, age=50)
# Letting num.diseases default to reference value
```

To examine interactions in a simpler way, you may want to group age into tertiles:

```
age.tertile ← cut2(age, g=3)
# For automatic ranges later, add age.tertile to datadist input
fit ← lrm(y ~ age.tertile * rcs(cholesterol))
```

Example output from these functions is shown in Chapter 10 and later chapters.

Note that type="terms" in predict scores each factor in a model with its fitted transformation. This may be used to compute, for example, rank correlation between the response and each transformed factor, treating it as 1 d.f.

When regression is done on principal components, one may use an ordinary linear model to decode "internal" regression coefficients for helping to understand the final model. Here is an example.

```
library(Design, T)
dd ← datadist(my.data)
options(datadist='dd')
pcfit ← princomp(~ pain.symptom1 + pain.symptom2 + sign1 +
                   sign2 + sign3 + smoking)
pc2 ← pcfit$scores[,1:2]                    # first 2 PCs
logistic.fit ← lrm(death ~ rcs(age,4) + pc2) # pc2 is a matrix var.
predicted.logit ← predict(logistic.fit)
linear.mod      ← ols(predicted.logit ~ rcs(age,4) + pain.symptom1 +
                     pain.symptom2 + sign1 + sign2 + sign3 + smoking)
# This model will have R-squared=1
nomogram(linear.mod, fun=function(x)1/(1+exp(-x)),
        funlabel="Probability of Death")       # can use fun=plogis
# 7 Axes showing effects of all predictors, plus a reading
# axis converting to predicted probability scale
```

In addition to many of the add-on functions described above, there are several other S functions that validate models. The first, predab.resample, is a general-purpose function that is used by functions for specific models described later. predab.resample computes estimates of optimism of, and bias-corrected estimates of a vector of indexes of predictive accuracy, for a model with a specified design matrix, with or without fast backward step-down of predictors. If bw=T, predab.resample prints a matrix of asterisks showing which factors were selected at each repetition, along with a frequency distribution of the number of factors retained across re-samples. The function has an optional parameter that may be specified to force the bootstrap algorithm to do sampling with replacement from clusters rather than from original records, which is useful when each subject has multiple records in the dataset. It also has a parameter that can be used to validate predictions in a subset of the records even though models are refit using all records.

The generic function `validate` invokes `predab.resample` with model-specific fits and measures of accuracy. The function `calibrate` invokes `predab.resample` to estimate bias-corrected model calibration and to plot the calibration curve. Model calibration is estimated at a sequence of predicted values.

6.4   Other Functions

For principal components analysis, S has the `princomp` (in S-PLUS only) and `prcomp` functions. Canonical correlations and canonical variates can be easily computed using the `cancor` function. There are many other S functions for examining associations and for fitting models. The `supsmu` function implements Friedman's "super smoother."[146] The `lowess` function implements Cleveland's two-dimensional smoother.[76] The `gam` function fits Hastie and Tibshirani's[191] generalized additive model for a variety of distributions. More is said about S-PLUS nonparametric additive multiple regression functions in Chapter 15. The `loess` function fits a multi-dimensional scatterplot smoother (the local regression model of Cleveland et al.[65]). `loess` provides approximate test statistics for normal or symmetrically distributed Y:

```
f ← loess(y ~ age * pressure)
plot(f)                          # cross-sectional plots
ages ← seq(20,70,length=40)
pressures ← seq(80,200,length=40)
pred ← predict(f, expand.grid(age=ages, pressure=pressures))
persp(ages, pressures, pred)     # 3-D plot
```

`loess` has a large number of options allowing various restrictions to be placed on the fitted surface.

S also has a wealth of software for tree-based modeling. Atkinson and Therneau's `rpart` recursive partitioning library and related functions implement classification and regression trees[48] algorithms for binary, continuous, and right-censored response variables (assuming an exponential distribution for the latter). `rpart` deals effectively with missing predictor values using surrogate splits. The S-PLUS-supplied function `tree` and related functions handle tree models for binary, continuous, and polytomous responses. `tree` deals with missing values by making new categories for missing values. For this it has to categorize continuous variables into quantile groups before growing the tree. The `Design` package has `validate.tree` for obtaining cross-validated mean squared errors and Somers' D_{xy} rank correlations (Brier score and ROC areas for probability models).

For displaying which variables tend to be missing on the same subjects, the `Hmisc` `naclus` function can be used (e.g., `plot(naclus(dataframename))` or `naplot(naclus(dataframename)))`). For characterizing what type of subjects have `NA`'s on a given predictor (or response) variable, a tree model whose response variable is `is.na(varname)` can be quite useful. To allow the other predictors to contain `NA`'s you can specify an `na.action` for the `tree` function as shown in the example below.

```
f ← tree(is.na(cholesterol) ∼ age + sex + trig + smoking,
         na.action=na.tree.replace)
plot(f)        # plots the decision tree
text(f)        # labels the tree
```

The `na.tree.replace` function categorizes continuous variables into quartiles and adds a new level ('`NA`') when a variable contains any `NA`'s.

6.5   Further Reading

[1]   Harrell and Goldstein[179] list components of statistical languages or packages and compare several popular packages for survival analysis capabilities.

Chapter 7

Case Study in Least Squares Fitting and Interpretation of a Linear Model

This chapter presents some of the stages of modeling, using a linear multiple regression model whose coefficients are estimated using ordinary least squares. The data are taken from the 1994 version of the *City and County Databook* compiled by the Geospatial and Statistical Data Center of the University of Virginia Library and available at `fisher.lib.virginia.edu/ccdb`. Most of the variables come from the U.S. Census[a]. Variables related to the 1992 U.S. presidential election were originally provided and copyrighted by the Elections Research Center and are taken from [365], with permission from the Copyright Clearance Center. The data extract analyzed here is available from this text's Web site (see Appendix). The data did not contain election results from the 25 counties of Alaska. In addition, two other counties had zero voters in 1992. For these the percent voting for each of the candidates was also set to missing. The 27 counties with missing percent votes were excluded when fitting the multivariable model.

The dependent variable is taken as the percentage of voters voting for the Democratic Party nominee for President of the U.S. in 1992, Bill Clinton, who received

---

[a]U.S. Bureau of the Census. 1990 Census of Population and Housing, Population and Housing Unit Counts, United States (CPH-2-1.), and Data for States and Counties, Population Division, July 1, 1992, Population Estimates for Counties, Including Components of Change, PPL-7.

43.0% of the vote according to this dataset. The Republican Party nominee George Bush received 37.4%, and the Independent candidate Ross Perot received 18.9% of the vote. Republican and Independent votes tended to positively correlate over the counties.

To properly answer questions about voting patterns of individuals, subject-level data are needed. Such data are difficult to obtain. Analyses presented here may shed light on individual tendencies but are formally a characterization of the 3141 counties (and selected other geographic regions) in the United States. As virtually all of these counties are represented in the analyses, the sample is in a sense the whole population so inferential statistics (test statistics and confidence bands) are not strictly required. These are presented anyway for illustration.

There are many aspects of least squares model fitting that are not considered in this chapter. These include assessment of *groups* of overly influential observations, and robust estimation. The reader should refer to one of the many excellent texts on linear models for more information on these and other methods dedicated to such models.

7.1   Descriptive Statistics

First we print basic descriptive statistics using the Hmisc library's describe function.[b]

```
> library(Hmisc,T);  library(Design,T)
> describe(counties[,-(1:4)])            # omit first 4 vars.
```

counties
15 Variables   3141 Observations

---

pop.density : 1992 pop per 1990 miles^2

n	missing	unique	Mean	.05	.10	.25	.50	.75	.90	.95
3141	0	541	222.9	2	4	16	39	96	297	725

lowest :   0   1   2   3   4
highest: 15609 17834 28443 32428 52432

---

pop : 1990 population

n	missing	unique	Mean	.05	.10	.25	.50	.75	.90	.95
3141	0	3078	79182	3206	5189	10332	22085	54753	149838	320167

lowest :   52   107   130   354   460
highest: 2410556 2498016 2818199 5105067 8863164

---

[b]For a continuous variable, describe stores frequencies for 100 bins of the variable. This information is shown in a histogram that is added to the text when the latex method is used on the object created by describe. The output produced here was created by latex(describe(counties[,-(1:4)], descript='counties')).

pop.change : % population change 1980-1992

n	missing	unique	Mean	.05	.10	.25	.50	.75	.90	.95
3141	0	768	6.501	-16.7	-13.0	-6.0	2.7	13.3	29.6	43.7

lowest : -34.4 -32.2 -31.6 -31.3 -30.2
highest: 146.5 152.2 181.7 191.4 207.7

---

age6574 : % age 65-74, 1990

n	missing	unique	Mean	.05	.10	.25	.50	.75	.90	.95
3141	0	153	8.286	4.9	5.7	6.9	8.2	9.5	10.9	11.9

lowest : 0.6 0.9 1.8 1.9 2.0, highest: 19.8 20.0 20.6 20.9 21.1

---

age75 : % age $\geq$ 75, 1990

n	missing	unique	Mean	.05	.10	.25	.50	.75	.90	.95
3141	0	144	6.578	3.1	3.9	5.0	6.3	7.9	9.9	11.3

lowest : 0.0 0.3 0.5 0.8 0.9, highest: 14.9 15.2 15.4 15.5 15.9

---

crime : serious crimes per 100,000 1991

n	missing	unique	Mean	.05	.10	.25	.50	.75	.90	.95
3141	0	2339	3008	0	286	1308	2629	4243	6157	7518

lowest :   0   39   40   41   44
highest: 13229 13444 14016 16031 20179

---

college : % with bachelor's degree or higher of those age$\geq$25

n	missing	unique	Mean	.05	.10	.25	.50	.75	.90	.95
3141	0	322	13.51	6.6	7.5	9.2	11.8	15.6	21.9	27.1

lowest : 0.0 3.7 4.0 4.1 4.2, highest: 49.8 49.9 52.3 52.8 53.4

---

income : median family income, 1989 dollars

n	missing	unique	Mean	.05	.10	.25	.50	.75	.90	.95
3141	0	2927	28476	19096	20904	23838	27361	31724	36931	41929

lowest : 10903 11110 11362 11502 12042
highest: 61988 62187 62255 62749 65201

---

farm : farm population, % of total, 1990

n	missing	unique	Mean	.05	.10	.25	.50	.75	.90	.95
3141	0	302	6.437	0.1	0.4	1.5	3.9	8.6	16.5	21.4

lowest : 0.0 0.1 0.2 0.3 0.4, highest: 50.9 54.6 55.0 65.8 67.6

---

democrat : % votes cast for democratic president

n	missing	unique	Mean	.05	.10	.25	.50	.75	.90	.95
3114	27	530	39.73	22.80	27.03	32.70	39.00	46.00	53.80	58.84

lowest : 6.8 9.5 12.9 13.0 13.6, highest: 79.2 79.4 79.6 82.8 84.6

---

republican : % votes cast for republican president

n	missing	unique	Mean	.05	.10	.25	.50	.75	.90	.95
3114	27	431	39.79	26.67	29.50	33.80	39.20	45.50	50.90	54.80

lowest : 9.1 12.9 13.1 13.6 13.9, highest: 68.0 68.1 69.1 72.2 75.0

Perot : % votes cast for Ross Perot

n	missing	unique	Mean	.05	.10	.25	.50	.75	.90	.95
3114	27	316	19.81	8.765	10.400	14.400	20.300	25.100	28.500	30.600

lowest :   3.2   3.3   3.4   3.6   3.7, highest: 37.7 39.0 39.8 40.4 46.9

---

white : % white, 1990

n	missing	unique	Mean	.05	.10	.25	.50	.75	.90	.95
3141	0	3133	87.11	54.37	64.44	80.43	94.14	98.42	99.32	99.54

lowest :   5.039   5.975 10.694 13.695 13.758
highest: 99.901 99.903 99.938 99.948 100.000

---

black : % black, 1990

n	missing	unique	Mean	.05	.10	.25	.50	.75
3141	0	3022	8.586	0.01813	0.04452	0.16031	1.49721	10.00701

.90	.95
30.72989	41.69317

lowest :   0.000000   0.007913   0.008597   0.009426   0.009799
highest: 79.445442 80.577171 82.145996 85.606544 86.235985

---

turnout : 1992 votes for president / 1990 pop x 100

n	missing	unique	Mean	.05	.10	.25	.50	.75	.90	.95
3116	25	3113	44.06	31.79	34.41	39.13	44.19	49.10	53.13	55.71

lowest :   0.000   7.075   14.968   16.230   16.673
highest: 72.899   75.027   80.466   89.720 101.927

Of note is the incredible skewness of population density across counties. This variable will cause problems when displaying trends graphically as well as possibly causing instability in fitting spline functions. Therefore we transform it by taking $\log_{10}$ after adding one to avoid taking the log of zero. We compute one other derived variable—the proportion of county residents with age of at least 65 years. Then the datadist function from the Design library is run to compute covariable ranges and settings for constructing graphs and estimating effects of predictors.

```
> older ← counties$age6574 + counties$age75
> label(older) ← '% age >= 65, 1990'
> pdensity ← logb(counties$pop.density+1, 10)
> label(pdensity) ← 'log 10 of 1992 pop per 1990 miles^2'

> dd ← datadist(counties)
> dd ← datadist(dd, older, pdensity)   # add 2 vars. not in data frame
> options(datadist='dd')
```

Next, examine how some of the key variables interrelate, using hierarchical variable clustering based on squared Spearman rank correlation coefficients as similarity measures.

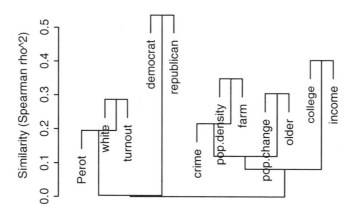

FIGURE 7.1: Variable clustering of some key variables in the `counties` dataset.

```
> v ← varclus(~ pop.density + pop.change + older + crime + college +
+              income + farm + democrat + republican + Perot +
+              white + turnout, data=counties)
> plot(v)                          # Figure 7.1
```

The percentage of voters voting Democratic is strongly related to the percentage voting Republican because of the strong negative correlation between the two. The Spearman ρ^2 between percentage of residents at least 25 years old who are college educated and median family income in the county is about 0.4.

Next we examine descriptive associations with the dependent variable, by stratifying separately by key predictors, being careful not to use this information in formulating the model because of the phantom degrees of freedom problem.

```
> s ← summary(democrat ~ pop.density + pop.change + older + crime +
+              college + income + farm + white + turnout,
+              data=counties)
> plot(s, cex.labels=.7)                    # Figure 7.2
```

There is apparently no "smoking gun" predictor of extraordinary strength although all variables except age and crime rate seem to have some predictive ability. The voter turnout (bottom variable) is a strong and apparently monotonic factor. Some of the variables appear to predict Democratic votes nonmonotonically (see especially population density). It will be interesting to test whether voter turnout is merely a reflection of the county demographics that, when adjusted for, negate the association between voter turnout and voter choice.

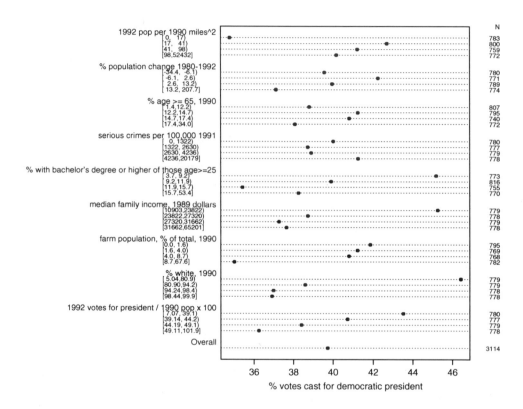

FIGURE 7.2: Percentage of votes cast for Bill Clinton stratified separately by quartiles of other variables. Sample sizes are shown in the right margin.

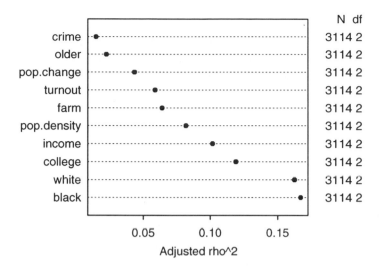

FIGURE 7.3: Strength of marginal relationships between predictors and response using generalized Spearman χ^2.

7.2 Spending Degrees of Freedom/Specifying Predictor Complexity

As described in Section 4.1, in the absence of subject matter insight we might spend degrees of freedom according to estimates of strengths of relationships without a severe "phantom d.f." problem, as long as our assessment is masked to the contributions of particular parameters in the model (e.g., linear vs. nonlinear effects). The following S-PLUS code computes and plots the nonmonotonic (quadratic in ranks) generalization of the Spearman rank correlation coefficient, separately for each of a series of prespecified predictor variables.

```
> s ← spearman2(democrat ~ pop.density + pop.change + older + crime +
+              college + income + farm + black + white + turnout,
+              data=counties, p=2)
> plot(s)                          # Figure 7.3
```

From Figure 7.3 we guess that lack of fit will be more consequential (in descending order of importance) for racial makeup, college education, income, and population density.

7.3   Fitting the Model Using Least Squares

A major issue for continuous Y is always the choice of the Y-transformation. When the raw data are percentages that vary from 30 to 70% all the way to nearly 0 or 100%, a transformation that expands the tails of the Y distribution, such as the arcsine square root, logit, or probit, often results in a better fit with more normally distributed residuals. The percentage of a county's voters who participated is centered around the median of 39% and does not have a very large number of counties near 0 or 100%. Residual plots were no more normal with a standard transformation than that from untransformed Y. So we use untransformed percentages.

We use the linear model

$$E(Y|X) = X\beta, \tag{7.1}$$

where β is estimated using ordinary least squares, that is, by solving for $\hat{\beta}$ to minimize $\sum(Y_i - X\hat{\beta})^2$. If we want to compute P-values and confidence limits using parametric methods we would have to assume that $Y|X$ is normal with mean $X\beta$ and constant variance σ^2 (the latter assumption may be dispensed with if we use a robust Huber–White or bootstrap covariance matrix estimate—see Section 9.5). This assumption is equivalent to stating the model as conditional on X,

$$Y = X\beta + \epsilon, \tag{7.2}$$

where ϵ is normally distributed with mean zero, constant variance σ^2, and residuals $Y - E(Y|X)$ are independent across observations.

To not assume linearity the Xs above are expanded into restricted cubic spline functions, with the number of knots specified according the estimated "power" of each predictor. Let us assume that the most complex relationship could be fitted adequately using a restricted cubic spline function with five knots. `crime` is thought to be so weak that linearity is forced. Note that the term "linear model" is a bit misleading as we have just made the model as nonlinear in X as desired.

We prespecify one second-order interaction, between `income` and `college`. To save d.f. we fit a "nondoubly nonlinear" restricted interaction as described in Equation 2.38, using the `Design` library's `%ia%` function. Default knot locations, using quantiles of each predictor's distribution, are chosen as described in Section 2.4.5.

```
> f ←   ols(democrat ~ rcs(pdensity,4) + rcs(pop.change,3) +
+            rcs(older,3) + crime + rcs(college,5) + rcs(income,4) +
+            rcs(college,5) %ia% rcs(income,4) +
+            rcs(farm,3) + rcs(white,5) + rcs(turnout,3))
> f
```

Linear Regression Model

Frequencies of Missing Values Due to Each Variable
  democrat pdensity pop.change older crime college income farm white turnout
        27   0   0   0   0   0   0   0   0   25

    n Model L.R. d.f.   R2 Sigma
 3114   2210   29 0.5082 7.592

Residuals:
    Min   1Q Median   3Q   Max
  -30.43 -4.978 -0.299 4.76 31.99

Coefficients:
	Value	Std. Error	t value	Pr(>|t|)
Intercept	6.258e+01	9.479e+00	6.602144	4.753e-11
pdensity	1.339e+01	9.981e-01	13.412037	0.000e+00
pdensity'	-1.982e+01	2.790e+00	-7.103653	1.502e-12
pdensity''	7.637e+01	1.298e+01	5.882266	4.481e-09
pop.change	-2.323e-01	2.577e-02	-9.013698	0.000e+00
pop.change'	1.689e-01	2.862e-02	5.900727	4.012e-09
older	5.037e-01	1.042e-01	4.833013	1.411e-06
older'	-5.134e-01	1.104e-01	-4.649931	3.460e-06
crime	1.652e-05	8.224e-05	0.200837	8.408e-01
college	5.205e-01	1.184e+00	0.439539	6.603e-01
college'	-8.738e-01	2.243e+01	-0.038962	9.689e-01
college''	7.330e+01	6.608e+01	1.109281	2.674e-01
college'''	-1.246e+02	5.976e+01	-2.084648	3.718e-02
income	1.714e-05	4.041e-04	0.042410	9.662e-01
income'	-6.372e-03	1.490e-03	-4.275674	1.963e-05
income''	1.615e-02	4.182e-03	3.861556	1.150e-04
college * income	0.525e-05	5.097e-05	-1.672504	9.453e-02
college * income'	7.729e-04	1.360e-04	5.684197	1.437e-08
college * income''	-1.972e-03	3.556e-04	-5.545263	3.183e-08
college' * income	-9.362e-05	8.968e-04	-0.104389	9.169e-01
college'' * income	-2.067e-03	2.562e-03	-0.806767	4.199e-01
college''' * income	3.934e-03	2.226e-03	1.767361	7.727e-02
farm	-5.305e-01	9.881e-02	-5.368650	8.521e-08
farm'	4.454e-01	1.838e-01	2.423328	1.544e-02
white	-3.533e-01	2.600e-02	-13.589860	0.000e+00
white'	2.340e-01	5.012e-02	4.668865	3.158e-06
white''	-1.597e+00	9.641e-01	-1.656138	9.780e-02
white'''	-1.740e+01	1.648e+01	-1.055580	2.912e-01
turnout	-7.522e-05	4.881e-02	-0.001541	9.988e-01
turnout'	1.692e-01	4.801e-02	3.524592	4.303e-04

```
Residual standard error: 7.592 on 3084 degrees of freedom
Adjusted R-Squared: 0.5036
```

The analysis discarded 27 observations (most of them from Alaska) having missing data, and used the remaining 3114 counties. The proportion of variation across counties explained by the model is $R^2 = 0.508$, with adjusted $R^2 = 0.504$. The estimate of σ (7.59%) is obtained from the unbiased estimate of σ^2. For the linear model the likelihood ratio statistic is $-n\log(1 - R^2)$, which here is $-3114\log(1 - 0.508^2) = 2210$ on 29 d.f. The ratio of observations to variables is 3114/29 or 107, so there is no issue with overfitting.[c]

In the above printout, primes after variable names indicate cubic spline components (see Section 2.4.4). The most compact algebraic form of the fitted model appears below, using Equation 2.26 to simplify restricted cubic spline terms.

```
> latex(f)
```

$$E(\text{democrat}) = X\beta, \quad \text{where}$$

$X\hat{\beta} =$

62.57849

$+ 13.38714\text{pdensity} - 3.487746(\text{pdensity} - 0.4771213)^3_+$

$+ 13.43985(\text{pdensity} - 1.39794)^3_+ - 10.82831(\text{pdensity} - 1.812913)^3_+$

$+ 0.8761998(\text{pdensity} - 2.860937)^3_+$

$- 0.2323114\text{pop.change} + 9.307077 \times 10^{-5}(\text{pop.change} + 13)^3_+$

$- 0.0001473909(\text{pop.change} - 2.7)^3_+ + 5.432011 \times 10^{-5}(\text{pop.change} - 29.6)^3_+$

$+ 0.5037175\text{older} - 0.004167098(\text{older} - 9.6)^3_+ + 0.007460448(\text{older} - 14.5)^3_+$

$- 0.003293351(\text{older} - 20.7)^3_+ + 1.651695 \times 10^{-5}\text{crime}$

$+ 0.5205324\text{college} - 0.002079334(\text{college} - 6.6)^3_+ + 0.17443(\text{college} - 9.45)^3_+$

$- 0.2964471(\text{college} - 11.8)^3_+ + 0.123932(\text{college} - 15)^3_+$

$+ 0.0001644174(\text{college} - 27.1)^3_+$

$+ 1.71383 \times 10^{-5}\text{income} - 1.222161 \times 10^{-11}(\text{income} - 19096)^3_+$

$+ 3.097825 \times 10^{-11}(\text{income} - 25437)^3_+ - 1.925238 \times 10^{-11}(\text{income} - 29887)^3_+$

$+ 4.957448 \times 10^{-13}(\text{income} - 41929)^3_+$

$+ \text{income}[-8.52499 \times 10^{-5}\text{college} - 2.22771 \times 10^{-7}(\text{college} - 6.6)^3_+$

$- 4.919284 \times 10^{-6}(\text{college} - 9.45)^3_+ + 9.360726 \times 10^{-6}(\text{college} - 11.8)^3_+$

$- 4.283218 \times 10^{-6}(\text{college} - 15)^3_+ + 6.454693 \times 10^{-8}(\text{college} - 27.1)^3_+]$

---

[c]This can also be assessed using the heuristic shrinkage estimate $(2210 - 29)/2210 = 0.987$, another version of which is proportional to the ratio of adjusted to ordinary R^2 as given on p. 64. The latter method yields $(3114 - 29 - 1)/(3114 - 1) \times 0.5036/0.5082 = 0.982$.

$+\text{college}[1.482526\times10^{-12}(\text{income}-19096)_+^3-3.781803\times10^{-12}(\text{income}-25437)_+^3$

$+2.368292\times10^{-12}(\text{income}-29887)_+^3-6.901521\times10^{-14}(\text{income}-41929)_+^3]$

$-0.5304876\text{farm}+0.00171818(\text{farm}-0.4)_+^3-0.002195452(\text{farm}-3.9)_+^3$

$+0.0004772722(\text{farm}-16.5)_+^3$

$-0.353288\text{white}+0.0001147081(\text{white}-54.37108)_+^3$

$-0.0007826866(\text{white}-82.81484)_+^3-0.008527786(\text{white}-94.1359)_+^3$

$+0.03878391(\text{white}-98.14566)_+^3-0.02958815(\text{white}-99.53718)_+^3$

$-7.522335\times10^{-5}\,\text{turnout}+0.0004826373(\text{turnout}-34.40698)_+^3$

$-0.001010226(\text{turnout}-44.18553)_+^3+0.000527589(\text{turnout}-53.13093)_+^3$

and $(x)_+ = x$ if $x > 0$, 0 otherwise.

Interpretation and testing of individual coefficients listed above is not recommended except for the coefficient of the one linear effect in the model (for crime) and for nonlinear effects when there is only one of them (i.e., for variables modeled with three knots). For crime, the two-tailed t-test of partial association resulted in $P = 0.8$. Other effects are better interpreted through predicted values as shown in Section 7.8.

7.4 Checking Distributional Assumptions

As mentioned above, if one wanted to use parametric inferential methods on the least squares parameter estimates, and to have confidence that the estimates are efficient, certain assumptions must be validated: (1) the residuals should have no systematic trend in central tendency against any predictor variable or against $\hat{Y}$; (2) the residuals should have the same dispersion for all levels of $\hat{Y}$ and of individual values of X; and (3) the residuals should have a normal distribution, both overall and for any subset in the X-space. Our first assessment addresses elements (1) and (2) by plotting the median and lower and upper quartiles of the residuals, stratified by intervals of $\hat{Y}$ containing 200 observations.[d]

```
> r ← resid(f)
> xYplot(r ~ fitted(f), method='quantile', nx=200,
+        ylim=c(-10,10), xlim=c(20,60),
+        abline=list(h=0, lwd=.5, lty=2),
+        aspect='fill')                    # Figure 7.4
```

No trends of concern are apparent in Figure 7.4; variability appears constant. This same kind of graph should be done with respect to the predictors. Figure 7.5 shows

[d]The number of observations is too large for a scatterplot.

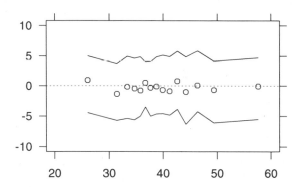

FIGURE 7.4: Quartiles of residuals from the linear model, stratifying $\hat{Y}$ into intervals containing 200 counties each. For each interval the x-coordinate is the mean predicted percentage voting Democratic over the counties in that interval. S-PLUS trellis graphics are used through the Hmisc library xYplot function.

the results for two of the most important predictors. Again, no aspect of the graphs causes concern.

```
> p1 ← xYplot(r ~ white, method='quantile', nx=200,
+               ylim=c(-10,10), xlim=c(40,100),
+               abline=list(h=0, lwd=.5, lty=2),
+               aspect='fill')

> p2 ← xYplot(r ~ pdensity, method='quantile', nx=200,
+               ylim=c(-10,10), xlim=c(0,3.5),
+               abline=list(h=0, lwd=.5, lty=2),
+               aspect='fill')

> print(p1, split=c(1,1,1,2), more=T)      # 1 column, 2 rows
> print(p2, split=c(1,2,1,2))              # Figure 7.5
```

For the assessment of normality of residuals we use q–q plots which are straight lines if normality holds. Figure 7.6 shows q–q plots stratified by quartiles of population density.

```
> qqmath(~r | cut2(pdensity,g=4))          # Figure 7.6
```

Each graph appears sufficiently linear to make us feel comfortable with the normality assumption should we need it to hold.

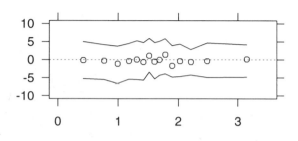

log 10 of 1992 pop per 1990 miles^2

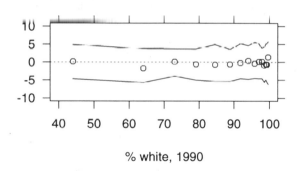

% white, 1990

FIGURE 7.5: Quartiles of residuals against population density (top panel) and % white (bottom panel).

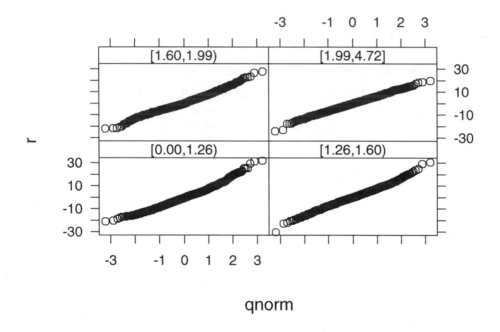

FIGURE 7.6:   Quantile–quantile plot for estimated residuals stratified by quartiles of population density.

7.5   Checking Goodness of Fit

Flexible specification of main effects (without assuming linearity) and selected interaction effects were built into the model. The principal lack of fit would be due to interactions that were not specified. To test the importance of all such (two-way, at least) interactions, including generalizing the income × college interaction, we can fit a linear model with all two-way interactions:

```
> f2 ← ols(democrat ~ (rcs(pdensity,4) + rcs(pop.change,3) +
+              rcs(older,3) + crime + rcs(college,5) + rcs(income,4) +
+              rcs(farm,3) + rcs(white,5) + rcs(turnout,3))^2)
> f2$stats

       n Model L.R. d.f.      R2 Sigma
    3114       2974  254 0.6152 6.975
```

The F test for goodness of fit can be done using this model's R^2 and that of the original model ($R^2 = 0.5082$ on 29 d.f.). The F statistic for testing two nested models is

$$F_{k,n-p-1} = \frac{\frac{R^2 - R_*^2}{k}}{\frac{1 - R^2}{n-p-1}}, \qquad (7.3)$$

where R^2 is from the full model, R_*^2 is from the submodel, p is the number of regression coefficients in the full model (excluding the intercept, here 254), and k is the d.f. of the full model minus the d.f. of the submodel (here, $254 - 29$). Here $F_{225,2860} = 3.54, P < 0.0001$, so there is strong statistical evidence of a lack of fit from some two-way interaction term. Subject matter input should have been used to specify more interactions likely to be important. At this point, testing a multitude of two-way interactions without such guidance is inadvisable, and we stay with this imperfect model. To gauge the impact of this decision on a scale that is more relevant than that of statistical significance, the median absolute difference in predicted values between our model and the all-two-way-interaction model is 2.02%, with 369 of the counties having predicted values differing by more than 5%.

7.6   Overly Influential Observations

Below are observations that are overly influential when considered singly. An asterisk is placed next to a variable when any of the coefficients associated with that variable changed by more than 0.3 standard errors upon removal of that observation. DFFITS is also shown.

```
> g ← update(f, x=T)      # add X to fit to get influence stats
> w ← which.influence(g, 0.3)
```

```
> dffits ← resid(g, 'dffits')
> show.influence(w, data.frame(counties, pdensity, older, dffits),
+                report=c('democrat','dffits'), id=county)
```

	Count	college	income	white	turnout	democrat	dffits
Jackson	4	* 5	*14767	100	38	17	-0.8
McCreary	4	* 5	*12223	99	40	31	-0.8
Taos	2	18	*20049	73	46	66	0.6
Duval	1	6	*15773	79	39	80	0.5
Loving	5	* 4	*30833	87	*90	21	-0.9
Starr	2	7	*10903	62	23	83	0.8
Menominee	5	* 4	*14801	* 11	30	60	-0.6

One can see, for example, that for Starr County, which has a very low median family income of \$10,903, at least one regression coefficient associated with income changes by more than 0.3 standard errors when that county is removed from the dataset. These influential observations appear to contain valid data and do not lead us to delete the data or change the model (other than to make a mental note to pay more attention to robust estimation in the future!).

7.7   Test Statistics and Partial R^2

Most of the partial F-statistics that one might desire are shown in Table 7.1.

```
> an ← anova(f)
> an^e
> plot(an, what='partial R2')                    # Figure 7.7
```

The 20 d.f. simultaneous test that no effects are nonlinear or interacting provides strong support for the need for complexity in the model. Every variable that was allowed to have a nonlinear effect on the percentage voting for Bill Clinton had a significant nonlinear effect. Even the nonlinear interaction terms are significant (the global test for linearity of interaction had $F_{5,3084} = 7.58$). college × income interaction is moderately strong. Note that voter turnout is still significantly associated with Democratic voting even after adjusting for county demographics ($F = 19.2$). Figure 7.7 is a good snapshot of the predictive power of all the predictors. It is very much in agreement with Figure 7.3; this is expected unless major confounding or collinearity is present.

---

[e]The output was actually produced using latex(an, dec.ss=0, dec.ms=0, dec.F=1, scientific=c(-6,6)).

TABLE 7.1: Analysis of Variance for democrat

	d.f.	PartialSS	MS	F	P
pdensity	3	18698	6233	108.1	< 0.0001
Nonlinear	2	4259	2130	36.9	< 0.0001
pop.change	2	8031	4016	69.7	< 0.0001
Nonlinear	1	2007	2007	34.8	< 0.0001
older	2	1387	694	12.0	< 0.0001
Nonlinear	1	1246	1246	21.6	< 0.0001
crime	1	2	2	0.0	0.8408
college (Factor+Higher Order Factors)	10	17166	1717	29.8	< 0.0001
All Interactions	6	2466	411	7.1	< 0.0001
Nonlinear (Factor+Higher Order Factors)	6	8461	1410	24.5	< 0.0001
income (Factor+Higher Order Factors)	9	12945	1438	25.0	< 0.0001
All Interactions	6	2466	411	7.1	< 0.0001
Nonlinear (Factor+Higher Order Factors)	4	3163	791	13.7	< 0.0001
college × income (Factor+Higher Order Factors)	6	2466	411	7.1	< 0.0001
Nonlinear	5	2183	437	7.6	< 0.0001
Nonlinear Interaction : f(A,B) vs. AB	5	2183	437	7.6	< 0.0001
Nonlinear Interaction in college vs. Af(B)	3	1306	435	7.6	< 0.0001
Nonlinear Interaction in income vs. Bg(A)	2	1864	932	16.2	< 0.0001
farm	2	7179	3590	62.3	< 0.0001
Nonlinear	1	339	339	5.9	0.0154
white	4	22243	5561	96.5	< 0.0001
Nonlinear	3	2508	836	14.5	< 0.0001
turnout	2	2209	1105	19.2	< 0.0001
Nonlinear	1	716	716	12.4	0.0004
TOTAL NONLINEAR	19	23231	1223	21.2	< 0.0001
TOTAL NONLINEAR + INTERACTION	20	37779	1889	32.8	< 0.0001
TOTAL	29	183694	6334	109.9	< 0.0001
ERROR	3084	177767	58		

7.8 Interpreting the Model

Our first task is to interpret the interaction surface relating education and income. This can be done with perspective plots (see Section 10.5) and image plots. Often it is easier to see patterns by making ordinary line graphs in which separate curves are drawn for levels of an interacting factor. No matter how interaction surfaces are drawn, it is advisable to suppress plotting regions where there are very few datapoints in the space of the two predictor variables, to avoid unwarranted extrapolation. The plot function for model fits created with the S-PLUS Design library in effect makes it easy to display interactions in many different ways, and to suppress poorly supported points for any of them. In Figure 7.8 is shown the estimated relationship between percentage college educated in the county versus percentage

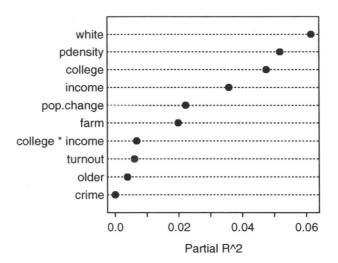

FIGURE 7.7: Partial R^2s for all of the predictors. For `college` and `income` partial R^2 includes the higher-order `college` × `income` interaction effect.

voting Democratic, with county median family income set to four equally spaced values between the 25th and 75th percentiles, and rounded. Curves are drawn for intervals of education in which there are at least 10 counties having median family income within $1650 of the median income represented by that curve.

```
> incomes ← seq(22900, 32800, length=4)
> show.pts ← function(college.pts, income.pt) {
+    s ← abs(income - income.pt) < 1650
+    # Compute 10th smallest and 10th largest % college
+    # educated in counties with median family income within
+    # $1650 of the target income
+    x ← college[s]
+    x ← sort(x[!is.na(x)])
+    n ← length(x)
+    low ← x[10]; high ← x[n-9]
+    college.pts >= low & college.pts <= high
+ }

> plot(f, college=NA, income=incomes,          # Figure 7.8
+        conf.int=F, xlim=c(0,35), ylim=c(30,55),
+        lty=1, lwd=c(.25,1.5,3.5,6), col=c(1,1,2,2),
+        perim=show.pts)
```

The interaction between the two variables is evidenced by the lessened impact of low education when income increases.

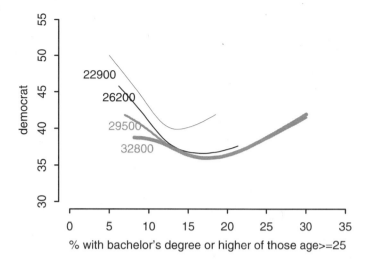

FIGURE 7.8: Predicted percentage voting Democratic as a function of college education (x-axis) and income (four levels used to label the curves) in the county. Other variables are set to overall medians.

Figure 7.9 shows the effects of all of the predictors, holding other predictors to their medians. All graphs are drawn on the same scale so that relative importance of predictors can be perceived. Nonlinearities are obvious.

```
> plot(f, ylim=c(20,70))                    # Figure 7.9
```

Another way to display effects of predictors is to use a device discussed in Section 5.3. We compute $\hat{Y}$ at the lower quartile of an X, holding all other Xs at their medians, then set the X of interest to its upper quartile and again compute $\hat{Y}$. By subtracting the two predicted values we obtain an estimate of the effects of predictors over the range containing one-half of the counties. The analyst should exercise more care than that used here in choosing settings for variables nonmonotonically related to Y.

```
> s ← summary(f)
> options(digits=4)
> plot(s)                                   # Figure 7.10
```

All predictor effects may be shown in a nomogram, which also allows predicted values to be computed. As two of the variables interact, it is difficult to use continuous axes for both, and the Design library's nomogram function does not allow this. We must specify the levels of one of the interacting factors so that separate scales can be drawn for each level.

```
> f <- Newlabels(f, list(turnout='voter turnout (%)'))
```

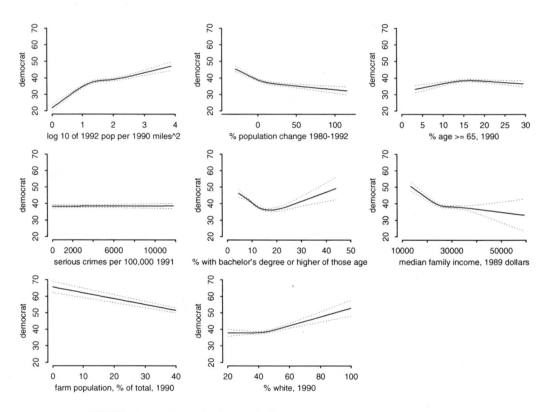

FIGURE 7.9: Partial effects of all county characteristics in the model.

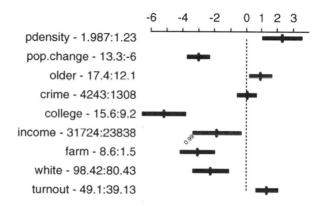

Adjusted to:college=11.8 income=27361

FIGURE 7.10: Summary of effects of predictors in the model using default ranges (interquartile). For variables that interact with other predictors, the settings of interacting factors are very important. For others, these settings are irrelevant for this graph. As an example, the effect of increasing population density from its first quartile (1.23) to its third quartile (1.987) is to add approximately an average of 2.3% voters voting Democratic. The 0.95 confidence interval for this mean effect is $[1.37, 3.23]$. This range of $1.987 - 1.23$ or 0.756 on the $\log_{10}$ population density scale corresponds to a $10^{0.756} = 5.7$-fold population increase.

TABLE 7.2

Characteristic	Points
Population density $10/\text{mile}^2$ $(log_{10} = 1)$	30
No population size change	27
Older age 5%	6
Median family income $29500	
and 40% college educated	27
Farm population 45%	37
White 90%	8
Voter turnout 40%	0

```
> nomogram(f, interact=list(income=incomes),
+          turnout=seq(30,100,by=10),
+          lplabel='estimated % voting Democratic',
+          cex.var=.8, cex.axis=.75)          # Figure 7.11
```

As an example, a county having the characteristics in Table 7.2 would derive the indicated approximate number of points. The total number of points is 135, for which we estimate a 38% vote for Bill Clinton. Note that the crime rate is irrelevant.

7.9 Problems

1. Picking up with the problems in Section 3.10 related to the SUPPORT study, begin to relate a set of predictors (age, sex, dzgroup, num.co, scoma, race, meanbp, pafi, alb) to total cost. Delete the observation having zero cost from all analyses.[f]

   (a) Compute mean and median cost stratified separately by all predictors (by quartiles of continuous ones; for S-Plus see the help file for the Hmisc summary.formula function). For categorical variables, compute P-values based on the Kruskal–Wallis test for group differences in costs.[g]

   (b) Decide whether to model costs or log costs. Whatever you decide, justify your conclusion and use that transformation in all later steps.

---

[f]In S-Plus issue the command attach(support[support$totcst > 0 | is.na(support$ totcst),]).

[g]You can use the Hmisc spearman2 function for this. If you use the built-in S-Plus function for the Kruskal–Wallis test note that you have to exclude any observations having missing values in the grouping variable. Note that the Kruskal–Wallis test and its two-sample special case, the Wilcoxon–Mann–Whitney test, tests in a general way whether the values in one group tend to be larger than values in another group.

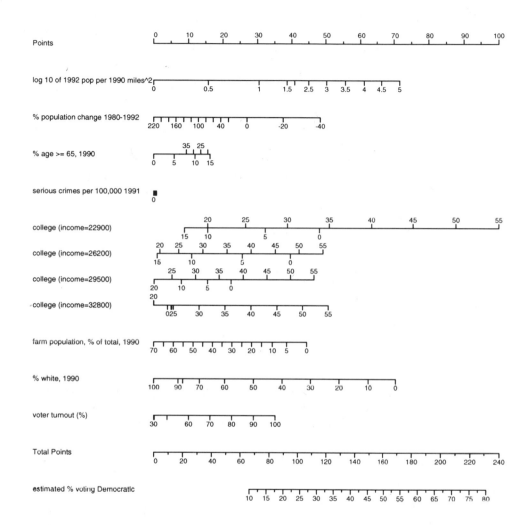

FIGURE 7.11: Nomogram for the full model for predicting the percentage of voters in a county who voted Democratic in the 1992 U.S. presidential election.

(c) Use all nonmissing data for each continuous predictor to make a plot showing the estimated relationship, superimposing nonparametric trend lines and restricted cubic spline fits (use five knots). If you used a log transformation, be sure to tell the nonparametric smoother to use the log of costs also. As the number of comorbidities and coma score have heavily tied values, splines may not work well unless knot locations are carefully chosen. For these two variables it may be better to use quadratic fits. You can define an S-PLUS function to help do all of this:

```
doplot ← function(predictor, type=c('spline','quadratic')) {
  type ← match.arg(type)
  r ← range(predictor, na.rm=T)
  xs ← seq(r[1], r[2], length=150)
  f ← switch(type,
             spline   = ols(log(totcst) ~ rcs(predictor, 5)),
             quadratic= ols(log(totcst) ~ pol(predictor, 2)))
  print(f)
  print(anova(f))
  plot(f, predictor=xs, xlab=label(predictor))
  plsmo(predictor, log(totcst), add=T, trim=0, col=3, lwd=3)
  scat1d(predictor)
  title(sub=paste('n=',f$stats['n']),adj=0)
  invisible()
}
doplot(pafi)
doplot(scoma, 'quadratic')
etc.
```

Note that the purpose of Parts (c) and (d) is to become more familiar with estimating trends without assuming linearity, and to compare parametric regression spline fits with nonparametric smoothers. These exercises should not be used in selecting the number of degrees of freedom to devote to each predictor in the upcoming multivariable model.

(d) For each continuous variable provide a test of association with costs and a test of nonlinearity, as well as adjusted R^2.

2. Develop a multivariable least squares regression model predicting the log of total hospital cost. For patients with missing costs but nonmissing charges, impute costs as you did in Problem 2b in Chapter 3. Consider the following predictors: age, sex, dzgroup, num.co, scoma, race (use all levels), meanbp, hrt, temp, pafi, alb.

(a) Graphically describe how the predictors interrelate, using squared Spearman correlation coefficients. Comment briefly on whether you think any of the predictors are redundant.

(b) Decide for which predictors you want to "spend" more than one degree of freedom, using subject–matter knowledge or by computing a measure (or generalized measure allowing nonmonotonic associations) of rank correlation between each predictor and the response. Note that rank correlations do not depend on how the variables are transformed (as long as transformations are monotonic).

(c) Depict whether and how the same patients tend to have missing values for the same groups of predictor and response variables.

(d) The dataset contains many laboratory measurements on patients. Measurements such as blood gases are not done on every patient. The PaO_2/FiO_2 ratio (variable `pafi`) is derived from the blood gas measurements. Using any method you wish, describe which types of patients are missing `pafi`, by considering other predictors that are almost never missing.

(e) Impute `race` using the most frequent category. Can you justify imputing a constant for `race` in this dataset?

(f) Physicians often decide not to order lab tests when they think it likely that the patient will have normal values for the test results. Previous analyses showed that this strategy worked well for `pafi` and `alb`. When these values are missing, impute them using "normal values," 333.3 and 3.5, respectively.

(g) Fit a model to predict cost (or a transformation of it) using all predictors. For continuous predictors assume a smooth relationship but allow it to be nonlinear. Choose the complexity to allow for each predictor's shape (i.e., degrees of freedom or knots) building upon your work in Part 2b. Quantify the ability of the model to discriminate costs. Do an overall test for whether any variables are associated with costs.

Here are some hints for using `Design` library functions effectively for this problem.

- Optionally `attach` the subset of the `support` data frame for which you will be able to get a nonmissing total hospital cost, that is, those observations for which either `totcst` or `charges` are not NA.
- Don't use new variable names when imputing NAs. You can always tell which observations have been imputed using the `is.imputed` function, assuming you use the `impute` function to do the imputations.
- Run `datadist` before doing imputations, so that quantiles of predictors are estimated on the basis of "real" data. You will need to update the `datadist` object only when variables are recoded (e.g., when categories are collapsed).

(h) Graphically assess the overall normality of residuals from the model. For the single most important predictor, assess whether there is a systematic trend in the residuals against this predictor.

(i) Compute partial tests of association for each predictor and a test of nonlinearity for continuous ones. Compute a global test of nonlinearity. Graphically display the ranking of importance of the predictors based on the partial tests.

(j) Display the shape of how each predictor relates to cost, setting other predictors to typical values (one value per predictor).

(k) For each predictor estimate (and either print or plot) how much $\hat{Y}$ changes when the predictor changes from its first to its third quartile, all other predictors held constant. For categorical predictors, compute differences in $\hat{Y}$ between all categories and the reference category. Antilog these differences to obtain estimated cost ratios.[h]

(l) Make a nomogram for the model, including a final axis that translates predictions to the original cost scale if needed (note that antilogging predictions from a regression model that assumes normality in log costs results in estimates of median cost). Use the nomogram to obtain a predicted value for a patient having values of all the predictors of your choosing. Compare this with the predicted value computed by either the `predict` or `Function` function in S-Plus.

(m) Use resampling to validate the R^2 and slope of predicted against observed response. Compare this estimate of R^2 to the adjusted R^2. Draw a validated calibration curve. Comment on the quality (potential "exportability") of the model.

(n) Refit the full model, excluding observations for which `pafi` was imputed. Plot the shape of the effect of `pafi` in this new model and comment on whether and how it differs from the shape of the `pafi` effect for the fit in which `pafi` was imputed.

Hints: Analyses (but not graph titles or interpretation) for Parts (a), (b), (c), (e), and (j) can be done using one S-Plus command each. Parts (f), (h), (i), (k), (l), and (n) can be done using two commands. Parts (d), (g), and (m) can be done using three commands. For part (h) you can use the `resid` and `qqnorm` functions or the pull-down 2-D graphics menu in Windows S-Plus. `plot.lm(fit object)` may also work, depending on how it handles `NA`s.

---

[h]There is an option on the pertinent S-Plus function to do that automatically when the differences are estimated.

Chapter 8

Case Study in Imputation and Data Reduction

The following case study illustrates these techniques:

1. missing data imputation using mean substitution, recursive partitioning, and customized regressions;

2. variable clustering;

3. data reduction using principal components analysis and pretransformations;

4. restricted cubic spline fitting using ordinary least squares, in the context of scaling; and

5. scaling/variable transformations using canonical variates and nonparametric additive regression.

8.1   Data

Consider the 506-patient prostate cancer dataset from Byar and Green.[60] The data are listed in [21, Table 46] and are available in ASCII form from StatLib (lib.-stat.cmu.edu) in the Datasets area or in S-PLUS transport format from this book's Web page. These data were from a randomized trial comparing four treatments for stage 3 and 4 prostate cancer, with almost equal numbers of patients on placebo and each of three doses of estrogen. Four patients had missing values on all of the following variables: wt, pf, hx, sbp, dbp, ekg, hg, bm; two of these patients were also missing sz. These patients are excluded from consideration. The ultimate goal of an analysis of the dataset might be to discover patterns in survival or to do an analysis of covariance to assess the effect of treatment while adjusting for patient heterogeneity. See Chapter 20 for such analyses. The data reduction and some of the imputations developed here are general and can be used for a variety of dependent variables.

The variable names, labels, and a summary of the data are printed below. This printout was obtained by the S-PLUS statement latex(describe(prostate)) (the describe and latex functions are in the Hmisc library; typing describe(prostate) will produce a standard printout).

prostate

18 Variables   502 Observations

---

patno : Patient Number

n	missing	unique	Mean	.05	.10	.25	.50	.75	.90	.95
502	0	502	251.7	26.05	51.10	126.25	251.50	376.75	451.90	479.95

lowest :   1   2   3   4   5, highest: 502 503 504 505 506

---

stage : Stage

n	missing	unique	Mean
502	0	2	3.424

3 (289, 58%), 4 (213, 42%)

---

rx : Treatment

n	missing	unique
502	0	4

placebo (127, 25%), 0.2 mg estrogen (124, 25%)
1.0 mg estrogen (126, 25%), 5.0 mg estrogen (125, 25%)

---

dtime : Months of Followup

n	missing	unique	Mean	.05	.10	.25	.50	.75	.90	.95
502	0	76	36.13	1.05	5.00	14.25	34.00	57.75	67.00	71.00

lowest :   0   1   2   3   4, highest: 72 73 74 75 76

---

status : Followup Status

n	missing	unique
502	0	10

alive (148, 29%), dead - prostatic ca (130, 26%)
dead - heart or vascular (96, 19%), dead - cerebrovascular (31, 6%)
dead - pulmonary embolus (14, 3%), dead - other ca (25, 5%)
dead - respiratory disease (16, 3%)
dead - other specific non-ca (28, 6%), dead - unspecified non-ca (7, 1%)
dead - unknown cause (7, 1%)

---

age : Age in Years

n	missing	unique	Mean	.05	.10	.25	.50	.75	.90	.95
501	1	41	71.46	56	60	70	73	76	78	80

lowest : 48 49 50 51 52, highest: 84 85 87 88 89

wt : Weight Index = wt(kg)-ht(cm)+200

n	missing	unique	Mean	.05	.10	.25	.50	.75	.90	.95
500	2	67	99.03	77.95	82.90	90.00	98.00	107.00	116.00	123.00

lowest : 69 71 72 73 74, highest: 136 142 145 150 152

pf : Performance Rating

n	missing	unique
502	0	4

normal activity (450, 90%), in bed < 50% daytime (37, 7%)
in bed > 50% daytime (13, 3%), confined to bed (2, 0%)

hx : History of Cardiovascular Disease

n	missing	unique	Sum	Mean
502	0	2	213	0.4243

sbp : Systolic Blood Pressure/10

n	missing	unique	Mean	.05	.10	.25	.50	.75	.90	.95
502	0	18	14.35	11	12	13	14	16	17	18

	8	9	10	11	12	13	14	15	16	17	18	19	20	21	22	23	24	30
Frequency	1	3	14	27	65	74	98	74	72	34	17	12	3	2	3	1	1	1
%	0	1	3	5	13	15	20	15	14	7	3	2	1	0	1	0	0	0

dbp : Diastolic Blood Pressure/10

n	missing	unique	Mean	.05	.10	.25	.50	.75	.90	.95
502	0	12	8.149	6	6	7	8	9	10	10

	4	5	6	7	8	9	10	11	12	13	14	18
Frequency	4	5	43	107	165	94	66	9	5	2	1	1
%	1	1	9	21	33	19	13	2	1	0	0	0

ekg : Electrocardiogram Code

n	missing	unique
494	8	7

normal (168, 34%), benign (23, 5%)
rhythmic disturb & electrolyte ch (51, 10%)
heart block or conduction def (26, 5%), heart strain (150, 30%)
old MI (75, 15%), recent MI (1, 0%)

hg : Serum Hemoglobin (g/100ml)

n	missing	unique	Mean	.05	.10	.25	.50	.75	.90	.95
502	0	91	13.45	10.2	10.7	12.3	13.7	14.7	15.8	16.4

lowest : 5.899 7.000 7.199 7.800 8.199
highest: 17.297 17.500 17.598 18.199 21.199

sz : Size of Primary Tumor (cm^2)

n	missing	unique	Mean	.05	.10	.25	.50	.75	.90	.95
497	5	55	14.63	2.0	3.0	5.0	11.0	21.0	32.0	39.2

lowest : 0 1 2 3 4, highest: 54 55 61 62 69

sg : Combined Index of Stage and Hist. Grade

n	missing	unique	Mean	.05	.10	.25	.50	.75	.90	.95
491	11	11	10.31	8	8	9	10	11	13	13

	5	6	7	8	9	10	11	12	13	14	15
Frequency	3	8	7	67	137	33	114	26	75	5	16
%	1	2	1	14	28	7	23	5	15	1	3

ap : Serum Prostatic Acid Phosphatase

n	missing	unique	Mean	.05	.10	.25	.50	.75	.90	.95
502	0	128	12.18	0.300	0.300	0.500	0.700	2.975	21.689	38.470

lowest :   0.09999   0.19998   0.29999   0.39996   0.50000
highest: 316.00000 353.50000 367.00000 596.00000 999.87500

bm : Bone Metastases

n	missing	unique	Sum	Mean
502	0	2	82	0.1633

sdate : Date on study Format: ddmmmyy

n	missing	unique	Mean	.05	.10	.25	.50	.75	.90
502	0	305	27Apr68	23May67	27Jun67	30Oct67	9Apr68	9Oct68	26Mar69

	.95
	13May69

lowest :   6Apr67 12Apr67 14Apr67 21Apr67 24Apr67
highest: 28May69 29May69   2Jun69   3Jun69 27Jun69

stage is defined by ap as well as X-ray results. Of the patients in stage 3, 0.92 have ap $\leq$ 0.8. Of those in stage 4, 0.93 have ap > 0.8. Since stage can be predicted almost certainly from ap, we do not consider stage in the regression analyses.

8.2   How Many Parameters Can Be Estimated?

There are 354 deaths among the 502 patients. If predicting survival time were of major interest, we could develop a reliable model if no more than about $354/15 = 24$ parameters were *examined* in modeling. Suppose that a full model with no interactions is fitted and that linearity is not assumed for any continuous predictors. Assuming age is almost linear, we could fit a restricted cubic spline function with three knots. For the other continuous variables, let us use five knots. For categorical predictors, the maximum number of degrees of freedom needed would be one less than the number of categories. For pf we could lump the last two categories since the last category has only 2 patients. Likewise, we could combine the last two

TABLE 8.1

Predictor	Number of Parameters
rx	3
age	2
wt	4
pf	2
hx	1
sbp	4
dbp	4
ekg	5
hg	4
sz	4
sg	4
ap	4
bm	1

levels of ekg. Table 8.1 lists the candidate predictors with the maximum number of parameters we consider for each.

8.3   Variable Clustering

The total number of parameters is 42, so some data reduction should be considered. We resist the temptation to take the "easy way out" using stepwise variable selection so that we can achieve a more stable modeling process and obtain variance estimates that are more fair. Before using a variable clustering procedure, note that ap is extremely skewed. To handle skewness, we use Spearman rank correlations for continuous variables (later we transform each variable using transcan, which will allow ordinary correlation coefficients to be used). After classifying ekg as "normal/benign" versus everything else, the Spearman correlations are as follows, with the S-PLUS code that produced them.   [1]

```
> ekg.norm ← ekg=="normal" | ekg=="benign"
> x ← cbind(stage, rx, age, wt, pf, hx, sbp, dbp, ekg.norm,
+               hg, sz, sg, ap, bm)
> # If no missing data, could have done cor(apply(x, 2, rank))
> rcorr(x, type="spearman")     # rcorr in Hmisc
```

TABLE 8.2

Cluster	Predictors
1	stage, sz, sg, ap, bm
2	sbp, dbp
3	hx, ekgnorm
4	hg
5	rx
6	age
7	pf
8	wt

```
          stage    rx   age    wt    pf    hx   sbp   dbp ekg.norm    hg    sz    sg    ap    bm
stage      1.00  0.02 -0.02 -0.10  0.12 -0.09 -0.01 -0.03    -0.02 -0.15  0.27  0.74  0.78  0.50
   rx      0.02  1.00  0.00 -0.06  0.00 -0.01 -0.09 -0.06    -0.01  0.05 -0.04 -0.01  0.09  0.09
  age     -0.02  0.00  1.00 -0.06  0.04  0.16  0.06 -0.11    -0.15 -0.15 -0.03 -0.04  0.01 -0.03
   wt     -0.10 -0.06 -0.06  1.00 -0.10  0.04  0.18  0.21    -0.01  0.26 -0.02 -0.08 -0.08 -0.18
   pf      0.12  0.00  0.04 -0.10  1.00  0.10  0.05 -0.02    -0.05 -0.15  0.09  0.13  0.10  0.23
   hx     -0.09 -0.01  0.16  0.04  0.10  1.00  0.12  0.03    -0.20 -0.02 -0.10 -0.16 -0.14 -0.08
  sbp     -0.01 -0.09  0.06  0.18  0.05  0.12  1.00  0.56    -0.14  0.07  0.06 -0.02 -0.03 -0.04
  dbp     -0.03 -0.06 -0.11  0.21 -0.02  0.03  0.56  1.00    -0.08  0.15 -0.03 -0.05 -0.04 -0.08
ekg.norm  -0.02 -0.01 -0.15 -0.01 -0.05 -0.20 -0.14 -0.08     1.00  0.01 -0.02  0.02  0.00 -0.04
   hg     -0.15  0.05 -0.15  0.26 -0.15 -0.02  0.07  0.15     0.01  1.00 -0.13 -0.12 -0.10 -0.25
   sz      0.27 -0.04 -0.03 -0.02  0.09 -0.10  0.06 -0.03    -0.02 -0.13  1.00  0.36  0.31  0.26
   sg      0.74 -0.01 -0.04 -0.08  0.13 -0.16 -0.02 -0.05     0.02 -0.12  0.36  1.00  0.64  0.39
   ap      0.78  0.09  0.01 -0.08  0.10 -0.14 -0.03 -0.04     0.00 -0.10  0.31  0.64  1.00  0.46
   bm      0.50  0.09 -0.03 -0.18  0.23 -0.08 -0.04 -0.08    -0.04 -0.25  0.26  0.39  0.46  1.00
```

For SAS, we could have used `PROC CORR SPEARMAN; VAR ...;`. Let us use the SAS VARCLUS procedure to group the predictors.[a] The `proportion=.75` option is specified to make VARCLUS break clusters as long as the first principal component for the cluster explains < 0.75 of the total variation of the cluster. This results in 11 clusters for the 14 predictors. We terminate splitting at 8 clusters, which explain just over 0.75 of the variation of the *total set* of predictors.

```
PROC RANK; VAR age wt sbp dbp hg sz sg ap;
PROC VARCLUS SHORT PROPORTION=.75;
    VAR stage rx age wt pf hx sbp dbp ekgnorm hg sz sg ap bm;
```

The resulting clusters are given in Table 8.2. Since treatment was randomized, it is fortunate that it was not clustered with another variable! Remember that we plan not to estimate a regression coefficient for `stage`, but are including it in the variable clustering to make sure it clusters sensibly.

---

[a]Note that had there been many missing values in the dataset, it would have been advisable to impute missings first. (Alternatively, one could compute a Spearman correlation matrix using pairwise deletion of missing values and pass this matrix to `PROC VARCLUS`.) Also, had variable transformations been highly nonmonotonic, it would have been better to transform variables before clustering them. This is demonstrated later.

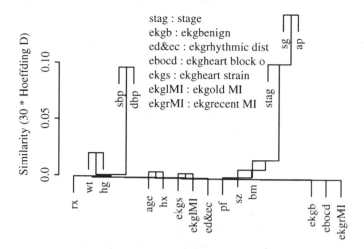

FIGURE 8.1: Hierarchical clustering using Hoeffding's D as a similarity measure. Dummy variables were used for the categorical variable ekg. Some of the dummy variables cluster together since they are by definition negatively correlated. Had normal EKG not been the reference level (and hence had no dummy variable in this example), it would have clustered with history of cardiovascular disease. Abbreviations are shown in the legend. Note that labels for automatically generated dummy variables are prefixed by the name of the original categorical variable.

As another approach to variable clustering, we perform a hierarchical cluster analysis based on a similarity matrix that contains pairwise Hoeffding D statistics.[203] D will detect nonmonotonic associations.

```
> rxn ← as.numeric(rx)      # don't use dummy variables
> pfn ← as.numeric(pf)
> vc ← varclus(∼ stage+rxn+age+wt+pfn+hx+sbp+dbp+ekg+hg+
+                sz+sg+ap+bm, sim='hoeffding')
> plot(vc, legend=T, maxlen=16)
```

The output is shown in Figure 8.1. The results are very similar to those from VARCLUS. We combine sbp and dbp, and tentatively combine ap, sg, sz, and bm.

8.4 Single Imputation Using Constants or Recursive Partitioning

Before proceeding to scaling variables that are clustered together, let us deal with the missing predictors in the dataset. The SAS PRINQUAL procedure can automatically impute all missing values while determining transformations of all predictors:

```
PROC PRINQUAL OUT=t METHOD=MGV; ID patno;
    TRANSFORM MSPLINE(sz sg ap sbp dbp age wt/nknots=4)
              SPLINE(hg/nknots=4)
              MONOTONE(pf)
              LINEAR(bm hx)
              OPSCORE(ekg);
```

Even though PRINQUAL found very good transformations of each variable, the imputed values were not sensible. Let us turn to tree models for imputation, assuming nearly monotonic transformations of variables begin imputed. Later we compare imputed values with those from transcan. For the small amount of missing data, we do not have to worry about major penalties for imputation in our final analyses. Since age has only one missing value, we replace that value with the mean (71.44). Likewise, replace the two missing wt values with the mean (99.03). sz has five missing values. The S-PLUS program below shows how Atkinson and Therneau's rpart function is used to build a prediction tree for sz, as well as how the missing age and wt values are replaced.

```
> fillin <- function(v, p)        {
> v.f <- ifelse(is.na(v), p, v)
> if(length(p)==1) label(v.f) <- paste(label(v),"with",
+                   sum(is.na(v)),
+                   "NAs replaced with",format(p))
>  else label(v.f) <- paste(label(v),"with",
+                   sum(is.na(v)),"NAs replaced")
>  v.f                            }

> spearman <- function(x, y)      {   # Also defined in Hmisc
+  notna <- !is.na(x+y)    # exclude NAs
+  cor(rank(x[notna]), rank(y[notna]))  }

> age.f <- fillin(age, 71.44)   # same as age.f <- impute(age, mean)
> wt.f  <- fillin(wt,  99.03)   # same as wt.f <- impute(wt, mean)

> library(rpart)
> f <- rpart(sz ~ stage+age+wt+pfn+hx+sbp+dbp+ekg+hg+sg+ap+bm,
+            control=rpart.control(minsplit=50))
> f
> p <- predict(f, prostate)
```

TABLE 8.3

Method	Patient ID:	48	74	131	158	485
rpart	sz:	10.4	10.4	10.4	17.8	24.0
transcan		7.4	6.0	6.0	24.7	20.2

TABLE 8.4

Method	Patient ID:	2	57	123	125	169	336	418	436	474	484	506
rpart	sg:	10.3	10.3	8.9	8.9	12.2	8.9	8.9	8.9	8.9	12.2	12.2
transcan		10.3	10.4	7.3	7.4	15.0	8.0	10.3	6.5	10.3	10.7	15.0

```
> # adding prostate in 2nd argument gets predictions on NAs
> spearman(p, sz)
> p[is.na(sz)]                    # prints replacements used
> sz.f ← fillin(sz, p)
> post(f, digits=3)              # makes PostScript graphic
> # Can also use plot(f); text(f)
```

Since **rpart** uses surrogate splits, it allows missing candidate predictors for sz. The tree fitted here first split on sg $\leq$ 10, with a surrogate split on **stage** when sg was missing. The next split was on ap $\leq$ 6.65. By not allowing a split if a node contained < 50 observations, we arrived at five terminal nodes, the smallest containing 24 observations. Except for surrogate splits, the tree is depicted in Figure 8.2. The predictions for this model had Spearman $\rho = 0.44$ with the actual values of sz. The imputed values are shown in Table 8.3.[b].

Next, use **rpart** to impute the 11 missing sg's.

```
> f ← rpart(sg ~ stage+age+wt+pfn+hx+sbp+dbp+ekg+hg+sz+ap+bm,
+            control=rpart.control(minsplit=50))
> f
> p ← predict(f,prostate)
> spearman(p,sg)
> p[is.na(sg)]
> sg.f ← fillin(sg, p)
```

The first split was on **stage**, then sz $\leq$ 24, with a surrogate split of hg < 15.65. The predictions had $\rho = 0.76$ with the observed. The imputed values are in Table 8.4.

For imputing the eight missing **ekg** values, we use a classification tree based on the most probable category. Because of difficulties in how the **tree** function handles

---

[b] An older version of **rpart** produced imputed values that were used after this point, so results will differ slightly from those obtained from the newer version.

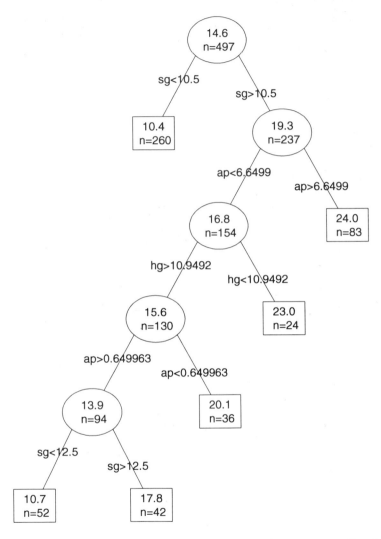

FIGURE 8.2: Tree model for imputing **sz**. Numbers in boxes are predicted values at terminal nodes; ovals are intermediate predictions.

missings, first use imputed values on candidate predictors, and set all missing `ekgs` to a new category.

```
> e ← na.include(ekg)              # Adds NA as a new level
> f ← tree(e ~ stage+age.f+wt.f+pfn+hx+sbp+dbp+hg+
+           sz.f+sg.f+ap+bm,
+           control=tree.control(nobs=502,mincut=50))
> f
> p ← predict(f)
> p ← (t(apply(-p, 1, order)))[,1]
> # Get level no. for most probable category
> p ← levels(e)[p]
> # Convert to character variable
> table(ekg,p)
> ekg[is.na(ekg)]                  # to get Patient IDs
> p[is.na(ekg)]
> ekg.f ← impute(ekg, p[is.na(ekg)])
> # last statement equivalent to following 3:
> # ekg.f ← ekg
> # ekg.f[is.na(ekg.f)] ← p[is.na(ekg.f)]
> # label(ekg.f) ← paste(label(ekg),"with 8 NAs replaced")
```

The first split is on `hx`. Within the "no history of cardiovascular disease" group, the first split is on `age`≤ 73, then there are splits based on `dbp` and `wt`. Within the positive history subset, the first split is again based on `age`≤ 73, then splits are made on `wt` and `hg`. Only the categories "normal" and "heart strain" (the most frequent observed categories) were predicted for the 502 patients. The imputed `ekgs` are in Table 8.5 (here n stands for normal, s stands for heart strain, r for rhythmic disturbance and electrolyte change, and b for heart block or conduction defect). `transcan-1` refers to the default operation of `transcan` in which categories are those whose transformed scores are closest to predicted scores, and `transcan-2` refers to `transcan` with `impcat='tree'`, in which recursive partitioning is used to build a classification tree (using the `tree` function), and the imputed categories are the most probable categories. "Category Probability" is the predicted probability for that most likely category. "`transcan-1` Cat. Prob." refers to the predicted probability from `tree` (again as called by `transcan`) for the category selected by `transcan`'s optimal scoring method.

8.5 Transformation and Single Imputation Using `transcan`

Now we turn to the scoring of the predictors to potentially reduce the number of regression parameters that are needed later. As mentioned before, this could have been done as a first step using, for example, the S-PLUS `transcan` function to

TABLE 8.5

Method Patient ID:	243	269	270	271	280	285	404	470
tree	n	n	n	n	n	n	n	s
transcan-1	n	s	r	b	r	n	n	r
transcan-2	n	n	n	n	n	s	s	s
Category Probability	0.62	0.34	0.34	0.34	0.34	0.38	0.38	0.40
transcan-1 Cat. Prob.	0.62	0.24	0.08	0.09	0.08	0.33	0.33	0.18

simultaneously impute missing data. The first principal component-based method, MTV in SAS `PROC PRINQUAL`, could also be used to derive transformations, especially once clustering is done so that the first component is representative of the cluster. Let us concentrate on MGV-type methods that do not require this. First, let's use `transcan` (see above for SAS `PROC PRINQUAL` statements that would estimate similar transformations).

```
> levels(ekg)  ← list(MI=c('old MI','recent MI'))
> # Combine last 2 levels
> pf.coded     ← as.integer(pf)
> # keep numeric version
> levels(pf)   ← levels(pf)[c(1,2,3,3)]
> # Combine last 2

> par(mfrow=c(4,3))
> prostate.transcan ← transcan(∼ sz + sg + ap + sbp + dbp +
+     age + wt + hg + ekg + pf + bm + hx,
+     imputed=T, transformed=T, impcat="tree")
```

The plotted output is shown in Figure 8.3. Note that at face value the transformation of `ap` was derived in a circular manner, since the combined index of stage and histologic grade, `sg`, uses in its stage component a cutoff on `ap`. However, if `sg` is omitted from consideration, the resulting transformation for `ap` does not change appreciably.

Imputed values from `transcan` are shown under those from `rpart` and `tree` in previous tables. In addition, `transcan` imputed the missing values of `age` to 71.7 and `wt` to 104 and 91.2.

```
> summary(prostate.transcan, long=T)  # print imputed values
                                       # on original scale


R-squared achieved in predicting each variable:

    sz    sg    ap   sbp   dbp   age    wt    hg   ekg    pf    bm    hx
 0.207 0.556 0.573 0.497 0.484 0.096 0.123 0.158 0.092 0.113 0.349 0.108
```

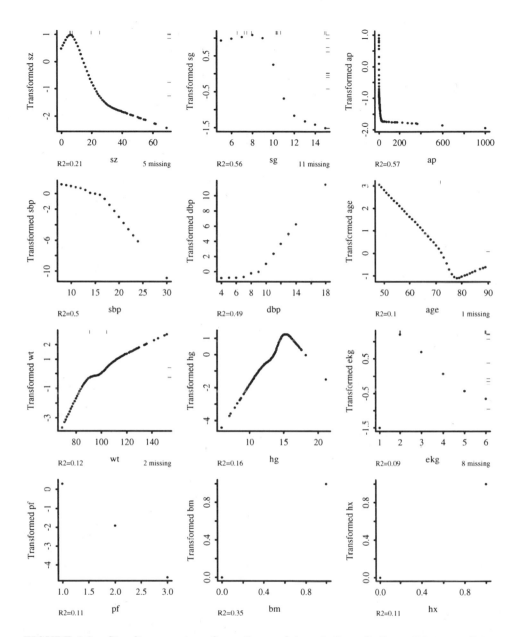

FIGURE 8.3: Simultaneous transformation and imputation of all candidate predictors using `transcan`. Horizontal tick marks at the right of plots indicate transformed values that are imputed for missing values. Tick marks above plots are imputed values on the original scale (jittered for `ekg`).

Adjusted R-squared:

sz	sg	ap	sbp	dbp	age	wt	hg	ekg	pf	bm	hx
0.18	0.541	0.559	0.48	0.467	0.065	0.094	0.13	0.059	0.086	0.331	0.083

Coefficients of canonical variates for predicting each (row) variable

	sz	sg	ap	sbp	dbp	age	wt	hg	ekg	pf	bm	hx
sz		0.66	0.20	0.33	0.33	-0.01	-0.01	0.11	-0.11	0.03	-0.36	0.34
sg	0.23		0.84	0.08	0.07	-0.02	0.01	-0.01	0.07	0.02	-0.20	0.14
ap	0.07	0.80		-0.11	-0.05	0.03	-0.02	0.01	-0.01	0.00	-0.83	-0.03
sbp	0.13	0.10	-0.14		-0.94	0.14	-0.09	0.03	-0.10	0.10	-0.03	-0.14
dbp	0.13	0.09	-0.06	-0.98		0.14	0.07	0.05	-0.03	0.04	0.03	-0.01
age	-0.02	-0.06	0.18	0.58	0.57		0.14	0.46	-0.43	-0.03	1.05	-0.76
wt	-0.02	0.06	-0.08	-0.31	0.23	0.12		0.51	0.06	0.21	-1.09	0.27
hg	0.13	-0.02	0.03	0.09	0.15	0.33	0.43		0.02	0.24	-1.53	-0.12
ekg	-0.20	0.38	-0.10	-0.42	-0.12	-0.41	0.04	0.04		-0.15	0.42	1.23
pf	0.04	0.08	0.02	0.36	0.14	-0.03	0.22	0.29	-0.13		-1.75	-0.46
bm	-0.02	-0.03	-0.13	0.00	0.00	0.03	-0.04	-0.06	0.01	-0.06		-0.02
hx	0.04	0.05	-0.01	-0.04	0.00	-0.06	0.02	-0.01	0.09	-0.04	-0.05	

Note that bm and hx are represented as binary variables, so their coefficients in the table of canonical variable coefficients are on a different scale. For the variables that were actually transformed, the coefficients are for standardized transformed variables (mean 0, variance 1). From examining the R^2s, age, wt, ekg, pf, and hx are not strongly related to other variables. Imputations for age, wt, ekg are thus relying more on the median or modal values from the marginal distributions. From the coefficients of first (standardized) canonical variates, sbp is predicted almost solely from dbp; bm is predicted mainly from ap, hg, and pf.

2

8.6   Data Reduction Using Principal Components

The response variable (here, time until death due to any cause) is not examined during data reduction. For instructional purposes, however, let us give in to the temptation by examining the model likelihood ratio χ^2 for a variety of data reductions. While doing this, let us also examine the worth of principal components (PCs). First, consider PCs on raw variables, expanding polytomous factors using dummy variables. The S-PLUS function princomp is used, after imputing missing raw values on the basis of the transcan output. In this series of analyses we ignore the treatment variable, rx.

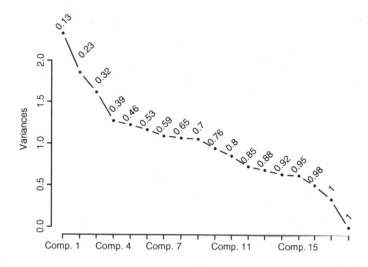

FIGURE 8.4: Variance of raw variables explained by principal components.

```
> w ← prostate.transcan

> sz  ← impute(w, sz)
> sg  ← impute(w, sg)
> age ← impute(w, age)
> wt  ← impute(w, wt)
> ekg ← impute(w, ekg)

> prin.raw ← princomp(~ sz + sg + ap + sbp + dbp + age + wt + hg +
+                            ekg + pf + bm + hx, cor=T) # use correlation matrix

> screeplot(prin.raw, var=1:18, style='lines', xlab='', srt=45)
```

The resulting plot shown in Figure 8.4 is called a "scree" plot [222, pp. 96–99, 104, 106].[c] It shows the variation explained by the first k principal components as k increases all the way to 18 parameters (no data reduction). It requires at least 14 of the 18 possible components to explain ≥ 0.9 of the variance, and the first 5 components explain 0.46 of the variance. Two of the 18 dimensions are almost totally redundant. Let us see how the PCs "explain" the times until death using the Cox regression[92] function from Design, cph, described in Chapter 19.

```
> library(Design, T)                         # get access to Design
```

---

[c]In older versions of S-PLUS scree plots were obtained using a plot function rather than screeplot.

```
> S ← Surv(dtime, status!="alive")      # two-column response var.

> pcs ← prin.raw$scores                 # pick off all PCs
> p1  ← pcs[,1]                          # pick off PC1
> cph(S ~ p1)


Cox Proportional Hazards Model

 cph(formula = S ~ p1)


 Obs Events Model L.R. d.f. P Score Score P    R2
 502    354         17.9   1 0  19.6        0 0.035


       coef se(coef)    z       p
 p1 -0.145   0.0326 -4.45 8.52e-06


> # L.R. is likelihood ratio Chi-square statistic

> p5  ← pcs[,1:5]                        # pick off PC1-PC5
> cph(S ~ p5)


 Obs Events Model L.R. d.f. P Score Score P    R2
 502    354         79.8   5 0  82.8        0 0.147


            coef se(coef)    z       p
 Comp. 1 -0.1572   0.0335 -4.699 2.61e-006
 Comp. 2 -0.2388   0.0400 -5.968 2.40e-009
 Comp. 3  0.1761   0.0427  4.121 3.77e-005
 Comp. 4  0.0253   0.0460  0.549 5.83e-001
 Comp. 5  0.1684   0.0468  3.599 3.20e-004


> p10 ← pcs[,1:10]                       # pick off PC1-PC10
> cph(S ~ p10)


 Obs Events Model L.R. d.f. P Score Score P    R2
 502    354         83.6  10 0  88.4        0 0.154


             coef se(coef)    z       p
 Comp. 1 -0.16135   0.0335 -4.812 1.49e-006
 Comp. 2 -0.23543   0.0394 -5.968 2.39e-009
 Comp. 3  0.18041   0.0431  4.184 2.86e-005
 Comp. 4  0.02254   0.0460  0.490 6.24e-001
 Comp. 5  0.16731   0.0473  3.538 4.04e-004
 Comp. 6  0.03895   0.0482  0.808 4.19e-001
 Comp. 7 -0.00817   0.0516 -0.158 8.74e-001
 Comp. 8 -0.06126   0.0541 -1.133 2.57e-001
```

```
Comp.  9   0.07202     0.0523  1.377 1.69e-001
Comp. 10   0.01168     0.0545  0.214 8.30e-001
```

Now we analyze all components except the last, which is redundant.

```
> pcs17 ← pcs[,-18]
> cph(S ∼ pcs17)


 Obs Events Model L.R. d.f. P Score Score P    R2
 502    354        97.8  17 0   102       0 0.177
```

```
> # Now analyze all variables with original (linear) coding +
> # dummy variables

> cph(S ∼ sz + sg + ap + sbp + dbp + age + wt + hg +
¦           ekg + pf + bm + hx)


 Obs Events Model L.R. d.f. P Score Score P    R2
 502    354        97.8  17 0   102       0 0.177
```

```
> # Next allow all variables to be modeled with smooth spline
> # functions so as to not assume linearity


> cph(S ∼ rcs(sz,5)+rcs(sg,5)+rcs(ap,5)+rcs(sbp,5)+rcs(dbp,5)+
+           rcs(age,3)+rcs(wt,5)+rcs(hg,5)+ekg+pf+hm+hx,
+           tol=1e-14)


 Obs Events Model L.R. d.f. P Score Score P    R2
 502    354        140   39 0   149       0 0.244
```

Next we repeat this process after transforming all predictors via transcan. Now we have only 12 degrees of freedom for the 12 predictors.

```
> prin.trans ← princomp(w$transformed, cor=T)
> screeplot(prin.trans, var=1:12, style='lines',
+            xlab='', srt=45)
```

The variance explained is depicted in Figure 8.5. It requires at least 9 of the 12 possible components to explain ≥ 0.9 of the variance, and the first 5 components explain 0.66 of the variance as opposed to 0.46 for untransformed variables. Now examine how the PCs on transformed variables relate to the outcomes.

```
> pcs ← prin.trans$scores
> p1  ← pcs[,1]
> cph(S ∼ p1)
```

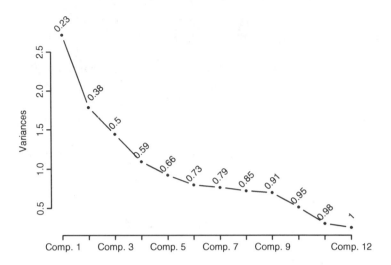

FIGURE 8.5: Variance of transformed variables explained by PCs.

```
Cox Proportional Hazards Model

cph(formula = S ~ p1)

 Obs Events Model L.R. d.f. P Score Score P    R2
 502   354        31.6    1 0 33.7        0 0.061


       coef se(coef)     z        p
 p1 -0.188   0.0326 -5.78 7.43e-09

> p5  ← pcs[,1:5]
> cph(S ~ p5)


 Obs Events Model L.R. d.f. P Score Score P    R2
 502   354        78.1    5 0 84.6        0 0.144


          coef se(coef)      z        p
Comp. 1 -0.1894   0.0317 -5.981 2.21e-09
Comp. 2 -0.1525   0.0407 -3.748 1.78e-04
Comp. 3 -0.2470   0.0452 -5.466 4.61e-08
Comp. 4  0.0881   0.0500  1.763 7.79e-02
Comp. 5 -0.0330   0.0548 -0.603 5.46e-01

> p10 ← pcs[,1:10]
> cph(S ~ p10)
```

```
Obs Events Model L.R. d.f. P Score Score P    R2
502   354         85.5   10 0  90.4       0 0.157
```

```
> # See how all PCs predict

> cph(S ~ pcs)
```

```
Obs Events Model L.R. d.f. P Score Score P    R2
502   354         85.9   12 0  90.7       0 0.157
```

Finally, see how PCs based on variable clusters perform.

```
> # First test PC1 cluster scores on raw variables (using dummies
> # for categorical ones)
> f ← princomp(~ sz+sg+ap+bm, cor=T)
> summary(f)
Importance of components:
```

	Comp. 1	Comp. 2	Comp. 3	Comp. 4
Standard deviation	1.351	0.985	0.812	0.739
Proportion of Variance	0.456	0.243	0.165	0.136
Cumulative Proportion	0.456	0.699	0.864	1.000

```
> tumor ← f$scores[,1]
> f      ← princomp(~ sbp+dbp, cor=T)
> summary(f)
Importance of components:
```

	Comp. 1	Comp. 2
Standard deviation	1.272	0.618
Proportion of Variance	0.809	0.191
Cumulative Proportion	0.809	1.000

```
> bp ← f$scores[,1]
> f ← princomp(~ hx+ekg, cor=T)
> summary(f)
```

Importance of components:

	Comp. 1	Comp. 2	Comp. 3	Comp. 4	Comp. 5	Comp. 6	Comp. 7
Standard deviation	1.253	1.143	1.075	1.038	1.03	0.916	0
Proportion of Variance	0.224	0.187	0.165	0.154	0.15	0.120	0
Cumulative Proportion	0.224	0.411	0.576	0.730	0.88	1.000	1

```
> cardiac ← f$scores[,1]


> cph(S ~ tumor + bp + cardiac + hg + age + pf + wt)
```

```
Obs Events Model L.R. d.f. P Score Score P    R2
502    354          77.2   8 0  81.7        0 0.143
```

	coef	se(coef)	z	p
tumor	0.15264	0.03886	3.928	8.57e-005
bp	-0.00661	0.04145	-0.159	8.73e-001
cardiac	-0.21334	0.04655	-4.583	4.58e-006
hg	-0.05896	0.02998	-1.967	4.92e-002
age	0.02199	0.00836	2.632	8.50e-003
pf=in bed < 50% daytime	0.48544	0.18784	2.584	9.76e-003
pf=in bed > 50% daytime	0.28128	0.29537	0.952	3.41e-001
wt	-0.00827	0.00444	-1.863	6.24e-002

```
> # Now use clusters on PCs of transformed variables
> # Use w again, which is a copy of prostate.transcan
> f ← princomp(w$transformed[,c("sz","sg","ap","bm")], cor=T)
> summary(f)
```

Importance of components:

	Comp. 1	Comp. 2	Comp. 3	Comp. 4
Standard deviation	1.541	0.871	0.774	0.5172
Proportion of Variance	0.594	0.190	0.150	0.0669
Cumulative Proportion	0.594	0.783	0.933	1.0000

```
> tumor ← f$scores[,1]
> f     ← princomp(w$transformed[,c("sbp","dbp")], cor=T)
> summary(f)
```

Importance of components:

	Comp. 1	Comp. 2
Standard deviation	1.293	0.572
Proportion of Variance	0.836	0.164
Cumulative Proportion	0.836	1.000

```
> bp ← f$scores[,1]
> f  ← princomp(w$transformed[,c("hx","ekg")], cor=T)
```

```
> summary(f)
```

Importance of components:

	Comp. 1	Comp. 2
Standard deviation	1.108	0.878
Proportion of Variance	0.614	0.386
Cumulative Proportion	0.614	1.000

TABLE 8.6

Predictors Used	d.f.	χ^2	AIC
PC_1	1	17.9	15.9
PC_{1-5}	5	79.8	69.8
PC_{1-10}	10	83.6	63.6
PC_{1-17}	17	97.8	63.8
All individual var., linear	17	97.8	63.8
All individual var., splines	39	140.0	62.0
PC_1 on transformed var.	1	31.6	29.6
PC_{1-5} on trans.	5	78.1	68.1
PC_{1-10} on trans.	10	85.5	65.5
PC_{1-12} on trans.	12	85.9	61.9
PCs on clusters of raw var.	8	77.2	61.2
PCs on clusters of trans.	7	81.1	67.1

```
> cardiac ← f$scores[,1]
> hg.t    ← w$transformed[,"hg"]      # pick off hg transformation column
> age.t   ← w$transformed[,"age"]
> pf.t    ← w$transformed[,"pf"]
> wt.t    ← w$transformed[,"wt"]
> cph(S ~ tumor + bp + cardiac + hg.t + age.t + pf.t + wt.t)

 Obs Events Model L.R. d.f. P Score Score P   R2
 502    354        81.1    7 0  86.8         0 0.149


          coef se(coef)    z        p
 tumor  0.1723   0.0367  4.688 2.76e-06
    bp -0.0251   0.0424 -0.594 5.53e-01
cardiac -0.2513  0.0516 -4.873 1.10e-06
  hg.t -0.1407   0.0554 -2.541 1.11e-02
 age.t -0.1034   0.0579 -1.787 7.39e-02
  pf.t -0.0933   0.0487 -1.918 5.51e-02
  wt.t -0.0910   0.0555 -1.639 1.01e-01

> # tumor and cardiac clusters seem to dominate
```

The results are summarized in Table 8.6. Again, AIC refers to $\chi^2 - 2\times$ d.f. As is usually the case, the later PCs are not very predictive. It must be emphasized that the 39 d.f. model with AIC = 62.0, which corresponds to maximum data analysis except that interactions were not examined, would be expected to have no worse predictive performance on independent data than a stepwise model based on screening all predictors against the response and discarding insignificant ones. When

TABLE 8.7

Factor	AIC		
	Original	Transformed	Optimum
sz	16.3	12.8	10.8
sg	13.0	17.0	14.4
ap	-1.7	13.8	17.4
sbp	-1.9	-1.9	-4.7
dbp	-0.3	1.0	3.0
age	10.9	9.1	12.7
wt	7.3	7.5	7.3
hg	14.4	19.1	16.4
ekg	7.0	8.8	7.0
pf	11.0	11.0	11.0

all variables are taken as a group, the transcan-transformed variables performed no better than the original variables. We have fitted many models for purposes of explication, but the best models appear to be those with a moderate amount of data reduction: the five PC models and the model based on first principal components of clusters of the transformed variables.

Table 8.6 demonstrates a common occurrence in data reduction and variable transformation. Better transformations benefit single summaries such as PC_1, but when the transformations are derived from examining the correlation pattern across predictors, the more principal components that are used the less it matters how variables were transformed. That is because we are attempting to use the same data for two purposes; redundancies in the data are used to drive both transformation estimation and formation of principal components.

8.7   Detailed Examination of Individual Transformations

Now examine Table 8.7 to see what individual transformations provide over the original scorings, and how they compare with "optimum" fits from dummy variable or spline expansions. Note that for transformed variables, d.f. is always 1. The fits used the subset of observations for which the variable was actually measured. The last column has χ^2 based on "optimum" fits using restricted cubic spline functions with five knots for continuous factors (yielding 4 d.f.), and dummy variables for categorical factors. Note that for ekg, the first χ^2 has five degrees of freedom while the last two have 1 degree of freedom. For pf, the first column used the 0–3 coding and has 1 d.f. The last column has 2 d.f. (after the infrequent code 3 was pooled with code 2). The transformations resulted in slightly worse predictive power than the original scorings for sz and age, slightly better power for sg, dbp, wt, hg, and

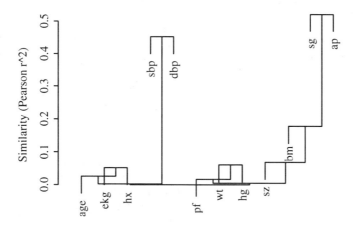

FIGURE 8.6: Hierarchical clustering using squared Pearson correlation of transformed variables as similarities.

ekg, and vastly better power for ap, the highly skewed variable. By comparing AIC in the second and third columns we see that the selftransformations were optimal for sz, sg, sbp, wt, hg, ekg and were deficient for ap, dbp, age. The optimum transformation of ap using a five-knot spline revealed that very low ap is associated with increasing mortality, in addition to very high ap. The optimum age transformation had an acceleration of risk after age 70, rather than a decreasing slope. But on the average we observed a common finding: transforming predictors based on their interrelationships is better than assuming linearity.

8.8   Examination of Variable Clusters on Transformed Variables

Let's stop and reexamine the variable clusters using the transformed variables, this time using squared Pearson correlations as similarity measures (since the transformations have handled skewness). We also score ekg numerically.

```
> plot(varclus(prostate.transcan$transformed, similarity="pearson"))
```

The resulting clusters shown in Figure 8.6 are similar to previous ones.

For a small dataset, we would need to represent the "extent of cancer" cluster with a summary score such as PC_1. For our 354-death dataset, we may desire to keep the four variables in this cluster separate, but use the transformed scores to reduce each variable to 1 d.f.

Again prematurely peeking at the response variable, we check to see if the PC_1 adequately weights the four variables.

```
> sz.t ← w$transformed[,'sz']
> sg.t ← w$transformed[,'sg']
> ap.t ← w$transformed[,'ap']
> f ← cph(S ~ tumor + sz.t + sg.t + ap.t)
> # omit bm (would cause singularity)
> anova(f, sz.t, sg.t, ap.t)   # pool effects of 3 var.
```

The fraction of variation explained by PC_1 of the four untransformed variables is 0.46. For the transformed variables it is 0.59. The anova test for adequacy of internal weights yielded $\chi^2 = 1.52$ with 3 d.f., $p = 0.68$, so we accept the null hypothesis of adequate weights. However, we must remember that the ap transformation could be improved. The model likelihood ratio χ^2 with 1 d.f. for tumor is 28.1.

Next consider how to combine the two blood pressure measurements. PC_1 of sbp,dbp explains 0.81 of the variation, and transcan increased this to only 0.84. However, PC_1 is not an adequate summary since either the transformed sbp or dbp adds significantly to it. Remembering that the original linear dbp was judged to be inadequate, we abandon data reduction for blood pressures. SAS PROC PRINQUAL, using monotonic spline transformations, stopped with the initial linear transformation when using the MTV option. PRINQUAL's MGV (maximum generalized variance) criterion found highly nonlinear transformations of both blood pressures.

8.9   Transformation Using Nonparametric Smoothers

The ACE nonparametric additive regression method of Breiman and Friedman[47] can be used to transform the predictors using the S-PLUS ace function, packaged for easy use with the transace function in the Hmisc library. transace does not impute data but merely does casewise deletion of missing values. Here transace is run after single imputation by transcan. To do an alternative one-iteration MGV-type analysis with some monotonicity restrictions, use the following. binary is used to tell transace which variables not to try to predict.

```
> x ← cbind(sz, sg, ap, sbp, dbp, age, wt, hg, ekg, pf, bm, hx)

> par(mfrow=c(5,2), bty="n")

> monotonic ← c("sz","sg","ap","sbp","dbp","age","pf")
> transace(x, monotonic, categorical="ekg", binary=c("bm","hx"))
```

Except for ekg, age, and for arbitrary sign reversals, the transformations in Figure 8.7 determined using transace were similar to those in Figure 8.3. The transcan transformation for ekg makes more sense.

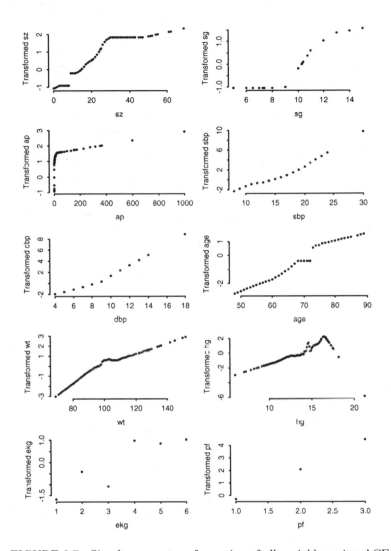

FIGURE 8.7: Simultaneous transformation of all variables using ACE.

8.10   Multiple Imputation

Every step that has been done so far used single imputation (unconditional means, conditional means, or most likely categories). With the relatively small extent of missing data in the prostate dataset, single imputation will not likely cause significant biases in the final regression coefficients or in their estimated variances. But let us develop multiple imputations to see how the imputed values vary around the single imputations, and to quantify differences in Cox model estimates from those obtained from single imputation.

In using multiple imputation we can now incorporate the response variable into prediction of X. When the response is censored this presents a problem. For the dataset at hand the smallest followup time for uncensored observations was 50 months. We categorize survival time using cutoffs of 12, 24, 36, and 48 months. The first category of the new variable signifies death before 12 months. The last category, signifying survival time of at least 48 months, is the only category of the newly constructed variable having a mixture of patients who lived and died; all patients in the other categories died. We obtain transformations (the same ones obtained using single imputation) and multiple imputations using transcan. Multiple imputations are obtained using the approximate Bayesian bootstrap by adding randomly drawn residuals to predicted mean transformed values, and then back-transforming.

```
> surv ← cut2(dtime, c(12,24,36,48))
> prostate.transcan.mi ←
+      transcan(∼ sz + sg + ap + sbp + dbp + age + wt + hg +
+      ekg + pf + bm + hx + surv, imputed=T, pl=F,
+      n.impute=10)
```

Let us examine the extent to which the response increased explained variation in the predictors over that provided by the other predictors alone.

```
> summary(prostate.transcan)

. . . .
Adjusted R-squared:

   sz    sg    ap   sbp   dbp   age    wt    hg   ekg    pf    bm    hx
 0.18 0.541 0.559 0.481 0.468 0.065 0.093 0.129 0.059 0.086 0.331 0.083
      . . . .

> summary(prostate.transcan.mi)

. . . .
Adjusted R-squared:

    sz    sg    ap  sbp   dbp   age    wt    hg   ekg    pf    bm    hx  surv
 0.184 0.544 0.558 0.48 0.465 0.072 0.096 0.137 0.067 0.091 0.328 0.101 0.132
```

The optimally numerically scored surv variable can be predicted from the others with an adjusted R^2 of 0.132. Using surv resulted in less variance in imputed values of most of the variables. The adjusted R^2 for some variables actually decreased because the additional variation explained was not enough to offset the additional d.f. from surv used in the predictions.

The 10 multiply imputed values are below. Single imputations have been added to the right of each table. These imputations were obtained from transcan using the default (impcat='score', which is the only method allowed for multiple imputation) instead of impcat='tree' which was used previously (this affects only the imputation of ekg). For ekg, imputations from impcat='tree' are also shown.

```
> prostate.transcan.mi$imputed

$sz:
         1     2     3     4     5     6     7     8     9    10
 48  17.1  6.00 20.7   6.0  6.00  6.0  6.00 17.8 12.7  2.98   7.4
 74   6.0  6.00  6.0   6.0  8.22  6.0  6.00  6.0  6.0  6.00   6.0
131   6.0  7.05  6.0   6.0  6.00 14.9  3.48  6.0  6.0  6.00   6.0
158  19.2 69.00 18.0  22.8 52.69 15.3 45.66 31.9 18.7 28.34  24.7
485  60.1 31.36 20.3   7.6  8.24  6.0 36.25 66.6 21.3  6.00  20.2

$sg:
          1     2     3     4     5     6     7     8     9    10
  2   9.99 11.01 10.75 11.8  8.01  7.28 10.3 10.5 10.12  6.86  10.3
 57  10.89 10.37 10.33 10.3  9.95 10.36 11.3 11.0 13.55  7.00  10.4
123   8.28  8.00  9.68  8.0 10.24  7.78 10.5 10.9 10.24 10.26   7.3
125   9.58 10.17  8.00  8.0  5.15  8.00  8.0  8.0  8.00  8.00   7.4
169  13.74 11.59 12.79 12.5 11.33 11.50 15.0 13.4 11.59 11.97  15.0
336   5.77 10.34  7.85  8.0  8.00 10.67  8.0  8.0  8.00 10.22   8.0
418  10.82 10.60 10.37 10.9 10.21 10.61 10.6 10.5  7.91  9.27  10.3
436   9.28  8.00  5.27 11.0  5.39  8.00 10.6  8.0  5.69  8.00   6.5
474  10.36  7.45 10.23 10.2 10.26 11.09 15.0 11.0  5.15 10.11  10.3
484  10.70  9.17 11.30 10.6  7.15 10.36 15.0 10.5 10.41 10.46  10.7
506  15.00 15.00 15.00 15.0 15.00 15.00 15.0 11.9 15.00 15.00  15.0

$age:
         1    2    3    4    5    6    7    8  9 10
 42  69.5 61.5 73.8 72.3 60.1 62.7 51.8 50.7 63 77   71.7

$wt:
          1     2     3    4   5   6   7     8   9  10
193  81.1 101.0 147.7 102 152 116 103  77.8 152 107   262.0
262 103.8  82.7  98.4 100 102 108 103 101.1 111 102    91.2
```

```
$ekg:
    1 2 3 4 5 6 7 8 9 10    score    tree
243 2 2 4 2 3 2 3 2 3  4      2        2
269 1 5 1 1 5 4 1 6 5  1      4        2
270 4 1 4 5 1 6 2 6 4  1      4        2
271 2 3 4 1 1 1 2 4 6  1      5        2
280 3 1 1 3 4 5 2 2 5  2      4        2
285 2 2 2 2 3 2 2 2 2  2      2        6
404 5 4 2 2 5 2 2 6 4  2      2        6
470 2 1 3 3 1 4 2 3 1  6      4        6
```

For continuous variables, the average of the multiple imputations approximately equals the single imputation, as by design. For `ekg` the pattern is less clear. We see many of the multiple imputations set to the most common category (2, normal).

Let us fit an abbreviated Cox model using both single and multiple imputation. Here age is modeled using a linear spline with a slope change at age 70, and tumor size is modeled using a restricted cubic spline with four knots. The `fit.mult.impute` function in the `Hmisc` library will in succession draw the 10 imputations created by `transcan(..., n.impute=10)`, average regression coefficients, and compute an imputation-adjusted variance–covariance matrix for $\hat{\beta}$. Thus Wald statistics are computed properly. Likelihood ratio and score χ^2 statistics are not shown because `fit.mult.impute` computes them only for the last filled-in dataset.

```
> f ← cph(S ~ rcs(sz,4) + lsp(age,70) + ekg)
> g ← fit.mult.impute(S ~ rcs(sz,4) + lsp(age,70) + ekg,
+                      cph, prostate.transcan.mi)


Variance Inflation Factors Due to Imputation:

  sz   sz'  sz''   age  age'  ekg=normal ekg=benign ekg=rhythmic...
 1.01 1.01 1.01  1.04  1.03      1.04       1.11         1.06
 ekg=heart block or conduction def ekg=heart strain
               1.09                    1.03
```

```
        > f
                                    coef se(coef)      z       p
                              sz  0.03184   0.0342  0.931 0.35200
                             sz' -0.15769   0.3179 -0.496 0.61992
                             sz''  0.26224  0.5120  0.512 0.60850
                             age -0.00963   0.0134 -0.721 0.47122
                            age'  0.08381   0.0257  3.260 0.00111
                     ekg=normal -0.30620   0.1666 -1.838 0.06602
                     ekg=benign -0.08995   0.2863 -0.314 0.75342
ekg=rhythmic disturb & electrolyte ch  0.23763   0.2075  1.145 0.25201
   ekg=heart block or conduction def -0.27564   0.2837 -0.972 0.33121
                  ekg=heart strain  0.17900   0.1623  1.103 0.27004
```

```
> g
```

	coef	se(coef)	z	p
sz	0.02790	0.0341	0.818	0.41339
sz'	-0.12211	0.3331	-0.367	0.71393
sz''	0.20293	0.5357	0.379	0.70484
age	-0.00616	0.0136	-0.452	0.65140
age'	0.07740	0.0260	2.979	0.00289
ekg=normal	-0.23881	0.1703	-1.403	0.16074
ekg=benign	-0.07517	0.2971	-0.253	0.80026
ekg=rhythmic disturb & electrolyte ch	0.24616	0.2116	1.163	0.24477
ekg=heart block or conduction def	-0.26791	0.2910	-0.920	0.35731
ekg=heart strain	0.19394	0.1648	1.177	0.23936

```
> anova(f)
```

Factor	Chi-Square	d.f.	P
sz	21.49	3	0.0001
Nonlinear	0.38	2	0.8287
age	21.93	2	<.0001
Nonlinear	10.63	1	0.0011
ekg	16.87	5	0.0047
TOTAL NONLINEAR	10.84	3	0.0126
TOTAL	59.08	10	<.0001

```
> anova(g)
```

Factor	Chi-Square	d.f.	P
sz	19.73	3	0.0002
Nonlinear	0.21	2	0.9011
age	20.48	2	<.0001
Nonlinear	8.88	1	0.0029
ekg	13.65	5	0.0180
TOTAL NONLINEAR	8.97	3	0.0297
TOTAL	54.70	10	<.0001

For this example, using survival time to assist in imputing the predictors did not result in a noticeable strengthening of effects. Here estimated regression coefficients are slightly smaller under multiple imputation on the whole. Introducing the right amount of randomness into the imputed values also resulted in appropriately larger standard errors.

8.11   Further Reading

[1]   Sauerbrei and Schumacher[364] used the bootstrap to demonstrate the variability of a standard variable selection procedure for the prostate cancer dataset.

[2]   · Schemper and Heinze[372] used logistic models to impute dichotomizations of the predictors for this dataset.

8.12   Problems

The Mayo Clinic conducted a randomized trial in primary biliary cirrhosis (PBC) of the liver between January 1974 and May 1984, to compare D-penicillamine with placebo. The drug was found to be ineffective [141, p. 2], and the trial was done before liver transplantation was common, so this trial constitutes a natural history study for PBC. Followup continued through July, 1986. For the 19 patients that did undergo transplant, followup time was censored at the day of transplant. 312 patients were randomized, and another 106 patients were entered into a registry. The nonrandomized patients have most of their laboratory values missing, except for bilirubin, albumin, and prothrombin time. 28 randomized patients had both serum cholesterol and triglycerides missing. The data, which consist of clinical, biochemical, serologic, and histologic information are listed in [141, pp. 359–375]. The PBC data are discussed and analyzed in [141, pp. 2–7, 102–104, 153–162], [114], [6] (a tree-based analysis which on its p. 480 mentions some possible lack of fit of the earlier analyses), and [244]. The data are stored in S-PLUS data frame pbc (see the Appendix) and are also available in StatLib in the datasets directory. Do the following steps using only the data on randomized patients and ignoring followup time, status, and drug.

1. Do an initial variable clustering based on ranks, using pairwise deletion of missing data. Comment on the potential for one-dimensional summaries of subsets of variables being adequate summaries of prognostic information.

2. cholesterol, triglycerides, platelets, and copper are missing on some patients. Impute them using one of the following methods: (possibly nonlinear) multiple regression, a canonical regression developed with the transformation/scaling analysis below, or recursive partitioning. Use some or all of the remaining predictors. Provide a correlation coefficient describing the usefulness of each imputation model. Provide the actual imputed values, specifying observation numbers. For all later analyses, use imputed values for missing values.

3. Perform a scaling/transformation analysis to better measure how the predictors interrelate and to possibly pretransform some of them. Use a transcan, ACE, or MGV-type analysis (or MTV if necessary). Repeat the variable clustering using the transformed scores and Pearson correlation or using an oblique rotation principal component analysis. Determine if the correlation structure (or variance explained by the first principal component) indicates whether it is possible to summarize multiple variables into single scores.

4. Do a principal component analysis of all transformed variables simultaneously. Make a graph of the number of components versus the cumulative proportion of explained variation. Repeat this for laboratory variables alone.

5. How well can variables (lab and otherwise) that are routinely collected (on nonrandomized patients) capture the information (variation) of the variables that are often missing? It would be helpful to explore the strength of interrelationships by

   (a) correlating two PC_1s obtained from untransformed variables,

   (b) correlating two PC_1s obtained from transformed variables,

   (c) correlating the best linear combination of one set of variables with the best linear combination of the other set, and

   (d) doing the same on transformed variables.

Chapter 9

Overview of Maximum Likelihood Estimation

9.1   General Notions—Simple Cases

In ordinary least squares multiple regression, the objective in fitting a model is to find the values of the unknown parameters that minimize the sum of squared errors of prediction. When the response variable is polytomous or is not observed completely, a more general objective to optimize is needed.

Maximum likelihood (ML) estimation is a general technique for estimating parameters and drawing statistical inferences in a variety of situations, especially nonstandard ones. Before laying out the method in general, ML estimation is illustrated with a standard situation, the one-sample binomial problem. Here, independent binary responses are observed and one wishes to draw inferences about an unknown parameter, the probability of an event in a population.

Suppose that in a population of individuals, each individual has the same probability P that an event occurs. We could also say that the event has already been observed, so that P is the prevalence of some condition in the population. For each individual, let $Y = 1$ denote the occurrence of the event and $Y = 0$ denote nonoccurrence. Then $\text{Prob}\{Y = 1\} = P$ for each individual. Suppose that a random sample of size 3 from the population is drawn and that the first individual had $Y = 1$, the second had $Y = 0$, and the third had $Y = 1$. The respective probabilities of these outcomes are P, $1 - P$, and P. The joint probability of observing the independent events $Y = 1, 0, 1$ is $P(1 - P)P = P^2(1 - P)$. Now the value of P is unknown, but we can solve for the value of P that makes the observed data $(Y = 1, 0, 1)$ *most likely to have occurred*. In this case, the value of P that maximizes $P^2(1 - P)$ is $P = 2/3$. This value for P is the *maximum likelihood estimate (MLE)* of the population probability.

Let us now study the situation of independent binary trials in general. Let the sample size be n and the observed responses be $Y_1, Y_2, \ldots, Y_n$. The joint probability of observing the data is given by

$$L = \prod_{i=1}^{n} P^{Y_i}(1 - P)^{1-Y_i}. \tag{9.1}$$

Now let s denote the sum of the Ys or the number of times that the event occurred $(Y_i = 1)$, that is the number of "successes." The number of nonoccurrences ("failures") is $n - s$. The likelihood of the data can be simplified to

$$L = P^s(1 - P)^{n-s}. \tag{9.2}$$

It is easier to work with the log of the likelihood function, and as is discussed later, the *log likelihood function* has certain desirable statistic properties. For the one-sample binary response problem, the log likelihood is

$$\log L = s \log(P) + (n - s) \log(1 - P). \tag{9.3}$$

The MLE of P is that value of P that maximizes L or $\log L$. Since $\log L$ is a smooth function of P, its maximum value can be found by finding the point at which $\log L$ has a slope of 0. The slope or first derivative of $\log L$, with respect to P, is

$$U(P) = \partial \log L / dP = s/P - (n - s)/(1 - P). \tag{9.4}$$

The first derivative of the log likelihood function with respect to the parameter(s), here $U(P)$, is called the *score function*. Equating this function to zero requires that $s/P = (n - s)/(1 - P)$. Multiplying both sides of the equation by $P(1 - P)$ yields $s(1 - P) = (n - s)P$ or that $s = (n - s)P + sP = nP$. Thus the MLE of P is $p = s/n$.

Another important function is called the *Fisher information* about the unknown parameters. The information function is the expected value of the negative of the curvature in $\log L$, which is the negative of the slope of the slope as a function of the parameter, or the negative of the second derivative of $\log L$. Motivation for consideration of the Fisher information is as follows. If the log likelihood function has a distinct peak, the sample provides information that allows one to readily discriminate between a good parameter estimate (the location of the obvious peak) and a bad one. In such a case the MLE will have good precision or small variance. If on the other hand the likelihood function is relatively flat, almost any estimate will do and the chosen estimate will have poor precision or large variance. The degree

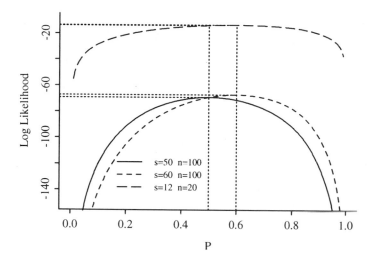

FIGURE 9.1: log likelihood functions for three one-sample binomial problems.

of peakedness of a function at a given point is the speed with which the slope is changing at that point, that is, the slope of the slope or second derivative of the function at that point.

Here, the information is

$$
\begin{aligned}
I(P) &= E\{-\partial^2 \log L/\partial P^2\} \\
&= E\{s/P^2 + (n-s)/(1-P)^2\} \\
&= nP/P^2 + n(1-P)/(1-P)^2 = n/[P(1-P)].
\end{aligned}
\tag{9.5}
$$

We estimate the information by substituting the MLE of P into $I(P)$, yielding $I(p) = n/[p(1-p)]$.

Figures 9.1, 9.2, and 9.3 depict, respectively, $\log L$, $U(P)$, and $I(P)$, all as a function of P. Three combinations of n and s were used in each graph. These combinations correspond to $p = .5, .6$, and $.6$, respectively.

In each case it can be seen that the value of P that makes the data most likely to have occurred (the value that maximizes L or $\log L$) is p given above. Also, the score function (slope of $\log L$) is zero at $P = p$. Note that the information function $I(P)$ is highest for P approaching 0 or 1 and is lowest for P near .5, where there is maximum uncertainty about P. Note also that while $\log L$ has the same shape for the $s = 60$ and $s = 12$ curves in Figure 9.1, the range of log L is much greater for the larger sample size. Figures 9.2 and 9.3 show that the larger sample size produces a sharper likelihood. In other words, with larger n, one can zero in on the true value of P with more precision.

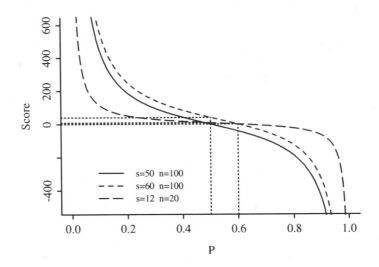

FIGURE 9.2: Score functions $(\partial L/\partial P)$.

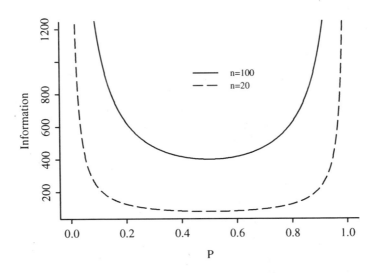

FIGURE 9.3: Information functions $(-\,\partial^2 \log L/\partial P^2)$.

In this binary response one-sample example let us now turn to inference about the parameter P. First, we turn to the estimation of the variance of the MLE, p. An estimate of this variance is given by the inverse of the information at $P = p$:

$$Var(p) = I(p)^{-1} = p(1 - p)/n. \tag{9.6}$$

Note that the variance is smallest when the information is greatest ($p = 0$ or 1).

The variance estimate forms a basis for confidence limits on the unknown parameter. For large n, the MLE p is approximately normally distributed with expected value (mean) P and variance $P(1 - P)/n$. Since $p(1 - p)$ is a consistent estimate of $P(1 - P)/n$, it follows that $p \pm z[p(1 - p)/n]^{1/2}$ is an approximate $1 - \alpha$ confidence interval for P if z is the $1 - \alpha/2$ critical value of the standard normal distribution.

9.2 Hypothesis Tests

Now let us turn to hypothesis tests about the unknown population parameter P — $H_0 : P = P_0$. There are three kinds of statistical tests that arise from likelihood theory.

9.2.1 Likelihood Ratio Test

This test statistic is the ratio of the likelihood at the hypothesized parameter values to the likelihood of the data at the maximum (i.e., at parameter values = MLEs). It turns out that $-2\times$ the log of this likelihood ratio has desirable statistical properties. The likelihood ratio test statistic is given by

$$
\begin{aligned}
LR &= -2\log(L \text{ at } H_0/L \text{ at MLEs}) \\
&= -2(\log L \text{ at } H_0) - [-2(\log L \text{ at MLEs})].
\end{aligned} \tag{9.7}
$$

The LR statistic, for large enough samples, has approximately a χ^2 distribution with degrees of freedom equal to the number of parameters estimated, if the null hypothesis is "simple," that is, doesn't involve any unknown parameters. Here LR has 1 d.f.

The value of $\log L$ at H_0 is

$$\log L(H_0) = s \log(P_0) + (n - s) \log(1 - P_0). \tag{9.8}$$

The maximum value of $\log L$ (at MLEs) is

$$\log L(P = p) = s \log(p) + (n - s) \log(1 - p). \tag{9.9}$$

For the hypothesis $H_0 : P = P_0$, the test statistic is

$$LR = -2\{s \log(P_0/p) + (n - s) \log[(1 - P_0)/(1 - p)]\}. \qquad (9.10)$$

Note that when p happens to equal P_0, $LR = 0$. When p is far from P_0, LR will be large. Suppose that $P_0 = 1/2$, so that H_0 is $P = 1/2$. For $n = 100, s = 50, LR = 0$. For $n = 100, s = 60$,

$$LR = -2\{60 \log(.5/.6) + 40 \log(.5/.4)\} = 4.03. \qquad (9.11)$$

For $n = 20, s = 12$,

$$LR = -2\{12 \log(.5/.6) + 8 \log(.5/.4)\} = .81 = 4.03/5. \qquad (9.12)$$

Therefore, even though the best estimate of P is the same for these two cases, the test statistic is more impressive when the sample size is five times larger.

9.2.2   Wald Test

The Wald test statistic is a generalization of a t- or z-statistic. It is a function of the difference in the MLE and its hypothesized value, normalized by an estimate of the standard deviation of the MLE. Here the statistic is

$$W = [p - P_0]^2/[p(1 - p)/n]. \qquad (9.13)$$

For large enough n, W is distributed as χ^2 with 1 d.f. For $n = 100, s = 50, W = 0$. For the other samples, W is, respectively, 4.17 and 0.83 (note $0.83 = 4.17/5$).

Many statistical packages treat $\sqrt{W}$ as having a t distribution instead of a normal distribution. As pointed out by Gould,[156] there is no basis for this outside ordinary linear models. In linear regression, a t distribution is used to penalize for the fact that the variance of $Y|X$ is estimated. In models such as the logistic model, there is no separate variance parameter to estimate. Gould has done simulations that show that the normal distribution provides more accurate P-values than the t for binary logistic regression.

9.2.3   Score Test

If the MLE happens to equal the hypothesized value P_0, P_0 maximizes the likelihood and so $U(P_0) = 0$. Rao's score statistic measures how far from zero the score function is when evaluated at the null hypothesis. The score function (slope or first derivative of $\log L$) is normalized by the information (curvature or second derivative of $-\log L$). The test statistic for our example is

$$S = U(P_0)^2/I(P_0), \qquad (9.14)$$

which formally does not involve the MLE, p. The statistic can be simplified as follows.

$$
\begin{aligned}
U(P_0) &= s/P_0 - (n-s)/(1-P_0) \\
I(P_0) &= s/P_0^2 + (n-s)/(1-P_0)^2 \\
S &= (s-nP_0)^2/[nP_0(1-P_0)] = n(p-P_0)^2/[P_0(1-P_0)].
\end{aligned}
\tag{9.15}
$$

Note that the numerator of S involves $s - nP_0$, the difference between the observed number of successes and the number of successes expected under H_0.

As with the other two test statistics, $S = 0$ for the first sample. For the last two samples S is, respectively, 4 and $.8 = 4/5$.

[1]

9.2.4 Normal Distribution—One Sample

Suppose that a sample of size n is taken from a population for a random variable Y that is known to be normally distributed with unknown mean μ and variance σ^2. Denote the observed values of the random variable by $Y_1, Y_2, \ldots, Y_n$. Now unlike the binary response case ($Y = 0$ or 1), we cannot use the notion of the probability that Y equals an observed value. This is because Y is continuous and the probability that it will take on a given value is zero. We substitute the *density function* for the probability. The density at a point y is the limit as d approaches zero of

$$
\text{Prob}\{y < Y \le y + d\}/d = [F(y+d) - F(y)]/d,
\tag{9.16}
$$

where $F(y)$ is the normal cumulative distribution function (for a mean of μ and variance of σ^2). The limit of the right-hand side of the above equation as d approaches zero is $f(y)$, the density function of a normal distribution with mean μ and variance σ^2. This density function is

$$
f(y) = (2\pi\sigma^2)^{-1/2} \exp\{-(y-\mu)^2/2\sigma^2\}.
\tag{9.17}
$$

The likelihood of observing the observed sample values is the joint density of the Ys. The log likelihood function here is a function of two unknowns, μ and σ^2.

$$
\log L = -.5n \log(2\pi\sigma^2) - .5 \sum_{i=1}^{n}(Y_i - \mu)^2/\sigma^2.
\tag{9.18}
$$

It can be shown that the value of μ that maximizes $\log L$ is the value that minimizes the sum of squared deviations about μ, which is the sample mean $\overline{Y}$. The MLE of σ^2 is

$$
s^2 = \sum_{i=1}^{n}(Y_i - \overline{Y})^2/n.
\tag{9.19}
$$

Recall that the sample variance uses $n - 1$ instead of n in the denominator. It can be shown that the expected value of the MLE of σ^2, s^2, is $[(n - 1)/n]\sigma^2$; in other words, s^2 is too small by a factor of $(n - 1)/n$ on the average. The sample variance is unbiased, but being unbiased does not necessarily make it a better estimator. The MLE has greater precision (smaller mean squared error) in many cases.

9.3   General Case

Suppose we need to estimate a vector of unknown parameters $B = \{B_1, B_2, \ldots, B_p\}$ from a sample of size n based on observations $Y_1, \ldots, Y_n$. Denote the probability or density function of the random variable Y for the ith observation by $f_i(y; B)$. The likelihood for the ith observation is $L_i(B) = f_i(Y_i; B)$. In the one-sample binary response case, recall that $L_i(B) = L_i(P) = P^{Y_i}[1 - P]^{1 - Y_i}$. The likelihood function, or joint likelihood of the sample, is given by

$$L(B) = \prod_{i=1}^{n} f_i(Y_i; B). \tag{9.20}$$

The log likelihood function is

$$\log L(B) = \sum_{i=1}^{n} \log L_i(B). \tag{9.21}$$

The MLE of B is that value of the vector B that maximizes $\log L(B)$ as a function of B. In general, the solution for B requires iterative trial-and-error methods as outlined later. Denote the MLE of B as $b = \{b_1, \ldots, b_p\}$. The *score vector* is the vector of first derivatives of $\log L(B)$ with respect to $B_1, \ldots, B_p$:

$$
\begin{aligned}
U(B) &= \{\partial/\partial B_1 \log L(B), \ldots, \partial/\partial B_p \log L(B)\} \\
&= (\partial/\partial B) \log L(B).
\end{aligned}
\tag{9.22}
$$

The Fisher *information matrix* is the $p \times p$ matrix whose elements are the negative of the expectation of all second partial derivatives of $\log L(B)$:

$$
\begin{aligned}
I^*(B) &= -\{E[(\partial^2 \log L(B)/\partial B_j \partial B_k)]\}_{p \times p} \\
&= -E\{(\partial^2/\partial B \partial B') \log L(B)\}.
\end{aligned}
\tag{9.23}
$$

The *observed information matrix* $I(B)$ is $I^*(B)$ without taking the expectation. In other words, observed values remain in the second derivatives:

$$I(B) = -(\partial^2/\partial B \partial B') \log L(B). \tag{9.24}$$

This information matrix is often estimated from the sample using the *estimated observed information* $I(b)$, by inserting b, the MLE of B, into the formula for $I(B)$.

Under suitable conditions, which are satisfied for most situations likely to be encountered, the MLE b for large samples is an optimal estimator (has as great a chance of being close to the true parameter as all other types of estimators) and has an approximate multivariate normal distribution with mean vector B and variance–covariance matrix $I^{*-1}(B)$, where C^{-1} denotes the inverse of the matrix C. (C^{-1} is the matrix such that $C^{-1}C$ is the identity matrix, a matrix with ones on the diagonal and zeros elsewhere. If C is a 1×1 matrix, $C^{-1} = 1/C$). A consistent estimator of the variance–covariance matrix is given by the matrix V, obtained by inserting b for B in $I(B) : V = I^{-1}(b)$.

9.3.1 Global Test Statistics

Suppose we wish to test the null hypothesis $H_0 : B = B^0$. The likelihood ratio test statistic is

$$
\begin{aligned}
LR &= -2\log(L \text{ at } H_0/L \text{ at MLEs}) \\
&= -2[\log L(B^0) - \log L(b)].
\end{aligned}
\tag{9.25}
$$

The corresponding Wald test statistic, using the estimated observed information matrix, is

$$
W = (b - B^0)'I(b)(b - B^0) = (b - B^0)'V^{-1}(b - B^0).
\tag{9.26}
$$

(A quadratic form $a'Va$ is a matrix generalization of a^2V.) Note that if the number of estimated parameters is $p = 1$, W reduces to $(b - B^0)^2/V$, which is the square of a z- or t-type statistic (estimate $-$ hypothesized value divided by estimated standard deviation of estimate).

The score statistic for H_0 is

$$
S = U'(B^0)I^{-1}(B^0)U(B^0).
\tag{9.27}
$$

Note that as before, S does not require solving for the MLE. For large samples, LR, W, and S have a χ^2 distribution with p d.f. under suitable conditions.

9.3.2 Testing a Subset of the Parameters

Let $B = \{B_1, B_2\}$ and suppose that we wish to test $H_0 : B_1 = B_1^0$. We are treating B_2 as a nuisance parameter. For example, we may want to test whether blood pressure and cholesterol are risk factors after adjusting for confounders age and sex. In that case B_1 is the pair of regression coefficients for blood pressure and cholesterol and B_2 is the pair of coefficients for age and sex. B_2 must be estimated to allow adjustment for age and sex, although B_2 is a nuisance parameter and is not of primary interest.

Let the number of parameters of interest be k so that B_1 is a vector of length k. Let the number of "nuisance" or "adjustment" parameters be q, the length of B_2 (note $k + q = p$).

Let b_2^* be the MLE of B_2 under the restriction that $B_1 = B_1^0$. Then the likelihood ratio statistic is

$$LR = -2[\log L \text{ at } H_0 - \log L \text{ at MLE}]. \qquad (9.28)$$

Now $\log L$ at H_0 is more complex than before because H_0 involves an unknown nuisance parameter B_2 that must be estimated. $\log L$ at H_0 is the maximum of the likelihood function for any value of B_2 but subject to the condition that $B_1 = B_1^0$. Thus

$$LR = -2[\log L(B_1^0, b_2^*) - \log L(b)], \qquad (9.29)$$

where as before b is the overall MLE of B. Note that LR requires maximizing two log likelihood functions. The first component of LR is a restricted maximum likelihood and the second component is the overall or unrestricted maximum.

LR is often computed by examining successively more complex models in a stepwise fashion and calculating the increment in likelihood ratio χ^2 in the overall model. The LR χ^2 for testing $H_0 : B_2 = 0$ when B_1 is not in the model is

$$LR(H_0 : B_2 = 0 | B_1 = 0) = -2[\log L(0, 0) - \log L(0, b_2^*)]. \qquad (9.30)$$

Here we are specifying that B_1 is not in the model by setting $B_1 = B_1^0 = 0$, and we are testing $H_0 : B_2 = 0$. (We are also ignoring nuisance parameters such as an intercept term in the test for $B_2 = 0$).

The LR χ^2 for testing $H_0 : B_1 = B_2 = 0$ is given by

$$LR(H_0 : B_1 = B_2 = 0) = -2[\log L(0, 0) - \log L(b)]. \qquad (9.31)$$

Subtracting LR χ^2 for the smaller model from that of the larger model yields

$$\begin{aligned} -2[\log L(0, 0) - \log L(b)] - -2[\log L(0, 0) - \log L(0, b_{2*})] \\ = -2[\log L(0, b_2^*) - \log L(b)], \end{aligned} \qquad (9.32)$$

which is the same as above (letting $B_1^0 = 0$).

For example, suppose successively larger models yield the LR χ^2s in Table 9.1. The LR χ^2 for testing for linearity in age (not adjusting for sex) against quadratic alternatives is $1010 - 1000 = 10$ with 1 d.f. The LR χ^2 for testing the added information provided by sex, adjusting for a quadratic effect of age, is $1013 - 1010 = 3$ with 1 d.f. The LR χ^2 for testing the joint importance of sex and the nonlinear (quadratic) effect of age is $1013 - 1000 = 13$ with 2 d.f.

To derive the Wald statistic for testing $H_0 : B_1 = B_1^0$ with B_2 being a nuisance parameter, let the MLE b be partitioned into $b = \{b_1, b_2\}$. We can likewise partition

TABLE 9.1

Variables (Parameters) in Model	$LR\ \chi^2$	Number of Parameters
Intercept, age	1000	2
Intercept, age, age^2	1010	3
Intercept, age, age^2, sex	1013	4

the estimated variance–covariance matrix V into

$$V = \begin{bmatrix} V_{11} & V_{12} \\ V_{12}' & V_{22} \end{bmatrix}. \tag{9.33}$$

The Wald statistic is

$$W = (b_1 - B_1^0)'V_{11}^{-1}(b_1 - B_1^0), \tag{9.34}$$

which when $k = 1$ reduces to (estimate-hypothesized value)$^2/$ estimated variance, with the estimates adjusted for the parameters in B_2.

Wald tests are also done by setting up a general linear contrast. $H_0 : CB = 0$ is tested by a Wald statistic of the form

$$W = (Cb)'(CVC')^{-1}(Cb), \tag{9.35}$$

where C is a contrast matrix that "picks off" the proper elements of B.

The score statistic for testing $H_0 : B_1 = B_1^0$ does not require solving for the full set of unknown parameters. Only the MLEs of B_2 must be computed, under the restriction that $B_1 = B_1^0$. This restricted MLE is b_2^* from above. Let $U(B_1^0, b_2^*)$ denote the vector of first derivatives of $\log L$ with respect to all parameters in B, evaluated at the hypothesized parameter values B_1^0 for the first k parameters and at the restricted MLE b_2^* for the last q parameters. (Since the last q estimates are MLEs, the last q elements of U are zero, so the formulas that follow simplify.) Let $I(B_1^0, b_2^*)$ be the observed information matrix evaluated at the same values of B as is U. The score statistic for testing $H_0 : B_1 = B_1^0$ is

$$S = U'(B_1^0, b_2^*)I^{-1}(B_1^0, b_2^*)U(B_1^0, b_2^*). \tag{9.36}$$

Under suitable conditions, the distribution of LR, W, and S can be adequately approximated by a χ^2 distribution with k d.f.

9.3.3   Which Test Statistics to Use When

At this point, one may ask why three types of test statistics are needed. The answer lies in the statistical properties of the three tests as well as in computational expense in different situations. From the standpoint of statistical properties, LR is the best statistic, followed by S and W. The major statistical problem with W is that it is sensitive to problems in the estimated variance–covariance matrix in the full model. For some models, most notably the logistic regression model,[193] the variance–covariance estimates can be too large as the effects in the model become very strong, resulting in values of W that are too small (or significance levels that are too large). W is also sensitive to the way the parameter appears in the model. For example, a test of $H_0 :$ log odds ratio $= 0$ will yield a different value of W than will $H_0 :$ odds ratio $= 1$.

Relative computational efficiency of the three types of tests is also an issue. Computation of LR and W requires estimating all p unknown parameters, and in addition LR requires re-estimating the last q parameters under that restriction that the first k parameters $= B_1^0$. Therefore, when one is contemplating whether a set of parameters should be added to a model, the score test is the easiest test to carry out. For example, if one were interested in testing all two-way interactions among 4 predictors, the score test statistic for $H_0 :$ "no interactions present" could be computed without estimating the $4 \times 3/2 = 6$ interaction effects. S would also be appealing for testing linearity of effects in a model—the nonlinear spline terms could be tested for significance after adjusting for the linear effects (with estimation of only the linear effects). Only parameters for linear effects must be estimated to compute S, resulting in fewer numerical problems such as lack of convergence of the Newton–Raphson algorithm.

The Wald tests are very easy to make after all the parameters in a model have been estimated. Wald tests are thus appealing in a multiple regression setup when one wants to test whether a given predictor or set of predictors is "significant." A score test would require re-estimating the regression coefficients under the restriction that the parameters of interest equal zero.

Likelihood ratio tests are used often for testing the global hypothesis that no effects are significant, as the log likelihood evaluated at the MLEs is already available from fitting the model and the log likelihood evaluated at a "null model" (e.g., a model containing only an intercept) is often easy to compute. Likelihood ratio tests should also be used when the validity of a Wald test is in question as in the example cited above.

Table 9.2 summarizes recommendations for choice of test statistics for various situations, based on both computational efficiency and statistical properties.

9.3.4   Example: Binomial—Comparing Two Proportions

Suppose that a binary random variable Y_1 represents responses for population 1 and Y_2 represents responses for population 2. Let $P_i = \text{Prob}\{Y_i = 1\}$ and assume that a random sample has been drawn from each population with respective sample

TABLE 9.2

Type of Test	Recommended Test Statistic
Global association	LR (S for large no. parameters)
Partial association	W (LR or S if problem with W)
Lack of fit, 1 d.f.	W or S
Lack of fit, > 1 d.f.	S
Inclusion of additional predictors	S

sizes n_1 and n_2. The sample values are denoted by $Y_{i1}, \ldots, Y_{in_i}, i = 1$ or 2. Let

$$s_1 = \sum_{j=1}^{n_1} Y_{1j} \qquad s_2 = \sum_{j=1}^{n_2} Y_{2j}, \tag{9.37}$$

the respective observed number of "successes" in the two samples. Let us test the null hypothesis $H_0 : P_1 = P_2$ based on the two samples.

The likelihood function is

$$L = \prod_{i=1}^{2} \prod_{j=1}^{n_i} P_i^{Y_{ij}} (1 - P_i)^{1 - Y_{ij}}$$

$$= \prod_{i=1}^{2} P_i^{s_i} (1 - P_i)^{n_i - s_i} \tag{9.38}$$

$$\log L = \sum_{i=1}^{2} \{ s_i \log(P_i) + (n_i - s_i) \log(1 - P_i) \}. \tag{9.39}$$

Under $H_0, P_1 = P_2 = P$, so

$$\log L(H_0) = s \log(P) + (n - s) \log(1 - P), \tag{9.40}$$

where $s = s_1 + s_2, n = n_1 + n_2$. The (restricted) MLE of this common P is $p = s/n$ and $\log L$ at this value is $s \log(p) + (n - s) \log(1 - p)$.

Since the original unrestricted log likelihood function contains two terms with separate parameters, the two parts may be maximized separately giving MLEs

$$p_1 = s_1/n_1 \quad \text{and} \quad p_2 = s_2/n_2. \tag{9.41}$$

Log L evaluated at these (unrestricted) MLEs is

$$\begin{aligned} \log L = \; & s_1 \log(p_1) + (n_1 - s_1) \log(1 - p_1) \\ + \; & s_2 \log(p_2) + (n_2 - s_2) \log(1 - p_2). \end{aligned} \tag{9.42}$$

The likelihood ratio statistic for testing $H_0 : P_1 = P_2$ is then

$$
\begin{aligned}
LR \quad = \quad & -2\{s\log(p) + (n - s)\log(1 - p) \\
- \quad & [s_1\log(p_1) + (n_1 - s_1)\log(1 - p_1) \\
+ \quad & s_2\log(p_2) + (n_2 - s_2)\log(1 - p_2)]\}.
\end{aligned}
\tag{9.43}
$$

This statistic for large enough n_1 and n_2 has a χ^2 distribution with 1 d.f. since the null hypothesis involves the estimation of one less parameter than does the unrestricted case. This LR statistic is the likelihood ratio χ^2 statistic for a 2×2 contingency table. It can be shown that the corresponding score statistic is equivalent to the Pearson χ^2 statistic. With the use of a computer program, the better LR statistic can be used routinely over the Pearson χ^2 for testing hypotheses in contingency tables.

9.4   Iterative ML Estimation

In most cases, one cannot explicitly solve for MLEs but must use trial-and-error numerical methods on a computer to solve for parameter values B that maximize $\log L(B)$ or yield a score vector $U(B) = 0$. One of the fastest and most applicable methods for maximizing a function is the Newton–Raphson method, which is based on approximating $U(B)$ by a linear function of B in a small region. A starting estimate b^0 of the MLE b is made. The linear approximation (a first-order Taylor series approximation)

$$
U(b) = U(b^0) - I(b^0)(b - b^0)
\tag{9.44}
$$

is equated to 0 and solved by b yielding

$$
b = b^0 + I^{-1}(b^0)U(b^0).
\tag{9.45}
$$

The process is continued in like fashion. At the ith step the next estimate is obtained from the previous estimate using the formula

$$
b^{i+1} = b^i + I^{-1}(b^i)U(b^i).
\tag{9.46}
$$

If the log likelihood actually worsened at b^{i+1}, "step halving" is used; b^{i+1} is replaced with $(b^i + b^{i+1})/2$. Further step halving is done if the log likelihood still is worse than the log likelihood at b^i. At that point, the original iterative strategy is resumed. The Newton–Raphson iterations continue until the $-2\log$ likelihood changes by only a small amount over the previous iteration (say .025). The reasoning behind this stopping rule is that estimates of B that change the $-2\log$ likelihood by less than this amount do not affect statistical inference since $-2\log$ likelihood is on the χ^2 scale.

The Newton–Raphson algorithm has the extra benefit that at the last iteration (letting b now denote the estimate of B at the last iteration), an estimate of the variance–covariance matrix of b ($I^{-1}(b)$) has already been computed.

3

9.5   Robust Estimation of the Covariance Matrix

The estimator for the covariance matrix of b found in Section 9.3 assumes that the model is correctly specified in terms of distribution, regression assumptions, and independence assumptions. The model may be incorrect in a variety of ways such as nonindependence (e.g., repeated measurements within subjects), lack of fit (e.g., omitted covariable, incorrect covariable transformation, omitted interaction), and distributional (e.g., Y has a Γ distribution instead of a normal distribution). Variances and covariances, and hence confidence intervals and Wald tests, will be incorrect when these assumptions are violated.

For the case in which the observations are independent and identically distributed but other assumptions are possibly violated, Huber[213] provided a covariance matrix estimator that is consistent. His "sandwich" estimator is given by

$$H = I^{-1}(b)[\sum_{i=1}^{n} U_i U_i']I^{-1}(b), \qquad (9.47)$$

where $I(b)$ is the observed information matrix (Equation 9.24) and U_i is the vector of derivatives, with respect to all parameters, of the log likelihood component for the ith observation (assuming the log likelihood can be partitioned into per-observation contributions). For the normal multiple linear regression case, H was derived by White:[451]

$$(X'X)^{-1}[\sum_{i=1}^{n}(Y_i - X_ib)^2 X_i X_i'](X'X)^{-1}, \qquad (9.48)$$

where X is the design matrix (including an intercept if appropriate) and X_i is the vector of predictors (including an intercept) for the ith observation. This covariance estimator allows for any pattern of variances of $Y|X$ across observations. Note that even though H improves the bias of the covariance matrix of b, it may actually have larger mean squared error than the ordinary estimate in some cases due to increased variance.[118, 356]

4

When observations are dependent within clusters, and the number of observations within clusters is very small in comparison to the total sample size, a simple adjustment to Equation 9.47 can be used to derive appropriate covariance matrix estimates (see Lin [280, p. 2237], Rogers,[356] and Lee et al. [274, Eq. 5.1, p. 246]). One merely accumulates sums of elements of U within clusters before computing cross-product terms:

$$H_c = I^{-1}(b)[\sum_{i=1}^{c}\{(\sum_{j=1}^{n_i} U_{ij})(\sum_{j=1}^{n_i} U_{ij})'\}]I^{-1}(b), \qquad (9.49)$$

where c is the number of clusters, n_i is the number of observations in the ith cluster, U_{ij} is the contribution of the jth observation within the ith cluster to the score vector, and $I(b)$ is computed as before ignoring clusters. For a model such as the Cox model which has no per-observation score contributions, special score residuals[274, 280, 283, 412] are used for U.

Bootstrapping can also be used to derive robust covariance matrix estimates[129, 130] in many cases, especially if covariances of b that are not conditional on X are appropriate. One merely generates approximately 200 samples with replacement from the original dataset, computes 200 sets of parameter estimates, and computes the sample covariance matrix of these parameter estimates. Sampling with replacement from entire clusters can be used to derive variance estimates in the presence of intracluster correlation.[136] Bootstrap estimates of the conditional variance–covariance matrix given X are harder to obtain and depend on the model assumptions being satisfied. The simpler unconditional estimates may be more appropriate for many nonexperimental studies where one may desire to "penalize" for the X being random variables. It is interesting that these unconditional estimates may be very difficult to obtain parametrically, since a multivariate distribution may need to be assumed for X.

⑤

The previous discussion addresses the use of a "working independence model" with clustered data. Here one estimates regression coefficients assuming independence of all records (observations). Then a sandwich or bootstrap method is used to increase standard errors to reflect some redundancy in the correlated observations. The parameter estimates will often be consistent estimates of the true parameter values, but they may be inefficient for certain cluster or correlation structures.

⑥

The **Design** library's robcov function computes the Huber robust covariance matrix estimator, and the **bootcov** function computes the bootstrap covariance estimator. Both of these functions allow for clustering of data.

9.6 Wald, Score, and Likelihood-Based Confidence Intervals

A $1 - \alpha$ confidence interval for a parameter β_i is the set of all values β_i^0 that if hypothesized would be accepted in a test of $H_0 : \beta_i = \beta_i^0$ at the α level. What test should form the basis for the confidence interval? The Wald test is most frequently used because of its simplicity. A two-sided $1 - \alpha$ confidence interval is $b_i \pm z_{1-\alpha/2}s$, where z is the critical value from the normal distribution and s is the estimated standard error of the parameter estimate b_i.[a] The problem with s discussed in Section 9.3.3 points out that Wald statistics may not always be a good basis. Wald-based confidence intervals are also symmetric even though the coverage probability may not be.[115] Score- and LR-based confidence limits have definite advantages. When Wald-type confidence intervals are appropriate, the analyst may consider insertion of robust covariance estimates (Section 9.5) into the confidence interval formulas (note that adjustments for heterogeneity and correlated observations are not available for score and LR statistics).

Wald– (asymptotic normality) based statistics are convenient for deriving confidence intervals for linear or more complex combinations of the model's parameters. As in Equation 9.35, the variance–covariance matrix of Cb, where C is an appropriate matrix and b is the vector of parameter estimates, is CVC', where V is the variance matrix of b. In regression models we commonly substitute a vector of predictors (and optional intercept) for C to obtain the variance of the linear predictor Xb as

$$\text{var}(Xb) = XVX'. \tag{9.50}$$

The confidence intervals just discussed are *pointwise* confidence intervals. For some promising techniques for constructing *simultaneous* confidence intervals over a whole range of an X_i, see Lane and DuMouchel[257] as well as the bootstrap method described below.

9.7   Bootstrap Confidence Regions

A more nonparametric method for computing confidence intervals for functions of the vector of parameters B can be based on the bootstrap. For each sample with replacement from the original dataset, one computes the MLE of B, b, and then the quantity of interest $g(b)$. Then the gs are sorted and the desired quantiles are computed. At least 1000 bootstrap samples will be needed for accurate assessment of outer confidence limits. This method is suitable for obtaining pointwise confidence bands for a nonlinear regression function, say, the relationship between age and the log odds of disease. At each of, say, 100 age values, the predicted logits are computed for each bootstrap sample. Then separately for each age point the 0.025 and 0.975 quantiles of 1000 estimates of the logit are computed to derive a 0.95

---

[a]This is the basis for confidence limits computed by the S-PLUS `Design` library's `plot.Design` and `summary.Design` functions. When the `robcov` function has been used to replace the information-matrix-based covariance matrix with a Huber robust covariance estimate with an optional cluster sampling correction, `plot.Design` and `summary.Design` are using a "robust" Wald statistic basis. When the `bootcov` function has been used to replace the model fit's covariance matrix with a bootstrap unconditional covariance matrix estimate, the two functions are computing confidence limits based on a normal distribution but using more nonparametric covariance estimates.

confidence band. Other more complex bootstrap schemes will achieve somewhat greater accuracy of confidence interval coverage,[130] and as described in Section 9.5 one can use variations on the basic bootstrap in which the predictors are considered fixed and/or cluster sampling is taken into account. The S-PLUS function `bootcov` in the `Design` library bootstraps model fits to obtain unconditional (with respect to predictors) bootstrap distributions with or without cluster sampling. `bootcov` will store a matrix of bootstrap regression coefficients so that the bootstrapped quantities of interest can be computed in one sweep of the coefficient matrix once bootstrapping is completed.

Tibshirani and Knight[417] developed a promising and easy to program approach for deriving simultaneous confidence sets that is likely to be useful for getting simultaneous confidence regions for the entire vector of model parameters, for population values for an entire sequence of predictor values, and for a set of regression effects (e.g., interquartile-range odds ratios for age for both sexes). The basic idea is that during the, say, 1000 bootstrap repetitions one stores the -2 log likelihood for each model fit, being careful to compute the likelihood at the current bootstrap parameter estimates but with respect to the *original* data matrix, not the bootstrap sample of the data matrix. To obtain an approximate simultaneous 0.95 confidence set one computes the 0.95 quantile of the -2 log likelihood values and determines which vectors of parameter estimates correspond to -2 log likelihoods that are at least as small as the 0.95 quantile of all -2 log likelihoods. Once the qualifying parameter estimates are found, the quantities of interest are computed from those parameter estimates and an outer envelope of those quantities is found.

As an example, 1000 sets of simulated random normal variate vectors, all independent and with mean 0 and variance 1, were generated, with 300 subjects per simulation. X values ranging from $1, 2, \ldots, 30$ were duplicated 10 times per simulation, and a five-knot restricted cubic spline was fitted between these Xs and the random Ys whereas the true population regression function is a flat line through the origin. The simultaneous confidence region was derived by computing, separately for each of 100 X values between 1 and 30, the overall minima and maxima of the qualifying spline fits. The simulations used Harrell's `rm.boot` function in the `Hmisc` library, which computes simultaneous confidence regions for repeated measurements data using spline functions to describe time trends. Five hundred bootstrap repetitions (sampling with replacement from regression residuals since X was considered fixed) were used for each of the 1000 samples. The number of times that the 0.95 confidence bands everywhere included the flat line was 905 so the estimated coverage probability is 0.905 (exact 0.95 confidence interval $[0.885, 0.922]$). The coverage is thus not exactly 0.95 as intended but it is close. The S-PLUS code for this simulation follows.

```
> null.in.region ← 0
> time ← rep(1:30, 10)
> for(i in 1:1000) {
+    y    ← rnorm(300)
```

```
+
+    f ← rm.boot(time, y, B=500, nk=5, bootstrap.type='x fixed')
+    g ← plot(f, ylim=c(-1,1), pointwise=F)
+ # The plot method for objects created by rm.boot returns
+ # coordinates of points that were plotted
+
+    null.in.region ← null.in.region +
+                     all(g$lower <=0 & g$upper >= 0)
+ }
> print(null.in.region)
```

Two functions that are associated with the Design library's bootcov function, bootplot and confplot, make it relatively easy to plot bootstrap distributions and pointwise and simultaneous regions for many regression models. As an example, consider 200 simulated x values from a log-normal distribution and simulate binary y from a true population binary logistic model given by

$$\text{Prob}(Y = 1|X = x) = \frac{1}{1 + \exp[-(1 + x/2)]}. \tag{9.51}$$

Not knowing the true model, a quadratic logistic model is fitted. The S-PLUS code needed to generate the data and fit the model is given below.

```
> library(Design,T)
> set.seed(191)

> x ← exp(rnorm(200))
> logit ← 1 + x/2
> y ← ifelse(runif(200) <= plogis(logit), 1, 0)
> dd ← datadist(x)
> options(datadist='dd')

> f ← lrm(y ~ pol(x,2), x=T, y=T)
> f
```

Frequencies of Responses
```
  0   1
 31 169
```

Obs	Max Deriv	Model L.R.	d.f.	P	C	Dxy	Gamma	Tau-a
200	0.001	6.37	2	0.0413	0.63	0.261	0.31	0.069

R2	Brier
0.054	0.128

	Coef	S.E.	Wald Z	P
Intercept	1.5031	0.4405	3.41	0.0006
x	-0.1245	0.6318	-0.20	0.8438
x^2	0.1190	0.1627	0.73	0.4644

```
> anova(f)
```

```
        Wald Statistics          Response: y

Factor      Chi-Square d.f.       P
x              2.31       2     0.315
  Nonlinear 0.54         1     0.464
TOTAL        2.31         2     0.315
```

Note the disagreement between the overall Wald χ^2 of 2.31 and the LR χ^2 of 6.37, which is a warning that the log likelihood function may be very nonquadratic, so normal theory-based confidence limits may not be appropriate. The `bootcov` function is used to do 1000 resamples to obtain bootstrap estimates of the covariance matrix of the regression coefficients as well as to save the 1000×3 matrix of regression coefficients. Then, because individual regression coefficients for x do not tell us much, we summarize the x-effect by computing the effect (on the logit scale) of increasing x from 1 to 5. First we plot the bootstrap distribution using a histogram and a kernel density estimator, then we compute nonparametric confidence limits by computing sample quantiles of the 1000 log odds ratios.

```
> b ← bootcov(f, B=1000, coef.reps=T)

> # Get x=5 : x=1 log odds ratio and its 0.95 confidence
> # limits using the information matrix and normal theory
> s ← summary(f, x=c(1,5))
> s
```

```
            Factor Low High Diff. Effect S.E. Lower 0.95 Upper 0.95
x                1   5    4     2.36  1.8    -1.17        5.89
  Odds Ratio 1   5    4    10.57  NA     0.31      360.84
```

```
> # Get 2-row design matrix for obtaining predicted values
> # for x = 1 and 5
> X ← predict(f, data.frame(x=c(1,5)), type='x')
> X
  Intercept x x^2
1         1 1   1
2         1 5  25
```

```
> # Plot distribution of x = 5:1 log odds ratios and
> # get 3 nonparametric bootstrap confidence intervals for them
> # Get X1*beta - X2*beta using (X1-X2)*beta
> conf ← c(.9, .95, .99)
```

```
> Xdif ← X[2,,drop=F] - X[1,,drop=F]
> Xdif
  Intercept x x^2
          0 4  24
```

```
> bootplot(b, X=Xdif, conf.int=conf, xlim=c(-2,12),
+          labels='x=5 : x=1 Log Odds Ratio')
+          mult.width=.5, breaks=c(seq(0,12,by=.5),70))
> # Defaults for mult.width, breaks did not do well here
```

The 1000 bootstrap estimates of the log odds ratio are computed easily using a single matrix multiplication, and we obtain the bootstrap estimate of the standard error of the log odds ratio by computing the sample standard deviation of the 1000 values. As indicated below, this standard deviation can also be obtained by using the summary function on the object returned by bootcov, as bootcov returns a fit object like one from lrm except with the bootstrap covariance matrix substituted for the information-based one.

```
> boot.log.odds.ratio ← b$boot.Coef %*% t(Xdif)
> sd ← sqrt(var(boot.log.odds.ratio))
> sd
3.55
> # This is the same as summary(b, x=c(1,5))[1,'S.E.']

> # Compare this s.d. with one from information matrix
> s[1,'S.E.']
1.8

> # Draw normal density that has same mean and s.d. as
> # bootstrap distribution
> z ← seq(-2,12,length=100)
> lines(z, dnorm(z, mean=mean(boot.log.odds.ratio), sd=sd), lty=2)

> crit ← qnorm((conf+1)/2)
> clim ← s[1,'Effect'] + c(-sd * crit, sd * crit)
> # Put triangles near x-axis for these C.L.
> w ← rep(-.005,2)
> points(clim, rep(w,3), pch=2)
> # Note: left confidence limits are off the scale

> # Add circles for traditional Wald-based C.L.
> points(s[1,c('Lower 0.95','Upper 0.95')], w, pch=1)
> s99 ← summary(f, x=c(1,5), conf.int=.99)
> points(s99[1,c('Lower 0.99','Upper 0.99')], w, pch=1)
> s90 ← summary(f, x=c(1,5), conf.int=.90)
> points(s90[1,c('Lower 0.9','Upper 0.9')], w, pch=1)
```

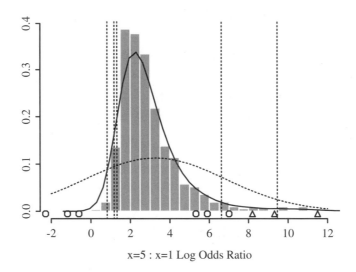

x=5 : x=1 Log Odds Ratio

FIGURE 9.4: Bootstrap distribution of the $x = 5 : x = 1$ log odds ratio from a quadratic logistic model with highly skewed x. The solid curve is a kernel density estimate, and the dashed curve is a normal density with the same mean and standard deviation as the bootstrapped values. Vertical lines indicate asymmetric $0.9, 0.95$, and 0.99 two-sided confidence limits for the log odds ratio based on quantiles of the bootstrap values. The upper 0.99 confidence limit of 18.99 is not shown with a line. Triangles indicate corresponding symmetric confidence limits obtained assuming normality of estimates but using the bootstrap estimate of the standard error. The left limits for these are off the scale because of the high variance of the bootstrap estimates. Circles indicate confidence limits based on the usual normal theory-information matrix method.

```
>  # Finally, compare with s.d. using Huber's sandwich
>  # covariance estimator (0.99)
>  summary(robcov(f), x=c(1,5))
```

	Factor	Low	High	Diff.	Effect	S.E.	Lower 0.95	Upper 0.95
x		1	5	4	2.36	0.99	0.43	4.29
Odds Ratio	1	5	4		10.57	NA	1.53	72.95

The resulting graph is shown in Figure 9.4. The high variance of the normal density resulted from some high outliers in the bootstrap values. This resulted in symmetric bootstrap confidence intervals that are too wide. The extreme asymmetry of nonparametric confidence limits based on quantiles of the bootstrap distribution, as indicated by the placement of the vertical lines, is apparent. These more accurate and robust confidence limits strongly disagree with symmetric confidence limits,

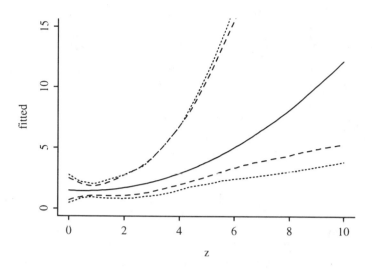

FIGURE 9.5: Simultaneous (outer dotted lines) and pointwise (inner dashed lines) 0.95 asymmetric bootstrap confidence bands for the regression function.

derived from normal theory using either information matrix or bootstrap standard deviations.

Now consider confidence bands for the true log odds that $y = 1$, across a sequence of x values (stored in the vector z below). First, the full design matrix corresponding to this sequence of x values is computed. This matrix is used to summarize the matrix of bootstrap regression coefficients.

```
> z ← seq(0, 10, length=100)
> X ← predict(f, data.frame(x=z), type='x')
> X[1:5,]
```

```
  Intercept    x      x^2
1         1 0.000 0.00000
2         1 0.101 0.01020
3         1 0.202 0.04081
4         1 0.303 0.09183
5         1 0.404 0.16325
```

```
> confplot(b, X, against=z, ylim=c(0,15))
> confplot(b, X, against=z, method='pointwise', add=T, lty.conf=3)
```

The results appear in Figure 9.5.

9.8   Further Use of the Log Likelihood

9.8.1   Rating Two Models, Penalizing for Complexity

Suppose that from a single sample two competing models were developed. Let the respective -2 log likelihoods for these models be denoted by L_1 and L_2, and let p_1 and p_2 denote the number of parameters estimated in each model. Suppose that $L_1 < L_2$. It may be tempting to rate model one as the "best" fitting or "best" predicting model. That model may provide a better fit for the data at hand, but if it required many more parameters to be estimated, it may not be better "for the money." If both models were applied to a new sample, model one's overfitting of the original dataset may actually result in a worse fit on the new dataset.

Akaike's information criterion (AIC[26, 433]) provides a method for penalizing the log likelihood achieved by a given model for its complexity to obtain a more unbiased assessment of the model's worth. The penalty is to subtract the number of parameters estimated from the log likelihood, or equivalently to add twice the number of parameters to the -2 log likelihood. The penalized log likelihood is analogous to Mallow's C_p in ordinary multiple regression. AIC would choose the model by comparing $L_1 + 2p_1$ to $L_2 + 2p_2$ and picking the model with the lower value. We use AIC in "adjusted χ^2" form: 9

$$AIC = LR\ \chi^2 - 2p. \tag{9.52}$$

Breiman [46, Section 1.3] and Chatfield [69, Section 4] discuss the fallacy of AIC and C_p for selecting from a series of nonprespecified models.

Schwarz[379] derived a different penalty using large-sample Bayesian properties of competing models. His Bayesian Information Criterion (BIC) chooses the model having the lowest value of $L + 1/2p\log n$ or the highest value of LR $\chi^2 - p\log n$. Kass and Raftery [231, p. 790] provide a nice review of this topic, stating that "AIC   10 picks the correct model asymptotically if the complexity of the true model grows with sample size" and that "AIC selects models that are too big even when the sample size is large." But they also cite other papers that show the existence of cases where AIC can work better than BIC. According to Buckland et al.,[55] BIC "assumes that a true model exists and is low-dimensional."

Hurvich and Tsai[215, 216] made an improvement in AIC that resulted in much better model selection for small n. They defined the corrected AIC as

$$AIC_C = LR\ \chi^2 - 2p[1 + \frac{p+1}{n-p-1}]. \tag{9.53}$$

In [215] they contrast asymptotically efficient model selection with AIC when the true model has infinitely many parameters with improvements using other indexes such as AIC_C when the model is finite.

One difficulty in applying the Schwarz, AIC_C, and related criteria is that with censored or binary responses it is not clear that the actual sample size n should be used in the formula.

9.8.2 Testing Whether One Model Is Better than Another

One way to test whether one model (A) is better than another (B) is to embed both models in a more general model $(A + B)$. Then a $LR \ \chi^2$ test can be done to test whether A is better than B by changing the hypothesis to test whether A adds predictive information to B $(H_0 : A + B > B)$ and whether B adds information to A $(H_0 : A + B > A)$. The approach of testing $A > B$ via testing $A + B > B$ and $A + B > A$ is especially useful for selecting from competing predictors such as a multivariable model and a subjective assessor.[91, 180, 276, 455]

Note that $LR \ \chi^2$ for $H_0 : A + B > B$ minus $LR \ \chi^2$ for $H_0 : A + B > A$ equals $LR \ \chi^2$ for $H_0 : A$ has no predictive information minus $LR \ \chi^2$ for $H_0 : B$ has no predictive information,[453] the difference in $LR \ \chi^2$ for testing each model (set of variables) separately. This gives further support to the use of two separately computed Akaike's information criteria for rating the two sets of variables.   11

See Section 9.8.4 for an example.

9.8.3 Unitless Index of Predictive Ability

The global likelihood ratio test for regression is useful for determining whether any predictor is associated with the response. If the sample is large enough, even weak associations can be "statistically significant." Even though a likelihood ratio test does not shed light on a model's predictive strength, the log likelihood (L.L.) can still be useful here. Consider the following L.L.s:

Best (lowest) possible -2 L.L.:
  $L^* = -2$ L.L. for a hypothetical model that perfectly predicts the outcome.

-2 L.L. achieved:
  $L = -2$ L.L. for the fitted model.

Worst -2 L.L.
  $L^0 = -2$ L.L. for a model that has no predictive information.

The last -2 L.L., for a "no information" model, is the -2 L.L. under the null hypothesis that all regression coefficients except for intercepts are zero. A "no information" model often contains only an intercept and some distributional parameters (a variance, for example).   12

The quantity $L^0 - L$ is LR, the log likelihood ratio statistic for testing the global null hypothesis that no predictors are related to the response. It is also the $-2 \log$

likelihood "explained" by the model. The best (lowest) -2 L.L. is L^*, so the amount of L.L. that is capable of being explained by the model is $L^0 - L^*$. The fraction of -2 L.L. explained that was capable of being explained is

$$(L^0 - L)/(L^0 - L^*) \quad = \quad LR/(L^0 - L^*). \tag{9.54}$$

The fraction of log likelihood explained is analogous to R^2 in an ordinary linear model, although Korn and Simon[248, 249] provide a much more precise notion.

Akaike's information criterion can be used to penalize this measure of association for the number of parameters estimated (p, say) to transform this unitless measure of association into a quantity that is analogous to the adjusted R^2 or Mallow's C_p in ordinary linear regression. We let R denote the square root of such a penalized fraction of log likelihood explained. R is defined by

$$R^2 = (LR - 2p)/(L_0 - L^*). \tag{9.55}$$

The R index can be used to assess how well the model compares to a "perfect" model, as well as to judge whether a more complex model has predictive strength that justifies its additional parameters. Had p been used in Equation 9.55 rather than $2p$, R^2 is negative if the log likelihood explained is less than what one would expect by chance. R will be the square root of $1 - 2p/(L_0 - L^*)$ if the model perfectly predicts the response. This upper limit will be near one if the sample size is large.

Partial R indexes can also be defined by substituting the -2 L.L. explained for a given factor in place of that for the entire model, LR. The "penalty factor" p becomes one. This index R_{partial} is defined by

$$R^2_{\text{partial}} = (LR_{\text{partial}} - 2)/(L_0 - L^*), \tag{9.56}$$

which is the (penalized) fraction of -2 log likelihood explained by the predictor. Here LR_{partial} is the log likelihood ratio statistic for testing whether the predictor is associated with the response, after adjustment for the other predictors. Since such likelihood ratio statistics are tedious to compute, the 1 d.f. Wald χ^2 can be substituted for the LR statistic (keeping in mind that difficulties with the Wald statistic can arise).

Liu and Dyer[293] and Cox and Wermuth[96] point out difficulties with the R^2 measure for binary logistic models. Cox and Snell[95] and Magee[298] used other analogies to derive other R^2 measures that may have better properties. For a sample of size n and a Wald statistic for testing overall association, they defined

$$\begin{aligned} R^2_{\text{W}} &= \frac{W}{n + W} \\ R^2_{\text{LR}} &= 1 - \exp(-LR/n) \\ &= 1 - \lambda^{2/n}, \end{aligned} \tag{9.57}$$

TABLE 9.3

Predictors Used	$LR\ \chi^2$	Adequacy
Coronary jeopardy score	42.6	0.74
Maximum % stenosis in each artery	51.8	0.90
Combined	57.5	1.00

where λ is the null model likelihood divided by the fitted model likelihood. In the case of ordinary least squares with normality both of the above indexes are equal to the traditional R^2. R^2_{LR} is equivalent to Maddala's index [297, Eq. 2.44]. Cragg and Uhler[97] and Nagelkerke[322] suggested dividing R^2_{LR} by its maximum attainable value

$$R^2_{\max} = 1 - \exp(-L^0/n) \tag{9.58}$$

to derive R^2_N which ranges from 0 to 1. This is the form of the R^2 index we use throughout.

For penalizing for overfitting, see Verweij and van Houwelingen[437] for a cross-validated R^2 that uses a cross-validated likelihood.   [13]

9.8.4   Unitless Index of Adequacy of a Subset of Predictors

log likelihoods are also useful for quantifying the predictive information contained in a subset of the predictors compared with the information contained in the entire set of predictors.[180] Let LR again denote the -2 log likelihood ratio statistic for testing the joint significance of the full set of predictors. Let LR^s denote the -2 log likelihood ratio statistic for testing the importance of the subset of predictors of interest, excluding the other predictors from the model. A measure of adequacy of the subset for predicting the response is given by

$$A = LR^s/LR. \tag{9.59}$$

A is then the proportion of log likelihood explained by the subset with reference to the log likelihood explained by the entire set. When $A = 1$, the subset contains all the predictive information found in the whole set of predictors; that is, the subset is adequate by itself and the additional predictors contain no independent information. When $A = 0$, the subset contains no predictive information by itself.

Califf et al.[62] used the A index to quantify the adequacy (with respect to prognosis) of two competing sets of predictors that each describe the extent of coronary artery disease. The response variable was time until cardiovascular death and the statistical model used was the Cox[92] proportional hazards model. Some of their results are reproduced in Table 9.3. A chance-corrected adequacy measure could be derived by squaring the ratio of the R-index for the subset to the R-index for the whole set. A formal test of superiority of X_1 = maximum % stenosis over

X_2 = jeopardy score can be obtained by testing whether X_1 adds to X_2 ($LR\ \chi^2 =$ 57.5 − 42.6 = 14.9) and whether X_2 adds to X_1 ($LR\ \chi^2 =$ 57.5 − 51.8 = 5.7). X_1 adds more to X_2 (14.9) than X_2 adds to X_1 (5.7). The difference 14.9 − 5.7 = 9.2 equals the difference in single factor χ^2 (51.8 − 42.6).[453]

9.9   Weighted Maximum Likelihood Estimation

It is commonly the case that data elements represent combinations of values that pertain to a set of individuals. This occurs, for example, when unique combinations of X and Y are determined from a massive dataset, along with the frequency of occurrence of each combination, for the purpose of reducing the size of the dataset to analyze. For the ith combination we have a *case weight* w_i that is a positive integer representing a frequency. Assuming that observations represented by combination i are independent, the likelihood needed to represent all w_i observations is computed simply by multiplying all of the likelihood elements (each having value L_i), yielding a total likelihood contribution for combination i of $L_i^{w_i}$ or a log likelihood contribution of $w_i \log L_i$. To obtain a likelihood for the entire dataset one computes the product over all combinations. The total log likelihood is $\sum w_i \log L_i$. As an example, the weighted likelihood that would be used to fit a weighted logistic regression model is given by

$$L = \prod_{i=1}^{n} P_i^{w_i Y_i}(1 - P_i)^{w_i(1-Y_i)}, \qquad (9.60)$$

where there are n combinations, $\sum_{i=1}^{n} w_i > n$, and P_i is Prob[$Y_i = 1|X_i$] as dictated by the model. Note that the correct likelihood function cannot be obtained by weighting the data and using an unweighted likelihood.

By a small leap one can obtain weighted maximum likelihood estimates from the above method even if the weights do not represent frequencies or even integers, as long as the weights are nonnegative. Nonfrequency weights are commonly used in sample surveys to adjust estimates back to better represent a target population when some types of subjects have been oversampled from that population. Analysts should beware of possible losses in efficiency when obtaining weighted estimates in sample surveys.[246, 247] Making the regression estimates conditional on sampling strata by including strata as covariables may be preferable to reweighting the strata. If weighted estimates must be obtained, the weighted likelihood function is generally valid for obtaining properly weighted parameter estimates. However, the variance–covariance matrix obtained by inverting the information matrix from the weighted likelihood will not be correct in general. For one thing, the sum of the weights may be far from the number of subjects in the sample. A rough approximation to the variance–covariance matrix may be obtained by first dividing each weight by $n/\sum w_i$ and then computing the weighted information matrix, where n is the number of actual subjects in the sample. ⌐14⌐

9.10   Penalized Maximum Likelihood Estimation

Maximizing the log likelihood provides the best fit to the dataset at hand, but this can also result in fitting noise in the data. For example, a categorical predictor with 20 levels can produce extreme estimates for some of the 19 regression parameters, especially for the small cells (see Section 4.5). A shrinkage approach will often result in regression coefficient estimates that while biased are lower in mean squared error and hence are more likely to be close to the true unknown parameter values. Ridge regression is one approach to shrinkage, but a more general and better developed approach is penalized maximum likelihood estimation,[161, 269, 436, 438] which is really a special case of Bayesian modeling with a Gaussian prior. Letting L denote the usual likelihood function and λ be a penalty factor, we maximize the penalized log likelihood given by

$$\log L - \frac{1}{2}\lambda \sum_{i=1}^{p}(s_i\beta_i)^2, \tag{9.61}$$

where $s_1, s_2, \ldots, s_p$ are scale factors chosen to make $s_i\beta_i$ unitless. Most authors standardize the data first and do not have scale factors in the equation, but Equation 9.61 has the advantage of allowing estimation of β on the original scale of the data. The usual methods (e.g., Newton–Raphson) are used to maximize 9.61.

The choice of the scaling constants has received far too little attention in the ridge regression and penalized MLE literature. It is common to use the standard deviation of each column of the design matrix to scale the corresponding parameter. For models containing nothing but continuous variables that enter the regression linearly, this is usually a reasonable approach. For continuous variables represented with multiple terms (one of which is linear), it is not always reasonable to scale each nonlinear term with its own standard deviation. For dummy variables, scaling using the standard deviation ($\sqrt{d(1-d)}$, where d is the mean of the dummy variable, i.e., the fraction of observations in that cell) is problematic since this will result in high prevalence cells getting more shrinkage than low prevalence ones because the high prevalence cells will dominate the penalty function.

An advantage of the formulation in Equation 9.61 is that one can assign scale constants of zero for parameters for which no shrinkage is desired.[161, 436] For example, one may have prior beliefs that a linear additive model will fit the data. In that case, nonlinear and nonadditive terms may be penalized.

For a categorical predictor having c levels, users of ridge regression often do not recognize that the amount of shrinkage and the predicted values from the fitted model depend on how the design matrix is coded. For example, one will get different predictions depending on which cell is chosen as the reference cell when constructing dummy variables. The setup in Equation 9.61 has the same problem. For example, if for a three-category factor we use category 1 as the reference cell and have parameters β_2 and β_3, the unscaled penalty function is $\beta_2^2 + \beta_3^2$. If category 3 were used as the reference cell instead, the penalty would be $\beta_3^2 + (\beta_2 - \beta_3)^2$. To get around this problem, Verweij and van Houwelingen[436] proposed using the penalty function $\sum_i^c (\beta_i - \overline{\beta})^2$, where $\overline{\beta}$ is the mean of all c βs. This causes shrinkage of all parameters toward the mean parameter value. Letting the first category be the reference cell, we use $c-1$ dummy variables and define $\beta_1 \equiv 0$. For the case $c = 3$ the sum of squares is $2[\beta_2^2 + \beta_3^2 - \beta_2\beta_3]/3$. For $c = 2$ the penalty is $\beta_2^2/2$. If no scale constant is used, this is the same as scaling β_2 with $\sqrt{2} \times$ the standard deviation of a binary dummy variable with prevalance of 0.5.

The sum of squares can be written in matrix form as $[\beta_2, \ldots, \beta_c]'(A-B)[\beta_2, \ldots, \beta_c]$, where A is a $c-1 \times c-1$ identity matrix and B is a $c-1 \times c-1$ matrix all of whose elements are $\frac{1}{c}$.

For general penalty functions such as that just described, the penalized log likelihood can be generalized to

$$\log L - \frac{1}{2}\lambda\beta'P\beta. \tag{9.62}$$

For purposes of using the Newton–Raphson procedure, the first derivative of the penalty function with respect to β is $-\lambda P\beta$, and the negative of the second derivative is λP.

Another problem in penalized estimation is how the choice of λ is made. Many authors use cross-validation. A limited number of simulation studies in binary logistic regression modeling has shown that for each λ being considered, at least 10-fold cross-validation must be done so as to obtain a reasonable estimate of predictive accuracy. Even then, a smoother[146] ("super smoother") must be used on the (λ, accuracy) pairs to allow location of the optimum value unless one is careful in choosing the initial subsamples and uses these same splits throughout. Simulation studies have shown that a modified AIC is not only much quicker to compute (since it requires no cross-validation) but performs better at finding a good value of λ (see below).

For a given λ, the effective number of parameters being estimated is reduced because of shrinkage. Gray [161, Eq. 2.9] and others estimate the effective degrees of freedom by computing the expected value of a global Wald statistic for testing association, when the null hypothesis of no association is true. The d.f. is equal to

$$\text{trace}[I(\hat{\beta}^P)V(\hat{\beta}^P)], \tag{9.63}$$

where $\hat{\beta}^P$ is the penalized MLE (the parameters that maximize Equation 9.61), I is the information matrix computed from ignoring the penalty function, and V is the covariance matrix computed by inverting the information matrix that included the second derivatives with respect to β in the penalty function.

Gray [161, Eq. 2.6] states that a better estimate of the variance–covariance matrix for $\hat{\beta}^P$ than $V(\hat{\beta}^P)$ is

$$V^* = V(\hat{\beta}^P)I(\hat{\beta}^P)V(\hat{\beta}^P). \tag{9.64}$$

Therneau (personal communication, 2000) has found in a limited number of simulation studies that V^* underestimates the true variances, and that a better estimate of the variance–covariance matrix is simply $V(\hat{\beta}^P)$, assuming that the model is correctly specified. This is the covariance matrix used by default in the **Design** library (the user can specifically request that the sandwich estimator be used instead) and is in fact the one Gray used for Wald tests.

Penalization will bias estimates of β, so hypothesis tests and confidence intervals using $\hat{\beta}^P$ may not have a simple interpretation. The same problem arises in score and likelihood ratio tests.

Equation 9.63 can be used to derive a modified AIC (see [436, Eq. 6] and [438, Eq. 7]) on the model χ^2 scale:

$$\text{LR } \chi^2 - 2 \times \text{ effective d.f.,} \tag{9.65}$$

where LR χ^2 is the likelihood ratio χ^2 for the penalized model, but ignoring the penalty function. If a variety of λ are tried and one plots the (λ, AIC) pairs, the λ that maximizes AIC will often be a good choice, that is, it is likely to be near the value of λ that maximizes predictive accuracy on a future dataset.

Several examples from simulated datasets have shown that using BIC to choose a penalty results in far too much shrinkage.

Note that if one does penalized maximum likelihood estimation where a set of variables being penalized has a negative value for the unpenalized $\chi^2 - 2 \times$ d.f., the value of λ that will optimize the overall model AIC will be ∞.

As an example, consider some simulated data $(n = 100)$ with one predictor in which the true model is $Y = X_1 + \epsilon$, where ϵ has a standard normal distribution and so does X_1. We use a series of penalties (found by trial and error) that give rise to sensible effective d.f., and fit penalized restricted cubic spline functions with five knots. We penalize two ways: all terms in the model including the coefficient of X_1, which in reality needs no penalty; and only the nonlinear terms. The following S-PLUS program, in conjunction with the **Design** library, does the job.

```
library(Design, T)
set.seed(191)
x1 ← rnorm(100)
y  ← x1 + rnorm(100)

pens ← df ← aic ← c(0,.07,.5,2,6,15)
par(mfrow=c(1,2))

for(penalize in 1:2) {
  for(i in 1:length(pens)) {
      f ← ols(y ~ rcs(x1,5), penalty=
              list(simple=if(penalize==1)pens[i] else 0,
                   nonlinear=pens[i]))
      plot(f, x1=seq(-2.5, 2.5, length=100), add=i>1)
```

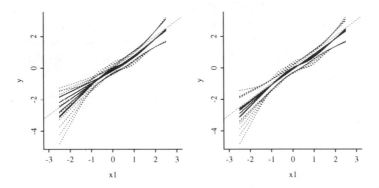

FIGURE 9.6: Penalized least squares estimates for an unnecessary five-knot restricted cubic spline function. In the left graph all parameters (except the intercept) are penalized. The effective d.f. are $4, 3.06, 2.59, 2.22, 1.99$, and 1.78. In the right graph, only parameters associated with nonlinear functions of X_1 are penalized. The effective d.f. are $4, 3.07, 2.60, 2.24, 2.04$, and 1.89.

```
        df[i] ← f$stats['d.f.']
        aic[i] ← f$stats['Model L.R.']-2*df[i]
    }
    abline(a=0,b=1,lty=2,lwd=1)
    print(rbind(df=df, aic=aic))
}
```

The plots are shown in Figure 9.6. The left graph corresponds to `penalty = list(simple=a, nonlinear=a)` in the S-PLUS program, meaning that all parameters except the intercept are shrunk by the same amount `a` (this would be more appropriate had there been multiple predictors). As effective d.f. get smaller (penalty factor gets larger), the regression fits get flatter (too flat for the largest penalties) and confidence bands get narrower. The right graph corresponds to `penalty=list(simple=0, nonlinear=a)`, causing only the cubic spline terms that are nonlinear in X_1 to be shrunk. As the amount of shrinkage increases (d.f. lowered), the fits become more linear and closer to the true regression line (longer dotted line). Again, confidence intervals become smaller.   16

9.11   Further Reading

1   Boos[42] has some nice generalizations of the score test.

2   See Marubini and Valsecchi [306, pp. 164–169] for an excellent description of the relationship between the three types of test statistics.

3   References [79, 340] have good descriptions of methods used to maximize $\log L$.

4   As Long and Ervin[294] argue, for small sample sizes, the usual Huber–White covariance estimator should not be used because there the residuals do not have constant variance even under homoscedasticity. They showed that a simple correction due to Efron and others can result in substantially better estimates. Lin and Wei,[283] Binder,[39] and Lin[280] have applied the Huber estimator to the Cox[92] survival model.

5   Feng et al.[136] showed that in the case of cluster correlations arising from repeated measurement data with Gaussian errors, the cluster bootstrap performs excellently even when the number of observations per cluster is large and the number of subjects is small.

6   Graubard and Korn[159] and Fitzmaurice[139] describe the kinds of situations in which the working independence model can be trusted.

7   Minkin,[317] Alho,[8] Doganaksoy and Schmee,[115] and Meeker and Escobar[311] discuss the need for LR and score-based confidence intervals. Alho found that score-based intervals are usually more tedious to compute, and provided useful algorithms for the computation of either type of interval (see also [311] and [306, p. 167]). Score and LR intervals require iterative computations and have to deal with the fact that when one parameter is changed (e.g., b_i is restricted to be zero), all other parameter estimates change. DiCiccio and Efron[113] provide a method for very accurate confidence intervals for exponential families that requires a modest amount of additional computation. Venzon and Moolgavkar provide an efficient general method for computing LR-based intervals.[435]

8   Carpenter and Bithell[63] have an excellent overview of several variations on the bootstrap for obtaining confidence limits.

9   van Houwelingen and le Cessie [433, Eq. 52] showed, consistent with AIC, that the average optimism in a mean logarithmic (minus log likelihood) quality score for logistic models is p/n.

10 Kass and Raftery have done several studies of BIC.[231] Smith and Spiegelhalter[390] and Laud and Ibrahim[259] discussed other useful generalizations of likelihood penalties. Zheng and Loh[464] studied several penalty measures, and found that AIC does not penalize enough for overfitting in the ordinary regression case.

11 Goldstein,[152] Willan et al.,[455] and Royston and Thompson[359] have nice discussions on comparing nonnested regression models. Schemper's method[371] is useful for testing whether a set of variables provides significantly greater information (using an R^2 measure) than another set of variables.

12 van Houwelingen and le Cessie [433, Eq. 22] recommended using $L/2$ (also called the Kullback–Leibler error rate) as a quality index.

13 Schemper[371] provides a bootstrap technique for testing for significant differences between correlated R^2 measures. Mittlböck and Schemper,[318] Schemper and Stare,[375] Korn and Simon,[248, 249] Menard,[312] and Zheng and Agresti[463] have excellent discussions about the pros and cons of various indexes of the predictive value of a model.

14 [39, 66, 282] provide good variance–covariance estimators from a weighted maximum likelihood analysis.

TABLE 9.4

Variables in Model	$LR \chi^2$
Age	100
Sex	108
Age, sex	111
Age^2	60
Age, age^2	102
Age, age^2, sex	115

15   Verweij and van Houwelingen [436, Eq. 4] derived another expression for d.f., but it requires more computation and did not perform any better than Equation 9.63 in choosing λ in several examples tested.

16   See van Houwelingen and Thorogood[131] for an approximate empirical Bayes approach to shrinkage. See Tibshirani[415] for the use of a nonsmooth penalty function that results in variable selection as well as shrinkage (see Section 4.3). Verweij and van Houwelingen[437] used a "cross-validated likelihood" based on leave-out-one estimates to penalize for overfitting. Wang and Taylor[444] presented some methods for carrying out hypothesis tests and computing confidence limits under penalization.

9.12   Problems

1. A sample of size 100 from a normal distribution with unknown mean and standard deviation (μ and σ) yielded the following log likelihood values when computed at two values of μ.

$$\log L(\mu = 10, \sigma = 5) = -800$$
$$\log L(\mu = 20, \sigma = 5) = -820.$$

What do you know about μ? What do you know about $\overline{Y}$?

2. Several regression models were considered for predicting a response. $LR \chi^2$ (corrected for the intercept) for models containing various combinations of variables are found in Table 9.4. Compute all possible meaningful $LR \chi^2$. For each, state the d.f. and an approximate p-value. State which $LR \chi^2$ involving only one variable is not very meaningful.

3. For each problem below, rank Wald, score, and LR statistics by overall statistical properties and then by computational convenience.

   (a) A forward stepwise variable selection is desired to determine a concise model that contains most of the independent information in all potential predictors.

(b) A test of independent association of each variable in a given model (each variable adjusted for the effects of all other variables in the given model) is to be obtained.

(c) A model that contains only additive effects is fitted. A large number of potential interaction terms are to be tested using a global (multiple d.f.) test.

Chapter 10

Binary Logistic Regression

10.1 Model

Binary responses are commonly studied in medical and epidemiologic research, for example, the presence or absence of a particular disease, death during surgery, and occurrence of ventricular fibrillation in a dog. Often one wishes to study how a set of predictor variables X is related to a dichotomous response variable Y. The predictors may describe such quantities as treatment assignment, dosage, risk factors, and year of treatment.

For convenience we define the response to be $Y = 0$ or 1, with $Y = 1$ denoting the occurrence of the event of interest. Often a dichotomous outcome can be studied by calculating certain proportions, for example, the proportion of deaths among females and the proportion among males. However, in many situations, there are multiple descriptors, or one or more of the descriptors are continuous. Without a statistical model, studying patterns such as the relationship between age and occurrence of a disease, for example, would require the creation of arbitrary age groups to allow estimation of disease prevalence as a function of age.

Letting X denote the vector of predictors $\{X_1, X_2, \ldots, X_k\}$, a first attempt at modeling the response might use the ordinary linear regression model

$$E\{Y|X\} = X\beta, \tag{10.1}$$

since the expectation of a binary variable Y is $\mathrm{Prob}\{Y = 1\}$. However, such a model by definition cannot fit the data over the whole range of the predictors since a purely linear model $\mathrm{E}\{Y|X\} = \mathrm{Prob}\{Y = 1|X\} = X\beta$ can allow $\mathrm{Prob}\{Y = 1\}$ to exceed 1

①

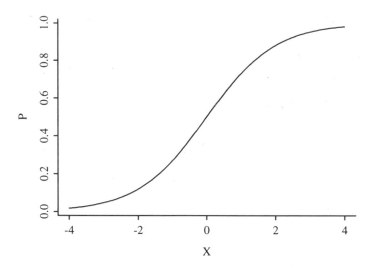

FIGURE 10.1: Logistic function.

or fall below 0. The statistical model that is generally preferred for the analysis of binary responses is instead the binary logistic regression model, stated in terms of the probability that $Y = 1$ given X, the values of the predictors:

$$\text{Prob}\{Y = 1|X\} = [1 + \exp(-X\beta)]^{-1}. \qquad (10.2)$$

As before, $X\beta$ stands for $\beta_0 + \beta_1 X_1 + \beta_2 X_2 + \ldots + \beta_k X_k$. The binary logistic regression model was developed primarily by Cox[89] and Walker and Duncan.[440]

The regression parameters β are estimated by the method of maximum likelihood (see below).

The function

$$P = [1 + \exp(-x)]^{-1} \qquad (10.3)$$

is called the logistic function. This function is plotted in Figure 10.1 for x varying from -4 to $+4$. This function has an unlimited range for x while P is restricted to range from 0 to 1. For future derivations it is useful to express x in terms of P. Solving the equation above for x by using

$$1 - P = \exp(-x)/[1 + \exp(-x)] \qquad (10.4)$$

yields the inverse of the logistic function:

$$x = \log[P/(1 - P)] = \log[\text{odds that } Y = 1 \text{ occurs}] = \text{logit}\{Y = 1\}. \qquad (10.5)$$

Other methods that have been used to analyze binary response data include the probit model, which writes P in terms of the cumulative normal distribution, and discriminant analysis. Probit regression, although assuming a similar shape to the logistic function for the regression relationship between $X\beta$ and Prob$\{Y = 1\}$, involves more cumbersome calculations, and there is no natural interpretation of its regression parameters. In the past, discriminant analysis has been the predominant method since it is the simplest computationally. However, not only does discriminant analysis assume the same regression model as logistic regression, but it also assumes that the predictors are each normally distributed and that jointly the predictors have a multivariate normal distribution. These assumptions are unlikely to be met in practice, especially when one of the predictors is a discrete variable such as sex group. When discriminant analysis assumptions are violated, logistic regression yields more accurate estimates.[170, 345] Even when discriminant analysis is optimal (i.e., when all its assumptions are satisfied) logistic regression is virtually as accurate as the discriminant model.[180]

The model used in discriminant analysis is stated in terms of the distribution of X given the outcome group Y, even though one is seldom interested in the distribution of the predictors per se. The discriminant model has to be inverted using Bayes' rule to derive the quantity of primary interest, Prob$\{Y = 1\}$. By contrast, the logistic model is a *direct probability model* since it is stated in terms of Prob$\{Y = 1|X\}$. Since the distribution of a binary random variable Y is completely defined by the true probability that $Y = 1$ and since the model makes no assumption about the distribution of the predictors, the logistic model makes no distributional assumptions whatsoever.

10.1.1 *Model Assumptions and Interpretation of Parameters*

Since the logistic model is a direct probability model, its only assumptions relate to the form of the regression equation. Regression assumptions are verifiable, unlike the assumption of multivariate normality made by discriminant analysis. The logistic model assumptions are most easily understood by transforming Prob$\{Y = 1\}$ to make a model that is linear in $X\beta$:

$$\begin{aligned}\text{logit}\{Y = 1|X\} &= \text{logit}(P) = \log[P/(1 - P)] \\ &= X\beta, \end{aligned} \tag{10.6}$$

where $P = \text{Prob}\{Y = 1|X\}$. Thus the model is a linear regression model in the log odds that $Y = 1$ since logit(P) is a weighted sum of the Xs. If all effects are additive (i.e., no interactions are present), the model assumes that for every predictor X_j,

$$\begin{aligned}\text{logit}\{Y = 1|X\} &= \beta_0 + \beta_1 X_1 + \ldots + \beta_j X_j + \ldots + \beta_k X_k \\ &= \beta_j X_j + C, \end{aligned} \tag{10.7}$$

where if all other factors are held constant, C is a constant given by

$$C = \beta_0 + \beta_1 X_1 + \ldots + \beta_{j-1} X_{j-1} + \beta_{j+1} X_{j+1} + \ldots + \beta_k X_k. \tag{10.8}$$

The parameter β_j is then the change in the log odds per unit change in X_j if X_j represents a single factor that is linear and does not interact with other factors and if all other factors are held constant. Instead of writing this relationship in terms of log odds, it could just as easily be written in terms of the odds that $Y = 1$:

$$\text{odds}\{Y = 1 | X\} = \exp(X\beta), \tag{10.9}$$

and if all factors other than X_j are held constant,

$$\text{odds}\{Y = 1 | X\} = \exp(\beta_j X_j + C) = \exp(\beta_j X_j) \exp(C). \tag{10.10}$$

The regression parameters can also be written in terms of *odds ratios*.

The odds that $Y = 1$ when X_j is increased by d, divided by the odds at X_j is

$$
\begin{aligned}
\frac{\text{odds}\{Y = 1 | X_1, X_2, \ldots, X_j + d, \ldots, X_k\}}{\text{odds}\{Y = 1 | X_1, X_2, \ldots, X_j, \ldots, X_k\}} \\
= \frac{\exp[\beta_j(X_j + d)] \exp(C)}{[\exp(\beta_j X_j) \exp(C)]} \\
= \exp[\beta_j X_j + \beta_j d - \beta_j X_j] = \exp(\beta_j d).
\end{aligned} \tag{10.11}
$$

Thus the effect of increasing X_j by d is to increase the odds that $Y = 1$ by a factor of $\exp(\beta_j d)$, or to increase the log odds that $Y = 1$ by an increment of $\beta_j d$. In general, the ratio of the odds of response for an individual with predictor variable values X^* compared to an individual with predictors X is

$$
\begin{aligned}
X^* : X \text{ odds ratio} &= \exp(X^*\beta) / \exp(X\beta) \\
&= \exp[(X^* - X)\beta].
\end{aligned} \tag{10.12}
$$

Now consider some special cases of the logistic multiple regression model. If there is only one predictor X and that predictor is binary, the model can be written

$$
\begin{aligned}
\text{logit}\{Y = 1 | X = 0\} &= \beta_0 \\
\text{logit}\{Y = 1 | X = 1\} &= \beta_0 + \beta_1.
\end{aligned} \tag{10.13}
$$

Here β_0 is the log odds of $Y = 1$ when $X = 0$. By subtracting the two equations above, it can be seen that β_1 is the difference in the log odds when $X = 1$ as compared to $X = 0$, which is equivalent to the log of the ratio of the odds when $X = 1$ compared to the odds when $X = 0$. The quantity $\exp(\beta_1)$ is the odds ratio for $X = 1$ compared to $X = 0$. Letting $P^0 = \text{Prob}\{Y = 1 | X = 0\}$ and

$P^1 = \text{Prob}\{Y = 1|X = 1\}$, the regression parameters are interpreted by

$$\begin{aligned}
\beta_0 &= \text{logit}(P^0) = \log[P^0/(1 - P^0)] \\
\beta_1 &= \text{logit}(P^1) - \text{logit}(P^0) \\
&= \log[P^1/(1 - P^1)] - \log[P^0/(1 - P^0)] \\
&= \log\{[P^1/(1 - P^1)]/[P^0/(1 - P^0)]\}.
\end{aligned} \tag{10.14}$$

Since there are only two quantities to model and two free parameters, there is no way that this two-sample model can't fit; the model in this case is essentially fitting two cell proportions. Similarly, if there are $g - 1$ dummy indicator Xs representing g groups, the ANOVA-type logistic model must always fit.

If there is one continuous predictor X, the model is

$$\text{logit}\{Y = 1|X\} = \beta_0 + \beta_1 X, \tag{10.15}$$

and without further modification (e.g., taking log transformation of the predictor), the model assumes a straight line in the log odds, or that an increase in X by one unit increases the odds by a factor of $\exp(\beta_1)$.

Now consider the simplest analysis of covariance model in which there are two treatments (indicated by $X_1 = 0$ or 1) and one continuous covariable (X_2). The simplest logistic model for this setup is

$$\text{logit}\{Y = 1|X\} = \beta_0 + \beta_1 X_1 + \beta_2 X_2, \tag{10.16}$$

which can be written also as

$$\begin{aligned}
\text{logit}\{Y = 1|X_1 = 0, X_2\} &= \beta_0 + \beta_2 X_2 \\
\text{logit}\{Y = 1|X_1 = 1, X_2\} &= \beta_0 + \beta_1 + \beta_2 X_2.
\end{aligned} \tag{10.17}$$

The $X_1 = 1 : X_1 = 0$ odds ratio is $\exp(\beta_1)$, independent of X_2. The odds ratio for a one-unit increase in X_2 is $\exp(\beta_2)$, independent of X_1.

This model, with no term for a possible interaction between treatment and covariable, assumes that for each treatment the relationship between X_2 and log odds is linear, and that the lines have equal slope; that is, they are parallel. Assuming linearity in X_2, the only way that this model can fail is for the two slopes to differ. Thus, the only assumptions that need verification are linearity and lack of interaction between X_1 and X_2.

To adapt the model to allow or test for interaction, we write

$$\text{logit}\{Y = 1|X\} = \beta_0 + \beta_1 X_1 + \beta_2 X_2 + \beta_3 X_3, \tag{10.18}$$

TABLE 10.1

| Without Risk Factor | | With Risk Factor | |
Probability	Odds	Odds	Probability
.2	.25	.5	.33
.5	1	2	.67
.8	4	8	.89
.9	9	18	.95
.98	49	98	.99

where the derived variable X_3 is defined to be $X_1 X_2$. The test for lack of interaction (equal slopes) is $H_0 : \beta_3 = 0$. The model can be amplified as

$$\begin{aligned}
\text{logit}\{Y = 1 | X_1 = 0, X_2\} &= \beta_0 + \beta_2 X_2 \\
\text{logit}\{Y = 1 | X_1 = 1, X_2\} &= \beta_0 + \beta_1 + \beta_2 X_2 + \beta_3 X_2 \\
&= \beta_0' + \beta_2' X_2,
\end{aligned} \qquad (10.19)$$

where $\beta_0' = \beta_0 + \beta_1$ and $\beta_2' = \beta_2 + \beta_3$. The model with interaction is therefore equivalent to fitting two separate logistic models with X_2 as the only predictor, one model for each treatment group. Here the $X_1 = 1 : X_1 = 0$ odds ratio is $\exp(\beta_1 + \beta_3 X_2)$.

10.1.2 Odds Ratio, Risk Ratio, and Risk Difference

As discussed above, the logistic model quantifies the effect of a predictor in terms of an odds ratio or log odds ratio. An odds ratio is a natural description of an effect in a probability model since an odds ratio *can* be constant. For example, suppose that a given risk factor doubles the odds of disease. Table 10.1 shows the effect of the risk factor for various levels of initial risk.

Since odds have an unlimited range, any positive odds ratio will still yield a valid probability. If one attempted to describe an effect by a risk ratio, the effect can only occur over a limited range of risk (probability). For example, a risk ratio of 2 can only apply to risks below .5; above that point the risk ratio must diminish. (Risk ratios are similar to odds ratios if the risk is small.) Risk differences have the same difficulty; the risk difference cannot be constant and must depend on the initial risk. Odds ratios, on the other hand, can describe an effect over the entire range of risk. An odds ratio can, for example, describe the effect of a treatment independently of covariables affecting risk. Figure 10.2 depicts the relationship between risk of a subject without the risk factor and the increase in risk for a variety of relative increases (odds ratios). The figure demonstrates how absolute risk increase is a function of the baseline risk of a subject. Risk increase will also be a function of factors that interact with the risk factor, that is,, factors that modify its relative effect. Once a model is developed for

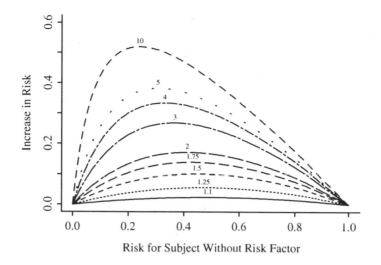

FIGURE 10.2: Absolute benefit as a function of risk of the event in a control subject and the relative effect (odds ratio) of the risk factor. The odds ratios are given for each curve.

estimating $\text{Prob}\{Y = 1|X\}$, this model can easily be used to estimate the absolute risk increase as a function of baseline risk factors as well as interacting factors. Let X_1 be a binary risk factor and let $A = \{X_2, \ldots, X_p\}$ be the other factors (which for convenience we assume do not interact with X_1) Then the estimate of $\text{Prob}\{Y = 1|X_1 = 1, A\} - \text{Prob}\{Y = 1|X_1 = 0, A\}$ is

$$\frac{1}{1 + \exp -[\hat{\beta}_0 + \hat{\beta}_1 + \hat{\beta}_2 X_2 + \ldots + \hat{\beta}_p X_p]}$$
$$- \frac{1}{1 + \exp -[\hat{\beta}_0 + \hat{\beta}_2 X_2 + \ldots + \hat{\beta}_p X_p]}$$
$$= \frac{1}{1 + (\frac{1-\hat{R}}{\hat{R}}) \exp(-\hat{\beta}_1)} - \hat{R}, \tag{10.20}$$

where $\hat{R}$ is the estimate of the baseline risk, $\text{Prob}\{Y = 1|X_1 = 0\}$. The risk difference estimate can be plotted against $\hat{R}$ or against levels of variables in A to display absolute risk increase against overall risk (Figure 10.2) or against specific subject characteristics.

③

10.1.3   Detailed Example

Consider the data in Table 10.2. A graph of the data, along with a fitted logistic model (described later) appears in Figure 10.3. The graph also displays proportions

TABLE 10.2

Females		Males	
Age	Response	Age	Response
37	0	34	1
39	0	38	1
39	0	40	0
42	0	40	0
47	0	41	0
48	0	43	1
48	1	43	1
52	0	43	1
53	0	44	0
55	0	46	0
56	0	47	1
57	0	48	1
58	0	48	1
58	1	50	0
60	0	50	1
64	0	52	1
65	1	55	1
68	1	60	1
68	1	61	1
70	1	61	1

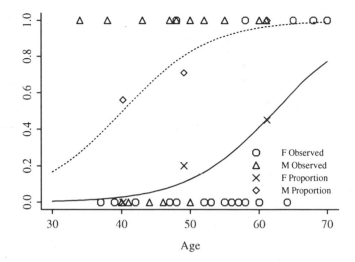

FIGURE 10.3: Data, subgroup proportions, and fitted logistic model.

of responses obtained by stratifying the data by sex and age group ($< 45, 45 - 54, \geq$ 55). The age points on the abscissa for these groups are the overall mean ages in the three age intervals (40.2, 49.1, and 61.1, respectively). Descriptive statistics (mostly printed by SAS PROC FREQ) for assessing the association between sex and response, age group and response, and age group and response stratified by sex are found below. Corresponding fitted logistic models, with sex coded as 0 — female, 1 = male are also given. Models were fitted first with sex as the only predictor, then with age as the (continuous) predictor, then with sex and age simultaneously.

First consider the relationship between sex and response, ignoring the effect of age.

TABLE OF SEX BY RESPONSE

SEX Frequency Row Pct	RESPONSE 0	1	Total	Odds/Log
F	14 70.00	6 30.00	20	6/14=.429 −.847
M	6 30.00	14 70.00	20	14/6=2.33 .847
Total	20	20	40	

M:F odds ratio = (14/6)/(6/14) = 5.44, log=1.695

STATISTICS FOR TABLE OF SEX BY RESPONSE

Statistic	DF	Value	Prob
Chi Square	1	6.400	0.011
Likelihood Ratio Chi-Square	1	6.583	0.010

Fitted Logistic Model

Parameter	Estimate	Std Err	Wald χ^2	P
β_0	-0.8472978	0.48795	3.015237	
β_1	1.6945956	0.69007	6.030474	0.0141

Note that the estimate of β_0, $\hat{\beta}_0$ is the log odds for females and that $\hat{\beta}_1$ is the log odds (M:F) ratio. $\hat{\beta}_0 + \hat{\beta}_1 = .847$, the log odds for males. The likelihood ratio test for H_0 : no effect of sex on probability of response is obtained as follows.

Log likelihood $(\beta_1 = 0)$: -27.727
Log likelihood (max) : -24.435
LR $\chi^2(H_0 : \beta_1 = 0)$: $-2(-27.727 - -24.435) = 6.584$.

(Note the agreement of the LR χ^2 with the contingency table likelihood ratio χ^2, and compare 6.584 with the Wald statistic 6.03.)

Next, consider the relationship between age and response, ignoring sex.

TABLE OF AGE BY RESPONSE

AGE Frequency Row Pct	RESPONSE 0	1	Total	Odds/Log
<45	8 61.5	5 38.4	13	5/8=.625 -.47
45–54	6 50.0	6 50.0	12	6/6=1 0
55+	6 40.0	9 60.0	15	9/6=1.5 .405
Total	20	20	40	

55+ : <45 odds ratio = (9/6)/(5/8) = 2.4, log=.875

Fitted Logistic Model

Parameter	Estimate	Std Err	Wald χ^2	P
β_0	-2.7338405	1.83752	2.213422	0.1368
β_1	0.0539798	0.03578	2.276263	0.1314

The estimate of β_1 is in rough agreement with that obtained from the frequency table. The $55+ \, : \, < 45$ log odds ratio is .875, and since the respective mean ages in the $55+$ and <45 age groups are 61.1 and 40.2, an estimate of the log odds ratio increase per year is $.875/(61.1 - 40.2) - .875/20.9 = .042$.

The likelihood ratio test for H_0 : no association between age and response is obtained as follows.

Log likelihood $(\beta_1 = 0)$: -27.727
Log likelihood (max)   : -26.511
LR $\chi^2(H_0 : \beta_1 = 0)$: $-2(-27.727 - -26.511) = 2.432$.

(Compare 2.432 with the Wald statistic 2.28.)

Next we consider the simultaneous association of age and sex with response.

SEX=F

AGE Frequency Row Pct	RESPONSE 0	1	Total
<45	4 100.0	0 0.0	4
45-54	4 80.0	1 20.0	5
55+	6 54.6	5 45.4	11
Total	14	6	20

```
                             SEX=M

        AGE            RESPONSE
        Frequency
        Row Pct         0          1      Total

        <45             4          5        9
                       44.4       55.6

        45-54           2          5        7
                       28.6       71.4

        55+             0          4        4
                        0.0      100.0


        Total           6         14       20
```

A logistic model for relating sex and age simultaneously to response is given below.

Fitted Logistic Model

Parameter	Estimate	Std Err	Wald χ^2	P
β_0	-9.8429426	3.67576	7.17057	0.0074
β_1 (sex)	3.4898280	1.19917	8.46928	0.0036
β_2 (age)	0.1580583	0.06164	6.57556	0.0103

Likelihood ratio tests are obtained from the information below.

Log likelihood $(\beta_1 = 0, \beta_2 = 0)$	:	-27.727
Log likelihood (max)	:	-19.458
Log likelihood $(\beta_1 = 0)$	:	-26.511
Log likelihood $(\beta_2 = 0)$	:	-24.435
LR χ^2 $(H_0 : \beta_1 = \beta_2 = 0)$	:	$-2(-27.727 - -19.458) = 16.538$
LR χ^2 $(H_0 : \beta_1 = 0)$ sex|age	:	$-2(-26.511 - -19.458) = 14.106$
LR χ^2 $(H_0 : \beta_2 = 0)$ age|sex	:	$-2(-24.435 - -19.458) = 9.954.$

The 14.1 should be compared with the Wald statistic of 8.47, and 9.954 should be compared with 6.58. The fitted logistic model is plotted separately for females and males in Figure 10.3. The fitted model is

$$\text{logit}\{\text{Response} = 1|\text{sex,age}\} = -9.84 + 3.49 \times \text{sex} + .158 \times \text{age}, \qquad (10.21)$$

where as before sex $= 0$ for females, 1 for males. For example, for a 40-year-old female, the predicted logit is $-9.84 + .158(40) = -3.52$. The predicted probability of a response is $1/[1 + \exp(3.52)] = .029$. For a 40-year-old male, the predicted logit is $-9.84 + 3.49 + .158(40) = -.03$, with a probability of .492.

10.1.4   Design Formulations

The logistic multiple regression model can incorporate the same designs as can ordinary linear regression. An analysis of variance (ANOVA) model for a treatment with k levels can be formulated with $k-1$ dummy variables. This logistic model is equivalent to a $2 \times k$ contingency table. An analysis of covariance logistic model is simply an ANOVA model augmented with covariables used for adjustment.

One unique design that is interesting to consider in the context of logistic models is a simultaneous comparison of multiple factors between two groups. Suppose, for example, that in a randomized trial with two treatments one wished to test whether any of 10 baseline characteristics are maldistributed between the two groups. If the 10 factors are continuous, one could perform a two-sample Wilcoxon–Mann–Whitney test or a t-test for each factor (if each is normally distributed). However, this procedure would result in multiple comparison problems and would also not be able to detect the combined effect of small differences across all the factors. A better procedure would be a multivariate test. The Hotelling T^2 test is designed for just this situation. It is a k-variable extension of the one-variable unpaired t-test. The T^2 test, like discriminant analysis, does assume multivariate normality of the k factors. This assumption is especially tenuous when some of the factors are polytomous. A better alternative is the global test of no regression from the logistic model. This test is valid because it can be shown that H_0 : mean X is the same for both groups (= H_0 : mean X does not depend on group = H_0 : mean $X|$ group = constant) is true if and only if H_0 : Prob$\{$group$|X\}$ = constant. Thus k factors can be tested simultaneously for differences between the two groups using the binary logistic model, which has far fewer assumptions than does the Hotelling T^2 test. The logistic global test of no regression (with k d.f.) would be expected to have greater power if there is nonnormality. Since the logistic model makes no assumption regarding the distribution of the descriptor variables, it can easily test for simultaneous group differences involving a mixture of continuous, binary, and nominal variables. In observational studies, such models for treatment received or exposure (propensity score models) hold great promise for adjusting for confounding.[82, 262, 353, 357, 358]

O'Brien[326] has developed a general test for comparing group 1 and group 2 for a single measurement. His test detects location and scale differences by fitting a logistic model for Prob$\{$Group 2$\}$ using X and X^2 as predictors.

For a randomized study where adjustment for confounding is seldom necessary, adjusting for covariables using a binary logistic model results in *increases* in standard errors of regression coefficients.[354] This is the opposite of what happens in linear regression where there is an unknown variance parameter that is estimated using the residual squared error. Fortunately, adjusting for covariables using logistic regression, by accounting for subject heterogeneity, will result in larger regression coefficients even for a randomized treatment variable. The increase in estimated regression coefficients more than offsets the increase in standard error.

10.2   Estimation

10.2.1   Maximum Likelihood Estimates

The parameters in the logistic regression model are estimated using the maximum likelihood (ML) method. The method is based on the same principles as the one-sample proportion example described earlier. The difference is that the general logistic model is not a single sample or a two-sample problem. The probability of response for the ith subject depends on a particular set of predictors X_i, and in fact the list of predictors may not be the same for any two subjects. Denoting the response and probability of response of the ith subject by Y_i and P_i, respectively, the model states that

$$P_i = \text{Prob}\{Y_i = 1 | X_i\} = [1 + \exp(-X_i\beta)]^{-1}. \tag{10.22}$$

The likelihood of an observed response Y_i given predictors X_i and the unknown parameters β is

$$P_i^{Y_i}[1 - P_i]^{1-Y_i}. \tag{10.23}$$

The joint likelihood of all responses $Y_1, Y_2, \ldots, Y_n$ is the product of these likelihoods for $i = 1, \ldots, n$. The likelihood and log likelihood functions are rewritten by using the definition of P_i above to allow them to be recognized as a function of the unknown parameters β. Except in simple special cases (such as the k-sample problem in which all Xs are dummy variables), the ML estimates (MLE) of β cannot be written explicitly. The Newton–Raphson method described earlier is usually used to solve iteratively for the list of values β that maximize the log likelihood. The MLEs are denoted by $\hat{\beta}$. The inverse of the estimated observed information matrix is taken as the estimate of the variance–covariance matrix of $\hat{\beta}$.

Under $H_0 : \beta_1 = \beta_2 = \ldots = \beta_k = 0$, the intercept parameter β_0 can be estimated explicitly and the log likelihood under this global null hypothesis can be computed explicitly. Under the global null hypothesis, $P_i = P = [1 + \exp(-\beta_0)]^{-1}$ and the MLE of P is $\hat{P} = s/n$ where s is the number of responses and n is the sample size. The MLE of β_0 is $\hat{\beta}_0 = \text{logit}(\hat{P})$. The log likelihood under this null hypothesis is

$$
\begin{aligned}
&\quad s \, \log(\hat{P}) + (n - s)\log(1 - \hat{P}) \\
&= \quad s \, \log(s/n) + (n - s)\log[(n - s)/n] \\
&= \quad s \, \log s + (n - s)\log(n - s) - n\log(n).
\end{aligned} \tag{10.24}
$$

4

10.2.2   Estimation of Odds Ratios and Probabilities

Once β is estimated, one can estimate any log odds, odds, or odds ratios. The MLE of the $X_j + 1 : X_j$ log odds ratio is $\hat{\beta}_j$, and the estimate of the $X_j + d : X_j$ log odds ratio is $\hat{\beta}_j d$, all other predictors remaining constant (assuming the absence of interactions involving X_j). For large enough samples, the MLEs are normally distributed with variances that are consistently estimated from the estimated variance–covariance matrix. Letting z denote the $1 - \alpha/2$ critical value of the standard normal distribution, a two-sided $1 - \alpha$ confidence interval for the log odds ratio for a one-unit increase in X_j is $[\hat{\beta}_j - zs, \hat{\beta}_j + zs]$, where s is the estimated standard error of $\hat{\beta}_j$. (Note that for $\alpha = .05$, i.e., for a 95% confidence interval, $z = 1.96$.)

A theorem in statistics states that the MLE of a function of a parameter is that same function of the MLE of the parameter. Thus the MLE of the $X_j + 1 : X_j$ odds ratio is $\exp(\hat{\beta}_j)$. Also, if a $1 - \alpha$ confidence interval of a parameter β is $[c, d]$ and $f(u)$ is a one-to-one function, a $1 - \alpha$ confidence interval of $f(\beta)$ is $[f(c), f(d)]$. Thus a $1 - \alpha$ confidence interval for the $X_j + 1 : X_j$ odds ratio is $\exp[\hat{\beta}_j \pm zs]$. Note that while the confidence interval for β_j is symmetric about $\hat{\beta}_j$, the confidence interval for $\exp(\beta_j)$ is not. By the same theorem just used, the MLE of $P_i = \text{Prob}\{Y_i = 1 | X_i\}$ is

$$\hat{P}_i = [1 + \exp(-X_i\hat{\beta})]^{-1}. \tag{10.25}$$

A confidence interval for P_i could be derived by computing the standard error of $\hat{P}_i$, yielding a symmetric confidence interval. However, such an interval would have the disadvantage that its endpoints could fall below zero or exceed one. A better approach uses the fact that for large samples $X\hat{\beta}$ is approximately normally distributed. An estimate of the variance of $X\hat{\beta}$ in matrix notation is XVX' where V is the estimated variance–covariance matrix of $\hat{\beta}$ (see Equation 9.50). This variance is the sum of all variances and covariances of $\hat{\beta}$ weighted by squares and products of the predictors. The estimated standard error of $X\hat{\beta}$, s, is the square root of this variance estimate. A $1 - \alpha$ confidence interval for P_i is then

$$\{1 + \exp[-(X_i\hat{\beta} \pm zs)]\}^{-1}. \tag{10.26}$$

10.3   Test Statistics

The likelihood ratio, score, and Wald statistics discussed earlier can be used to test any hypothesis in the logistic model. The likelihood ratio test is generally preferred. When true parameters are near the null values all three statistics usually agree. The Wald test has a significant drawback when the true parameter value is very far from the null value. In such case the standard error estimate becomes too large. As $\hat{\beta}_j$ increases from 0, the Wald test statistic for $H_0 : \beta_j = 0$ becomes larger, but after a certain point it becomes smaller. The statistic will eventually drop to zero if $\hat{\beta}_j$ becomes infinite.[193] Infinite estimates can occur in the logistic model especially when there is a binary predictor whose mean is near 0 or 1. Wald statistics are especially problematic in this case. For example, if 10 out of 20 males had a disease and 5 out of 5 females had the disease, the female : male odds ratio is infinite and so is the logistic regression coefficient for sex. If such a situation occurs, the likelihood ratio or score statistic should be used instead of the Wald statistic.

For k-sample (ANOVA-type) logistic models, logistic model statistics are equivalent to contingency table χ^2 statistics. As exemplified in the logistic model relating sex to response described previously, the global likelihood ratio statistic for all dummy variables in a k-sample model is identical to the contingency table (k-sample binomial) likelihood ratio χ^2 statistic. The score statistic for this same situation turns out to be identical to the $k-1$ degree of freedom Pearson χ^2 for a $k \times 2$ table.

As mentioned in Section 2.6, it can be dangerous to interpret individual parameters, make pairwise treatment comparisons, or test linearity if the overall test of association for a factor represented by multiple parameters is insignificant.

10.4 Residuals

Several types of residuals can be computed for binary logistic model fits. Many of these residuals are used to examine the influence of individual observations on the fit. One type of residual, the *partial residual* is useful for directly assessing how each predictor should be transformed. For the ith observation, the partial residual for the jth element of X is defined by   [6]

$$r_{ij} = \hat{\beta}_j X_{ij} + \frac{Y_i - \hat{P}_i}{\hat{P}_i(1 - \hat{P}_i)}, \tag{10.27}$$

where X_{ij} is the value of the jth variable in the ith observation, Y_i is the corresponding value of the response, and $\hat{P}_i$ is the predicted probability that $Y_i = 1$. A smooth plot (using, e.g., loess) of X_{ij} against r_{ij} will provide an estimate of how X_j should be transformed, adjusting for the other Xs (using their current transformations). Typically one tentatively models X_j linearly and checks the smoothed plot for linearity. A U-shaped relationship in this plot, for example, indicates that a squared term or spline function needs to be added for X_j. This approach does assume additivity of predictors.   [7]

10.5 Assessment of Model Fit

As the logistic regression model makes no distributional assumptions, only the assumptions of linearity and additivity need to be verified (in addition to the usual assumptions about independence of observations and inclusion of important covariables). In ordinary linear regression there is no global test for lack of model fit unless there are replicate observations at various settings of X. This is because ordinary regression entails estimation of a separate variance parameter σ^2. In logistic regression there are global tests for goodness of fit. Unfortunately, some of the most frequently used ones are inappropriate. For example, it is common to see a deviance test of goodness of fit based on the "residual" log likelihood, with P-values obtained from a χ^2 distribution with $n - p$ d.f. This P-value is inappropriate since the deviance does not have an asymptotic χ^2 distribution, due to the facts that the number of parameters estimated is increasing at the same rate as n and the expected cell frequencies are far below five (by definition).

Hosmer and Lemeshow[209] have developed a commonly used test for goodness of fit for binary logistic models based on grouping into deciles of predicted probability and performing an ordinary χ^2 test for the mean predicted probability against the observed fraction of events (using 8 d.f. to account for evaluating fit on the model development sample). The Hosmer–Lemeshow test is fairly dependent on the choice of how predictions are grouped[208] and it is not clear that the choice of the number of groups should be independent of n. Hosmer et al.[208] have compared a number of global goodness of fit tests for binary logistic regression. They concluded that the simple unweighted sum of squares test of Copas[86] as modified by le Cessie and van Houwelingen[268] is as good as any. They used a normal Z-test for the sum of squared errors ($n \times B$, where B is the Brier index in Equation 10.35). This test takes into account the fact that one cannot obtain a χ^2 distribution for the sum of squares. It also takes into account the estimation of β. It is not yet clear for which types of lack of fit this test has reasonable power.

More power for detecting lack of fit is expected to be obtained from testing specific alternatives to the model. In the model

$$\text{logit}\{Y = 1 | X\} = \beta_0 + \beta_1 X_1 + \beta_2 X_2, \tag{10.28}$$

where X_1 is binary and X_2 is continuous, one needs to verify that the log odds is related to X_1 and X_2 according to Figure 10.4.

The simplest method for validating that the data are consistent with the no interaction linear model involves stratifying the sample by X_1 and quantile groups (e.g., deciles) of X_2.[181] Within each stratum the proportion of responses $\hat{P}$ is computed and the log odds calculated from $\log[\hat{P}/(1 - \hat{P})]$. The number of quantile groups should be such that there are at least 20 subjects in each $X_1 \times X_2$ group. Otherwise, probabilities cannot be estimated precisely enough to allow trends to be seen above "noise" in the data. Since at least 3 X_2 groups must be formed to allow assessment of linearity, the total sample size must be at least $2 \times 3 \times 20 = 120$ for this method to work at all. Figure 10.5 demonstrates this method for a large sample size of 3504 subjects stratified by sex and deciles of age. Linearity is apparent for males while there is evidence for slight interaction between age and sex since the age trend for females appears curved.

The subgrouping method requires relatively large sample sizes and does not use continuous factors effectively. The ordering of values is not used at all between intervals, and the estimate of the relationship for a continuous variable has lit-

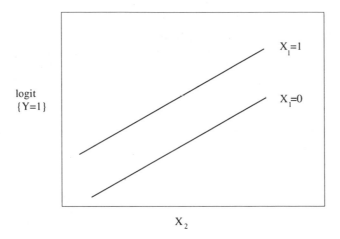

FIGURE 10.4: Logistic regression assumptions for one binary and one continuous predictor.

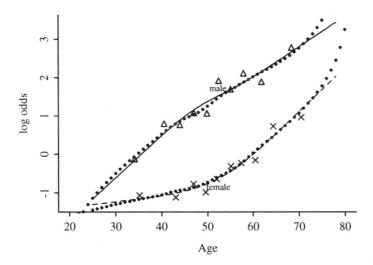

FIGURE 10.5: Logit proportions of significant coronary artery disease by sex and deciles of age for $n = 3504$ patients, with spline fits (smooth curves). Spline fits are for $k = 4$ knots at age $= 36, 48, 56$, and 68 years, and interaction between age and sex is allowed. Smooth nonparametric estimates are shown as dotted curves. Data courtesy of the Duke Cardiovascular Disease Databank.

tle resolution. Also, the method of grouping chosen (e.g., deciles vs. quintiles vs. rounding) can alter the shape of the plot.

In this dataset with only two variables, it is efficient to use a nonparametric smoother for age, separately for males and females. Nonparametric smoothers, such as loess[76] used here, work well for binary response variables (see Section 2.4.6); the logit transformation is made on the smoothed probability estimates. The smoothed estimates are shown in Figure 10.5.

⑧

When there are several predictors, the restricted cubic spline function is better for estimating the true relationship between X_2 and logit$\{Y = 1\}$ for continuous variables without assuming linearity. By fitting a model containing X_2 expanded into $k - 1$ terms, where k is the number of knots, one can obtain an estimate of the function of X_2 that should be used linearly in the model as described in general in Section 2.4:

$$\begin{aligned} \text{logit}\{Y = 1|X\} &= \hat{\beta}_0 + \hat{\beta}_1 X_1 + \hat{\beta}_2 X_2 + \hat{\beta}_3 X_2' + \hat{\beta}_4 X_2'' \\ &= \hat{\beta}_0 + \hat{\beta}_1 X_1 + f(X_2), \end{aligned} \tag{10.29}$$

where X_2' and X_2'' are constructed spline variables (when $k = 4$) as described in Section 2.4. Plotting the estimated spline function $f(X_2)$ versus X_2 will estimate how the effect of X_2 should be modeled. If the sample is sufficiently large, the spline function can be fitted separately for $X_1 = 0$ and $X_1 = 1$, allowing detection of even unusual interaction patterns. A formal test of linearity in X_2 is obtained by testing $H_0 : \beta_3 = \beta_4 = 0$.

For testing interaction between X_1 and X_2 (after a needed transformation may have been applied), frequently a product term (e.g., $X_1 X_2$) can be added to the model and its coefficient tested. A more general simultaneous test of linearity and lack of interaction for a two-variable model in which one variable is binary (or is assumed linear) is obtained by fitting the model

$$\begin{aligned} \text{logit}\{Y = 1|X\} &= \beta_0 + \beta_1 X_1 + \beta_2 X_2 + \beta_3 X_2' + \beta_4 X_2'' \\ &+ \beta_5 X_1 X_2 + \beta_6 X_1 X_2' + \beta_7 X_1 X_2'' \end{aligned} \tag{10.30}$$

and testing $H_0 : \beta_3 = \ldots = \beta_7 = 0$. This formulation allows the shape of the X_2 effect to be completely different for each level of X_1. There is virtually no departure from linearity and additivity that cannot be detected from this expanded model formulation. The most computationally efficient test for lack of fit is the score test (e.g., X_1 and X_2 are forced into a tentative model and the remaining variables are candidates in SAS PROC LOGISTIC). Figure 10.5 also depicts a fitted spline logistic model with $k = 4$, allowing for general interaction between age and sex as parameterized above. The fitted function, after expanding the restricted cubic spline function for simplicity (see Equation 2.26) is $X\hat{\beta} = -3.92 + 1.10 \times 10^{-1}\text{age} - 7.98 \times 10^{-5}(\text{age} - 36)_+^3 + 2.57 \times 10^{-4}(\text{age} - 48)_+^3 - 2.16 \times 10^{-4}(\text{age} - 56)_+^3 + 3.84 \times 10^{-5}(\text{age} - 68)_+^3 + 2.23\{\text{female}\} + \{\text{female}\}[-9.49 \times 10^{-2}\text{age} + 1.41 \times 10^{-4}(\text{age} -$

TABLE 10.3

Model / Hypothesis	Likelihood Ratio χ^2	d.f.	P	Formula
a: sex, age (linear, no interaction)	766.0	2		
b: sex, age, age × sex	768.2	3		
c: sex, spline in age	769.4	4		
d: sex, spline in age, interaction	782.5	7		
H_0 : no age × sex interaction given linearity	2.2	1	.14	$(b - a)$
H_0 : age linear | no interaction	3.4	2	.18	$(c - a)$
H_0 : age linear, no interaction	16.6	5	.005	$(d - a)$
H_0 : age linear, product form interaction	14.4	4	.006	$(d - b)$
H_0 : no interaction, allowing for nonlinearity in age	13.1	3	.004	$(d - c)$

$36)_+^3 - 2.94 \times 10^{-4}(\text{age} - 48)_+^3 + 1.13 \times 10^{-4}(\text{age} - 56)_+^3 + 3.93 \times 10^{-5}(\text{age} - 68)_+^3]$. Note the good agreement between the empirical estimates of log odds and the spline fits and nonparametric estimates in this large dataset.

An analysis of log likelihood for this model and various submodels is found in Table 10.3. The χ^2 for global tests is corrected for the intercept and the degrees of freedom does not include the intercept.

This analysis confirms the first impression from the graph, namely, that age × sex interaction is present but it is not of the form of a simple product between age and sex (change in slope). In the context of a linear age effect, there is no significant product interaction effect ($P = .14$). Without allowing for interaction, there is no significant nonlinear effect of age ($P = .18$). However, the general test of lack of fit with 5 d.f. indicates a significant departure from the linear additive model ($P = .005$).

In Figure 10.6, data from 2332 patients who underwent cardiac catheterization at Duke University Medical Center and were found to have significant ($\geq 75\%$) diameter narrowing of at least one major coronary artery were analyzed (the dataset is available from the Web site). The relationship between the time from the onset of symptoms of coronary artery disease (e.g., angina, myocardial infarction) to the probability that the patient has severe (three-vessel disease or left main disease— tvdlm) coronary disease was of interest. There were 1129 patients with tvdlm. A logistic model was used with the duration of symptoms appearing as a restricted cubic spline function with $k = 3, 4, 5$, and 6 equally spaced knots in terms of quantiles between .05 and .95. The best fit for the number of parameters was chosen using Akaike's information criterion (AIC), computed in Table 10.4 as the model likelihood ratio χ^2 minus twice the number of parameters in the model aside from

TABLE 10.4

k	Model χ^2	AIC
0	99.23	97.23
3	112.69	108.69
4	121.30	115.30
5	123.51	115.51
6	124.41	114.51

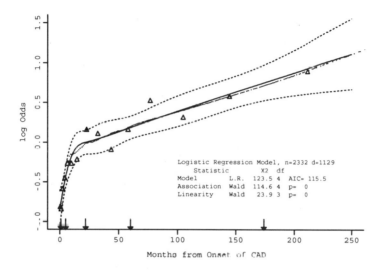

FIGURE 10.6: Estimated relationship between duration of symptoms and the log odds of severe coronary artery disease for $k = 5$. Knots are marked with arrows. Solid line is spline fit; dotted line is a nonparametric "super-smoothed" estimate.

the intercept. The linear model is denoted $k = 0$. Figure 10.6 displays the spline fit for $k = 5$. The triangles represent subgroup estimates obtained by dividing the sample into groups of 150 patients. For example, the leftmost triangle represents the logit of the proportion of tvdlm in the 150 patients with the shortest duration of symptoms, versus the mean duration in that group. A Wald test of linearity, with 3 d.f., showed highly significant nonlinearity ($\chi^2 = 23.92$ with 3 d.f.). The plot of the spline transformation suggests a log transformation, and when log (duration of symptoms in months + 1) was fitted in a logistic model, the log likelihood of the model (119.33 with 1 d.f.) was virtually as good as the spline model (123.51 with 4 d.f.); the corresponding Akaike information criteria are 117.33 and 115.51. To check for adequacy in the log transformation, a five-knot restricted cubic spline function was fitted to $\log_{10}(\text{months} + 1)$, as displayed in Figure 10.7. There is some evidence

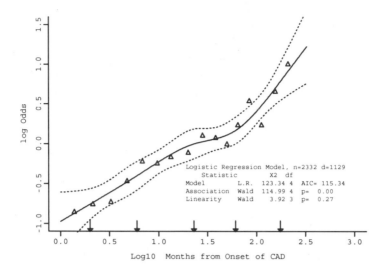

FIGURE 10.7: Assessing adequacy of log transformed predictor.

for lack of fit on the right, but the Wald χ^2 for testing linearity yields $P = .27$. The fitted logistic model that is linear in log duration is shown in Figure 10.8.

If the model contains two continuous predictors, they may both be expanded with spline functions in order to test linearity or to describe nonlinear relationships. Testing interaction is more difficult here, but one can attempt to reduce the variables to two transformed variables, in which case interaction can be approximated by a single product of the two new variables. If X_1 is continuous, the same method can be used after grouping X_1 into quantile groups. Consider the subset of 2258 (1490 with disease) of the 3504 patients used in Figure 10.5 who have serum cholesterol measured. A logistic model for predicting significant coronary disease was fitted with age in tertiles (modeled with two dummy variables), sex, age × sex interaction, four-knot restricted cubic spline in cholesterol, and age tertile × cholesterol interaction. A previous analysis had found the sex × cholesterol interaction to be insignificant. Except for the sex adjustment this model is equivalent to fitting three separate spline functions in cholesterol, one for each age tertile. The fitted model is shown in Figure 10.9 for cholesterol and age tertile against logit of significant disease. Significant age × cholesterol interaction is apparent from the figure and is suggested by the Wald χ^2 statistic (10.03) that follows. Note that the test for linearity of the interaction with respect to cholesterol is very insignificant ($\chi^2 = 2.40$ on 4 d.f.), but we retain it for now. The fitted function is $X\hat{\beta} = -0.342 + 0.372\{\text{age} \in [48, 57)\} + 4.798\{\text{age} \in [57, 82]\} - 1.54\{\text{female}\} + 2.29 \times 10^{-3}\text{chol} + 1.62 \times 10^{-6}(\text{chol} - 160)_+^3 - 4.90 \times 10^{-6}(\text{chol} - 208)_+^3 + 3.76 \times 10^{-6}(\text{chol} - 243)_+^3 - 4.83 \times 10^{-7}(\text{chol} - 319)_+^3 + \{\text{female}\}[-0.696\{\text{age} \in [48, 57)\} - 0.750\{\text{age} \in [57, 82]\}] + \{\text{age} \in [48, 57)\}[3.09 \times$

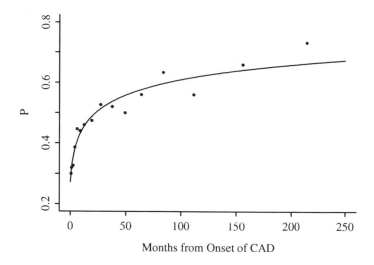

FIGURE 10.8:   Fitted linear logistic model in $\log_{10}(\text{duration} + 1)$, with subgroup estimates using groups of 150 patients. Fitted equation is $\text{logit}(\texttt{tvdlm}) = -.9809 + .7122 \log_{10}(\text{months} + 1)$.

$10^{-3}\text{chol} - 1.01 \times 10^{-6}(\text{chol} - 160)_{+}^{3} + 3.37 \times 10^{-6}(\text{chol} - 208)_{+}^{3} - 2.80 \times 10^{-6}(\text{chol} - 243)_{+}^{3} + 4.45 \times 10^{-7}(\text{chol} - 319)_{+}^{3}] + \{\text{age} \in [57, 82]\}[-1.57 \times 10^{-2}\text{chol} + 7.60 \times 10^{-7}(\text{chol} - 160)_{+}^{3} - 1.47 \times 10^{-6}(\text{chol} - 208)_{+}^{3} + 5.59 \times 10^{-7}(\text{chol} - 243)_{+}^{0} + 1.52 \times 10^{-7}(\text{chol} - 319)_{+}^{3}].$

Wald Statistics

Factor	χ^2	d.f.	P
age.tertile (Main+Interactions)	112.62	10	0.0000
All Interactions	22.37	8	0.0043
sex (Main+Interactions)	328.90	3	0.0000
All Interactions	9.61	2	0.0082
cholesterol (Main+Interactions)	94.01	9	0.0000
All Interactions	10.03	6	0.1234
Nonlinear (Main+Interactions)	10.30	6	0.1124
age.tertile * sex	9.61	2	0.0082
age.tertile * cholesterol	10.03	6	0.1232
Nonlinear Interaction : $f(A, B)$ vs. AB	2.40	4	0.6635
TOTAL NONLINEAR	10.30	6	0.1124
TOTAL INTERACTION	22.37	8	0.0043
TOTAL NONLINEAR+INTERACTION	30.12	10	0.0008
TOTAL	404.94	14	0.0000

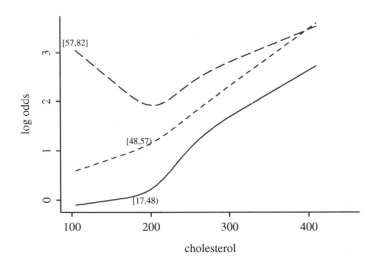

FIGURE 10.9: Log odds of significant coronary artery disease modeling age with two dummy variables.

Before fitting a parametric model that allows interaction between age and cholesterol, let us use the local regression model of Cleveland et al.[65] discussed in Section 2.4.6. This nonparametric smoothing method is not meant to handle binary Y, but it can still provide useful graphical displays in the binary case. Figure 10.10 depicts the fit from a local regression model predicting $Y = 1 = $ significant coronary artery disease. Predictors are sex (modeled parametrically with a dummy variable), age, and cholesterol, the last two fitted nonparametrically. The effect of not explicitly modeling a probability is seen in the figure, as the predicted probabilities exceeded 1. Because of this we do not take the logit transformation but leave the predicted values in raw form. However, the overall shape is in agreement with Figure 10.9.

Chapter 2 discussed linear splines, which can be used to construct linear spline surfaces by adding all cross-products of the linear variables and spline terms in the model. With a sufficient number of knots for each predictor, the linear spline surface can fit a wide variety of patterns. However, it requires a large number of parameters to be estimated. For the age–sex–cholesterol example, a linear spline surface is fitted for age and cholesterol, and a sex × age spline interaction is also allowed. Figure 10.11 shows a fit that placed knots at quartiles of the two continuous variables. The fitted model is $X\hat{\beta} = -1.83 + 0.0232$ age $+ 0.0759$(age $- 46)_+ - 0.0025$(age $- 52)_+ + 2.2722$(age $- 59)_+ + 3.02$\{female\} $- 0.0177$ chol $+ 0.1139$(chol $- 196)_+ - 0.1310$(chol$-224)_+ +0.0651$(chol$-259)_+ +$\{female\}$[-0.1124$age$+0.0852$(age$-46)_+ - 0.0302$(a ge$-52)_+ +0.1761$(age$-59)_+] +$age$[0.000577$chol-0.002857(chol$-196)_+ + 0.003818$ (chol $- 224)_+ - 0.002052$ (chol $- 259)_+] + ($age $- 46)_+[-0.000936$ chol $+ 0.006433$ (chol $- 196)_+ - 0.011469$ (chol $- 224)_+ + 0.007563$ (chol $- 259)_+] + ($age $-$

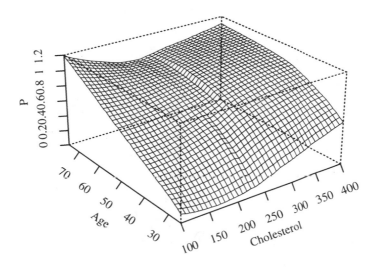

FIGURE 10.10:   Local regression fit for the probability of significant coronary disease versus age and cholesterol for males, based on the S-PLUS **loess** function.[65]

$52)_+[0.000433\ \text{chol} - 0.003699(\text{chol} - 196)_+ + 0.008150(\text{chol} - 224)_+ - 0.007152(\text{chol} - 259)_+] + (\text{age} - 59)_+[-0.012360\ \text{chol} + 0.015039\ (\text{chol} - 196)_+ \quad 0.006702\ (\text{chol} - 224)_+ + 0.007519\ (\text{chol} - 259)_+]$.

Chapter 2 also discussed an extension of the restricted cubic spline model to a smooth function of two predictors, $f(X_1, X_2)$. Since this function allows for general interaction between X_1 and X_2, the two-variable cubic spline is a powerful tool for displaying and testing interaction, assuming the sample size warrants estimating $2(k-1) + (k-1)^2$ parameters for a rectangular grid of $k \times k$ knots. Unlike the linear spline surface, the cubic surface is smooth. It also requires fewer parameters in most situations. The general cubic model with $k = 4$ (ignoring the sex effect here) is

$$
\begin{aligned}
& \beta_0 + \beta_1 X_1 + \beta_2 X_1' + \beta_3 X_1'' + \beta_4 X_2 + \beta_5 X_2' + \beta_6 X_2'' + \beta_7 X_1 X_2 \\
+ \quad & \beta_8 X_1 X_2' + \beta_9 X_1 X_2'' + \beta_{10} X_1' X_2 + \beta_{11} X_1' X_2' \\
+ \quad & + \beta_{12} X_1' X_2'' + \beta_{13} X_1'' X_2 + \beta_{14} X_1'' X_2' + \beta_{15} X_1'' X_2'',
\end{aligned} \tag{10.31}
$$

where X_1', X_1'', X_2', and X_2'' are restricted cubic spline component variables for X_1 and X_2 for $k = 4$. A general test of interaction with 9 d.f. is $H_0 : \beta_7 = \ldots = \beta_{15} = 0$. A test of adequacy of a simple product form interaction is $H_0 : \beta_8 = \ldots = \beta_{15} = 0$ with 8 d.f. A 13 d.f. test of linearity and additivity is $H_0 : \beta_2 = \beta_3 = \beta_5 = \beta_6 = \beta_7 = \beta_8 = \beta_9 = \beta_{10} = \beta_{11} = \beta_{12} = \beta_{13} = \beta_{14} = \beta_{15} = 0$.

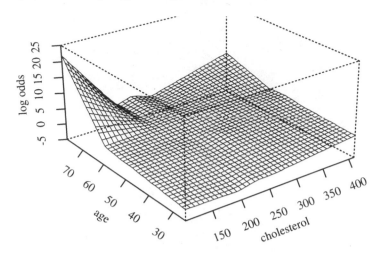

FIGURE 10.11: Linear spline surface for males, with knots for age at $46, 52$, and 59 and knots for cholesterol at $196, 224$, and 259 (quartiles).

Figure 10.12 depicts the fit of this model. There is excellent agreement with Figures 10.9 and 10.11, including an increased (but probably insignificant) risk with low cholesterol for age ≥ 57. The fitted function is $X\hat{\beta} = -6.41 + 0.16606$ age $- 0.00067(\text{age} - 36)^3_+ + 0.00543(\text{age} - 48)^3_+ - 0.00727(\text{age} - 56)^3_+ + 0.00251(\text{age} - 68)^3_+ + 2.87\{\text{female}\} + 9.79 \times 10^{-3}\text{chol} + 1.96 \times 10^{-6}(\text{chol} - 160)^3_+ - 7.16 \times 10^{-6}(\text{chol} - 208)^3_+ + 6.35 \times 10^{-6}(\text{chol} - 243)^3_+ - 1.16 \times 10^{-6}(\text{chol} - 319)^3_+ + \{\text{female}\}[-1.09 \times 10^{-1}\text{age} + 7.52 \times 10^{-5}(\text{age} - 36)^3_+ + 1.50 \times 10^{-4}(\text{age} - 48)^3_+ - 4.50 \times 10^{-4}(\text{age} - 56)^3_+ + 2.25 \times 10^{-4}(\text{age} - 68)^3_+] + \text{age}[-2.80 \times 10^{-4}\text{chol} + 2.68 \times 10^{-9}(\text{chol} - 160)^3_+ + 3.03 \times 10^{-8}(\text{chol} - 208)^3_+ - 4.99 \times 10^{-8}(\text{chol} - 243)^3_+ + 1.69 \times 10^{-8}(\text{chol} - 319)^3_+] + \text{age}'[3.41 \times 10^{-3}\text{chol} - 4.02 \times 10^{-7}(\text{chol} - 160)^3_+ + 9.71 \times 10^{-7}(\text{chol} - 208)^3_+ - 5.79 \times 10^{-7}(\text{chol} - 243)^3_+ + 8.79 \times 10^{-9}(\text{chol} - 319)^3_+] + \text{age}''[-2.90 \times 10^{-2}\text{chol} + 3.04 \times 10^{-6}(\text{chol} - 160)^3_+ - 7.34 \times 10^{-6}(\text{chol} - 208)^3_+ + 4.36 \times 10^{-6}(\text{chol} - 243)^3_+ - 5.82 \times 10^{-8}(\text{chol} - 319)^3_+].$

Statistics for testing age $\times$ cholesterol components of this fit follow.

Wald Statistics

Factor	χ^2	d.f.	P
age * cholesterol	12.95	9	0.1649
Nonlinear Interaction : $f(A, B)$ vs. AB	7.27	8	0.5078
$f(A, B)$ vs. $Af(B) + Bg(A)$	5.41	4	0.2480
Nonlinear Interaction in age vs. $Af(B)$	6.44	6	0.3753
Nonlinear Interaction in cholesterol vs. $Bg(A)$	6.27	6	0.3931

None of the nonlinear interaction components is significant, but we again retain them.

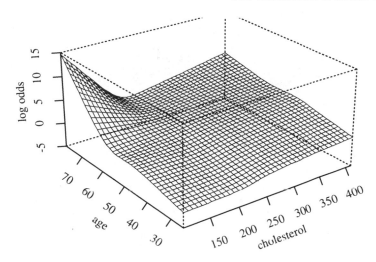

FIGURE 10.12: Restricted cubic spline surface in two variables, each with $k = 4$ knots.

The general interaction model can be restricted to be of the form

$$f(X_1, X_2) = f_1(X_1) + f_2(X_2) + X_1 g_2(X_2) + X_2 g_1(X_1) \qquad (10.32)$$

by removing the parameters $\beta_{11}, \beta_{12}, \beta_{14}$, and β_{15} from the model. The previous table of Wald statistics included a test of adequacy of this reduced form ($\chi^2 = 5.41$ on 4 d.f., $P = .248$). The resulting fit is in Figure 10.13, and the fitted equation is $X\hat{\beta} = -7.2 + 2.96\{\text{female}\} + 1.64 \times 10^{-1}\text{age} + 7.23 \times 10^{-5}(\text{age} - 36)_+^3 - 1.06 \times 10^{-4}(\text{age} - 48)_+^3 - 1.63 \times 10^{-5}(\text{age} - 56)_+^3 + 4.99 \times 10^{-5}(\text{age} - 68)_+^3 + 1.48 \times 10^{-2}\text{chol} + 1.21 \times 10^{-6}(\text{chol} - 160)_+^3 - 5.50 \times 10^{-6}(\text{chol} - 208)_+^3 + 5.50 \times 10^{-6}(\text{chol} - 243)_+^3 - 1.21 \times 10^{-6}(\text{chol} - 319)_+^3 + \text{age}[-2.90 \times 10^{-4}\text{chol} + 9.28 \times 10^{-9}(\text{chol} - 160)_+^3 + 1.70 \times 10^{-8}(\text{chol} - 208)_+^3 - 4.43 \times 10^{-8}(\text{chol} - 243)_+^3 + 1.79 \times 10^{-8}(\text{chol} - 319)_+^3] + \text{chol}[-5.52 \times 10^{-7}(\text{age} - 36)_+^3 + 7.97 \times 10^{-7}(\text{age} - 48)_+^3 + 1.45 \times 10^{-7}(\text{age} - 56)_+^3 - 3.89 \times 10^{-7}(\text{age} - 68)_+^3] + \{\text{female}\}[-1.11 \times 10^{-1}\text{age} + 8.03 \times 10^{-5}(\text{age} - 36)_+^3 + 1.35 \times 10^{-4}(\text{age} - 48)_+^3 - 4.40 \times 10^{-4}(\text{age} - 56)_+^3 + 2.24 \times 10^{-4}(\text{age} - 68)_+^3]$. The fit is similar to the former one except that the climb in risk for low-cholesterol older subjects is less pronounced.

Wald Statistics

Factor	χ^2	d.f.	P
age * cholesterol	10.83	5	0.0548
Nonlinear Interaction : $f(A, B)$ vs. AB	3.12	4	0.5372
Nonlinear Interaction in age vs. $Af(B)$	1.60	2	0.4496
Nonlinear Interaction in cholesterol vs. $Bg(A)$	1.64	2	0.4399

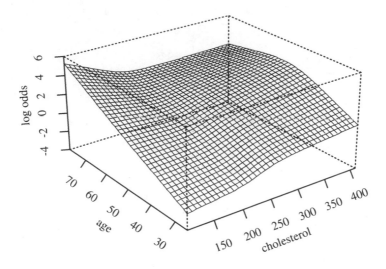

FIGURE 10.13: Restricted cubic spline fit with age $\times$ spline(cholesterol) and cholesterol $\times$ spline(age).

The test for nonlinear interaction is now more concentrated ($P = .54$ with 4 d.f.). Figure 10.14 accordingly depicts a fit that allows age and cholesterol to have nonlinear main effects, but restricts the interaction to be a product between (untransformed) age and cholesterol. The function agrees substantially with the previous fit. The fitted equation is $X\hat{\beta} = -7.36 + 1.82 \times 10^{-1} \text{age} - 5.18 \times 10^{-5} (\text{age} - 36)_+^3 + 8.45 \times 10^{-5} (\text{age} - 48)_+^3 - 2.91 \times 10^{-6} (\text{age} - 56)_+^3 - 2.99 \times 10^{-5} (\text{age} - 68)_+^3 + 2.8\{\text{female}\} + 1.39 \times 10^{-2} \text{chol} + 1.76 \times 10^{-6} (\text{chol} - 160)_+^3 - 4.88 \times 10^{-6} (\text{chol} - 208)_+^3 + 3.45 \times 10^{-6} (\text{chol} - 243)_+^3 - 3.26 \times 10^{-7} (\text{chol} - 319)_+^3 - 0.00034 \text{ age} \times \text{chol} + \{\text{female}\}[-1.07 \times 10^{-1} \text{age} + 7.71 \times 10^{-5} (\text{age} - 36)_+^3 + 1.15 \times 10^{-4} (\text{age} - 48)_+^3 - 3.98 \times 10^{-4} (\text{age} - 56)_+^3 + 2.05 \times 10^{-4} (\text{age} - 68)_+^3]$.

The Wald test for age $\times$ cholesterol interaction yields $\chi^2 = 7.99$ with 1 d.f., $P = .005$. These analyses favor the nonlinear model with simple product interaction in Figure 10.14 as best representing the relationships among cholesterol, age, and probability of prognostically severe coronary artery disease. A nomogram depicting this model is shown in Figure 10.21.

Using this simple product interaction model, Figure 10.15 displays predicted cholesterol effects at the mean age within each age tertile. Substantial agreement with Figure 10.9 is apparent.

The partial residuals discussed in Section 10.4 can be used to check logistic model fit (although it may be difficult to deal with interactions). As an example, reconsider the "duration of symptoms" fit in Figure 10.6. Figure 10.16 displays "loess smoothed" and raw partial residuals for the original and log-transformed variable.

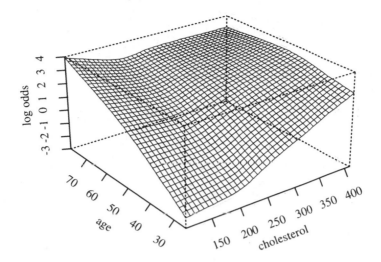

FIGURE 10.14:   Spline fit with nonlinear effects of cholesterol and age and a simple product interaction.

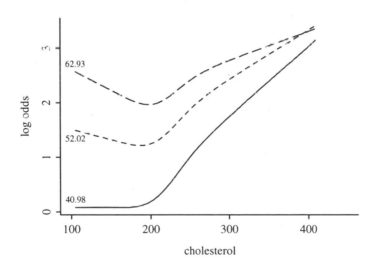

FIGURE 10.15:   Predictions from linear interaction model with mean age in tertiles indicated.

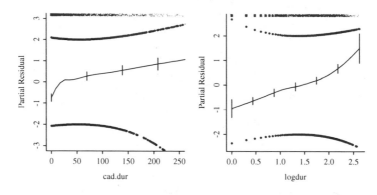

FIGURE 10.16: Partial residuals for duration and $\log_{10}(\text{duration}+1)$. Data density shown at top of each plot.

TABLE 10.5: Merits of Methods for Checking Logistic Model Assumptions

Method	Choice Required	Assumes Additivity	Uses Ordering of X	Low Variance	Good Resolution on X
Stratification	Intervals				
Smoother on X_1 stratifying on X_2	Bandwidth		x (not on X_2)	x (if min. strat.)	x (X_1)
Smooth partial residual plot	Bandwidth	x	x	x	x
Spline model for all Xs	Knots	x	x	x	x

The latter provides a more linear relationship, especially where the data are most dense.

Table 10.5 summarizes the relative merits of stratification, nonparametric smoothers, and regression splines for determining or checking binary logistic model fits.

10.6 Collinearity

The variance inflation factors (VIFs) discussed in Section 4.6 can apply to any regression fit. [106, 446] These VIFs allow the analyst to isolate which variable(s) are responsible for highly correlated parameter estimates. Recall that, in general, collinearity is not a large problem compared to nonlinearity and overfitting.

10.7   Overly Influential Observations

Pregibon[342] developed a number of regression diagnostics that apply to the family of regression models of which logistic regression is a member. Influence statistics based on the "leave-out-one" method use an approximation to avoid having to refit the model n times for n observations. This approximation uses the fit and covariance matrix at the last iteration and assumes that the "weights" in the weighted least squares fit can be kept constant, yielding a computationally feasible one-step estimate of the leave-out-one regression coefficients.

Hosmer and Lemeshow [210, pp. 149–170] discuss many diagnostics for logistic regression and show how the final fit can be used in any least squares program that provides diagnostics. A new dependent variable to do this is defined as

$$Z_i = X\hat{\beta} + \frac{Y_i - \hat{P}_i}{V_i}, \tag{10.33}$$

where $V_i = \hat{P}_i(1 - \hat{P}_i)$, and $\hat{P}_i = [1 + \exp -X\hat{\beta}]^{-1}$ is the predicted probability that $Y_i - 1$. The $V_i, i = 1, 2, \ldots, n$ are used as weights in an ordinary weighted least squares fit of X against Z. This least squares fit will provide regression coefficients identical to b. The new standard errors will be off from the actual logistic model ones by a constant.

As discussed in Section 4.8, the standardized change in the regression coefficients upon leaving out each observation in turn (DFBETAS) is one of the most useful diagnostics, as these can pinpoint which observations are influential on each part of the model. After carefully modeling predictor transformations, there should be no lack of fit due to improper transformations. However, as the white blood count example in Section 4.8 indicates, it is commonly the case that extreme predictor values can still have too much influence on the estimates of coefficients involving that predictor.

In the age–sex–response example of Section 10.1.3, both DFBETAS and DFFITS identified the same influential observations. The observation given by age = 48 sex = female response = 1 was influential for both age and sex, while the observation age = 34 sex = male response = 1 was influential for age and the observation age = 50 sex = male response = 0 was influential for sex. It can readily be seen from Figure 10.3 that these points do not fit the overall trends in the data. However, as these data were simulated from a population model that is truly linear in age and additive in age and sex, the apparent influential observations are just random occurrences. It is unwise to assume that in real data all points will agree with overall trends. Removal of such points would bias the results, making the model apparently more predictive than it will be prospectively. See Table 10.6.

TABLE 10.6

Females				Males			
DFBETAS			DFFITS	DFBETAS			DFFITS
Intercept	Age	Sex		Intercept	Age	Sex	
0.0	0.0	0.0	0	0.5	-0.5	-0.2	2
0.0	0.0	0.0	0	0.2	-0.3	0.0	1
0.0	0.0	0.0	0	-0.1	0.1	0.0	-1
0.0	0.0	0.0	0	-0.1	0.1	0.0	-1
-0.1	0.1	0.1	0	-0.1	0.1	-0.1	-1
-0.1	0.1	0.1	0	0.0	0.0	0.1	0
0.7	-0.7	-0.8	3	0.0	0.0	0.1	0
-0.1	0.1	0.1	0	0.0	0.0	0.1	0
-0.1	0.1	0.1	0	0.0	0.0	-0.2	-1
-0.1	0.1	0.1	0	0.1	-0.1	-0.2	-1
-0.1	0.1	0.1	0	0.0	0.0	0.1	0
-0.1	0.0	0.1	0	-0.1	0.1	0.1	0
-0.1	0.0	0.1	0	-0.1	0.1	0.1	0
0.1	0.0	-0.2	1	0.3	-0.3	-0.4	-2
0.0	0.0	0.1	-1	-0.1	0.1	0.1	0
0.1	-0.2	0.0	-1	-0.1	0.1	0.1	0
-0.1	0.2	0.0	1	-0.1	0.1	0.1	0
-0.2	0.2	0.0	1	0.0	0.0	0.0	0
-0.2	0.2	0.0	1	0.0	0.0	0.0	0
-0.2	0.2	0.1	1	0.0	0.0	0.0	0

10.8   Quantifying Predictive Ability

The test statistics discussed above allow one to test whether a factor or set of factors is related to the response. If the sample is sufficiently large, a factor that grades risk from .01 to .02 may be a significant risk factor. However, that factor is not very useful in predicting the response for an individual subject. There is controversy regarding the appropriateness of R^2 from ordinary least squares in this setting.[96, 293] The generalized R^2_N index of Nagelkerke[322] and Cragg and Uhler[97] described in Section 9.8.3 can be useful for quantifying the predictive strength of a model:

$$R^2_N = \frac{1 - \exp(-\text{LR}/n)}{1 - \exp(-L^0/n)},\tag{10.34}$$

where LR is the global log likelihood ratio statistic for testing the importance of all p predictors in the model and L^0 is the -2 log likelihood for the null model.

Linnet[287] advocates quadratic and logarithmic probability scoring rules for measuring predictive performance for probability models. Linnet shows how to bootstrap such measures to get bias-corrected estimates and how to use bootstrapping to compare two correlated scores. The quadratic scoring rule is Brier's score, frequently used in judging meteorologic forecasts[23, 52]:

$$B = \frac{1}{n}\sum_{i=1}^{n}(\hat{P}_i - Y_i)^2,\tag{10.35}$$

where $\hat{P}_i$ is the predicted probability and Y_i the corresponding observed response for the ith observation.

A unitless index of the strength of the rank correlation between predicted probability of response and actual response is a more interpretable measure of the fitted model's predictive discrimination. One such index is the probability of concordance, c, between predicted probability and response. The c index, which is derived from the Wilcoxon–Mann–Whitney two-sample rank test, is computed by taking all possible pairs of subjects such that one subject responded and the other did not. The index is the proportion of such pairs with the responder having a higher predicted probability of response than the nonresponder.

Bamber[27] and Hanley and McNeil[173] have shown that c is identical to a widely used measure of diagnostic discrimination, the area under a "receiver operating characteristic" (ROC) curve. A value of c of .5 indicates random predictions, and a value of 1 indicates perfect prediction (i.e., perfect separation of responders and nonresponders). A model having c greater than roughly .8 has some utility in predicting the responses of individual subjects. The concordance index is also related to another widely used index, Somers' D_{xy} rank correlation[393] between predicted probabilities and observed responses, by the identity

$$D_{xy} = 2(c - .5). \tag{10.36}$$

D_{xy} is the difference between concordance and discordance probabilities. When $D_{xy} = 0$, the model is making random predictions. When $D_{xy} = 1$, the predictions are perfectly discriminating. These rank-based indexes have the advantage of being insensitive to the prevalence of positive responses.

12

A commonly used measure of predictive ability for binary logistic models is the fraction of correctly classified responses. Here one chooses a cutoff on the predicted probability of a positive response and then predicts that a response will be positive if the predicted probability exceeds this cutoff. There are a number of reasons why this measure should be avoided.

1. It's highly dependent on the cutpoint chosen for a "positive" prediction.

2. You can add a highly significant variable to the model and have the percentage classified correctly actually decrease. Classification error is a very insensitive and statistically inefficient measure[180, 433] since if the threshold for "positive" is, say 0.75, a prediction of 0.99 rates the same as one of 0.751.

3. It gets away from the purpose of fitting a logistic model. A logistic model is a model for the probability of an event, not a model for the occurrence of the event. For example, suppose that the event we are predicting is the probability of being struck by lightning. Without having any data, we would predict that you won't get struck by lightning. However, you might develop an interesting model that discovers real risk factors that yield probabilities of being struck that range from 0.000000001 to 0.001.

4. If you make a classification rule from a probability model, you are being presumptuous. Suppose that a model is developed to assist physicians in diagnosing a disease. Physicians sometimes say that they want a binary decision model, but when you study their behavior you'll find that if you give them a probability, they will apply different thresholds for treating different patients or for ordering other diagnostic tests. Even though the age of the patient may be a strong predictor of the probability of disease, the physician will often use a lower threshold of disease likelihood for treating a young patient. This usage is above and beyond how age affects the likelihood.

5. van Houwelingen and le Cessie[433] demonstrated a peculiar property that occurs when you try to obtain an honest estimate of classification error using cross-validation. The cross-validated error rate corrects the apparent error rate only if the predicted probability is exactly $1/2$ or is $1/2 \pm 1/(2n)$. The cross-validation estimate of optimism is "zero for n even and negligibly small

for n odd." Better measures of error rate such as the Brier score and logarithmic scoring rule do not have this problem. They also have the nice property of being maximized when the predicted probabilities are the population probabilities.[287]

13

10.9   Validating the Fitted Model

The major cause of unreliable models is overfitting the data. The methods described in Section 5.2 can be used to assess the accuracy of models fairly. If a sample has been held out and never used to study associations with the response, indexes of predictive accuracy can now be estimated using that sample. More efficient is cross-validation, and bootstrapping is the most efficient validation procedure. As discussed earlier, bootstrapping does not require holding out any data, since all aspects of model development (stepwise variable selection, tests of linearity, estimation of coefficients, etc.) are revalidated on samples taken with replacement from the whole sample.

Cox[90] proposed and Harrell and Lee[183] and Miller et al.[315] further developed the idea of fitting a new binary logistic model to a new sample to estimate the relationship between the predicted probability and the observed outcome in that sample. This fit provides a simple calibration equation that can be used to quantify unreliability (lack of calibration) and to calibrate the predictions for future use. This logistic calibration also leads to indexes of unreliability (U), discrimination (D), and overall quality ($Q = D - U$) which are derived from likelihood ratio tests[183]. Q is a logarithmic scoring rule, which can be compared with Brier's index (Equation 10.35). See [433] for many more ideas.

With bootstrapping we do not have a separate validation sample for assessing calibration, but we can estimate the overoptimism in assuming that the final model needs no calibration, that is, it has overall intercept and slope corrections of 0 and 1, respectively. As discussed in Section 5.2, refitting the model

$$P_c = \text{Prob}\{Y = 1|X\hat{\beta}\} = [1 + \exp-(\gamma_0 + \gamma_1 X\hat{\beta})]^{-1} \qquad (10.37)$$

(where P_c denotes the actual calibrated probability and the original predicted probability is $\hat{P} = [1 + \exp(-X\hat{\beta})]^{-1}$) in the original sample will always result in $\gamma = (\gamma_0, \gamma_1) = (0, 1)$, since a logistic model will always "fit" the training sample when assessed overall. We thus estimate γ by using Efron's[124] method to estimate the overoptimism in $(0, 1)$ to obtain bias-corrected estimates of the true calibration. Simulations have shown this method produces an efficient estimate of γ.[176]

A good set of indexes to estimate for summarizing a model validation is the c or D_{xy} indexes and measures of calibration. In addition, the overoptimism in the indexes may be reported to quantify the amount of overfitting present. The

TABLE 10.7: Validation of Two-Variable Logistic Model

Index	Original Sample	Training Sample	Test Sample	Optimism	Corrected Index
D_{xy}	0.70	0.70	0.67	0.03	0.66
R^2	0.45	0.47	0.43	0.04	0.41
Intercept	0.00	0.00	0.00	0.00	0.00
Slope	1.00	1.00	0.91	0.09	0.91
E_{max}	0.00	0.00	0.02	0.02	0.02
D	0.39	0.42	0.36	0.06	0.33
U	-0.05	-0.05	0.02	-0.07	0.02
Q	0.44	0.47	0.35	0.12	0.32
B	0.16	0.15	0.17	-0.02	0.18

estimate of γ can be used to draw a calibration curve by plotting $\hat{P}$ on the x-axis and $\hat{P}_c = [1 + \exp -(\gamma_0 + \gamma_1 L)]^{-1}$ on the y-axis, where $L = \text{logit}(\hat{P})$.[90, 183] An easily interpreted index of unreliability, E_{max}, follows immediately from this calibration model:

$$E_{max}(a, b) = \max_{a \leq \hat{P} \leq b} |\hat{P} - \hat{P}_c|, \qquad (10.38)$$

the maximum error in predicted probabilities over the range $a \leq \hat{P} \leq b$. In some cases, we would compute the maximum absolute difference in predicted and calibrated probabilities over the entire interval, that is, use $E_{max}(0, 1)$. The null hypothesis $H_0 : E_{max}(0, 1) = 0$ can easily be tested by testing $H_0 : \gamma_0 = 0, \gamma_1 = 1$ as above. Since E_{max} does not weight the discrepancies by the actual distribution of predictions, it may be preferable to compute the average absolute discrepancy over the actual distribution of predictions (or to use a mean squared error, incorporating the same calibration function).

If stepwise variable selection is being done, a matrix depicting which factors are selected at each bootstrap sample will shed light on how arbitrary is the selection of "significant" factors. See Section 5.2 for reasons to compare full and stepwise model fits.

As an example using bootstrapping to validate the calibration and discrimination of a model, consider the data in Section 10.1.3. Using 80 samples with replacement, we first validate the additive model with age and sex forced into every model. The optimism-corrected discrimination and calibration statistics produced by `validate` (see Section 10.11) are in Table 10.7.

The apparent Somers' D_{xy} is 0.70, and the bias-corrected D_{xy} is 0.66. The slope shrinkage factor is 0.91. The maximum absolute error in predicted probability is estimated to be 0.02.

We next allow for step-down variable selection at each resample. For illustration purposes only, we use a suboptimal stopping rule based on significance of *individual*

TABLE 10.8: Validation of Two-Variable Stepwise Model

Index	Original Sample	Training Sample	Test Sample	Optimism	Corrected Index
D_{xy}	0.70	0.71	0.66	0.05	0.64
R^2	0.45	0.50	0.42	0.07	0.38
Intercept	0.00	0.00	0.04	-0.04	0.04
Slope	1.00	1.00	0.86	0.14	0.86
E_{max}	0.00	0.00	0.04	0.04	0.04
D	0.39	0.45	0.36	0.09	0.30
U	-0.05	-0.05	0.02	-0.07	0.02
Q	0.44	0.50	0.34	0.16	0.27
B	0.16	0.15	0.18	-0.03	0.19

variables at the $\alpha = 0.10$ level. Of the 80 repetitions, both age and sex were selected in 76. Age alone was selected in 1, sex alone in 2, and neither variable in 1 sample. The validation statistics are in Table 10.8.

The apparent Somers' D_{xy} is 0.70 for the original stepwise model (which actually retained both age and sex), and the bias-corrected D_{xy} is 0.64, slightly worse than the more correct model which forced in both variables. The calibration was also slightly worse as reflected in the slope correction factor estimate of 0.86 versus 0.91.

Next, five additional candidate variables are considered. These variables are random uniform variables, $r1$, $r5$ on the $[0, 1]$ interval, so in truth they have no association with the response. The initial model fit is as follows.

```
Obs Max Deriv Model L.R. d.f.     P   C  Dxy Gamma Tau-a   R2
 40   0.00039         21      7 0.0044 0.88 0.75  0.75  0.39  0.41
```

```
               Coef    S.E. Wald Z     P
Intercept -12.5937 4.98756 -2.53  0.0116
      age   0.1946 0.08022  2.43  0.0153
      sex   4.4041 1.65375  2.66  0.0077
       x1   1.7710 1.91092  0.93  0.3540
       x2  -0.1205 1.76278 -0.07  0.9455
       x3  -1.0918 1.60198 -0.68  0.4955
       x4   2.7479 1.65950  1.66  0.0978
       x5  -1.9737 2.22335 -0.89  0.3747
```

Using step-down variable selection with the same stopping rule as before, the "final" model on the original sample correctly deleted $x1, \ldots, x5$. Of the 80 bootstrap repetitions, 15 samples yielded a singularity or nonconvergence in either the full-model fit or after step-down variable selection. Of the 65 successful repetitions, the frequencies of the number of factors selected are shown in Table 10.9. The first 15 patterns of factors selected are listed in Table 10.10. Overall, age was selected

TABLE 10.9

Number of Factors Selected	0	1	2	3	4	5
Frequency	38	3	6	9	5	4

TABLE 10.10: Variables Selected in First 15 Resamples

age	sex	x1	x2	x3	x4	x5
x	x					
x	x				x	
x						
x	x					
x	x	x			x	x
x	x				x	
x	x			x		

TABLE 10.11: Validation of Model With Five Noise Variables

Index	Original Sample	Training Sample	Test Sample	Optimism	Corrected Index
D_{xy}	0.70	0.32	0.26	0.05	0.64
R^2	0.45	0.23	0.17	0.06	0.39
Intercept	0.00	0.00	-0.03	0.03	-0.03
Slope	1.00	1.00	0.85	0.15	0.85
E_{max}	0.00	0.00	0.04	0.04	0.04
D	0.39	0.21	0.13	0.07	0.32
U	-0.05	-0.05	0.03	-0.08	0.03
Q	0.44	0.26	0.10	0.15	0.29
B	0.16	0.20	0.23	-0.03	0.19

in 23 samples, sex in 27, and the next most common was $x4$ with 17. Note that $x4$ is the most significant of the 5 xs at $P = 0.098$, just significant at the cutoff value of 0.10. (After deleting insignificant x's, the P-value of $x4$ dropped to 0.21.) Validation statistics are in Table 10.11.

You can see that the stepwise modeling of age, sex, and $x1, \ldots, x5$ produces the worst model of the three methods, with $D_{xy} = 0.64$, slope = 0.85, and maximum prediction error 0.04. Figure 10.17 depicts the calibration (reliability) curves for the three strategies using the corrected intercept and slope estimates in the above tables as γ_0 and γ_1, and the logistic calibration model $P_c = [1 + \exp -(\gamma_0 + \gamma_1 L)]^{-1}$, where P_c is the "actual" or calibrated probability, L is logit($\hat{P}$), and $\hat{P}$ is the predicted probability. The shape of the calibration curves (driven by slopes < 1) is typical of overfitting—low predicted probabilities are too low and high predicted probabilities are too high. Predictions near the overall prevalence of the outcome tend to be calibrated even when overfitting is present. "Honest" calibration curves may also be estimated using nonparametric smoothers in conjunction with bootstrapping and cross-validation (see Section 10.11).

10.10   Describing the Fitted Model

Once the proper variables have been modeled and all model assumptions have been met, the analyst needs to present and interpret the fitted model. There are at least three ways to proceed. The coefficients in the model may be interpreted. For each variable, the change in log odds for a sensible change in the variable value (e.g., interquartile range) may be computed. Also, the odds ratio or factor by which the odds increases for a certain change in a predictor, holding all other predictors constant, may be displayed. Table 10.12 contains such summary statistics for the full age $\times$ cholesterol interaction surface fit described in Section 10.5.

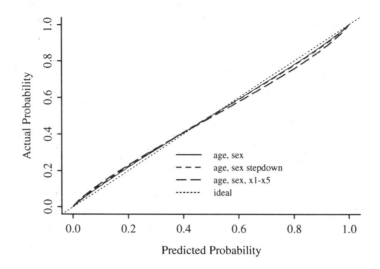

FIGURE 10.17: Estimated logistic calibration (reliability) curves obtained by bootstrapping three modeling strategies.

TABLE 10.12

Factor	Low	High	Δ	Effect	S.E.	Lower 0.95	Upper 0.95
age	46	59	13	0.90	0.21	0.49	1.32
Odds Ratio	46	59	13	2.47		1.63	3.74
cholesterol	196	259	63	0.79	0.18	0.44	1.15
Odds Ratio	196	259	63	2.21		1.55	3.17
sex – female:male	1	2		−2.46	0.15	−2.75	−2.16
Odds Ratio	1	2		0.09		0.06	0.12

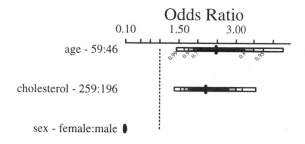

Adjusted to:age=52 sex=male cholesterol=224

FIGURE 10.18: Odds ratios and confidence bars, using quartiles of age and cholesterol for assessing their effects on the odds of coronary disease.

The outer quartiles of age are 46 and 59 years, so the "half-sample" odds ratio for age is 2.47, with 0.95 confidence interval $[1.63, 3.74]$ when sex is male and cholesterol is set to its median. The effect of increasing cholesterol from 196 (its lower quartile) to 259 (its upper quartile) is to increase the log odds by 0.79 or to increase the odds by a factor of 2.21. Since there are interactions allowed between age and sex and between age and cholesterol, each odds ratio in the above table depends on the setting of at least one other factor. The results are shown graphically in Figure 10.18. The shaded confidence bars show various levels of confidence and do not pin the analyst down to, say, 0.95.

For those used to thinking in terms of odds or log odds, the preceding description may be sufficient. Many prefer instead to interpret the model in terms of predicted probabilities instead of odds. If the model contains only a single predictor (even if several spline terms are required to represent that predictor), one may simply plot the predictor against the predicted response. Such a plot is shown in Figure 10.19 which depicts the fitted relationship between age of diagnosis and the probability of acute bacterial meningitis (ABM) as opposed to acute viral meningitis (AVM), based on an analysis of 422 cases from Duke University Medical Center.[394] The data may be found on the Web site. A linear spline function with knots at 1, 2, and 22 years was used to model this relationship. When the model contains more than one predictor, one may graph the predictor against log odds, and barring interactions, the shape of this relationship will be independent of the level of the other predictors. When displaying the model on what is usually a more interpretable scale, the probability scale, a difficulty arises in that unlike log odds the relationship between one predictor and the probability of response depends on the levels of all other factors. For example, in the model

$$\text{Prob}\{Y = 1|X\} = \{1 + \exp[-(\beta_0 + \beta_1 X_1 + \beta_2 X_2)]\}^{-1} \qquad (10.39)$$

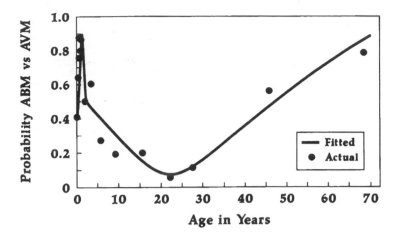

FIGURE 10.19: Linear spline fit for probability of bacterial versus viral meningitis as a function of age at onset[394]. Copyright 1989, American Medical Association. Reprinted by permission.

there is no way to factor out X_1 when examining the relationship between X_2 and the probability of a response. For the two-predictor case one can plot X_2 versus predicted probability for each level of X_1. When it is uncertain whether to include an interaction in this model, consider presenting graphs for two models (with and without interaction terms included) as was done in [450].

When three factors are present, one could draw a separate graph for each level of X_3, a separate curve on each graph for each level of X_1, and vary X_2 on the x-axis. Instead of this, or if more than three factors are present, a good way to display the results may be to plot "adjusted probability estimates" as a function of one predictor, adjusting all other factors to constants such as the mean. For example, one could display a graph relating serum cholesterol to probability of myocardial infarction or death, holding age constant at 55, sex at 1 (male), and systolic blood pressure at 120 mmHg.

The final method for displaying the relationship between several predictors and probability of response is to construct a nomogram.[28, 172] A nomogram not only sheds light on how the effect of one predictor on the probability of response depends on the levels of other factors, but it allows one to quickly estimate the probability of response for individual subjects. The nomogram in Figure 10.20 allows one to predict the probability of acute bacterial meningitis (given the patient has either viral or bacterial meningitis) using the same sample as in Figure 10.19. Here there are four continuous predictor values, none of which are linearly related to log odds of bacterial meningitis: age at admission (expressed as a linear spline function), month of admission (expressed as |month − 8|), cerebrospinal fluid glucose/blood glucose ratio (linear effect truncated at .6; that is, the effect is the glucose ratio if it is $\le$ .6, and .6 if it exceeded .6), and the cube root of the total number of polymorphonuclear leukocytes in the cerebrospinal fluid.

[14]

The model associated with Figure 10.14 is depicted in what could be called a "precision nomogram" in Figure 10.21. Discrete cholesterol levels were required because of the interaction between two continuous variables.

10.11   S-PLUS Functions

The general S-PLUS statistical modeling functions[65] described in Section 6.2 work with the lrm function written by Harrell for fitting binary and ordinal logistic regression models. lrm has several options for doing penalized maximum likelihood estimation, with special treatment of categorical predictors so as to shrink all estimates (including the reference cell) to the mean. The following example fits a logistic model containing predictors age, blood.pressure, and sex, with age fitted with a smooth five-knot restricted cubic spline function and a different shape of the age relationship for males and females.

```
fit ← lrm(death ~ blood.pressure + sex * rcs(age,5))
anova(fit)
plot(fit, age=NA, sex=NA)
```

The pentrace function makes it easy to check the effects of a sequence of penalties. The following code fits an unpenalized model and plots the AIC and Schwarz BIC for a variety of penalties so that approximately the best cross-validating model can be chosen (and so we can learn how the penalty relates to the effective degrees of freedom). Here we elect to only penalize the nonlinear or nonadditive parts of the model.

```
f ← lrm(death ~ rcs(age,5)*treatment + lsp(sbp,c(120,140)),
        x=T,y=T)
plot(pentrace(f, penalty=list(nonlinear=seq(.25,10,by=.25))))
```

See Sections 9.8.1 and 9.10 for more information.

Figure 10.5 was created using

```
f ← lrm(sigdz ~ rcs(age,4)*sex)
options(digits=3)
latex(f, inline=T)
plot(f, age=NA, sex=NA, conf.int=F)
pl ← function(x,y,pch) {
  z ← cut2(x, g=10)
  mx ← tapply(x, z, mean)
  my ← tapply(y, z, mean)
  points(mx, log(my/(1-my)), pch=pch)
  z ← lowess(x,y,iter=0)
```

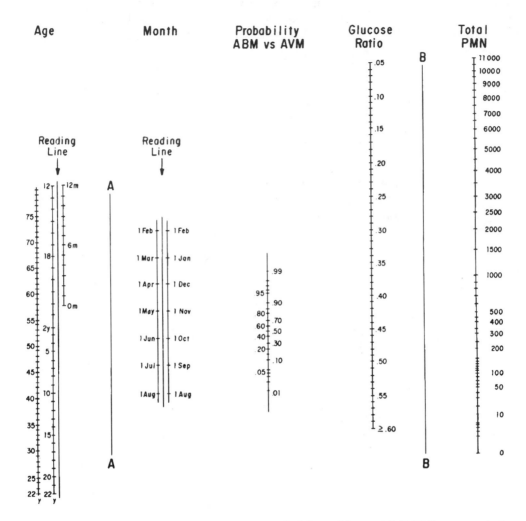

FIGURE 10.20: Nomogram for estimating probability of bacterial (ABM) versus viral (AVM) meningitis. Step 1, place ruler on reading lines for patient's age and month of presentation and mark intersection with line A; step 2, place ruler on values for glucose ratio and total polymorphonuclear leukocyte (PMN) count in cerebrospinal fluid and mark intersection with line B; step 3, use ruler to join marks on lines A and B, then read off the probability of ABM versus AVM.[394] Copyright 1989, American Medical Association. Reprinted by permission.

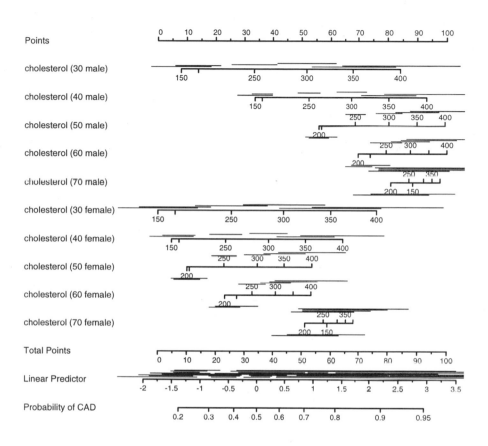

FIGURE 10.21: Nomogram relating age, sex, and cholesterol to the log odds and to the probability of significant coronary artery disease. Select one axis corresponding to sex and to age $\in \{30, 40, 50, 60, 70\}$. There is linear interaction between age and sex and between age and cholesterol. 0.70 and 0.90 confidence intervals are shown (0.90 in gray). Note that for the "Linear Predictor" scale there are various lengths of confidence intervals near the same value of $X\hat{\beta}$, demonstrating that the standard error of $X\hat{\beta}$ depends on the individual X values. Also note that confidence intervals corresponding to smaller patient groups (e.g., females) are wider.

```
      points(z$x,log(z$y/(1-z$y)))
}
pl(age[sex=="male"  ], sigdz[sex=="male"  ], pch=2)
pl(age[sex=="female"], sigdz[sex=="female"], pch=4)
```

The `rcspline.plot` function in Harrell's `Hmisc` library does not allow for interactions as does `lrm`, but it can provide detailed output for checking spline fits. This function plots the estimated spline regression and confidence limits, placing summary statistics on the graph. If there are no adjustment variables, `rcspline.plot` can also plot two alternative estimates of the regression function: proportions or logit proportions on grouped data, and a nonparametric estimate. The nonparametric regression estimate is based on smoothing the binary responses and taking the logit transformation of the smoothed estimates, if desired. The smoothing uses the "super smoother" of Friedman[146] implemented in the S-PLUS function `supsmu`.[308] Figures 10.6 and 10.7 were drawn by the commands

```
attach(acath[acath$sigdz==1,])
rcspline.plot(cad.dur, tvdlm, m=150)
rcspline.plot(log10(cad.dur+1), tvdlm, m=150)
```

and Figure 10.9, the table of statistics, and the typeset fitted function were created with the S-PLUS commands that follow:

```
age.tertile ← cut2(age, g=3)
fit ← lrm(sigdz ~ age.tertile * sex +
            age.tertile * rcs(cholesterol, 4))
anova(fit)
plot(fit, cholesterol=NA, age.tertile=NA, conf.int=F)
latex(fit,inline=T,var=c("age","sex","chol"))
```

Figure 10.11 was created with

```
fit ← lrm(y ~ lsp(age,c(46,52,59)) *
              (sex + lsp(cholesterol,c(196,224,259))))
plot(fit, cholesterol=NA, age=NA)
```

Figure 10.12 and the table of statistics were produced by

```
fit ← lrm(sigdz ~ rcs(age,4) * sex +
          rcs(age,4) * rcs(cholesterol,4),
          tol=1e-14)
anova(fit)
plot(fit, cholesterol=NA, age=NA)
```

Figures 10.13 and 10.14, respectively, were produced by the following fits:

```
fit2 ← lrm(sigdz ~ rcs(age,4) * sex +  rcs(cholesterol,4) +
                  rcs(age,4) %ia% rcs(cholesterol,4))
fit3 ← lrm(sigdz ~ rcs(age,4) * sex + rcs(cholesterol,4) +
              age %ia% cholesterol)
```

Figure 10.15 was produced by

```
mean.age ← tapply(age, age.tertile, mean)
plot(fit3, cholesterol=NA, age=mean.age, sex="male", conf.int=F)
```

The `nomogram` function automatically draws nomograms for `lrm` and other model fits. The nomogram in Figure 10.21 was produced by the following (`plogis` is the built-in S-PLUS logistic cumulative distribution function).

```
nomogram(fit, cholesterol=seq(150,400,by=50),
         interact=list(age=seq(30,70,by=10)),
         lp.at=seq(-2,3.5,by=.5), conf.int=T, conf.lp="all",
         fun=plogis, funlabel="Probability of CAD",
         fun.at=c(seq(.1,.9,by=.1),.95,.99),
         varname.label=F, ia.space=1, xfrac=.46)
```

The `residuals` function for `lrm` and the `which.influence` function can be used to check predictor transformations as well as to analyze overly influential observations in binary logistic regression. Figure 10.16 was produced by

```
f ← lrm(tvdlm ~ cad.dur, x=T, y=T)
resid(f, "partial", pl='loess')
scat1d(cad.dur)                    # scat1d in Hmisc: rug plot
logdur ← log10(cad.dur+1)
f ← lrm(tvdlm ~ logdur, x=T, y=T)
resid(f, 'partial', pl='loess')
scat1d(logdur)
```

In the example in Section 10.7 a cutoff of 0.4 was used instead of the default 0.2 for DFBETAS because of the small sample size:

```
f ← lrm(response ~ age + sex, x=T, y=T)
print(cbind(resid(f, "dfbetas"), resid(f, "dffits")))
which.influence(f, .4)
```

The `residuals.lrm` function will also perform the unweighted sum of squares test for global goodness of fit described in Section 10.5.

The `validate` function when used on an object created by `lrm` does resampling validation of a logistic regression model, with or without backward step-down variable deletion. It provides bias-corrected Somers' D_{xy} rank correlation, R^2_N index, the intercept and slope of an overall logistic calibration equation, the maximum absolute difference in predicted and calibrated probabilities E_{max}, the discrimination index D [(model L.R. $\chi^2 - 1)/n$], the unreliability index U = (difference in -2 log likelihood between uncalibrated $X\beta$ and $X\beta$ with overall intercept and slope calibrated to test sample)/n, and the overall quality index $Q = D - U$.[183] The "corrected" slope can be thought of as a shrinkage factor that takes overfitting into account. See `predab.resample` in Section 6.2 for the list of resampling methods. `validate` is called by the following, with default values shown.

```
fit ← lrm(response ~ terms, x=T, y=T)
validate(fit, method="boot", B=40,
        bw=F, rule="aic", type="residual", sls=0.05, aics=0,
        pr=F, Dxy.method="somers2", emax.lim=c(0,1))
```

The tables of statistics in Section 10.9 were produced by the following S-PLUS program.

```
f ← lrm(response ~ age + sex, x=T, y=T)
validate(f, B=80)
validate(f, B=80, bw=T, rule="p", sls=.1, type="individual")

.Random.seed ← c(17, 23,  3,  8, 55,  2, 25, 54, 15,  4, 61,  0)
# The previous statement allows the random variables to be regenerated
n  ← length(age)
x1 ← runif(n)
x2 ← runif(n)
x3 ← runif(n)
x4 ← runif(n)
x5 ← runif(n)
f ← lrm(response ~ age+sex+x1+x2+x3+x4+x5,x=T,y=T)
validate(f, B=80, bw=T, rule="p", sls=.1, type="individual")
```

The `calibrate` function produces bootstrapped or cross-validated calibration curves for logistic and linear models. The "apparent" calibration accuracy is estimated using a nonparametric smoother relating predicted probabilities to observed binary outcomes. The nonparametric estimate is evaluated at a sequence of predicted probability levels. Then the distances from the 45° line are compared with the differences when the current model is evaluated back on the whole sample (or omitted sample for cross-validation). The differences in the differences are estimates of overoptimism. After averaging over many replications, the predicted-value-specific differences are then subtracted from the apparent differences and an adjusted calibration curve is obtained. Unlike `validate`, `calibrate` does not assume a linear logistic calibration. For an example, see the end of Section 11. `calibrate` will print the mean absolute calibration error, the 0.9 quantile of the absolute error, and the mean squared error, all over the observed distribution of predicted values.

The `val.prob` function is used to compute measures of discrimination and calibration of predicted probabilities for a separate sample from the one used to derive the probability estimates. Thus `val.prob` is used in external validation and data-splitting. The function computes similar indexes as `validate` plus the Brier score and a statistic for testing for unreliability or $H_0 : \gamma_0 = 0, \gamma_1 = 1$.

```
val.prob(p, y, logit, pl=T, smooth=T,
    xlab="Predicted Probability",
    lim=c(0, 1), m, g, cuts, emax.lim=c(0,1),
    legendloc=c(.44,.44), statloc=c(0,1),
    riskdist="calibrated")
```

In the following example of `val.prob`, a logistic model is fitted on 100 observations simulated from the actual model given by

$$\text{Prob}\{Y = 1|X_1, X_2, X_3\} = \frac{1}{1 + \exp[-(-1 + 2X_1)]}, \qquad (10.40)$$

where X_1 is a random uniform $[0, 1]$ variable. Hence X_2 and X_3 are irrelevant. After fitting a linear additive model in X_1, X_2, and X_3, the coefficients are used to predict $\text{Prob}\{Y = 1\}$ on a separate sample of 100 observations. The S-PLUS program follows.

```
.Random.seed ← c( 53, 37, 31, 22, 51,  0, 63, 22, 46, 62,  9,  1)
n ← 200
x1 ← runif(n)
x2 ← runif(n)
x3 ← runif(n)
logit ← 2*(x1-.5)
P ← 1/(1+exp(-logit))
y ← ifelse(runif(n)<=P, 1, 0)
d ← data.frame(x1,x2,x3,y)
f ← lrm(y ~ x1 + x2 + x3, subset=1:100)
pred.logit ← predict(f, d[101:200,])
phat ← 1/(1+exp(-pred.logit))
val.prob(phat, y[101:200], m=20, cex=.5)
```

The output is shown in Figure 10.22.

The estimates of regression effects and odds ratios in Section 10.10 and Figure 10.18 were produced by the statement

```
fsum ← summary(f)
fsum
plot(fsum)
```

The S-PLUS built-in function `glm`, a very general modeling function, can fit binary logistic models. The response variable *must* be coded 0/1 for `glm` to work. `glmD` is a slight modification of the built-in `glm` function that allows fits to use `Design` methods.

```
# Set to use traditional dummy variable codings of factor variables
# lrm always uses this coding
 options(contrasts=c("contr.treatment","contr.poly"))
# options() is unnecessary if library(Design) is in effect
 f ← glmD(sick ~ rcs(age,5)*treatment, family=binomial)
```

The `loess` function was used to get the local least squares fit shown in Figure 10.10.

```
sx ← unclass(sex)-1   # for loess, need to code as numeric
                      # so not fit separate function for each sex
```

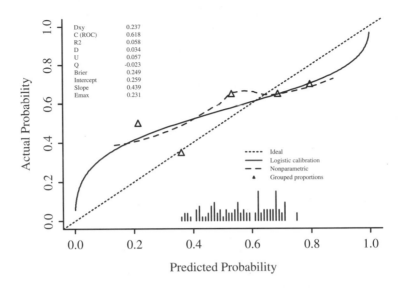

FIGURE 10.22: Validation of a logistic model in a test sample of size $n = 100$. The calibrated risk distribution (histogram of logistic-calibrated probabilities) is shown.

```
f ← loess(sigdz ~ age * (sx + cholesterol), na.action=na.omit,
          control=loess.control(trace.hat="approximate"),
          parametric="sx", drop.square="sx")
# sx is fitted as linear terms, trace.hat specified for speed

ages  ← seq(25,75,length=40)
chols ← seq(100,400,length=40)
p ← drop(predict(f, expand.grid(cholesterol=chols,
                                age=ages, sx=0)))
# drop sex dimension of grid since held to 1 value
persp(chols, ages, p, xlab="Cholesterol",
      ylab="Age", zlab="P", box=T)
# Could use plot(f, which.plots=c("cholesterol", "age")) to get coplots
```

10.12   Further Reading

[1]   See [400] for modeling strategies specific to binary logistic regression.

[2]   See [432] for a nice review of logistic modeling.

[3]   See [387] for a review of measures of effect for binary outcomes.

[4]   Pregibon[343] developed a modification of the log likelihood function that when maximized results in a fit that is resistant to overly influential and outlying observations.

[5] See Hosmer and Lemeshow[211] for methods of testing for a difference in the observed event proportion and the predicted event probability (average of predicted probabilities) for a group of heterogeneous subjects.

[6] See Hosmer and Lemeshow,[210] Kay and Little,[234] and Collett [79, pp. 121–4, 133–8]. Landwehr et al.[256] proposed the partial residual (see also Fowlkes[143]).

[7] See Berk and Booth[35] for other partial-like residuals.

[8] See [234] for an example comparing a smoothing method with a parametric logistic model fit.

[9] See Collett [79, pp. 146–160] and Pregibon[343] for more information about influence statistics. Pregibon's resistant estimator of β handles overly influential *groups* of observations and allows one to estimate the weight that an observation contributed to the fit after making the fit robust. Observations receiving low weight are partially ignored but are not deleted.

[10] Buyse[59] showed that in the case of a single categorical predictor, the ordinary R^2 has a ready interpretation in terms of variance explained for binary responses. Menard[312] studied various indexes for binary logistic regression. He criticized R_N^2 for being too dependent on the proportion of observations with $Y = 1$.

[11] [85, 433] have more pertinent discussion of probability accuracy scores.

[12] Copas[83] demonstrated how ROC areas can be misleading when applied to different responses having greatly different prevalences. He proposed another approach, the logit rank plot.

[13] Hand[171] contains much information about assessing classification accuracy. Mittlböck and Schemper[318] have an excellent review of indexes of explained variation for binary logistic models. See also Korn and Simon[249] and Zheng and Agresti.[463]

[14] Pryor et al.[346] presented nomograms for a 10-variable logistic model. One of the variables was sex, which interacted with some of the other variables. Evaluation of predicted probabilities was simplified by the construction of separate nomograms for females and males. Seven terms for discrete predictors were collapsed into one weighted point score axis in the nomograms, and age by risk factor interactions were captured by having four age scales.

10.13 Problems

1. Consider the age–sex–response example in Section 10.1.3. This dataset is available from the text's Web site in the Datasets area.

   (a) Duplicate the analyses done in Section 10.1.3.

   (b) For the model containing both age and sex, test H_0 : logit response is linear in age versus H_a : logit response is quadratic in age. Use the best test statistic.

(c) Using a Wald test, test H_0 : no age $\times$ sex interaction. Interpret all parameters in the model.

(d) Plot the estimated logit response as a function of age and sex, with and without fitting an interaction term.

(e) Perform a likelihood ratio test of H_0 : model containing only age and sex is adequate versus H_a : model is inadequate. Here, "inadequate" may mean nonlinearity (quadratic) in age or presence of an interaction.

(f) Assuming no interaction is present, test H_0 : model is linear in age versus H_a : model is nonlinear in age. Allow "nonlinear" to be more general that quadratic. (Hint: use a restricted cubic spline function with knots at age=39, 45, 55, 64 years.)

(g) Plot age against the estimated spline transformation of age (the transformation that would make age fit linearly). You can set the sex and intercept terms to anything you choose. Also plot Prob{response $= 1 \mid$ age, sex} from this fitted restricted cubic spline logistic model.

2. Consider a binary logistic regression model using the following predictors: age (years), sex, race (white, African-American, Hispanic, Oriental, other), blood pressure (mmHg). The fitted model is given by

logit Prob$[Y = 1 \mid X] = X\hat{\beta} = -1.36 + .03(\text{race} = \text{African-American})$
$- .04(\text{race} = \text{hispanic}) + .05(\text{race} = \text{oriental}) - .06(\text{race} = \text{other})$
$+ .07|\text{blood pressure} - 110| + .3(\text{sex} = \text{male}) - .1\text{age} + .002\text{age}^2 +$
$(\text{sex} = \text{male})[.05\text{age} - .003\text{age}^2].$

(a) Compute the predicted logit (log odds) that $Y = 1$ for a 50-year-old female Hispanic with a blood pressure of 90 mmHg. Also compute the odds that $Y = 1$ (Prob$[Y = 1]$/Prob$[Y = 0]$) and the estimated probability that $Y = 1$.

(b) Estimate odds ratios for each nonwhite race compared to the reference group (white), holding all other predictors constant. Why can you estimate the relative effect of race for all types of subjects without specifying their characteristics?

(c) Compute the odds ratio for a blood pressure of 120 mmHg compared to a blood pressure of 105, holding age first to 30 years and then to 40 years.

(d) Compute the odds ratio for a blood pressure of 120 mmHg compared to a blood pressure of 105, all other variables held to unspecified constants. Why is this relative effect meaningful without knowing the subject's age, race, or sex?

(e) Compute the estimated risk difference in changing blood pressure from 105 mmHg to 120 mmHg, first for age $= 30$ then for age $= 40$, for a white female. Why does the risk difference depend on age?

(f) Compute the relative odds for males compared to females, for age = 50 and other variables held constant.

(g) Same as the previous question but for females : males instead of males : females.

(h) Compute the odds ratio resulting from increasing age from 50 to 55 for males, and then for females, other variables held constant. What is wrong with the following question: What is the relative effect of changing age by one year?

Chapter 11

Logistic Model Case Study 1: Predicting Cause of Death

11.1   Preparation for Modeling

Consider the randomized trial of estrogen for treatment of prostate cancer[60] described in Chapter 8. In this trial, larger doses of estrogen reduced the effect of prostate cancer but at the cost of increased risk of cardiovascular death. Kay[233] did a formal analysis of the competing risks for cancer, cardiovascular, and other deaths. It can also be quite informative to study how treatment and baseline variables relate to the cause of death for those patients who died.[258] We subset the original dataset of those patients dying from prostate cancer ($n = 130$), heart or vascular disease ($n = 96$), or cerebrovascular disease ($n = 31$). Our goal is to predict cardiovascular death (cvd, $n = 127$) given the patient died from either cvd or prostate cancer. Of interest is whether the time to death has an effect on the cause of death, and whether the importance of certain variables depends on the time of death. We also need to formally test whether the data reductions and pretransformations in Chapter 8 are adequate for predicting cause of death.

In S-PLUS, first obtain the desired subset of the data and do some preliminary calculations.[a]

---

[a]Note that this case study used results from an earlier version of **transcan** that provided different imputed values for **ekg** than those derived in Section 8.5. Also, the ordering of levels of **ekg** is different here.

```
> library(Design, T)
> "%in%" ← function(a,b) match(a, b, nomatch=0) > 0
> # A better version of %in% is in Hmisc
> subset ← prostate$status %in% c("dead - heart or vascular",
+     "dead - cerebrovascular","dead - prostatic ca")
> attach(prostate[subset,])
>
> levels(ekg)[levels(ekg) %in% c("old MI","recent MI")] ← "MI"
> pf.lin ← as.integer(pf)-1    # recode to 0-3
> levels(pf) ← levels(pf)[c(1:3,3)]
> levels(pf) ← abbreviate(levels(pf))
> # Can also do levels(pf) ← edit(levels(pf)) or use merge.levels()
>
> # Fill in missings with imputed values from transcan
> w ← prostate.transcan[subset,]
>
> sz  ← impute(w, sz)        # invokes impute.transcan
> sg  ← impute(w, sg)
> age ← impute(w, age)
> wt  ← impute(w, wt)
> ekg ← impute(w, ekg)
```

```
> cvd ← status %in% c("dead - heart or vascular",
+                     "dead - cerebrovascular")
> ekg.norm ← ekg %in% c("normal","benign")
> # Abbreviate levels of ekg for shorter printouts later
> levels(ekg) ← abbreviate(levels(ekg))
>
> # Get variables transformed by transcan
> sz.t  ← w[,"sz"]
> sg.t  ← w[,"sg"]
> ap.t  ← w[,"ap"]
> sbp.t ← w[,"sbp"]
> dbp.t ← w[,"dbp"]
> age.t ← w[,"age"]
> wt.t  ← w[,"wt"]
> hg.t  ← w[,"hg"]
> ekg.t ← w[,"ekg"]
> pf.t  ← w[,"pf"]
```

11.2 Regression on Principal Components, Cluster Scores, and Pretransformations

We first examine the performance of data reduction in predicting the cause of death, just as we did for survival time in Sections 8.6 to 8.8. The first analyses assess how well principal components (on raw and transformed variables) predicts the cause of death.

```
> pcs ← prin.raw$scores[subset,]
> # print.raw was created previously
> p1  ← pcs[,1]
> lrm(cvd ∼ p1)
```

```
Logistic Regression Model

lrm(formula = cvd ∼ p1)

Frequencies of Responses
 FALSE TRUE
   130  127
```

Obs	Max Deriv	Model L.R.	d.f.	P	C	Dxy	Gamma	Tau-a	R2
257	1e-11	64.4	1	0	0.782	0.563	0.564	0.283	0.296

	Coef	S.E.	Wald Z	P
Intercept	0.1016	0.1419	0.72	0.474
p1	0.7628	0.1152	6.62	0.000

```
> p5  ← pcs[,1:5]
> lrm(cvd ∼ p5)
```

Obs	Max Deriv	Model L.R.	d.f.	P	C	Dxy	Gamma	Tau-a	R2
257	2e-07	93.4	5	0	0.827	0.654	0.655	0.328	0.406

	Coef	S.E.	Wald Z	P
Intercept	0.05461	0.1565	0.35	0.727
Comp. 1	0.82032	0.1249	6.57	0.000
Comp. 2	0.01249	0.1198	0.10	0.917
Comp. 3	0.62448	0.1303	4.79	0.000
Comp. 4	0.17810	0.1278	1.39	0.164
Comp. 5	0.16383	0.1649	0.99	0.320

(Other output not shown)

```
> p10 ← pcs[,1:10]
```

```
> lrm(cvd ~ p10)


 Obs Max Deriv Model L.R.  d.f.  P     C    Dxy  Gamma Tau-a   R2
 257    1e-06        114    10 0 0.855 0.709  0.71 0.356 0.478


> p17 <- pcs[,1:17]        # last component was redundant (singular)
> lrm(cvd ~ p17)


 Obs Max Deriv Model L.R.  d.f.  P     C    Dxy  Gamma Tau-a   R2
 257    1e-06        138    17 0 0.886 0.772 0.773 0.387 0.554



> # Look at predictive power of all untransformed variables
> # (with dummy variable expansions of categorical variables)
> lrm(cvd ~ sz + sg + ap + sbp + dbp + age + wt + hg +
+           ekg + pf + bm + hx)


 Obs Max Deriv Model L.R.  d.f.  P     C    Dxy  Gamma Tau-a   R2
 257    5e-05        138    17 0 0.886 0.772 0.773 0.387 0.554


> # Now test fullest model (allow all variables to be transformed
> # as directed by the response variable)
> lrm(cvd ~ rcs(sz,5) + rcs(sg,5) + rcs(ap,5) +
+           rcs(sbp,5) + rcs(dbp,5) + rcs(age,3) +
+           rcs(wt,5) + rcs(hg,5) + ekg + pf + bm + hx,
+           tol=1e-14)


 Obs Max Deriv Model L.R.  d.f.  P     C    Dxy  Gamma Tau-a   R2
 257    2e-05        161    39 0 0.908 0.816 0.816 0.409 0.621


> # Now get predictive ability of PCs based on transformed variables
> pcs <- prin.trans$scores[subset,]
> p1  <- pcs[,1]
> lrm(cvd ~ p1)


 Obs Max Deriv Model L.R.  d.f.  P     C    Dxy  Gamma Tau-a   R2
 257    3e-13        74.5    1 0 0.802 0.604 0.605 0.303 0.336


> p5   <- pcs[,1:5]
> lrm(cvd ~ p5)


 Obs Max Deriv Model L.R.  d.f.  P     C    Dxy  Gamma Tau-a   R2
 257    1e-10        101     5 0 0.837 0.674 0.675 0.338 0.434


> p10 <- pcs[,1:10]
> lrm(cvd ~ p10)
```

TABLE 11.1

Predictors Used	d.f.	χ^2	AIC
PC_1	1	64	62
PC_{1-5}	5	93	83
PC_{1-10}	10	114	94
PC_{1-17}	17	138	104
All individual var., linear	17	138	104
All individual var., splines	39	161	83
PC_1 on transformed var.	1	74	72
PC_{1-5} on trans.	5	101	91
PC_{1-10} on trans.	10	114	94
PC_{1-12} on trans.	12	123	99
PCs on clusters of trans.	7	103	89

```
Obs Max Deriv Model L.R. d.f. P     C   Dxy Gamma Tau-a    R2
257     2e-09         114   10 0 0.856 0.713 0.714 0.358 0.479


> lrm(cvd ~ pcs)


Obs Max Deriv Model L.R. d.f. P     C   Dxy Gamma Tau-a    R2
257     3e-07         123   12 0 0.868 0.737 0.738  0.37 0.508


> # Test cluster summary scores based on PCs of transformed variables
> tumor    ← tumor[subset]
> bp       ← bp[subset]
> cardiac ← cardiac[subset]
> lrm(cvd ~ tumor + bp + cardiac + hg.t + age.t + pf.t + wt.t)


Obs Max Deriv Model L.R. d.f. P    C  Dxy Gamma Tau-a    R2
257     3e-10         103    7 0 0.84 0.68 0.681 0.341 0.439
```

These results are summarized in Table 11.1[b].

Now test for adequacy of the data reduction of individual variables.

```
> # Test adequacy of summarizing transformed sbp, dbp by PC1
> lrm(cvd ~ bp + sbp.t)
```

---

[b] Note that lines 4 and 5 have the same number of degrees of freedom by accident. **princomp** assigns a parameter to all levels of the *first* categorical variable (here, **ekg**) whereas the logistic model fit took the first level to be the reference cell. Furthermore, there was an empty cell not used in this subset of subjects, which reduced the number of d.f. back to 17 for the exhaustive set of principal components.

```
Frequencies of Responses
FALSE TRUE
  130   127
```

```
Obs Max Deriv Model L.R. d.f.     P     C   Dxy Gamma Tau-a   R2
257     2e-08        15.2    2 5e-04 0.596 0.192 0.199 0.096 0.076
```

```
              Coef   S.E. Wald Z     P
Intercept 0.01552 0.1305 0.12    0.9053
       bp 1.03418 0.3353 3.08    0.0020
    sbp.t 0.78270 0.3581 2.19    0.0288
```

```
> # Accept adequacy of PC1 even with P=.0288
> # (approx. adequacy = 1 - 2.19^2/15.2=0.68)
> # Test adequacy of PC1 vs. response-driven transformations of
> # sbp, dbp
> f ← lrm(cvd ~ bp + rcs(sbp,3) + rcs(dbp,3))
```

```
> anova(f,sbp,dbp)
```

```
                    Wald Statistics        Response: cvd
```

```
         Factor     Chi-Square d.f.      P
sbp                   1.47       2     0.479
 Nonlinear            0.14       1     0.704
dbp                   0.35       2     0.840
 Nonlinear            0.32       1     0.571
TOTAL NONLINEAR       0.59       2     0.743
TOTAL                 4.09       4     0.393
```

We see that the bp summary is (almost) sufficient with respect to internal weights and internal transformations.

```
> # Test adequacy of summarizing sz, sg, ap, bm with PC1
> f ← lrm(cvd ~ tumor + sz.t + sg.t + ap.t)
> anova(f, sz.t, sg.t, ap.t)
```

```
                    Wald Statistics        Response: cvd
```

```
Factor     Chi-Square d.f.      P
sz.t          5.76       1     0.0164
sg.t          9.54       1     0.0020
ap.t          1.27       1     0.2605
TOTAL        11.41       3     0.0097
```

```
> # Test adequacy of pretransformations of individual variables
```

```
> f ← lrm(cvd ~ sz.t + sg.t + ap.t + bm +
+          rcs(sz,3) + rcs(sg, 3) + rcs(ap, 3))
> anova(f, sz, sg, ap)
```

| Wald Statistics   Response: cvd

Factor	Chi-Square	d.f.	P
sz	5.27	2	0.0718
Nonlinear	0.69	1	0.4066
sg	0.50	2	0.7789
Nonlinear	0.12	1	0.7310
ap	2.34	2	0.3111
Nonlinear	0.36	1	0.5474
TOTAL NONLINEAR	1.08	3	0.7826
TOTAL	8.41	6	0.2098

A global summary of the tumor size/extent of disease variables is not adequate. However, transformations of individual size/extent variables are adequate, so we stay with them for now. Now examine adequacy of transformations for all other variables (combined).

```
> # Test adequacy of pretransformations for age, wt, pf, ekg, hg
> # For pf, test to see if linear coding adds to transformed var.
> # For ekg, see if normal/benign adds anything
> f ← lrm(cvd ~ age.t + wt.t + pf.t + ekg.t + hg.t +
+          rcs(age,3) + rcs(wt,3) + pf.lin +
|          ekg.norm | rcs(hg,3))
> anova(f, age, wt, pf.lin, ekg.norm, hg)
```

| Wald Statistics   Response: cvd

Factor	Chi-Square	d.f.	P
age	7.03	2	0.0298
Nonlinear	1.45	1	0.2288
wt	0.53	2	0.7687
Nonlinear	0.45	1	0.5017
pf.lin	5.12	1	0.0237
ekg.norm	1.01	1	0.3149
hg	1.13	2	0.5674
Nonlinear	0.00	1	0.9899
TOTAL NONLINEAR	1.86	3	0.6026
TOTAL	15.87	8	0.0443

Note that the age transformation is significantly inadequate, but not if we adjust for multiple tests of inadequacy. The fitted age relationship becomes flat at age = 73; the pretransformation is flat at age = 80. Both transformations are linear up to that point. The inadequacy of pf.t is hard to understand since it is so nearly linear. The overall test of adequacy is marginal.

11.3   Fit and Diagnostics for a Full Model, and Interpreting Pretransformations

Next we fit a full model. Dose of estrogen is modeled as a linear trend with additional dummy variables for the last two doses. These allow for a simple test of linearity of dose.

```
> # First convert levels to numeric dose values
> levels(rx) ← c(0, .2, 1, 5)
> # Save the full fit in f.full, with design matrix and
> # response vector for later bootstrapping
> # (to penalize for all variables examined)
> f.full ← lrm(cvd ~ scored(rx) + rcs(dtime,5) + age.t +
+                wt.t + pf.t + hx + bp + ekg.t +
+                sz.t + sg.t + ap.t + bm + hg.t,
+                x=T, y=T)
> # Wald statistics for rx are suspect (very high s.e.),
> #  but confirmed by LR
> stats ← f.full$stats
> stats
 Obs Max Deriv Model L.R. d.f. P    C  Dxy Gamma Tau-a   R2
 257  2.88e-06        133   18 0 0.88 0.76 0.761 0.382 0.54
> shrink ← (stats["Model L.R."]-stats["d.f."])/stats["Model L.R."]
> cat("Expected shrinkage factor:",format(shrink),"\n\n")
Expected shrinkage factor: 0.865


> anova(f.full)
```

	Wald Statistics		Response: cvd
Factor	Chi-Square	d.f.	P
rx	5.60	3	0.1329
Nonlinear	2.59	2	0.2734
dtime	10.10	4	0.0388
Nonlinear	9.02	3	0.0291
age.t	3.76	1	0.0526
wt.t	1.58	1	0.2086
pf.t	1.35	1	0.2454
hx	10.68	1	0.0011
bp	6.33	1	0.0119
ekg.t	0.25	1	0.6179
sz.t	12.45	1	0.0004
sg.t	10.56	1	0.0012
ap.t	2.30	1	0.1295
bm	0.01	1	0.9231
hg.t	0.00	1	0.9691

```
TOTAL NONLINEAR 11.49        5    0.0425
TOTAL           69.42       18    0.0000
```

The total likelihood ratio χ^2 for the model is 133 with 18 d.f., justifying further analysis. The van Houwelingen–Le Cessie heuristic shrinkage estimate (Equation 4.1) is 0.87, indicating that this model (or models derived from variable selection) will validate on new data about 13% worse than on this dataset.

To allow for model misspecification, the Huber "sandwich" estimator (Section 9.5) can be substituted for the usual information matrix-based estimate. Then Wald tests, confidence limits, and the like can be based on the robust covariance matrix.

```
> # First save usual variances for later comparison
> vars ← diag(f.full$var)
> # Replace variance matrix with Huber robust estimates
> f.full ← robcov(f.full)
> ratio ← vars/diag(f.full$var)
> names(ratio) ← names(f.full$coef)
> ratio
 Intercept rx rx=1  rx=5 dtime dtime' dtime''  dtime'''  age.t wt.t
      1.11  1     1 0.999  0.96  0.948    0.945     0.946   1.13 1.26
  pf.t    hx    bp ekg.t sz.t sg.t  ap.t    bm hg.t
 0.833 0.974 0.647 0.949 1.04 0.97 0.969 0.744 1.04
```

```
> anova(f.full)
```

	Wald Statistics		Response: cvd
Factor	Chi-Square	d.f.	P
rx	5.40	3	0.1450
Nonlinear	2.44	2	0.2954
dtime	11.92	4	0.0179
Nonlinear	10.13	3	0.0175
age.t	4.24	1	0.0395
wt.t	2.00	1	0.1577
pf.t	1.12	1	0.2889
hx	10.40	1	0.0013
bp	4.10	1	0.0429
ekg.t	0.24	1	0.6271
sz.t	12.91	1	0.0003
sg.t	10.24	1	0.0014
ap.t	2.23	1	0.1356
bm	0.01	1	0.9336
hg.t	0.00	1	0.9685
TOTAL NONLINEAR	12.88	5	0.0245
TOTAL	85.92	18	0.0000

The variances differ by a factor of 0.65 to 1.26, and the Wald statistics do not change substantially. There is little indirect evidence for extra unexplained variation or general lack of fit. Next look for overly influential observations, expecting to find some on this relatively small dataset used to fit 18 regression parameters.

```
> W ← which.influence(f.full, .4)
> nam ← names(W)
> df  ← data.frame(status,dtime,age,age.t,pf,pf.t,sbp,dbp,bp)
> for(i in 1:length(nam)) {
+    cat("\nInfluential observations for effect of",nam[i],"\n");
+    print(df[W[[i]],,drop=F])
+ }


Influential observations for effect of Intercept
               status dtime age age.t   pf pf.t sbp dbp     bp
120 dead - prostatic ca     0  77 -1.06 nact 0.312  12   7 -0.972


Influential observations for effect of dtime
               status dtime age age.t   pf pf.t sbp dbp     bp
120 dead - prostatic ca     0  77 -1.06 nact 0.312  12   7 -0.972


Influential observations for effect of age.t
                 status dtime age age.t      pf  pf.t sbp dbp    bp
194 dead - cerebrovascular    42  48  3.06 ib<50%d -1.91  14  10 0.674


Influential observations for effect of pf.t
                     status dtime age age.t      pf  pf.t sbp dbp    bp
 55      dead - prostatic ca    51  78 -1.10 ib>50%d -4.63  18   8 0.867
190 dead - heart or vascular    26  75 -0.72 ib>50%d -4.63  12   7 -0.972
489      dead - prostatic ca    12  80 -1.04 ib>50%d -4.63  14   7 -0.554


Influential observations for effect of bp
               status dtime age  age.t   pf pf.t sbp dbp   bp
435 dead - prostatic ca     6  74 -0.448 nact 0.312  20  10 2.88
```

This did not identify any values that are obviously worthy of further examination. The anovas above showed that rx is not important or that a nonlinear transformation of dose is an overkill. Let us model rx as a linear trend and examine this full model in more detail.

```
> dose ← as.numeric(levels(rx))[rx]
>
> # Save predictor distributional characteristics for
> # summary and plot
> ddist ← datadist(rx,dtime,dose,age.t,wt.t,pf.t,hx,bp,ekg.t,
+                  sz.t,sg.t,ap.t,bm,hg.t,age,wt,pf,sbp,dbp,
+                  ekg,sz,sg,ap,hg)
```

```
> options(datadist="ddist")
>
> # Create functions that transform each variable
> # Note that for variables having some imputed values (such
> #   as sg), .sg(sg) does not precisely match sg.t for the
> #   imputed sg. This is because transcan uses an approximate
> #   method to back-solve for imputed values on the original
> #   scale.
> options(digits=5)
> # To accurately represent function coefficients for
> # categorical variables
>
> Function(prostate.transcan)
Function for transforming sz stored as .sz
Function for transforming sg stored as .sg
Function for transforming ap stored as .ap
Function for transforming sbp stored as .sbp
Function for transforming dbp stored as .dbp
Function for transforming age stored as .age
Function for transforming wt stored as .wt
Function for transforming hg stored as .hg
Function for transforming ekg stored as .ekg
Function for transforming pf stored as .pf
Function for transforming bm stored as .bm
Function for transforming hx stored as .hx

> # Print some of the functions created
> .ap
function(x)
0.534483832307 + 1.23045508923 * x - 17.6773170413 *
pmax(x - 0.299987792969, 0)^3 + 38.0864642779 *
pmax(x - 0.5, 0)^3 - 20.7495230436 *
pmax(x - 0.699951171875, 0)^3 +
0.340359155722 * pmax(x - 2.2998046875, 0)^3 +
1.6651303286e-05 * pmax(x - 38.469921875, 0)^3
> .pf
function(x)
{
  x <- unclass(x)
  0.3116 * (x == 1) - 1.9107 * (x == 2) -
  4.6348 * (x == 3)
}
> .bm
function(x)
x

> # Use these transformation functions so that plots and
```

```
> # odds ratios will be on the original, easier to
> # interpret, scale

> f ← lrm(cvd ∼ dose + rcs(dtime,5) + .age(age) + .wt(wt) +
+           .pf(pf) + hx + bp + .ekg(ekg) + .sz(sz) + .sg(sg) +
+           .ap(ap) + bm + .hg(hg))
> f
```

. . . .

```
Frequencies of Responses
FALSE TRUE
  130   127


Obs Max Deriv Model L.R. d.f. P      C   Dxy Gamma Tau-a    R2
257     2e-06     130.42   16 0 0.876 0.752 0.753 0.378 0.531

                Coef     S.E. Wald Z       P
Intercept   0.40159 0.67715   0.59  0.5531
     dose   0.14880 0.08467   1.76  0.0789
    dtime  -0.13162 0.08681  -1.52  0.1295
   dtime'   0.96357 0.77641   1.24  0.2146
  dtime''  -1.86885 1.95525  -0.96  0.3392
 dtime'''   0.49337 1.98838   0.25  0.8040
      age  -0.39263 0.17894  -2.19  0.0282
       wt  -0.21849 0.17870  -1.22  0.2214
       pf   0.19551 0.16302   1.20  0.2304
       hx   1.16047 0.35969   3.23  0.0013
       bp   0.50871 0.19836   2.56  0.0103
      ekg  -0.07218 0.18430  -0.39  0.6953
       sz   0.59249 0.16984   3.49  0.0005
       sg   0.80243 0.24810   3.23  0.0012
       ap   0.32452 0.22776   1.42  0.1542
       bm   0.01606 0.47466   0.03  0.9730
       hg  -0.02024 0.17678  -0.11  0.9088


> specs(f, long=T)
```

	Transformation	Assumption	Parameters	d.f.
dose		asis		1
dtime		rcspline	1.8 12 24 36 56.2	4
age	.age(age)	asis		1
wt	.wt(wt)	asis		1
pf	.pf(pf)	asis		1
hx		asis		1
bp		asis		1

```
ekg  .ekg(ekg)        asis                      1
 sz  .sz(sz)          asis                      1
 sg  .sg(sg)          asis                      1
 ap  .ap(ap)          asis                      1
 bm                   asis                      1
 hg  .hg(hg)          asis                      1
```

```
                 dose dtime  age    wt       pf hx    bp  ekg    sz
Low:effect        0.0    11 70.0  89.0           0 -0.65        6.0
Adjust to         0.2    24 73.0  97.0 nact      0 -0.23 nrml 14.0
High:effect       5.0    37 76.0 106.0           1  0.13       24.7
Low:prediction    0.0     1 56.0  76.0 nact      0 -1.07 nrml  2.0
High:prediction   5.0    58 80.0 125.0 ib>50%d   1  2.34 MI   46.0
Low               0.0     0 48.0  71.0 nact      0 -1.43 nrml  0.0
High              5.0    71 88.0 152.0 ib>50%d   1  6.95 MI   69.0
                   sg       ap bm   hg
Low:effect        9.00   0.600  0 12.0
Adjust to        11.00   1.100  0 13.6
High:effect      12.00   7.000  1 14.6
Low:prediction    7.96   0.200  0  9.3
High:prediction  14.04  54.976  1 16.5
Low               5.00   0.100  0  5.9
High             15.00 999.875  1 21.2
```

```
> anova(f)
```

```
                 Wald Statistics        Response: cvd


Factor      Chi-Square d.f.       P
dose          3.09       1    0.0789
dtime        10.21       4    0.0370
 Nonlinear    9.19       3    0.0268
age           4.81       1    0.0282
wt            1.50       1    0.2214
pf            1.44       1    0.2304
hx           10.41       1    0.0013
bp            6.58       1    0.0103
ekg           0.15       1    0.6953
sz           12.17       1    0.0005
sg           10.46       1    0.0012
ap            2.03       1    0.1542
bm            0.00       1    0.9730
hg            0.01       1    0.9088
TOTAL        68.50      16    0.0000
```

```
> # Get odds ratios for default ranges of predictors
> # Except for pretesting on rx, these have proper confidence intervals
> #   unlike reduced model found with fastbw below
> options(digits=2)
> f.summ ← summary(f)
> f.summ
```

```
                Effects                   Response : cvd

                Factor    Low    High   Diff. Effect S.E. Lower Upper
dose                    0.000   5.000   5.000   0.74  0.42 -0.09  1.57
  Odds Ratio            0.000   5.000   5.000   2.10    NA  0.92  4.83
dtime                  11.000  37.000  26.000   1.02  0.52  0.00  2.05
  Odds Ratio           11.000  37.000  26.000   2.79    NA  1.00  7.74
age                    70.000  76.000   6.000   0.50  0.23  0.05  0.96
  Odds Ratio           70.000  76.000   6.000   1.66    NA  1.06  2.60
wt                     89.000 106.000  17.000  -0.21  0.17 -0.54  0.13
  Odds Ratio           89.000 106.000  17.000   0.81    NA  0.58  1.13
hx                      0.000   1.000   1.000   1.16  0.36  0.46  1.87
  Odds Ratio            0.000   1.000   1.000   3.19    NA  1.58  6.46
bp                     -0.645   0.129   0.774   0.39  0.15  0.09  0.69
  Odds Ratio           -0.645   0.129   0.774   1.48    NA  1.10  2.00
sz                      6.000  24.687  18.687  -1.32  0.38 -2.06 -0.58
  Odds Ratio            6.000  24.687  18.687   0.27    NA  0.13  0.56
sg                      9.000  12.000   3.000  -1.74  0.54 -2.79 -0.68
  Odds Ratio            9.000  12.000   3.000   0.18    NA  0.06  0.50
ap                      0.600   7.000   6.400  -0.66  0.46 -1.57  0.25
  Odds Ratio            0.600   7.000   6.400   0.52    NA  0.21  1.28
bm                      0.000   1.000   1.000   0.02  0.47 -0.91  0.95
  Odds Ratio            0.000   1.000   1.000   1.02    NA  0.40  2.58
hg                     12.000  14.600   2.600  -0.03  0.30 -0.61  0.55
  Odds Ratio           12.000  14.600   2.600   0.97    NA  0.54  1.73
pf - ib<50%d:nact       1.000   2.000     NA  -0.43  0.36 -1.14  0.28
  Odds Ratio            1.000   2.000     NA   0.65    NA  0.32  1.32
pf - ib>50%d:nact       1.000   3.000     NA  -0.97  0.81 -2.55  0.61
  Odds Ratio            1.000   3.000     NA   0.38    NA  0.08  1.85
ekg - bngn:nrml         1.000   2.000     NA  -0.04  0.09 -0.22  0.15
  Odds Ratio            1.000   2.000     NA   0.96    NA  0.80  1.16
ekg - rd&ec:nrml        1.000   3.000     NA  -0.08  0.21 -0.50 0.33
  Odds Ratio            1.000   3.000     NA   0.92    NA  0.61  1.40
ekg - hbocd:nrml        1.000   4.000     NA  -0.12  0.30 -0.72  0.48
  Odds Ratio            1.000   4.000     NA   0.89    NA  0.49  1.61
ekg - hrst:nrml         1.000   5.000     NA  -0.14  0.35 -0.81  0.54
  Odds Ratio            1.000   5.000     NA   0.87    NA  0.44  1.72
ekg - MI:nrml           1.000   6.000     NA  -0.20  0.50 -1.18  0.78
  Odds Ratio            1.000   6.000     NA   0.82    NA  0.31  2.19
```

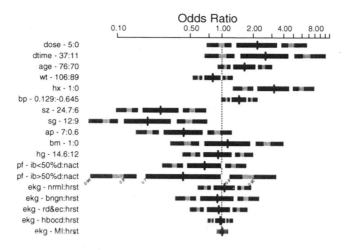

FIGURE 11.1: Interquartile-range odds ratios for continuous predictors and simple odds ratios for categorical predictors. Numbers at left are upper quartile : lower quartile or current group : reference group. The shaded bars represent 0.7, 0.8, 0.9, 0.95, 0.99 confidence limits. The intervals are drawn on the log odds ratio scale and labeled on the odds ratio scale. Ranges are on the original scale, even for transformed variables.

```
> plot(f.summ, log=T)
```

Confidence bars for these interquartile-range odds ratios are shown in Figure 11.1.

```
> # Plot effects for selected predictors on a common scale
> par(mfrow=c(2,2))
> plot(f, dtime=NA, ref.zero=T, ylim=c(-2,2))
> scat1d(dtime)
> plot(f, age=NA,   ref.zero=T, ylim=c(-2,2))
> scat1d(age)
> plot(f, sz=NA,    ref.zero=T, ylim=c(-2,2))
> scat1d(sz)
> # For probability scale, take control of adjustment values by
> # specifying an age
> plot(f, sz=NA, age=75, dose=0, fun=plogis,
+       # or fun=function(x)1/(1+exp(-x))
+       ylab="Predicted Probability of CVD", ylim=c(0,1))
```

The fitted relationships for three predictors are found in Figure 11.2. For this model, obtain predicted probabilities of cvd for selected settings of predictors (three ages, others set to constants).

```
> pred ← predict(f, expand.grid(age=c(60,70,80), dtime=10,
```

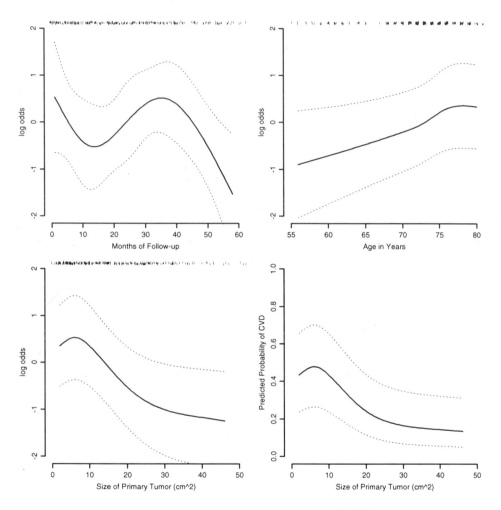

FIGURE 11.2: Relationships of important predictors to log odds or probability of cardiovascular death, with data densities (one-dimensional scatterplots) for the first three graphs.

```
+                    dose=0, wt=mean(wt),
+                    pf="nact", hx=1, bp=median(bp),
+                    ekg=mean(ekg="nrml"), sz=median(sz),
+                    sg=median(sg), ap=median(ap), bm=0,
+                    hg=median(hg)), type="fitted")
> # Use of the gendata function might have helped here
> pred
    1    2    3
0.32 0.44 0.58
```

11.4 Describing Results Using a Reduced Model

Now use fast backward step-down (with total residual AIC as the stopping rule) to identify the variables that explain the bulk of the cause of death. Later validation will take this screening of variables into account.

```
> fastbw(f)

 Deleted Chi-Sq d.f.      P Residual d.f.      P   AIC
 bm       0.00   1   0.9730  0.00    1   0.9730 -2.00
 hg       0.02   1   0.9003  0.02    2   0.9916 -3.98
 ekg      0.15   1   0.6947  0.17    3   0.9821 -5.83
 pf       1.60   1   0.2002  1.77    4   0.7782 -6.23
 wt       1.28   1   0.2587  3.04    5   0.6931 -6.96
 ap       1.84   1   0.1748  4.89    6   0.5586 -7.11
 dose     2.60   1   0.1072  7.48    7   0.3806 -6.52
 age      4.49   1   0.0341 11.97    8   0.1525 -4.03
 bp       3.97   1   0.0464 15.94    9   0.0682 -2.06

Approximate Estimates After Deleting Factors

              Coef   S.E.  Wald Z        P
Intercept   0.8626 0.6368  1.3546 1.755e-01
    dtime  -0.1672 0.0856 -1.9535 5.077e-02
   dtime'   1.2637 0.7624  1.6574 9.744e-02
  dtime''  -2.5964 1.9205 -1.3519 1.764e-01
 dtime'''   1.1929 1.9541  0.6104 5.416e-01
      hx    0.9223 0.3409  2.7059 6.813e-03
      sz    0.5157 0.1665  3.0973 1.953e-03
      sg    1.0007 0.1948  5.1363 2.801e-07

Factors in Final Model

[1] dtime hx    sz    sg
```

Delete `dtime` since the shape of its effect is hard to understand. With the reduced model, give `dose` one more chance, coded as high dose versus other levels.

```
> high ← dose==5
> lrm(cvd ~ high + .age(age) + hx + .sz(sz) + .sg(sg))
```

```
Logistic Regression Model
```

```
lrm(formula = cvd ~ high + .age(age) + hx + .sz(sz) + .sg(sg))
```

```
Frequencies of Responses
 FALSE TRUE
   130  127
```

```
Obs Max Deriv Model L.R. d.f. P     C   Dxy Gamma Tau-a   R2
257      6e-11          104  5 0 0.844 0.689  0.69 0.346 0.442
```

```
              Coef   S.E. Wald Z     P
Intercept -0.3032 0.2565  -1.18  0.2372
     high  0.5339 0.3597   1.48  0.1378
      age -0.3806 0.1632  -2.33  0.0197
       hx  1.0080 0.3130   3.22  0.0013
       sz  0.4954 0.1530   3.24  0.0012
       sg  0.9730 0.1758   5.53  0.0000
```

Since this reduced model is more workable, take the opportunity to see if dose of estrogen is important for some level of the important factors. Also check to see if the important variables interact with each other (even though the model validation below does not penalize for this look).

```
> anova(lrm(cvd ~ dose*(.age(age)+hx+.sz(sz)+.sg(sg))))
```

Factor	Chi-Square	d.f.	P
dose (Factor+Higher Order Factors)	5.68	5	0.3390
All Interactions	3.07	4	0.5463
age (Factor+Higher Order Factors)	7.47	2	0.0238
All Interactions	2.60	1	0.1068
hx (Factor+Higher Order Factors)	11.01	2	0.0041
All Interactions	0.14	1	0.7055
sz (Factor+Higher Order Factors)	10.49	2	0.0053
All Interactions	0.22	1	0.6378
sg (Factor+Higher Order Factors)	28.64	2	0.0000
All Interactions	0.20	1	0.6549
dose * age (Factor+Higher Order Factors)	2.60	1	0.1068
dose * hx (Factor+Higher Order Factors)	0.14	1	0.7055
dose * sz (Factor+Higher Order Factors)	0.22	1	0.6378

```
dose * sg  (Factor+Higher Order Factors)    0.20      1     0.6549
TOTAL INTERACTION                           3.07      4     0.5463
TOTAL                                      65.52      9     0.0000
```

```
> # Then test if they interact with each other
> anova(lrm(cvd ~ (.age(age) + hx + .sz(sz) + .sg(sg))^2))
```

```
                        Wald Statistics        Response: cvd


                               Factor    Chi-Square d.f.       P
age  (Factor+Higher Order Factors)          7.29      4     0.1212
 All Interactions                           3.09      3     0.3778
hx  (Factor+Higher Order Factors)          11.77      4     0.0191
 All Interactions                           1.19      3     0.7557
sz  (Factor+Higher Order Factors)          12.64      4     0.0132
 All Interactions                           1.38      3     0.7098
sg  (Factor+Higher Order Factors)          32.68      4     0.0000
 All Interactions                           2.91      3     0.4064
age * hx  (Factor+Higher Order Factors)     0.14      1     0.7046
age * sz  (Factor+Higher Order Factors)     0.35      1     0.5540
age * sg  (Factor+Higher Order Factors)     2.90      1     0.0885
hx * sz  (Factor+Higher Order Factors)      1.10      1     0.2945
hx * sg  (Factor+Higher Order Factors)      0.02      1     0.8918
sz * sg  (Factor+Higher Order Factors)      0.01      1     0.9211
TOTAL INTERACTION                           3.97      6     0.6801
TOTAL                                      66.01     10     0.0000
```

No important interactions of either type are seen. Next, we fit a final reduced model, even though we dare not use P-values or confidence intervals from this model. Use the original age, tumor size, and stage/grade variables for easier explanation.

```
> f.reduced ← lrm(cvd ~ rcs(age,4) + hx + rcs(sz,5) + rcs(sg,4))
> f.reduced
```

```
Logistic Regression Model
```

```
lrm(formula = cvd ~ rcs(age, 4) + hx + rcs(sz, 5) + rcs(sg, 4))
```

```
Frequencies of Responses
 FALSE TRUE
   130  127
 Obs Max Deriv Model L.R. d.f. P      C   Dxy Gamma Tau-a     R2
 257     9e-07         119  11 0 0.859 0.718 0.719  0.36  0.493
```

```
                  Coef     S.E. Wald Z      P
Intercept -14.7134 5.91484 -2.49  0.0129
      age   0.2227 0.08697  2.56  0.0105
     age'  -0.2430 0.13509 -1.80  0.0720
    age''   2.3459 1.57174  1.49  0.1356
       hx   1.0253 0.32707  3.13  0.0017
       sz  -0.3506 0.15683 -2.24  0.0254
      sz'   4.8942 2.54040  1.93  0.0540
     sz''  -9.7360 5.21523 -1.87  0.0619
    sz'''   5.9056 3.53952  1.67  0.0952
       sg   0.3929 0.28431  1.38  0.1670
      sg'  -4.2341 1.29450 -3.27  0.0011
     sg''  18.8451 5.66775  3.32  0.0009
```

```
> anova(f.reduced)
```

```
                  Wald Statistics            Response: cvd

        Factor    Chi-Square d.f.      P
   age               9.96       3   0.0189
    Nonlinear        3.44       2   0.1791
   hx                9.83       1   0.0017
   sz               16.48       4   0.0024
    Nonlinear        4.00       3   0.2615
   sg               29.44       3   0.0000
    Nonlinear       11.06       2   0.0040
   TOTAL NONLINEAR  17.79       7   0.0129
   TOTAL            67.65      11   0.0000
```

Age and tumor size can be modeled linearly. Plot the estimated sg relationship, then simplify it.

```
> par(mfrow=c(2,2))
> # plot sg using full range (not many subjects at sg=5,6,7)
> plot(f.reduced, sg=5:15, adj.subtitle=F, ylim=c(-2,2), ref.zero=T)
> scat1d(sg)
> # Force sg relationship to be flat in the tails, age,sz=linear
> f.reduced ← lrm(cvd ~ age + hx + sz + pmax(pmin(sg,12),8))
> f.reduced$stats
 Obs Max Deriv Model L.R. d.f. P    C   Dxy Gamma Tau-a    R2
 257  2.77e-09       105    4 0 0.847 0.694 0.695 0.348 0.446
> anova(f.reduced)
```

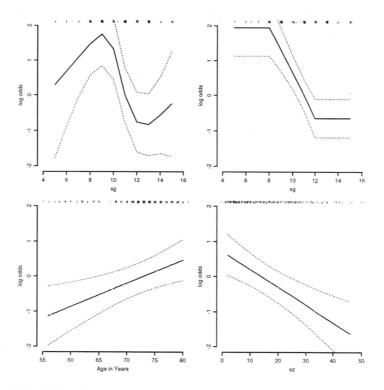

FIGURE 11.3: Spline fit and simplified fit (constrained to be monotonic) for stage/grade.

```
        Wald Statistics              Response: cvd

Factor    Chi-Square d.f.       P
age          8.00     1      0.0047
hx           9.86     1      0.0017
sz          13.83     1      0.0002
sg          26.05     1      0.0000
TOTAL       64.26     4      0.0000
```

```
> plot(f.reduced, sg=5:15, adj.subtitle=F, ylim=c(-2,2), ref.zero=T)
> scat1d(sg)
> plot(f.reduced, age=NA,  adj.subtitle=F, ylim=c(-2,2), ref.zero=T)
> scat1d(age)
> plot(f.reduced, sz=NA,   adj.subtitle=F, ylim=c(-2,2), ref.zero=T)
> scat1d(sz)
```

The plots produced from this code are in Figure 11.3. Next display this reduced model in more readable form.

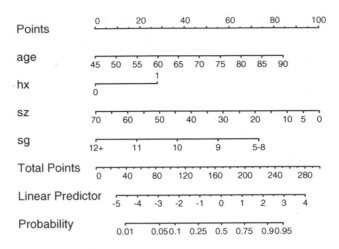

FIGURE 11.4: Nomogram calculating $X\hat{\beta}$ and $\hat{P}$ for cardiovascular death as the cause of death. For each predictor, read the points assigned on the 0–100 scale and add these points. Read the result on the "Total Points" scale and then read the corresponding predictions below it.

```
> latex(f.reduced)
```

$$\text{Prob}\{\text{cvd}\} = \frac{1}{1 + \exp(-X\beta)},$$

where

$$X\hat{\beta} =$$
$$2.39 + 0.0663\,\text{age} + 0.981\,\text{hx} - 0.0507\,\text{sz} - 0.647\,\max(\min(\text{sg}, 12), 8).$$

It is readily seen from this model that older patients, patients with a history of heart disease, and patients with less extensive prostate cancer are those more likely to die from cardiovascular causes rather than from cancer. It is interesting that dose of estrogen does not play a role here. A nomogram for obtaining predictions from the model and for understanding the fit is obtained by the following commands. The result is in Figure 11.4.

```
> nomogram(f.reduced, fun=plogis,
+           funlabel="Probability",
+           fun.at=c(.01,.05,.1,.25,.5,.75,.9,.95,.99), xfrac=.45)
```

11.5 Approximating the Full Model Using Recursive Partitioning

Here we use a regression tree to approximate the full model to make it easier to understand. First grow a very large tree (down to four observations allowing to be cut), using the full model's predicted probability as the dependent variable. For each terminal node, show the distribution of the full model's predicted probabilities to show the residual variation.

```
> pred.full ← predict(f.full, type="fitted")
>
> options(digits=5)
> sg ← round(sg,1)      # make tree use shorter labels
> ap ← round(ap,2)      # really do this in a separate step to not
> hg ← round(hg,1)      # destroy original values
> g  ← tree(pred.full ~ rx + dtime + age + wt + pf +
+              hx + sbp + dbp + ekg + sz + sg + ap + bm + hg,
+              control=tree.control(nobs=257, mindev=0, mincut=4))
> tree.screens()
> plot(g, type="u")
> text(g, digits=1)
> pred.tree ← predict(g)
> pred.full.grouped ← cut2(pred.full, seq(0,1,by=.01))
> tile.tree(g, pred.full.grouped)
```

From Figure 11.5 you can see much variation in full-model predicted probabilities (approximation error) for nodes that terminated early, especially when the predictions are in the midprobability range.

Now study how limiting the number of terminal nodes relates to both the error in predicting the full model prediction and to the error (Brier score) in predicting the actual cause of death. Let us also examine the apparent and 10-fold cross-validated Brier score for regression tree models developed from scratch (but using transcan imputations) to predict actual outcomes.

```
> nodes ← 45
> mean.error ← brier ← numeric(nodes)
> for(i in 1:nodes) {
+   pred ← if(i==1) mean(pred.full) else {
+     g.subset ← prune.tree(g, best=i)
+     predict(g.subset)
+   }
+   mean.error[i] ← mean(abs(pred-pred.full))
+   brier[i] ← mean((pred-cvd)^2)
> }
>
> plot(1:nodes, mean.error, xlab="Number of Nodes",
```

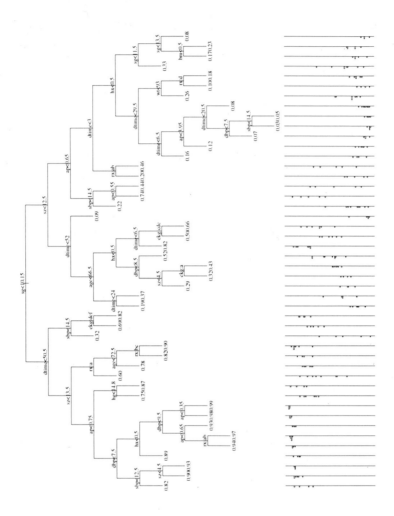

FIGURE 11.5: Regression tree approximating the regression model's predicted probability of cardiovascular death. Numbers at terminal nodes are predicted probabilities. Levels of categorical variables are abbreviated as a, b, ... The frequency bar charts at the bottom correspond to actual full-model predicted probabilities ranging from 0 to 1.0 by increments of 0.01 (0 is farthest from the tree).

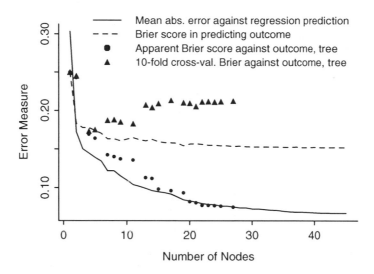

FIGURE 11.6: Approximation accuracy and predictive accuracy of tree models as a function of the number of terminal nodes, and apparent and actual accuracy of regression tree models for actual outcomes as a function of the amount of pruning. The bootstrap estimate of the Brier score for the full regression model is 0.173 which in this case equals the cross-validated Brier score for the best tree model for all possible number of nodes. The best tree model against the outcome had four nodes and $D_{xy} = 0.568$, which was not as good as the 11-node tree model (the tree with the optimum cross-validated D_{xy}) with $D_{xy} = 0.604$ (note the D_{xy} does not penalize for calibration error). The bootstrap estimate of D_{xy} for the full regression model is 0.673.

```
+        ylab="Error Measure", type="l")
> lines(1:nodes, brier, lty=3)
> f.cart ← tree(cvd ∼ rx + dtime + age + wt + pf +
>               hx + sbp + dbp + ekg + sz + sg + ap + bm + hg)
> w ← validate(f.cart)   # function not shown here
> points(w$size, w$mse.app, pch=183)
> points(w$size, w$mse.val, pch=17)
> legend(2.5,.335,
+        c('Mean absolute error in predicting regression prediction',
+          'Brier score in predicting outcome',
+          'Apparent Brier score against outcome, tree'
+          '10-fold cross-val. Brier against outcome, tree'),
+        lty=c(1,3,0,0),marks=c(-1,-1,16,17),bty='n',mkh=.07)
```

Note that from Figure 11.6, the more closely the tree model approximates the full model, the more accurate it is in predicting actual outcomes, although the curve is more shallow after about 15 nodes. Even when the predictive accuracy for a tree approximation is adequate overall, there may still be major discrepancies for individual patients (usually ones having rare predictor values). For this problem, the best cross-validating tree model had about the same Brier score as the full regression model (estimated using bootstrapping, below).

11.6   Validating the Reduced Model

Before validating the reduced model, let us examine the potential our modeling process has for overfitting and for finding spurious associations by estimating how well a model predicts when the response variable is randomly permuted.

```
> validate(f.full, B=20, method="random")
```

	index.orig	training	test	optimism	index.corrected	n
Dxy	0.75990	0.30395	-0.0174	0.3214	0.4385	20
R2	0.53999	0.09394	0.0392	0.0547	0.4853	20
Intercept	0.00000	0.00000	-0.0263	0.0263	-0.0263	20
Slope	1.00000	1.00000	-0.1077	1.1077	-0.1077	20
Emax	0.00000	0.00000	1.0000	1.0000	1.0000	20
D	0.51526	0.06935	0.0264	0.0429	0.4724	20
U	-0.00778	-0.00778	0.1030	-0.1108	0.1030	20
Q	0.52305	0.07713	-0.0766	0.1537	0.3693	20
B	0.14198	0.23220	0.2681	-0.0359	0.1778	20

One can achieve (averaging over 20 permutations) a D_{xy} of 0.30 when there are no associations just by fitting 18 parameters plus an intercept. The randomization estimate of optimism is 0.32, yielding a corrected D_{xy} of 0.44 for the full model fit (without variable selection). This estimate of D_{xy} is too low compared to the bootstrap estimate; the randomization method is more of a teaching tool than one that yields accurate estimates of optimism. With customary variable selection ($P = 0.05$ using individual tests instead of residual χ^2 test), no significant variables were selected in 13 out of 20 permutations and one or two variables were selected in 7 permutations. The estimate of optimism of D_{xy} is 0.03; that is, variable selection can sometimes work well when *all* variables represent noise.

```
> validate(f.full, B=20, method="random", bw=T, type="individual",
+          rule="p", sls=.05)
```

```
        Frequencies of Numbers of Factors Retained

   0 1 2
  13 6 1
```

	index.orig	training	test	optimism	index.corrected	n
Dxy	0.73131	0.06862	0.03542	0.03320	0.6981	20
R2	0.50655	0.01535	0.04792	-0.03257	0.5391	20
Intercept	0.00000	0.00000	-0.01114	0.01114	-0.0111	20
Slope	1.00000	1.00000	1.00981	-0.00981	1.0098	20
Emax	0.00000	0.00000	0.00410	0.00410	0.0041	20
D	0.47398	0.00791	0.03600	-0.02809	0.5021	20
U	-0.00778	-0.00778	0.03834	-0.04612	0.0383	20
Q	0.48176	0.01569	-0.00234	0.01803	0.4637	20
B	0.14750	0.24708	0.25123	-0.00415	0.1516	20

Next use the bootstrap to validate the full model fit.

```
> validate(f.full, B=50)
```

	index.orig	training	test	optimism	index.corrected	n
Dxy	0.75990	0.80906	0.7222	0.0869	0.6730	50
R2	0.53999	0.60671	0.4901	0.1166	0.4234	50
Intercept	0.00000	0.00000	-0.0305	0.0305	-0.0305	50
Slope	1.00000	1.00000	0.7507	0.2493	0.7507	50
Emax	0.00000	0.00000	0.0690	0.0690	0.0690	50
D	0.51526	0.60427	0.4545	0.1497	0.3655	50
U	-0.00778	-0.00778	0.0290	-0.0368	0.0290	50
Q	0.52305	0.61205	0.4255	0.1865	0.3365	50
B	0.14198	0.12373	0.1549	-0.0312	0.1732	50

The estimated optimism in D_{xy} is 0.087, and the bias-corrected D_{xy} is 0.67. Estimated shrinkage is 0.75, worse than that predicted by the simple estimator (0.87).

Now use the bootstrap to validate the reduced model. We do this by validating the full model with step-down variable deletion repeated for each bootstrap repetition.

```
> validate(f.full, B=50, bw=T)
```

Factors Retained in Backwards Elimination

rx	dtime	age.t	wt.t	pf.t	hx	bp	ekg.t	sz.t	sg.t	ap.t	bm	hg.t
*	*	*	*		*		*	*		*		
	*				*			*	*			
					*			*	*			
					*			*	*			
		*						*	*			
*			*		*	*	*	*		*	*	*
			*		*	*			*			
					*				*			
		*			*			*	*			
*					*			*	*	*		

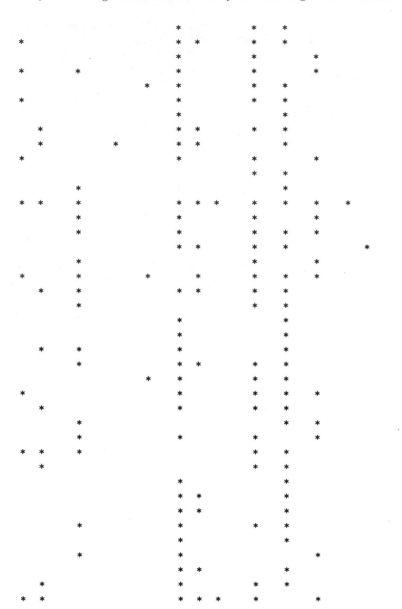

Frequencies of Numbers of Factors Retained

```
2  3   4   5  6 7 8 10
8  13  12  11 1 2 1  2
```

	index.orig	training	test	optimism	index.corrected	n
Dxy	0.70563	0.72170	0.6553	0.0664	0.6392	50
R2	0.46884	0.49178	0.4084	0.0834	0.3854	50
Intercept	0.00000	0.00000	0.0022	-0.0022	0.0022	50
Slope	1.00000	1.00000	0.8266	0.1734	0.8266	50
Emax	0.00000	0.00000	0.0429	0.0429	0.0429	50
D	0.42938	0.45813	0.3624	0.0957	0.3337	50
U	-0.00778	-0.00778	0.0141	-0.0219	0.0141	50
Q	0.43716	0.46591	0.3483	0.1176	0.3196	50
B	0.15479	0.14870	0.1697	-0.0210	0.1758	50

The factors that are consistently selected across the resamples are the same factors deemed important by the step-down algorithm. The D_{xy} for the reduced model is overoptimistic by 0.07. A good estimate of D_{xy} that would be obtained by a future independent validation is 0.64. The corresponding R^2 value, penalized for estimating regression coefficients and for variable selection, is 0.39. The estimated calibration curve is

$$\mathrm{Prob}\{cvd = 1\} = \frac{1}{1 + \exp[-(0.002 + 0.827L)]}, \tag{11.1}$$

where L is the logit of the predicted probability of cvd. This curve provides an estimate of the maximum error in predicted probability to be $E_{max} = 0.043$. This estimate would be larger if we hadn't assumed a linear-logistic calibration function (0.065, see below). The shrunken estimates will likely yield more accurate predictions for future cases.

Let us estimate an honest calibration curve (Figure 11.7) without assuming a linear logistic calibration. We also superimpose the linear logistic calibration.

```
> cal ← calibrate(f.full, B=50, bw=T)
> plot(cal)
> pred ← seq(.02,.98,by=.02)
> logistic.cal ← 1/(1+exp(-(.0022+.8266*log(pred/(1-pred)))))
> points(pred, logistic.cal, pch=183)
```

Compared to the validation of the full model, the step-down model has less optimism, but it started with a smaller D_{xy} due to loss of information from moderately important variables. The improvement in optimism was not enough to offset the effect of eliminating variables. If shrinkage were used with the full model, it would have better calibration and discrimination than the reduced model, since shrinkage does not diminish D_{xy}.

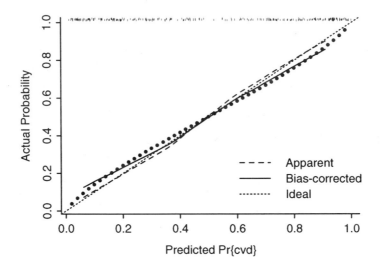

FIGURE 11.7: Bootstrap calibration curve using a smooth nonparametric calibration estimator (**loess**), along with linear logistic calibration curve estimated by bootstrapping an intercept and slope correction (dots).

Chapter 12

Logistic Model Case Study 2: Survival of Titanic Passengers

This case study demonstrates the development of a binary logistic regression model to describe patterns of survival in passengers on the *Titanic*, based on passenger age, sex, ticket class, and the number of family members accompanying each passenger. Nonparametric regression is also used. Since many of the passengers had missing ages, multiple imputation is used so that the complete information on the other variables can be efficiently utilized.

Titanic passenger data were gathered by many researchers. Primary references are the *Encyclopedia Titanica* at `www.encyclopedia-titanica.org` and Eaton and Haas.[122] Titanic survival patterns have been analyzed previously[109, 204, 386] but without incorporation of individual passenger ages. Thomas Cason of the University of Virginia compiled and interpreted the data from the World Wide Web. One thousand three hundred nine of the passengers are represented in the dataset, which is available from this text's Web site under the name `titanic3`.

12.1   Descriptive Statistics

First we obtain basic descriptive statistics on key variables.[a]

```
> library(Hmisc,T); library(Design,T)
> # List of names of variables to analyze
> v ← c('pclass','survived','age','sex','sibsp','parch')
> describe(titanic3[,v])
```

titanic3
6 Variables   1309 Observations

---

pclass : Passenger Class

```
   n missing unique
1309       0      3
```

1st (323, 25%), 2nd (277, 21%), 3rd (709, 54%)

---

survived : Survived

```
   n missing unique Sum  Mean
1309 0         2     500 0.382
```

---

age : Age (Year)

```
   n missing unique  Mean  .05 .10 .25 .50 .75 .90 .95
1046 263        98   29.88  5  14  21  28  39  50  57
```

```
lowest :   0.1667   0.3333   0.4167   0.6667   0.7500
highest: 70.5000 71.0000 74.0000 76.0000 80.0000
```

---

sex : Sex

```
   n missing unique
1309       0      2
```

female (466, 36%), male (843, 64%)

---

sibsp : Number of Siblings/Spouses Aboard

```
   n missing unique   Mean
1309 0         7      0.4989
```

	0	1	2	3	4	5	8
Frequency	891	319	42	20	22	6	9
%	68	24	3	2	2	0	1

---

parch : Number of Parents/Children Aboard

```
   n missing unique  Mean
1309 0         8     0.385
```

	0	1	2	3	4	5	6	9
Frequency	1002	170	113	8	6	6	2	2
%	77	13	9	1	0	0	0	0

---

[a]The output shown here actually used `latex(describe(titanic3[,v], descript=`
`'titanic3'))`.

Next, we obtain access to the needed variables and observations, and save data distribution characteristics for plotting and for computing predictor effects. There are not many passengers having more than 3 siblings or spouses or more than 3 children, so we truncate two variables at 3 for the purpose of estimating stratified survival probabilities.

```
> dd ← datadist(titanic3[,v])
> # describe distributions of variables to Design
> options(datadist='dd')
> attach(titanic3[,v])
> options(digits=2)
> s ← summary(survived ~ age + sex + pclass +
+                cut2(sibsp,0:3) + cut2(parch,0:3))
> s     # usual print
> w ← latex(s)          # create LATEX code for Table 12.1
> plot(s)               # convert table to dot plot (Figure 12.1)
```

Note the large number of missing ages. Also note the strong effects of sex and passenger class on the probability of surviving. The age effect does not appear to be very strong, because as we show later, much of the effect is restricted to age < 21 years for one of the sexes. The effects of the last two variables are unclear as the estimated proportions are not monotonic in the values of these descriptors. Although some of the cell sizes are small, we can show four-way empirical relationships with the fraction of surviving passengers by creating four cells for sibsp × parch combinations and by creating two age groups. We suppress proportions based on fewer than 25 passengers in a cell. Results are shown in Figure 12.2.

```
> agec ← ifelse(age<21,'child','adult')
> sibsp.parch ←
+   paste(ifelse(sibsp==0,'no sib/spouse','sib/spouse'),
+   ifelse(parch==0,'no parent/child','parent/child'),
+   sep=' / ')
> g ← function(y) if(length(y) < 25) NA else mean(y)
> s ← summarize(survived,
+   llist(agec, sex, pclass, sibsp.parch),g)
> # llist, summarize, Dotplot in Hmisc library


> Dotplot(pclass ~ survived | sibsp.parch*agec,
+         groups=sex, data=s, pch=1:2,
+         xlab='Proportion Surviving')   # Figure 12.2
> Key(.09,-.065)
```

Note that none of the effects of sibsp or parch for common passenger groups appear strong on an absolute risk scale.

TABLE 12.1: Survived $N = 1309$

	N	survived
Age		
[0.167,21.000)	249	0.46
[21.000,28.000)	255	0.38
[28.000,39.000)	277	0.40
[39.000,80.000]	265	0.39
Missing	263	0.28
Sex		
female	466	0.73
male	843	0.19
Passenger Class		
1st	323	0.62
2nd	277	0.43
3rd	709	0.26
Number of Siblings/Spouses Aboard		
0	891	0.35
1	319	0.51
2	42	0.45
[3,8]	57	0.16
Number of Parents/Children Aboard		
0	1002	0.34
1	170	0.59
2	113	0.50
[3,9]	24	0.29
Overall		
	1309	0.38

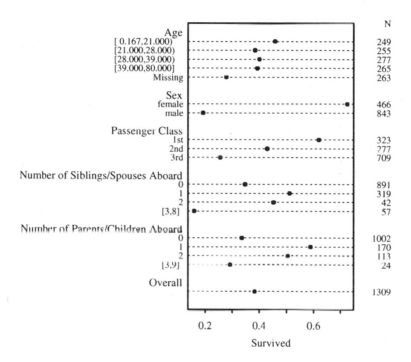

FIGURE 12.1: Univariable summaries of Titanic survival.

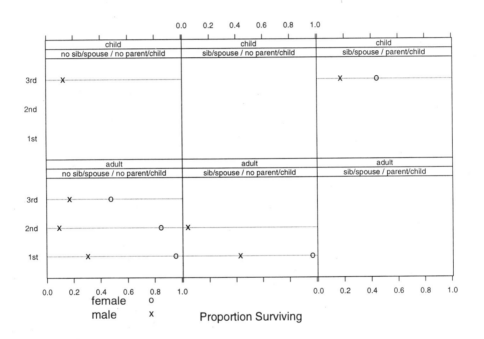

FIGURE 12.2: Multiway summary of Titanic survival.

12.2   Exploring Trends with Nonparametric Regression

As described in Section 2.4.6, the `loess` smoother has excellent performance when the response is binary, as long as outlier detection is turned off. Here we use the `plsmo` function in the `Hmisc` library to obtain and plot the `loess` fit. `plsmo` uses the "no iteration" option for the `lowess` function when the response is binary, and it has several useful options, including the ability to indicate locations of raw data points using "moving rug plots."

```
> par(mfrow=c(2,2))      # To create Figure 12.3
> plsmo(age, survived, datadensity=T)
> plsmo(age, survived, group=sex, datadensity=T)
> plsmo(age, survived, group=pclass, datadensity=T)
> plsmo(age, survived, group=interaction(pclass,sex),
+        datadensity=T, lty=c(1,1,1,2,2,2),
+        label.curves=list(keys=rep(1:3,2)))
```

Figure 12.3 shows much of the story of passenger survival patterns. "Women and children first" seems to be true except for women in third class. It is interesting that there is no real cutoff for who is considered a child. For men, the younger the greater chance of surviving. The interpretation of the effects of the "number of relatives"-type variables will be more difficult, as their definitions are a function of age. Figure 12.4 shows these relationships.

```
> par(mfrow=c(1,2))    # Figure 12.4
> plsmo(age, survived, group=cut2(sibsp,0:2), datadensity=T)
> plsmo(age, survived, group=cut2(parch,0:2), datadensity=T)
```

12.3   Binary Logistic Model With Casewise Deletion of Missing Values

What follows is the standard analysis based on eliminating observations having any missing data. We develop an initial somewhat saturated logistic model, allowing for a flexible nonlinear age effect that can differ in shape for all six sex × class strata. The `sibsp` and `parch` variables do not have sufficiently dispersed distributions to allow for us to model them nonlinearly. Also, there are too few passengers with nonzero values of these two variables in sex × `pclass` × age strata to allow us to model complex interactions involving them. The meaning of these variables does depend on the passenger's age, so we consider only age interactions involving `sibsp` and `parch`.

```
> f1 ← lrm(survived ~ sex*pclass*rcs(age,5) +
+            rcs(age,5)*(sibsp + parch))
> anova(f1)    # actually used latex(anova(f1)) to get Table 12.2
```

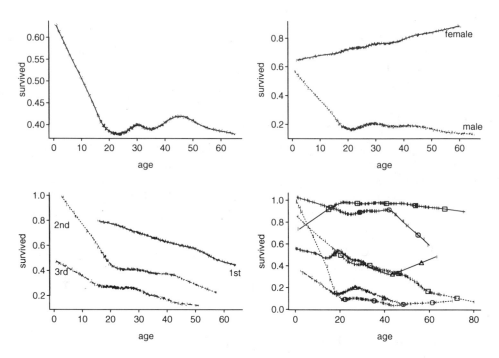

FIGURE 12.3: Nonparametric regression (loess) estimates of the relationship between age and the probability of surviving the Titanic. The top left panel shows unstratified estimates. The top right panel depicts relationships stratified by sex. The bottom left and right panels show, respectively, estimates stratified by class and by the cross-classification of sex and class of the passenger. Tick marks are drawn at actual age values for each stratum. In the bottom right panel, solid lines correspond to females and dotted lines to males. First class is depicted by squares, second class by circles, and third class by triangles.

TABLE 12.2: Wald Statistics for survived

	χ^2	d.f.	P
sex (Factor+Higher Order Factors)	187.15	15	< 0.0001
All Interactions	59.74	14	< 0.0001
pclass (Factor+Higher Order Factors)	100.10	20	< 0.0001
All Interactions	46.51	18	0.0003
age (Factor+Higher Order Factors)	56.20	32	0.0052
All Interactions	34.57	28	0.1826
Nonlinear (Factor+Higher Order Factors)	28.66	24	0.2331
sibsp (Factor+Higher Order Factors)	19.67	5	0.0014
All Interactions	12.13	4	0.0164
parch (Factor+Higher Order Factors)	3.51	5	0.6217
All Interactions	3.51	4	0.4761
sex × pclass (Factor+Higher Order Factors)	42.43	10	< 0.0001
sex × age (Factor+Higher Order Factors)	15.89	12	0.1962
Nonlinear (Factor+Higher Order Factors)	14.47	9	0.1066
Nonlinear Interaction : f(A,B) vs. AB	4.17	3	0.2441
pclass × age (Factor+Higher Order Factors)	13.47	16	0.6385
Nonlinear (Factor+Higher Order Factors)	12.92	12	0.3749
Nonlinear Interaction : f(A,B) vs. AB	6.88	6	0.3324
age × sibsp (Factor+Higher Order Factors)	12.13	4	0.0164
Nonlinear	1.76	3	0.6235
Nonlinear Interaction : f(A,B) vs. AB	1.76	3	0.6235
age × parch (Factor+Higher Order Factors)	3.51	4	0.4761
Nonlinear	1.80	3	0.6147
Nonlinear Interaction : f(A,B) vs. AB	1.80	3	0.6147
sex × pclass × age (Factor+Higher Order Factors)	8.34	8	0.4006
Nonlinear	7.74	6	0.2581
TOTAL NONLINEAR	28.66	24	0.2331
TOTAL INTERACTION	75.61	30	< 0.0001
TOTAL NONLINEAR + INTERACTION	79.49	33	< 0.0001
TOTAL	241.93	39	< 0.0001

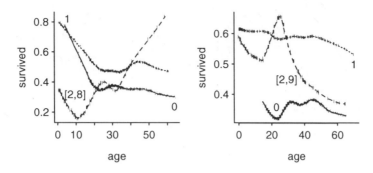

FIGURE 12.4: Relationship between age and survival stratified by number of siblings or spouses on board (left panel) or by number of parents or children of passengers on board (right panel).

Three-way interactions are clearly insignificant ($P = 0.4$) in Table 12.2. So is parch ($P = 0.6$ for testing the combined main effect + interaction effects for parch, i.e., whether parch is important for any age). These effects would be deleted in almost all bootstrap resamples had we bootstrapped a variable selection procedure using $\alpha = 0.1$ for retention of terms, so we can safely ignore these terms for future steps. The model not containing those terms is fitted below. The ^2 in the model formula means to expand the terms in parentheses to include all main effects and second-order interactions.

```
> f ← lrm(survived ∼ (sex + pclass + rcs(age,5))^2 +
+              rcs(age,5)*sibsp)
> f
```

```
Frequencies of Responses
  0   1
619 427
```

```
Frequencies of Missing Values Due to Each Variable
 survived sex pclass age sibsp parch
    0    0      0 263     0     0
```

Obs	Max Deriv	Model L.R.	d.f.	P	C	Dxy	Gamma	Tau-a	R2	Brier
1046	6e-006	554	26	0	0.88	0.76	0.76	0.37	0.56	0.13

	Coef	S.E.	Wald Z	P
Intercept	3.30746	1.84266	1.79	0.0727
sex=male	-1.14781	1.08782	-1.06	0.2914

```
              pclass=2nd   6.73087 3.96166  1.70  0.0893
              pclass=3rd  -1.64369 1.82988 -0.90  0.3691
                     age   0.08860 0.13455  0.66  0.5102
                    age'  -0.74099 0.65128 -1.14  0.2552
                   age''   4.92642 4.00468  1.23  0.2186
                  age'''  -6.61296 5.41003 -1.22  0.2216
                   sibsp  -1.04461 0.34414 -3.04  0.0024
 sex=male * pclass=2nd   -0.76822 0.70827 -1.08  0.2781
 sex=male * pclass=3rd    2.15200 0.62140  3.46  0.0005
        sex=male * age   -0.21911 0.07215 -3.04  0.0024
       sex=male * age'    1.08422 0.38862  2.79  0.0053
      sex=male * age''   -6.55781 2.65108 -2.47  0.0134
     sex=male * age'''    8.37161 3.85324  2.17  0.0298
      pclass=2nd * age   -0.54459 0.26526 -2.05  0.0401
      pclass=3rd * age   -0.16335 0.13083 -1.25  0.2118
     pclass=2nd * age'    1.91559 1.01892  1.88  0.0601
     pclass=3rd * age'    0.82045 0.60914  1.35  0.1780
    pclass=2nd * age''   -8.95448 5.50269 -1.63  0.1037
    pclass=3rd * age''   -5.42760 3.64751 -1.49  0.1367
   pclass=2nd * age'''    9.39265 6.95595  1.35  0.1769
   pclass=3rd * age'''    7.54036 4.85185  1.55  0.1202
           age * sibsp    0.03571 0.03398  1.05  0.2933
          age' * sibsp   -0.04665 0.22126 -0.21  0.8330
         age'' * sibsp    0.55743 1.66797  0.33  0.7382
        age''' * sibsp   -1.19370 2.57112 -0.46  0.6425

> anova(f)    # Table 12.3
```

This is a very powerful model (ROC area $= C = 0.88$); the survival patterns are easy to detect. The Wald ANOVA in Table 12.3 indicates especially strong sex and pclass effects ($\chi^2 = 199$ and 109, respectively). There is a very strong sex × pclass interaction and a strong age × sibsp interaction, considering the strength of sibsp overall.

Let us examine the shapes of predictor effects. With so many interactions in the model we need to obtain predicted values at least for all combinations of sex and pclass. For sibsp we consider only two of its possible values.

```
> for(sx in c('female','male'))
+   plot(f, age=NA, pclass=NA, sex=sx,           # Fig. 12.5
+        fun=plogis, ylim=c(0,1), add=sx=='male',
+        conf.int=F, col=if(sx=='female')1 else 2,
+        adj.subtitle=F, lty=1)
> plot(f, sibsp=NA, age=c(10,15,20,50), conf.int=F) # Fig. 12.6
```

Note the agreement between the lower right-hand panel of Figure 12.3 with Figure 12.5. This results from our use of similar flexibility in the parametric and nonparametric approaches (and similar effective degrees of freedom). The estimated

TABLE 12.3: Wald Statistics for `survived`

	χ^2	d.f.	P
sex (Factor+Higher Order Factors)	199.42	7	< 0.0001
All Interactions	56.14	6	< 0.0001
pclass (Factor+Higher Order Factors)	108.73	12	< 0.0001
All Interactions	42.83	10	< 0.0001
age (Factor+Higher Order Factors)	47.04	20	0.0006
All Interactions	24.51	16	0.0789
Nonlinear (Factor+Higher Order Factors)	22.72	15	0.0902
sibsp (Factor+Higher Order Factors)	19.95	5	0.0013
All Interactions	10.99	4	0.0267
sex × pclass (Factor+Higher Order Factors)	35.40	2	< 0.0001
sex × age (Factor+Higher Order Factors)	10.08	4	0.0391
Nonlinear	8.17	3	0.0426
Nonlinear Interaction : f(A,B) vs. AB	8.17	3	0.0426
pclass × age (Factor+Higher Order Factors)	6.86	8	0.5516
Nonlinear	6.11	6	0.4113
Nonlinear Interaction : f(A,B) vs. AB	6.11	6	0.4113
age × sibsp (Factor+Higher Order Factors)	10.99	4	0.0267
Nonlinear	1.81	3	0.6134
Nonlinear Interaction : f(A,B) vs. AB	1.81	3	0.6134
TOTAL NONLINEAR	22.72	15	0.0902
TOTAL INTERACTION	67.58	18	< 0.0001
TOTAL NONLINEAR + INTERACTION	70.68	21	< 0.0001
TOTAL	253.18	26	< 0.0001

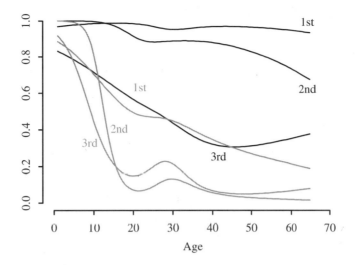

FIGURE 12.5: Effects of predictors on probability of survival of Titanic passengers, estimated for zero siblings or spouses. Lines for females are black; males are drawn using gray scale.

effect of `sibsp` as a function of age is shown in Figure 12.6. Note that children having many siblings apparently had lower survival. Married adults had slightly higher survival than unmarried ones.

There will never be another Titanic, so we do not need to validate the model for prospective use. But we use the bootstrap to validate the model anyway, in an effort to detect whether it is overfitting the data. We do not penalize the calculations that follow for having examined the effect of `parch` or for testing three-way interactions, in the belief that these tests would replicate well.

```
> f ← update(f, x=T, y=T)
> # x=T,y=T adds raw data to fit object so can bootstrap
> set.seed(131)                    # so can replicate resamples
> options(digits=2)
> validate(f, B=80)
```

	index.orig	training	test	optimism	index.corrected	n
Dxy	0.7560	0.7742	0.7417	0.0325	0.7235	80
R2	0.5545	0.5800	0.5293	0.0507	0.5039	80
Intercept	0.0000	0.0000	-0.0505	0.0505	-0.0505	80
Slope	1.0000	1.0000	0.8806	0.1194	0.8806	80
Emax	0.0000	0.0000	0.0368	0.0368	0.0368	80
B	0.1303	0.1251	0.1340	-0.0089	0.1392	80

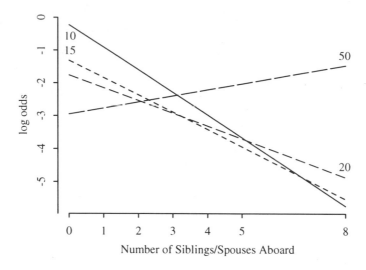

FIGURE 12.6: Effect of number of siblings and spouses on the log odds of surviving, for third class males. Numbers next to lines are ages in years.

```
> cal ← calibrate(f, B=80)       # Figure 12.7
> plot(cal)
```

The output of validate indicates minor overfitting. Overfitting would have been worse had the risk factors not been so strong. The closeness of the calibration curve to the 45° line in Figure 12.7 demonstrates excellent validation on an absolute probability scale. But the extent of missing data casts some doubt on the validity of this model, and on the efficiency of its parameter estimates.

12.4 Examining Missing Data Patterns

The first step to dealing with missing data is understanding the patterns of missing values. To do this we use the Hmisc library's naclus and naplot functions, and the recursive partitioning library of Atkinson and Therneau. Below naclus tells us which variables tend to be missing on the same persons, and it computes the proportion of missing values for each variable. The rpart function derives a tree to predict which types of passengers tended to have age missing.

```
> na.patterns ← naclus(titanic3)
> library(rpart)
> who.na ← rpart(is.na(age) ~ sex + pclass + survived +
+                 sibsp + parch, minbucket=15)
> par(mfrow=c(2,2))
```

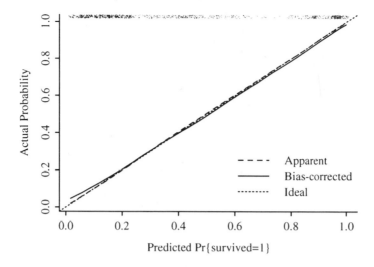

FIGURE 12.7: Bootstrap overfitting-corrected loess nonparametric calibration curve for casewise deletion model. Rug plot at top of graph indicates the distribution of predicted probabilities.

```
> naplot(na.patterns, 'na per var')
> plot(na.patterns)
> plot(who.na); text(who.na)      # Figure 12.8
> par(mfrow=c(1,1))                # Reset to 1x1 plot setup
```

We see in Figure 12.8 that age tends to be missing on the same passengers as the body bag identifier, and that it is missing in only 0.09 of first or second class passengers. The category of passengers having the highest fraction of missing ages is third class passengers having no parents or children on board. Below we use Hmisc's summary.formula function to plot simple descriptive statistics on the fraction of missing ages, stratified by other variables. We see that without adjusting for other variables, age is slightly more missing on nonsurviving passengers.

```
> plot(summary(is.na(age) ~ sex + pclass + survived +
+              sibsp + parch))   # Figure 12.9
```

Let us derive a logistic model to predict missingness of age, to see if the survival bias maintains after adjustment for the other variables.

```
> m ← lrm(is.na(age) ~ sex * pclass + survived + sibsp + parch)
> m
```

```
Frequencies of Responses
 FALSE TRUE
  1046  263
```

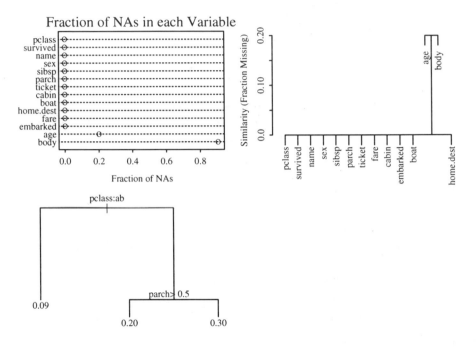

FIGURE 12.8: Patterns of missing data. Upper left panel shows the fraction of observations missing on each predictor. Upper right panel depicts a hierarchical cluster analysis of missingness combinations. The similarity measure shown on the Y-axis is the fraction of observations for which both variables are missing. Lower left panel shows the result of recursive partitioning for predicting is.na(age). The only strong pattern found by the rpart function was due to passenger class.

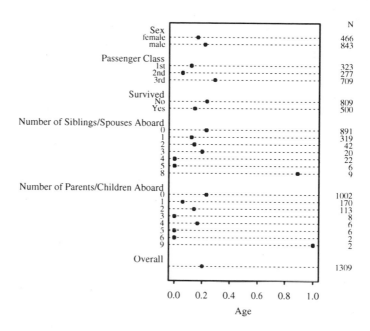

FIGURE 12.9: Univariable descriptions of proportion of passengers with missing age.

```
Obs Max Deriv Model L.R. d.f. P   C  Dxy Gamma Tau-a   R2 Brier
1309   5e-006          115   8  0 0.7 0.41 0.45  0.13 0.13 0.15
```

	Coef	S.E.	Wald Z	P
Intercept	-2.20299	0.36412	-6.05	0.0000
sex=male	0.64395	0.39526	1.63	0.1033
pclass=2nd	-1.00793	0.66578	-1.51	0.1300
pclass=3rd	1.61242	0.35962	4.48	0.0000
survived	-0.18058	0.18280	-0.99	0.3232
sibsp	0.04353	0.07372	0.59	0.5548
parch	-0.35261	0.12529	-2.81	0.0049
sex=male * pclass=2nd	0.13467	0.75451	0.18	0.8583
sex=male * pclass=3rd	-0.85628	0.42144	-2.03	0.0422

```
> anova(m)    # Table 12.4
```

Fortunately, after controlling for other variables, Table 12.4 provides evidence that nonsurviving passengers are no more likely to have age missing. The only important predictors of missingness are `pclass` and `parch` (the more parents or children the passenger has on board, the less likely age was to be missing).

TABLE 12.4: Wald Statistics for `is.na(age)`

	χ^2	d.f.	P
sex (Factor+Higher Order Factors)	5.61	3	0.1324
All Interactions	5.58	2	0.0614
pclass (Factor+Higher Order Factors)	68.43	4	< 0.0001
All Interactions	5.58	2	0.0614
survived	0.98	1	0.3232
sibsp	0.35	1	0.5548
parch	7.92	1	0.0049
sex $\times$ pclass (Factor+Higher Order Factors)	5.58	2	0.0614
TOTAL	82.90	8	< 0.0001

12.5   Single Conditional Mean Imputation

We first try single conditional mean imputation, allowing age to be transformed nonlinearly, using the `transcan` function. Note that for this type of imputation it would cause a major bias to include Y in the imputation model. For this dataset, the default spline transformation for age derived by `transcan` is curved for young passengers, resulting in mean imputed ages that do not match stratified sex $\times$ class $\times$ `parch` means of nonmissing ages. So we constrain age to be linear in the imputation model, implying that imputations use actual cell means but smoothed by an additivity assumption.

```
> xtrans ← transcan(∼ I(age) + sex + pclass + sibsp + parch,
+                   imputed=T, pl=F)
> summary(xtrans)
```

R-squared achieved in predicting each variable:

```
   age   sex pclass sibsp parch
 0.258 0.078  0.244 0.241 0.288
```

Adjusted R-squared:

```
   age   sex pclass sibsp parch
 0.254 0.074   0.24 0.238 0.285
```

Coefficients of canonical variates for predicting each (row) variable

```
            age   sex pclass sibsp parch
     age        -0.89  6.13 -1.81 -2.77
     sex -0.02         0.56  0.10  0.71
  pclass  0.08  0.26         0.07  0.25
   sibsp -0.02  0.04  0.07         0.87
   parch -0.03  0.29  0.22  0.75
```

Summary of imputed values

age
```
  n missing unique  Mean   .05   .10   .25   .50   .75   .90   .95
263 0           24  28.41 16.76 21.66 26.17 28.04 28.04 42.92 42.92
```

```
lowest :  7.563  9.425 14.617 16.479 16.687
highest: 33.219 34.749 38.588 41.058 42.920
```

Starting estimates for imputed values:

```
 age sex pclass sibsp parch
  28   2      3     0     0
```

```
> # Look at mean imputed values by sex,pclass and observed means
> # age.i is age, filled in with conditional mean estimates

> age.i ← impute(xtrans, age)

> i ← is.imputed(age.i)
> tapply(age.i[i], list(sex[i],pclass[i]), mean)

        1st  2nd  3rd
female 38.1 27.1 22.4
  male 40.7 29.7 25.0

> tapply(age, list(sex,pclass), mean, na.rm=T)

        1st  2nd  3rd
female   37 27.5 22.2
  male   41 30.8 26.0
```

Now we develop a logistic model using the single-imputed ages, to at least avoid deletion of good data.

```
> dd    ← datadist(dd, age.i)
> f.si ← lrm(survived ~ (sex + pclass + rcs(age.i,5))^2 +
+              rcs(age.i,5)*sibsp)
> f.si
```

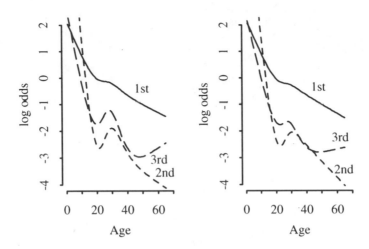

FIGURE 12.10: Predicted log odds of survival for males from fit using casewise deletion (left panel) and single conditional mean imputation (right panel). sibsp is set to zero for these predicted values.

```
Frequencies of Responses
   0   1
 809 500


 Obs Max Deriv Model L.R. d.f. P   C  Dxy Gamma Tau-a   R2 Brier
 1309    0.0004         641   26 0 0.86 0.72  0.73  0.34 0.53  0.13


 . . . . . . .

     > par(mfrow=c(1,2))      # Figure 12.10
     > plot(f,     age=NA,   pclass=NA, ylim=c(-4,2),
     +      conf.int=F, adj.subtitle=F)
     > plot(f.si, age.i=NA, pclass=NA, ylim=c(-4,2),
     +      conf.int=F, adj.subtitle=F)
     > anova(f.si)            # Table 12.5
```

We see a substantial increase in the likelihood ratio χ^2 (now 641) compared with the no-imputation model, due to the increase in sample size. There is a very slight drop in the C index. Wald statistics appear in Table 12.5. Figure 12.10 shows predicted values from the casewise deletion model and the single imputation model.

TABLE 12.5: Wald Statistics for `survived`

	χ^2	d.f.	P
sex (Factor+Higher Order Factors)	245.53	7	< 0.0001
All Interactions	52.80	6	< 0.0001
pclass (Factor+Higher Order Factors)	112.02	12	< 0.0001
All Interactions	36.77	10	0.0001
age.i (Factor+Higher Order Factors)	49.25	20	0.0003
All Interactions	25.53	16	0.0610
Nonlinear (Factor+Higher Order Factors)	19.86	15	0.1772
sibsp (Factor+Higher Order Factors)	21.74	5	0.0006
All Interactions	12.25	4	0.0156
sex × pclass (Factor+Higher Order Factors)	30.25	2	< 0.0001
sex × age.i (Factor+Higher Order Factors)	8.95	4	0.0622
Nonlinear	5.63	3	0.1308
Nonlinear Interaction : f(A,B) vs. AB	5.63	3	0.1308
pclass × age.i (Factor+Higher Order Factors)	6.04	8	0.6427
Nonlinear	5.44	6	0.4882
Nonlinear Interaction : f(A,B) vs. AB	5.44	6	0.4882
age.i × sibsp (Factor+Higher Order Factors)	12.25	4	0.0156
Nonlinear	2.04	3	0.5639
Nonlinear Interaction : f(A,B) vs. AB	2.04	3	0.5639
TOTAL NONLINEAR	19.86	15	0.1772
TOTAL INTERACTION	66.83	18	< 0.0001
TOTAL NONLINEAR + INTERACTION	69.48	21	< 0.0001
TOTAL	305.58	26	< 0.0001

12.6   Multiple Imputation

Multiple imputation is expected to arrive at less biased estimates as well as providing an estimate of the variance–covariance matrix of $\hat{\beta}$ penalized for imputation. With multiple imputation, survival status can be used to impute missing ages, so the age relationship will not be as attenuated as with single conditional mean imputation.

In the first try at transcan for multiple imputation, the age effect was curved for older passengers, resulting in what appeared to be too many imputed ages over 70 years. transcan was rerun forcing age to behave linearly. The resulting multiply imputed ages had a similar distribution to the actual nonmissing ones.

```
> set.seed(17)            # so can reproduce the random draws
> xtrans ← transcan(~ I(age) + sex + pclass +
+                       sibsp + parch + survived,
+                       n.impute=5, pl=F,
+                       trantab=T, imputed=T)


> summary(xtrans)

Adjusted R-squared achieved in predicting each variable:

  age sex pclass sibsp parch survived
 0.28 0.3   0.33  0.25  0.29     0.37


Coefficients of canonical variates for predicting each (row) variable

             age    sex pclass sibsp parch survived
      age           0.37  6.76  -2.17 -2.48 -5.37
      sex   0.00         -0.10   0.15  0.21  1.95
   pclass   0.07 -0.09          0.12  0.16  1.26
    sibsp  -0.03  0.18  0.15          0.84 -0.65
    parch  -0.03  0.22  0.18   0.75        0.29
 survived  -0.01  0.23  0.16  -0.06  0.03

Summary of imputed values

age
     n missing unique  Mean   .05   .10   .25   .50   .75   .90   .95
  1315 0         1006  28.96  6.88 12.27 19.38 27.80 37.94 47.73 52.95

lowest :   0.1667  0.5826  0.6028  0.6567  0.9990
highest: 68.9805 70.5000 72.2900 73.8221 74.0000
```

```
Starting estimates for imputed values:

age sex pclass sibsp parch survived
 28   2      3     0     0        0
```

```
> # Print the 5 imputations for the first 10 passengers having missing age
> xtrans$imputed$age[1:10,]
      1  2  3  4  5
 16  37 49 46 48 49
 38  45 32 50 40 26
 41  42 36 67 29 43
 47  48 60 30 49 42
 60  57 39 38 48 45
 70  38 32 31 30 18
 71  42 40 62 41 54
 75  40 42 34 44 29
 81  33 38 46 63 62
107  49 38 47 37 37
```

transcan has now developed five imputations for each missing age, by taking random draws from the residuals from the predicted transformed age values. We now fit logistic models for five completed datasets. The fit.mult.impute function fits five models and examines the within– and between–imputation variances to compute an imputation-corrected variance–covariance matrix that is stored in the fit object f.mi. fit.mult.impute will also average the five $\hat{\beta}$ vectors, storing the result in f.mi$coefficients. The function also prints the ratio of imputation-corrected variances to average ordinary variances.

```
> f.mi ← fit.mult.impute(survived ~ (sex + pclass + rcs(age,5))^2 +
+                        rcs(age,5)*sibsp,
+                        lrm, xtrans)
```

```
Variance Inflation Factors Due to Imputation:

Intercept sex=male pclass=2nd pclass=3rd age age' age'' age''' sibsp
        1      1.1          1          1   1    1   1.1    1.1   1.3
sex=male * pclass=2nd sex=male * pclass=3rd sex=male * age
                    1                     1              1.2
sex=male * age' sex=male * age'' sex=male * age''' pclass=2nd * age
           1.1              1.1               1.1                1
pclass=3rd * age pclass=2nd * age' pclass=3rd * age' pclass=2nd * age''
               1                 1                 1                  1
pclass=3rd * age'' pclass=2nd * age''' pclass=3rd * age''' age * sibsp
               1.1                   1                 1.1         1.3
age' * sibsp age'' * sibsp age''' * sibsp
         1.3          1.3            1.3
```

```
> f.mi
```

```
Frequencies of Responses
  0   1
809 500
```

```
  Obs Max Deriv Model L.R. d.f.  P    C  Dxy Gamma Tau-a   R2 Brier
 1309    2e-007       662   26  0 0.87 0.74 0.75  0.35 0.54  0.13
```

. . . . .

We see a further increase in likelihood ratio χ^2 due to multiple imputation being able to use relationships with the response variable to better impute missing ages. Now get Wald statistics for all effects in the model, adjusted for multiple imputation.

```
> anova(f.mi)    # Table 12.6
```

The Wald χ^2 for age is reduced by accounting for imputation but is increased by using patterns of association with survival status to impute missing age. Now examine the fitted age relationship using multiple as opposed to single imputation.

```
> par(mfrow=c(1,2))      # Figure 12.11
> plot(f.si, age.i=NA, pclass=NA, ylim=c(-4,2),
+      conf.int=F, adj.subtitle=F)
> plot(f.mi, age=NA,   pclass=NA, ylim=c(-4,2),
+      conf.int=F, adj.subtitle=F)
> par(mfrow=c(1,1))
```

12.7 Summarizing the Fitted Model

In this section we depict the model fitted using multiple imputation, by computing odds ratios and by showing various predicted values. For age, the odds ratio for an increase from 1 year old to 30 years old is computed, instead of the default odds ratio based on outer quartiles of age. The estimated odds ratios are very dependent on the levels of interacting factors, so Figure 12.12 depicts only one of many patterns.

```
> s ← summary(f.mi, age=c(1,30), sibsp=0:1)
> # override default ranges for 3 variables
> plot(s, log=T)                  # Figure 12.12
```

Now compute estimated probabilities of survival for a variety of settings of the predictors.

TABLE 12.6: Wald Statistics for survived

	χ^2	d.f.	P
sex (Factor+Higher Order Factors)	237.33	7	< 0.0001
All Interactions	53.50	6	< 0.0001
pclass (Factor+Higher Order Factors)	116.29	12	< 0.0001
All Interactions	37.18	10	0.0001
age (Factor+Higher Order Factors)	46.58	20	0.0007
All Interactions	23.78	16	0.0944
Nonlinear (Factor+Higher Order Factors)	20.12	15	0.1673
sibsp (Factor+Higher Order Factors)	17.81	5	0.0032
All Interactions	8.03	4	0.0905
sex × pclass (Factor+Higher Order Factors)	32.15	2	< 0.0001
sex × age (Factor+Higher Order Factors)	10.06	4	0.0394
Nonlinear	7.73	3	0.0520
Nonlinear Interaction : f(A,B) vs. AB	7.73	3	0.0520
pclass × age (Factor+Higher Order Factors)	5.68	8	0.6828
Nonlinear	5.16	6	0.5240
Nonlinear Interaction : f(A,B) vs. AB	5.16	6	0.5240
age × sibsp (Factor+Higher Order Factors)	8.03	4	0.0905
Nonlinear	1.31	3	0.7256
Nonlinear Interaction : f(A,B) vs. AB	1.31	3	0.7256
TOTAL NONLINEAR	20.12	15	0.1673
TOTAL INTERACTION	64.94	18	< 0.0001
TOTAL NONLINEAR + INTERACTION	67.84	21	< 0.0001
TOTAL	291.66	26	< 0.0001

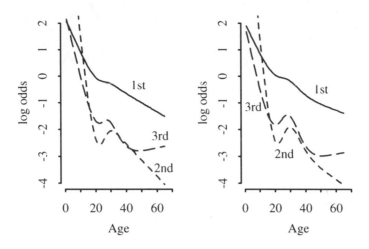

FIGURE 12.11: Predicted log odds of survival for males from fit using single conditional mean imputation again (left panel) and multiple random draw imputation (right panel). Both sets of predictions are for `sibsp` = 0.

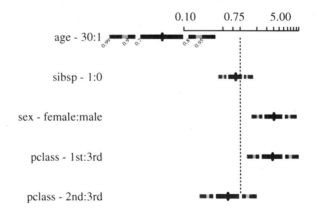

Adjusted to:sex=male pclass=3rd age=28 sibsp=0

FIGURE 12.12: Odds ratios for some predictor settings.

```
> phat ← predict(f.mi, combos ←
+  expand.grid(age=c(2,21,50),sex=levels(sex),pclass=levels(pclass),
+                  sibsp=0), type='fitted')
> options(digits=1)
> data.frame(combos, phat)
```

```
   age    sex pclass sibsp phat
1    2 female    1st     0 0.97
2   21 female    1st     0 0.98
3   50 female    1st     0 0.97
4    2   male    1st     0 0.85
5   21   male    1st     0 0.50
6   50   male    1st     0 0.26
7    2 female    2nd     0 1.00
8   21 female    2nd     0 0.90
9   50 female    2nd     0 0.83
10   2   male    2nd     0 1.00
11  21   male    2nd     0 0.07
12  50   male    2nd     0 0.03
13   2 female    3rd     0 0.78
14  21 female    3rd     0 0.58
15  50 female    3rd     0 0.36
16   2   male    3rd     0 0.80
17  21   male    3rd     0 0.14
18  50   male    3rd     0 0.05
```

We can also get predicted values by creating an S-PLUS function that will evaluate the model on demand.

```
> pred.logit ← Function(f.mi)

> pred.logit
function(sex = "male", pclass = "3rd", age = 28, sibsp = 0)
{
    3.440147 - 1.4381326 * (sex == "male") + 6.296592 * (pclass ==
        "2nd") - 2.0779809 * (pclass == "3rd") + 0.082134387 * age -
        0.00025084004 * pmax(age - 5, 0)^3 + 0.0016482259 * pmax(
        age - 21, 0)^3 - 0.0022035565 * pmax(age - 28, 0)^3 +
        0.00088444824 * pmax(age - 37, 0)^3 - 7.8277628e-005 *
        pmax(age - 56, 0)^3 - 0.92513167 * sibsp + (sex == "male") *
        (-0.58477831 * (pclass == "2nd") + 1.9845306 * (pclass ==
        "3rd")) + (sex == "male") * (-0.19813189 * age +
        0.00035992445 * pmax(age - 5, 0)^3 - 0.0022232117 * pmax(
        age - 21, 0)^3 + 0.002898667 * pmax(age - 28, 0)^3 -
        0.0011424428 * pmax(age - 37, 0)^3 + 0.00010706304 * pmax(
        age - 56, 0)^3) + (pclass == "2nd") * (-0.52315032 * age +
        0.00066960929 * pmax(age - 5, 0)^3 - 0.0030561012 * pmax(
```

```
        age - 21, 0)^3 + 0.0031229941 * pmax(age - 28, 0)^3 -
        0.0007700192 * pmax(age - 37, 0)^3 + 3.3517068e-005 * pmax(
        age - 56, 0)^3) + (pclass == "3rd") * (-0.13015825 * age +
        0.00024102399 * pmax(age - 5, 0)^3 - 0.0015255584 * pmax(
        age - 21, 0)^3 + 0.002044236 * pmax(age - 28, 0)^3 -
        0.00084927821 * pmax(age - 37, 0)^3 + 8.9576665e-005 *
        pmax(age - 56, 0)^3) + sibsp * (0.031980533 * age -
        1.679181e-005 * pmax(age - 5, 0)^3 + 0.00015089349 * pmax(
        age - 21, 0)^3 - 0.00030324003 * pmax(age - 28, 0)^3 +
        0.0002139911 * pmax(age - 37, 0)^3 - 4.4852752e-005 * pmax(
        age - 56, 0)^3)
}
> # Note: if don't define sibsp to pred.logit, default to 0
> plogis(pred.logit(age=c(2,21,50), sex='male', pclass='3rd'))

[1] 0.80 0.14 0.05
```

A nomogram could be used to obtain predicted values manually, but this is not feasible when so many interaction terms are present. For S-PLUS 2000 on Windows/NT we can compose a menu dialog for entering passenger characteristics and obtaining predicted survival probabilities. First use the Hmisc dataRep function to create an object summarizing how well different types of subjects are represented in the dataset. For matching on sibsp we only demand that we match on the presence or absence of accompanying family members. The object created by dataRep is later used by the graphical interface. Then the Design library's Dialog function creates the user interface to enter data and obtain predictions, shown in Figure 12.13.

```
> drep <- dataRep( ~ roundN(age,10) + sex + pclass +
+                    roundN(sibsp, clip=0:1))
> Dialog(fitPar('f.mi', lp=F, fun=list('Prob[Survival]'=plogis)),
+         limits='data', basename='Titanic',
+         vary=list(sex=c('female','male')), datarep=drep)
> runmenu.Titanic()
```

12.8   Problems

1. Use the 1000-patient SUPPORT dataset to develop a multivariable binary logistic model predicting the probability that a patient dies in the hospital. Consider the following predictors: age, sex, dzgroup, num.co, scoma, race (use all levels), meanbp, hrt, temp, pafi, alb.

   (a) Using one or two S-PLUS commands, make a single chart (if it's too busy make two) showing proportions of hospital death stratified by all of the predictors, one at a time. For continuous predictors use quartiles.

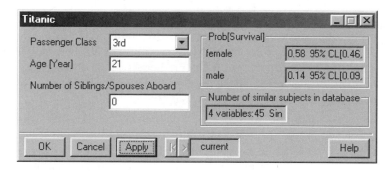

FIGURE 12.13: Graphical user interface for deriving and plotting $\hat{P}$ and 0.95 C.L.

(b) Compute the proportion of hospital deaths stratified by sex. Compute the odds of death stratified by sex, take logs, and then compute the difference in log odds of death due to sex and antilog this to get the sex odds ratio. Compare this with the sex odds ratio from a 2×2 table where logs are not used.

(c) Considering only the age variable, make two plots, one relating age non-parametrically to the proportion of deaths using a statement such as plsmo(age,hospdead) (plsmo is in the Hmisc library). Then make a similar plot to check whether the age effect is linear on the log odds scale. You can use a fun argument to plsmo to do this, for example, fun=qlogis or fun=function(p) log(p/(1-p)).

(d) Impute race using the most frequent category and pafi and alb using "normal" values. For any remaining NAs exclude observations while fitting models.

(e) Fit a model to predict the response using all predictors. For continuous ones assume a smooth relationship but allow it to be nonlinear. Quantify the ability of the model to discriminate patients who lived from those who died. Do an overall test for whether any variables are associated with in-hospital mortality.

(f) Compute partial tests of association for each predictor and a test of nonlinearity for continuous ones. Compute a global test of nonlinearity. Graphically display the ranking of importance of the predictors.

(g) Display the shape of how each predictor relates to the log odds of hospital death, setting other predictors to typical values (one value per predictor).

(h) For each predictor estimate (and either print or plot) the odds ratio associated with the predictor changing from its first to its third quartile, all other predictors held constant. For categorical predictors, compute odds ratios with respect to the reference category.

(i) Make a nomogram for the model, including a final axis that translates predictions to the probability scale. Use the nomogram to obtain a predicted probability for a patient having values of all the predictors of your choosing. Compare this with the predicted value computed by either the `predict` or `Function` functions. For the latter two be sure to translate predicted logits to predicted probabilities.

(j) Use resampling to validate the Somers' D_{xy} rank correlation between predicted probability of death and the binary life/death response. Also validate the Brier score, generalized R^2, and slope shrinkage coefficient, all using a single S-PLUS statement. Draw a validated calibration curve. Comment on the quality (potential "exportability") of the model.

(k) Refit the full model, excluding observations for which `pafi` was imputed. Plot the shape of the effect of `pafi` in this new model and comment on whether and how it differs from the shape of the `pafi` effect for the fit in which `pafi` was imputed.

2. Analyze the Mayo Clinic primary biliary cirrhosis dataset described in Section 8.12 to develop and test a model for the probability that a patient survives three years, even though such a binary analysis discards valuable data. For alive patients that were not followed for three years, set the three-year status to missing (even though this method may introduce some bias). You can either validate the final model using bootstrapping or cross-validation, or set aside a random portion (you choose the portion and the randomization) that is used *only* for validation (but beware of the problem of having too few events in training and test samples!). Use only randomized patients.

(a) Make a dot chart summarizing how each predictor relates to the response, without adjusting for the other predictors.

(b) Assess the nature of the marginal association of each continuous predictor with the log odds of dying (you may use imputations done previously or exclude observations with missing data since you are examining variables one at a time). Use restricted cubic spline fits and smooth nonparametric regression. For the latter, pay attention to the distribution of each predictor when interpreting the estimated relationship. Use a common y-axis scale for all the plots so that relative importance of different predictors can be gauged. Make a test of H_0 : predictor is not associated with outcome versus H_a : predictor is associated (by a smooth function). The test should have more than 1 d.f. Make a formal test of linearity of each predictor.

(c) Based on the distribution of the binary response variable, what's your estimate of the maximum total degrees of freedom the model can have on the right-hand side of the regression equation and still be expected to be reliable?

(d) To reduce the dimensionality of the problem, display how potential predictor variables interrelate, using a squared rank correlation coefficient as the basis for quantifying the relationships. Choose one predictor from groups of predictors that have even moderate relationships.

(e) For the remaining variables, determine the number of missing values, the proportion of patients that are missing on the same predictors (or graph patterns of missingness that include this), and what kinds of patients have missing values for predictors that are missing on more than 20 patients.

(f) When subject matter knowledge is available that allows you to rank the likely strength of each predictor, it is a good idea to allow potentially strong predictors to have more complexity, that is, more parameters in the model (e.g., more knots). When such subject matter knowledge is not available, it can also be good idea to allow more parameters for predictors that have more promise, when judged by a test that does not assume a simple linear or 1:1 monotonic relationship between X and Y (see Section 4.1). For remaining continuous predictors, decide how many knots to allow or decide to force linearity on the basis of an unadjusted nonparametric test relating the predictor to the response. For example, the `Hmisc` `spearman2` function can test for association between two variables while allowing general U-shaped relationships if you use `spearman2(response ~ x, 2)`. This function provides a kind of generalized Spearman's ρ^2 between y and both the ranks of x and the square of the ranks of x. Compute this ρ^2 for all remaining continuous predictors. Force linearity for predictors having very weak ρ^2 (e.g., $\rho^2 \leq 0.02$; you choose the cutpoint), use three-knot restricted cubic splines for predictors having mediocre ρ^2 (e.g., .02 to .08), four knots for, say, .08 to .15, and allow five knots when, say, $\rho^2 > 0.15$.

(g) For multivariable modeling, impute missing values for the reduced set of predictors. Describe the method used for imputation, and the reason you chose it (including expediency).

(h) Of the predictors you are considering, compare the pretransformations determined earlier (without using outcome status), with optimal transformations obtained using death (i.e., those obtained in the previous part), using AIC and optionally using graphs. Comment on the adequacy of each pretransformation. Also make a formal test of the adequacy of each pretransformation (again, for each predictor separately), using Wald, score, or likelihood ratio tests. If the data reduction in Problem 1 in Section 8.12 resulted in combining multiple predictors, test the adequacy of this data reduction also.

(i) Develop a model that incorporates all remaining predictors. Depending on the previous step, this model will use pretransformations, spline-expanded predictors, or summary measures that combine variables. For numerical reasons you may have to use only three knots in this joint model when using spline expansions. Again test the importance and the linearity (if not using a pretransformation) of each predictor. Use more knots if this gives a better fit according to AIC.

(j) If the resulting model includes variables that were not routinely measured in nonrandomized patients, compare the ROC area or D_{xy} indexes of that model with the best model which excludes those variables.

(k) Of the factors that remain, make a joint (simultaneous) test of all two-way interactions involving such factors. Also make Wald or score tests of the individual interaction effects. For both of these, test for linearity of interactions. Include any clearly significant interaction terms in the final model, simplifying interactions if warranted by the linearity tests.

(l) Locate overly influential observations with respect to each predictor in this model. If needed, curtail predictor ranges and refit the model.

(m) If using S, use the `robcov` or `bootcov` function to get alternative estimates of the standard errors of regression coefficients.

(n) Interpret the final model by making at least two graphs in which an important continuous variable is on the x-axis, predicted probability is on the y-axis, separate curves are drawn for various levels of one or two other factors, and any other factors in the model are adjusted to specified constants. Also state the model in simplest mathematical form and compute some meaningful odds ratios.

(o) For the final model, validate the accuracy of the model in the test sample or by bootstrapping or cross-validating on the entire sample, repeating as many of the intermediate steps as possible. For bootstrapping or cross-validation, summarize the variability of the variable selection process. For data-splitting, you can predict the probability of response for each subject in the test sample and divide the predictions into $0 - .1, .1 - .2, \ldots, .9 - 1.0$ and then compute the proportion of responses in each interval.

Chapter 13

Ordinal Logistic Regression

13.1 Background

Many medical and epidemiologic studies incorporate an ordinal response variable. In some cases an ordinal response Y represents levels of a standard measurement scale such as severity of pain (none, mild, moderate, severe). In other cases, ordinal responses are constructed by specifying a hierarchy of separate endpoints. For example, clinicians may specify an ordering of the severity of several component events and assign patients to the worst event present from among none, heart attack, disabling stroke, and death. Still another use of ordinal response methods is the application of rank-based methods to continuous responses so as to obtain robust inferences. For example, the proportional odds model described later allows for a continuous Y and is really a generalization of the Wilcoxon–Mann–Whitney rank test.

There are many variations of logistic models used for predicting an ordinal response variable Y. All of them have the advantage that they do not assume a spacing between levels of Y. In other words, the same regression coefficients and P-values result from an analysis of a response variable having levels $0, 1, 2$ when the levels are recoded $0, 1, 20$. Thus ordinal models use only the rank-ordering of values of Y.

In this chapter we consider two of the most popular ordinal logistic models, the proportional odds (PO) form of an ordinal logistic model[440] and the forward continuation ratio (CR) ordinal logistic model.[135]

13.2   Ordinality Assumption

A basic assumption of all commonly used ordinal regression models is that the response variable behaves in an ordinal fashion with respect to each predictor. Assuming that a predictor X is linearly related to the log odds of some appropriate event, a simple way to check for ordinality is to plot the mean of X stratified by levels of Y. These means should be in a consistent order. If for many of the Xs, two adjacent categories of Y do not distinguish the means, that is evidence that those levels of Y should be pooled.

One can also estimate the mean or expected value of $X|Y = j$ $(E(X|Y = j))$ given that the ordinal model assumptions hold. This is a useful tool for checking those assumptions, at least in an unadjusted fashion. For simplicity, assume that X is discrete, and let $P_{jx} = \Pr(Y = j|X = x)$ be the probability that $Y = j$ given $X = x$ that is dictated from the model being fitted, with X being the only predictor in the model. Then

$$
\begin{aligned}
\Pr(X = x|Y = j) &= \Pr(Y = j|X = x)\Pr(X = x)/\Pr(Y = j) \\
E(X|Y = j) &= \sum_{x} x P_{jx}\Pr(X = x)/\Pr(Y = j),
\end{aligned}
\tag{13.1}
$$

and the expectation can be estimated by

$$
\hat{E}(X|Y = j) = \sum_{x} x \hat{P}_{jx} f_x/g_j,
\tag{13.2}
$$

where $\hat{P}_{jx}$ denotes the estimate of P_{jx} from the fitted one-predictor model (for inner values of Y in the PO models, these probabilities are differences between terms given by Equation 13.4 below), f_x is the frequency of $X = x$ in the sample of size n, and g_j is the frequency of $Y = j$ in the sample. This estimate can be computed conveniently without grouping the data by X. For n subjects let the n values of X be $x_1, x_2, \ldots, x_n$. Then

$$
\hat{E}(X|Y = j) = \sum_{i=1}^{n} x_i \hat{P}_{jx_i}/g_j.
\tag{13.3}
$$

Note that if one were to compute differences between conditional means of X and the conditional means of X given PO, and if furthermore the means were conditioned on $Y \geq j$ instead of $Y = j$, the result would be proportional to means of score residuals defined later in Equation 13.6.

13.3   Proportional Odds Model

13.3.1   Model

The most commonly used ordinal logistic model was described in Walker and Duncan[440] and later called the *proportional odds (PO) model* by McCullagh.[309] The PO model is best stated as follows, for a response variable having levels $0, 1, 2, \ldots, k$:

$$\Pr[Y \geq j | X] = \frac{1}{1 + \exp[-(\alpha_j + X\beta)]}, \qquad (13.4)$$

where $j = 1, 2, \ldots, k$. Some authors write the model in terms of $Y \leq j$. Our formulation makes the model coefficients consistent with the binary logistic model. There are k intercepts (αs). For fixed j, the model is an ordinary logistic model for the event $Y \geq j$. By using a common vector of regression coefficients β connecting probabilities for varying j, the PO model allows for parsimonious modeling of the distribution of Y.

There is a nice connection between the PO model and the Wilcoxon–Mann–Whitney two-sample test: when there is a single predictor X_1 that is binary, the numerator of the score test for testing $H_0 : \beta_1 = 0$ is proportional to the two-sample test statistic [452, pp. 2258-2259].

13.3.2   Assumptions and Interpretation of Parameters

There is an implicit assumption in the PO model that the regression coefficients (β) are independent of j, the cutoff level for Y. One could say that there is no $X \times Y$ interaction if PO holds. For a specific Y-cutoff j, the model has the same assumptions as the binary logistic model (Section 10.1.1). That is, the model in its simplest form assumes the log odds that $Y \geq j$ is linearly related to each X and that there is no interaction between the Xs.

In designing clinical studies, one sometimes hears the statement that an ordinal outcome should be avoided since statistical tests of patterns of those outcomes are hard to interpret. In fact, one interprets effects in the PO model using ordinary odds ratios. The difference is that a single odds ratio is assumed to apply equally to *all* events $Y \geq j, j = 1, 2, \ldots, k$. If linearity and additivity hold, the $X_m + 1 : X_m$ odds ratio for $Y \geq j$ is $\exp(\beta_m)$, whatever the cutoff j.

Sometimes it helps in interpreting the model to estimate the mean Y as a function of one or more predictors, even though this assumes a spacing for the Y-levels.

13.3.3   Estimation

The PO model is fitted using MLE on a somewhat complex likelihood function that is dependent on differences in logistic model probabilities. The estimation process forces the αs to be in descending order.

13.3.4   Residuals

Schoenfeld residuals[377] are very effective[157] in checking the proportional hazards assumption in the Cox[92] survival model. For the PO model one could analogously compute each subject's contribution to the first derivative of the log likelihood function with respect to β_m, average them separately by levels of Y, and examine trends in the residual plots as in Section 19.5.2. A few examples have shown that such plots are usually hard to interpret. Easily interpreted score residual plots for the PO model can be constructed, however, by using the fitted PO model to predict a series of binary events $Y \geq j, j = 1, 2, \ldots, k$, using the corresponding predicted probabilities

$$\hat{P}_{ij} = \frac{1}{1 + \exp[-(\hat{\alpha}_j + X_i\hat{\beta})]}, \tag{13.5}$$

where X_i stands for a vector of predictors for subject i. Then, after forming an indicator variable for the event currently being predicted ($[Y_i \geq j]$), one computes the score (first derivative) components U_{im} from an ordinary binary logistic model:

$$U_{im} = X_{im}([Y_i \geq j] - \hat{P}_{ij}), \tag{13.6}$$

for the subject i and predictor m. Then, for each column of U, plot the mean $\bar{U}_{\cdot m}$ and confidence limits, with Y (i.e., j) on the x-axis. For each predictor the trend against j should be flat if PO holds. [a] In binary logistic regression, *partial residuals* are very useful as they allow the analyst to fit linear effects for all the predictors but then to nonparametrically estimate the true transformation that each predictor requires (Section 10.4). The partial residual is defined as follows, for the ith subject and mth predictor variable.[79, 256]

$$r_{im} = \hat{\beta}_m X_{im} + \frac{Y_i - \hat{P}_i}{\hat{P}_i(1 - \hat{P}_i)}, \tag{13.7}$$

where

$$\hat{P}_i = \frac{1}{1 + \exp[-(\alpha + X_i\hat{\beta})]}. \tag{13.8}$$

A smoothed plot (e.g., using the moving linear regression algorithm in loess[76]) of X_{im} against r_{im} provides a nonparametric estimate of how X_m relates to the log

---

[a]If $\hat{\beta}$ were derived from separate binary fits, all $\bar{U}_{\cdot m} \equiv 0$.

relative odds that $Y = 1|X_m$. For ordinal Y, we just need to compute binary model partial residuals for all cutoffs j:

$$r_{im} = \hat{\beta}_m X_{im} + \frac{[Y_i \geq j] - \hat{P}_{ij}}{\hat{P}_{ij}(1 - \hat{P}_{ij})}, \tag{13.9}$$

then to make a plot for each m showing smoothed partial residual curves for all j, looking for similar shapes and slopes for a given predictor for all j. Each curve provides an estimate of how X_m relates to the relative log odds that $Y \geq j$. Since partial residuals allow examination of predictor transformations (linearity) while simultaneously allowing examination of PO (parallelism), partial residual plots are generally preferred over score residual plots for ordinal models.

13.3.5 Assessment of Model Fit

Peterson and Harrell[335] developed score and likelihood ratio tests for testing the PO assumption. The score test is used in the SAS LOGISTIC procedure,[363] but its extreme anticonservatism in many cases can make it unreliable.[335]

[3]

For determining whether the PO assumption is likely to be satisfied for each predictor separately, there are several graphics that are useful. One is the graph comparing means of $X|Y$ with and without assuming PO, as described in Section 13.2 (see Figure 14.2 for an example). Another is the simple method of stratifying on each predictor and computing the logits of all proportions of the form $Y \geq j, j = 1, 2, \ldots, k$. When proportional odds holds, the differences in logits between different values of j should be the same at all levels of X, because the model dictates that $\text{logit}(Y \geq j|X) - \text{logit}(Y \geq i|X) = \alpha_j - \alpha_i$, for any constant X. An example of this is in Figure 13.1.

Chapter 14 has many examples of graphics for assessing fit of PO models. Regarding assessment of linearity and additivity assumptions, splines, partial residual plots, and interaction tests are among the best tools.

13.3.6 Quantifying Predictive Ability

The R_N^2 coefficient is really computed from the model LR χ^2 (χ^2 added to a model containing only the k intercept parameters) to describe the model's predictive power. The Somers' D_{xy} rank correlation between $X\hat{\beta}$ and Y is an easily interpreted measure of predictive discrimination. Since it is a rank measure, it does not matter which intercept α is used in the calculation. The probability of concordance, c, is also a useful measure. Here one takes all possible pairs of subjects having differing Y values and computes the fraction of such pairs for which the values of $X\hat{\beta}$ are in the same direction as the two Y values. c could be called a generalized ROC area in this setting. As before, $D_{xy} = 2(c - 0.5)$. Note that D_{xy},

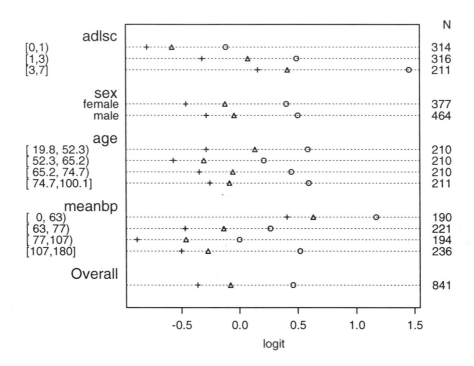

FIGURE 13.1: Checking PO assumption separately for a series of predictors. The cir-
cle, triangle, and plus sign correspond to $Y \geq 1, 2, 3$, respectively. PO is checked by
examining the vertical constancy of distances between any two of these three symbols.
Response variable is the severe functional disability scale sfdm2 from the 1000-patient
SUPPORT dataset, with the last two categories combined because of low frequency of
coma/intubation.

c, and the Brier score B can easily be computed for various dichotomizations of Y, to investigate predictive ability in more detail.

13.3.7 Validating the Fitted Model

The PO model is validated much the same way as the binary logistic model (see Section 10.9). For estimating an overfitting-corrected calibration curve (Section 10.11) one estimates $\Pr(Y \geq j | X)$ using one j at a time.

13.3.8 S-PLUS Functions

The Design library's lrm function fits the PO model directly, assuming that the levels of the response variable (e.g., the levels of a factor variable) are listed in the proper order. If the response is numeric, lrm assumes the numeric codes properly order the responses. If it is a character vector and is not a factor, lrm assumes the correct ordering is alphabetic. Of course ordered variables in S-PLUS are appropriate response variables for ordinal regression.

The S-PLUS functions popower and posamsize (in the Hmisc library) compute power and sample size estimates for ordinal responses using the proportional odds model.

The function plot.xmean.ordinaly in Design computes and graphs the quantities described in Section 13.2. It plots simple Y-stratified means overlaid with $\hat{E}(X|Y = j)$, with j on the x-axis. The $\hat{E}$s are computed for both PO and continuation ratio ordinal logistic models.

The Hmisc library's summary.formula function is also useful for assessing the PO assumption. Figure 13.1 was produced using the following code.

```
attach(support)
sfdm ← as.integer(sfdm2) - 1
sf ← function(y)
  c('Y>=1'=qlogis(mean(y >= 1)), 'Y>=2'=qlogis(mean(y >= 2)),
    'Y>=3'=qlogis(mean(y >= 3)))
s ← summary(sfdm ~ adlsc + sex + age + meanbp, fun=sf)
plot(s, which=1:3, pch=1:3, xlab='logit', vnames='names',
    main='', width.factor=1.5)
```

Generic Design functions such as validate, calibrate, and nomogram work with PO model fits from lrm as long as the analyst specifies which intercept(s) to use.

13.4   Continuation Ratio Model

13.4.1   Model

Unlike the PO model, which is based on *cumulative* probabilities, the continuation ratio (CR) model is based on *conditional* probabilities. The (forward) CR model[24, 36, 135] is stated as follows for $Y = 0, \ldots, k$.

$$
\begin{aligned}
\Pr(Y = j | Y \geq j, X) &= \frac{1}{1 + \exp[-(\theta_j + X\gamma)]} \\
\mathrm{logit}(Y = 0 | Y \geq 0, X) &= \mathrm{logit}(Y = 0 | X) \\
&= \theta_0 + X\gamma \qquad (13.10) \\
\mathrm{logit}(Y = 1 | Y \geq 1, X) &= \theta_1 + X\gamma \\
&\cdots \\
\mathrm{logit}(Y = k - 1 | Y \geq k - 1, X) &= \theta_{k-1} + X\gamma.
\end{aligned}
$$

The CR model has been said to be likely to fit ordinal responses when subjects have to "pass through" one category to get to the next. The CR model is a discrete version of the Cox proportional hazards model. The discrete hazard function is defined as $\Pr(Y = j | Y \geq j)$.

13.4.2   Assumptions and Interpretation of Parameters

The CR model assumes that the vector of regression coefficients, γ, is the same regardless of which conditional probability is being computed.

One could say that there is no $X \times$ condition interaction if the CR model holds. For a specific condition $Y \geq j$, the model has the same assumptions as the binary logistic model (Section 10.1.1). That is, the model in its simplest form assumes that the log odds that $Y = j$ conditional on $Y \geq j$ is linearly related to each X and that there is no interaction between the Xs.

A single odds ratio is assumed to apply equally to *all* conditions $Y \geq j, j = 0, 1, 2, \ldots, k - 1$. If linearity and additivity hold, the $X_m + 1 : X_m$ odds ratio for $Y = j$ is $\exp(\beta_m)$, whatever the conditioning event $Y \geq j$.

To compute $\Pr(Y > 0 | X)$ from the CR model, one only needs to take one minus $\Pr(Y = 0 | X)$. To compute other unconditional probabilities from the CR model, one must multiply the conditional probabilities. For example, $\Pr(Y > 1 | X) = \Pr(Y > 1 | X, Y \geq 1) \times \Pr(Y \geq 1 | X) = [1 - \Pr(Y = 1 | Y \geq 1, X)][1 - \Pr(Y = 0 | X)] = [1 - 1/(1 + \exp[-(\theta_1 + X\gamma)])][1 - 1/(1 + \exp[-(\theta_0 + X\gamma)])]$.

13.4.3 Estimation

Armstrong and Sloan[24] and Berridge and Whitehead[36] showed how the CR model can be fitted using an ordinary binary logistic model likelihood function, after certain rows of the X matrix are duplicated and a new binary Y vector is constructed. For each subject, one constructs separate records by considering successive conditions $Y \geq 0, Y \geq 1, \ldots, Y \geq k - 1$ for a response variable with values $0, 1, \ldots, k$. The binary response for each applicable condition or "cohort" is set to 1 if the subject failed at the current "cohort" or "risk set," that is, if $Y = j$ where the cohort being considered is $Y \geq j$. The constructed cohort variable is carried along with the new X and Y. This variable is considered to be categorical and its coefficients are fitted by adding $k - 1$ dummy variables to the binary logistic model. For ease of computation, the CR model is restated as follows, with the first cohort used as the reference cell.

$$\Pr(Y = j | Y \geq j, X) = \frac{1}{1 + \exp[-(\alpha + \theta_j + X\gamma)]}. \qquad (13.11)$$

Here α is an overall intercept, $\theta_0 \equiv 0$, and $\theta_1, \ldots, \theta_{k-1}$ are increments from α.

13.4.4 Residuals

To check CR model assumptions, binary logistic model partial residuals are again valuable. We separately fit a sequence of binary logistic models using a series of binary events and the corresponding applicable (increasingly small) subsets of subjects, and plot smoothed partial residuals against X for all of the binary events. Parallelism in these plots indicates that the CR model's constant γ assumptions are satisfied.

13.4.5 Assessment of Model Fit

The partial residual plots just described are very useful for checking the constant slope assumption of the CR model. The next section shows how to test this assumption formally. Linearity can be assessed visually using the smoothed partial residual plot, and interactions between predictors can be tested as usual.

13.4.6 Extended CR Model

The PO model has been extended by Peterson and Harrell[335] to allow for unequal slopes for some or all of the Xs for some or all levels of Y. This partial PO model requires specialized software, and with the demise of SAS Version 5 PROC LOGIST, software is not currently available. The CR model can be extended similarly. In S-PLUS notation, the ordinary CR model is specified as

```
y ~ cohort + X1 + X2 + X3 + ... ,
```

with `cohort` denoting a polytomous variable. The CR model can be extended to allow for some or all of the βs to change with the cohort or Y-cutoff.[24] Suppose that nonconstant slope is allowed for `X1` and `X2`. The S-PLUS notation for the extended model would be

```
y ~ cohort*(X1 + X2) + X3
```

The extended CR model is a discrete version of the Cox survival model with time-dependent covariables.

There is nothing about the CR model that makes it fit a given dataset better than other ordinal models such as the PO model. The real benefit of the CR model is that using standard binary logistic model software one can flexibly specify how the equal-slopes assumption can be relaxed.

13.4.7 Role of Penalization in Extended CR Model

As demonstrated in the upcoming case study, penalized MLE is invaluable in allowing the model to be extended into an unequal-slopes model insofar as the information content in the data will support. Faraway[134] has demonstrated how all data-driven steps of the modeling process increase the real variance in "final" parameter estimates, when one estimates variances without assuming that the final model was prespecified. For ordinal regression modeling, the most important modeling steps are (1) choice of predictor variables, (2) selecting or modeling predictor transformations, and (3) allowance for unequal slopes across Y-cutoffs (i.e., non-PO or non-CR). Regarding Steps (2) and (3) one is tempted to rely on graphical methods such as residual plots to make detours in the strategy, but it is very difficult to estimate variances or to properly penalize assessments of predictive accuracy for subjective modeling decisions. Regarding (1), shrinkage has been proven to work better than stepwise variable selection when one is attempting to build a main-effects model. Choosing a shrinkage factor is a well-defined, smooth, and often a unique process as opposed to binary decisions on whether variables are "in" or "out" of the model. Likewise, instead of using arbitrary subjective (residual plots) or objective (χ^2 due to `cohort` × covariable interactions, i.e., nonconstant covariable effects), shrinkage can systematically allow model enhancements insofar as the information content in the data will support, through the use of differential penalization. Shrinkage is a solution to the dilemma faced when the analyst attempts to choose between a parsimonious model and a more complex one that fits the data. Penalization does not require the analyst to make a binary decision, and it is a process that can be validated using the bootstrap.

13.4.8   Validating the Fitted Model

Validation of statistical indexes such as D_{xy} and model calibration is done using techniques discussed previously, except that certain problems must be addressed. First, when using the bootstrap, the resampling must take into account the existence of multiple records per subject that were created to use the binary logistic likelihood trick. That is, sampling should be done with replacement from *subjects* rather than *records*. Second, the analyst must isolate which event to predict. This is because when observations are expanded in order to use a binary logistic likelihood function to fit the CR model, several different events are being predicted simultaneously. Somers' D_{xy} could be computed by relating $X\hat{\gamma}$ (ignoring intercepts) to the ordinal Y, but other indexes are not defined so easily. The simplest approach here would be to validate a single prediction for $\Pr(Y = j | Y \geq j, X)$, for example. The simplest event to predict is $\Pr(Y = 0 | X)$, as this would just require subsetting on all observations in the first cohort level in the validation sample. It would also be easy to validate any one of the later conditional probabilities. The validation functions described in the next section allow for such subsetting, as well as handling the cluster sampling. Specialized calculations would be needed to validate an unconditional probability such as $\Pr(Y \geq 2 | X)$.

13.4.9   S-Plus Functions

The `cr.setup` function in `Design` returns a list of vectors useful in constructing a dataset used to trick a binary logistic function such as `lrm` into fitting CR models. The `subs` vector in this list contains observation numbers in the original data, some of which are repeated. Here is an example.

```
u ← cr.setup(Y)              # Y is original ordinal response vector
attach(mydata[u$subs,])      # mydata is the original dataset
                             # mydata[i,] subscripts the input data,
                             # using duplicate values of i for repeats
y       ← u$y                # constructed binary responses
cohort  ← u$cohort           # cohort or risk set categories

f ← lrm(y ~ cohort*age + sex)
```

Since the `lrm` and `pentrace` functions have the capability to penalize different parts of the model by different amounts, they are valuable for fitting extended CR models in which the `cohort` × predictor interactions are allowed to be only as important as the information content in the data will support. Simple main effects can be unpenalized or slightly penalized as desired.

The `validate` and `calibrate` functions for `lrm` allow specification of subject identifiers when using the bootstrap, so the samples can be constructed with replacement from the original subjects. In other words, cluster sampling is done from the expanded records. This is handled internally by the `predab.resample` function. These functions also allow one to specify a subset of the records to use in the validation, which makes it especially easy to validate the part of the model used to predict $\Pr(Y = 0|X)$.

The `plot.xmean.ordinaly` function is useful for checking the CR assumption for single predictors, as described earlier.

13.5   Further Reading

[1]   See [5, 18, 19, 24, 25, 36, 44, 45, 78, 88, 164, 168, 192, 242, 309, 335, 380, 452, 459] for some excellent background references, applications, and extensions to the ordinal models.

[2]   Anderson and Philips [19, p. 29] proposed methods for constructing properly spaced response values given a fitted PO model.

[3]   The simplest demonstration of this is to consider a model in which there is a single predictor that is totally independent of a nine-level response Y, so PO *must* hold. A PO model is fitted in SAS using:

```
DATA test;
DO i=1 to 50;
y=FLOOR(RANUNI(151)*9);
x=RANNOR(5);
OUTPUT;
END;
PROC LOGISTIC; MODEL y=x;
```

The score test for PO was $\chi^2 = 56$ on 7 d.f., $P < 0.0001$. This problem results from some small cell sizes in the distribution of Y.[335] The P-value for testing the regression effect for X was 0.76.

13.6   Problems

Test for the association between disease group and total hospital cost in SUPPORT, without imputing any missing costs (exclude the one patient having zero cost).

1. Use the Kruskal–Wallis rank test.

2. Use the proportional odds ordinal logistic model generalization of the Wilcoxon–Mann–Whitney Kruskal–Wallis Spearman test. Group total cost into 20 quantile groups so that only 19 intercepts will need to be in the model, not one less than the number of subjects (this would have taken the program too long to fit the model). Use the likelihood ratio χ^2 for this and later steps.

3. Use a binary logistic model to test for association between disease group and whether total cost exceeds the median of total cost. In other words, group total

cost into two quantile groups and use this binary variable as the response. What is wrong with this approach?

4. Instead of using only two cost groups, group cost into 3, 4, 5, 6, 8, 10, and 12 quantile groups. Describe the relationship between the number of intervals used to approximate the continuous response variable and the efficiency of the analysis. How many intervals of total cost, assuming that the ordering of the different intervals is used in the analysis, are required to avoid losing significant information in this continuous variable?

5. If you were selecting one of the rank-based tests for testing the association between disease and cost, which of any of the tests considered would you choose?

6. Why do all of the tests you did have the same number of degrees of freedom for the hypothesis of no association between dzgroup and totcst?

7. What is the advantage of a rank-based test over a parametric test based on log(cost)?

Chapter 14

Case Study in Ordinal Regression, Data Reduction, and Penalization

This case study is taken from Harrell et al.[199] which described a World Health Organization study[303] in which vital signs and a large number of clinical signs and symptoms were used to develop a predictive model for an ordinal response. This response consists of laboratory assessments of diagnosis and severity of illness related to pneumonia, meningitis, and sepsis. Much of the modeling strategy given in Chapter 4 was used to develop the model, with additional emphasis on penalized maximum likelihood estimation (Section 9.10). The following laboratory data are used in the response: cerebrospinal fluid (CSF) culture from a lumbar puncture (LP), blood culture (BC), arterial oxygen saturation (SaO_2, a measure of lung dysfunction), and chest X-ray (CXR). The sample consisted of 4552 infants aged 90 days or less.

This case study covers these topics:

1. definition of the ordinal response (Section 14.1);

2. scoring and clustering of clinical signs (Section 14.2);

3. testing adequacy of weights specified by subject-matter specialists and assessing the utility of various scoring schemes using a tentative ordinal logistic model (Section 14.3);

4. assessing the basic ordinality assumptions and examining the PO and CR assumptions separately for each predictor (Section 14.4);

5. deriving a tentative PO model using cluster scores and regression splines (Section 14.5);

6. using residual plots to check PO, CR, and linearity assumptions (Section 14.6);

7. examining the fit of a CR model (Section 14.7);

8. utilizing an extended CR model to allow some or all of the regression coefficients to vary with cutoffs of the response level as well as to provide formal tests of constant slopes (Section 14.8);

9. using penalized maximum likelihood estimation to improve accuracy (Section 14.9);

10. approximating the full model by a submodel and drawing a nomogram on the basis of the submodel (Section 14.10); and

11. validating the ordinal model using the bootstrap (Section 14.11).

14.1   Response Variable

To be a candidate for BC and CXR, an infant had to have a clinical indication for one of the three diseases, according to prespecified criteria in the study protocol ($n = 2398$). Blood work-up (but not necessarily LP) and CXR was also done on a random sample intended to be 10% of infants having no signs or symptoms suggestive of infection ($n = 175$). Infants with signs suggestive of meningitis had LP done. All 4552 infants received a full physical exam and standardized pulse oximetry to measure SaO_2. The vast majority of infants getting CXR had the X-rays interpreted by three independent radiologists.

The analyses that follow are not corrected for verification bias[465] with respect to BC, LP, and CXR, but Section 14.1 has some data describing the extent of the problem.

Patients were assigned to the worst qualifying outcome category. Table 14.1 shows the definition of the ordinal outcome variable Y and shows the distribution of Y by the lab work-up strategy.

The effect of verification bias is a false negative fraction of 0.03 for $Y = 2$, from comparing the detection fraction of zero for $Y = 2$ in the "Not Indicated" group with the observed positive fraction of 0.03 in the random sample that was fully worked up. The extent of verification bias in $Y = 1$ is $0.05 - 0.04 = 0.01$. These biases are ignored in this analysis.

TABLE 14.1: Ordinal Outcome Scale

Outcome Level Y	Definition	n	Fraction in Outcome Level		
			BC, CXR Indicated ($n = 2398$)	Not Indicated ($n = 1979$)	Random Sample ($n = 175$)
0	None of the below	3551	0.63	0.96	0.91
1	$90\% \leq SaO_2 < 95\%$ or CXR+	490	0.17	0.04^a	0.05
2	BC+ or CSF+ or $SaO_2 < 90\%$	511	0.21	0.00^b	0.03

$^a SaO_2$ was measured but CXR was not done

$^b Assumed$ zero since neither BC nor LP were done.

14.2   Variable Clustering

Forty-seven clinical signs were collected for each infant. Most questionnaire items were scored as a single variable using equally spaced codes, with 0 to 3 representing, for example, sign not present, mild, moderate, severe. The resulting list of clinical signs with their abbreviations is given in Table 14.2. The signs are organized into clusters as discussed later.

Here, **hx** stands for history, **ausc** for auscultation, and **hxprob** for history of problems. Two signs (**qcr, hcm**) were listed twice since they were later placed into two clusters each.

Next, hierarchical clustering was done using the matrix of squared Spearman rank correlation coefficients as the similarity matrix. The **varclus** S-PLUS function was used as follows.

```
> vclust ← varclus(∼ illd + hlt + slpm + slpl + wake + convul+ hfa +
+                  hfb + hfe  + hap + hcl  + hcm  + hcs  + hdi + fde +
+                  chi + twb  + ldy + apn  + lcw  + nfl  + str + gru +
+                  coh + ccy  + jau + omph + csd  + csa  + aro + qcr +
+                  con + att  + mvm + afe  + absu + stu  + deh + dcp +
+                  crs + abb  + abk + whz  + hdb  + smi2 + abd + conj +
+                  oto + puskin)
> plot(vclust)
```

The output appears in Figure 14.1. This output served as a starting point for clinicians to use in constructing more meaningful clinical clusters. The clusters in Table 14.2 were the consensus of the clinicians who were the investigators in the WHO study. Prior subject matter knowledge plays a key role at this stage in the analysis.

TABLE 14.2: Clinical Signs

Cluster Name	Sign Abbreviation	Name of Sign	Values
bul.conv	abb	bulging fontanele	0-1
	convul	hx convulsion	0-1
hydration	abk	sunken fontanele	0-1
	hdi	hx diarrhoea	0-1
	deh	dehydrated	0-2
	stu	skin turgor	0-2
	dcp	digital capilliary refill	0-2
drowsy	hcl	less activity	0-1
	qcr	quality of crying	0-2
	csd	drowsy state	0-2
	slpm	sleeping more	0-1
	wake	wakes less easily	0-1
	aro	arousal	0-2
	mvm	amount of movement	0-2
agitated	hcm	crying more	0-1
	slpl	sleeping less	0-1
	con	consolability	0-2
	csa	agitated state	0-1
crying	hcm	crying more	0-1
	hcs	crying less	0-1
	qcr	quality of crying	0-2
	smi2	smiling ability $\times$ age $>$ 42 days	0-2
reffort	nfl	nasal flaring	0-3
	lcw	lower chest in-drawing	0-3
	gru	grunting	0-2
	ccy	central cyanosis	0-1
stop.breath	hap	hx stop breathing	0-1
	apn	apnea	0-1
ausc	whz	wheezing	0-1
	coh	cough heard	0-1
	crs	crepitation	0-2
hxprob	hfb	fast breathing	0-1
	hdb	difficulty breathing	0-1
	hlt	mother report resp. problems	none, chest, other
feeding	hfa	hx abnormal feeding	0-3
	absu	sucking ability	0-2
	afe	drinking ability	0-2
labor	chi	previous child died	0-1
	fde	fever at delivery	0-1
	ldy	days in labor	1-9
	twb	water broke	0-1
abdominal	adb	abdominal distension	0-4
	jau	jaundice	0-1
	omph	omphalitis	0-1
fever.ill	illd	age-adjusted no. days ill	
	hfe	hx fever	0-1
pustular	conj	conjunctivitis	0-1
	oto	otoscopy impression	0-2
	puskin	pustular skin rash	0-1

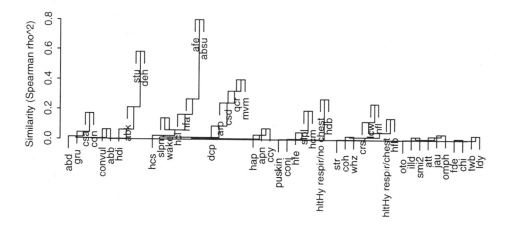

FIGURE 14.1: Hierarchical variable clustering using Spearman ρ^2 as a similarity measure for all pairs of variables. Note that since the `hlt` variable was nominal, it is represented by two dummy variables here.

14.3 Developing Cluster Summary Scores

The clusters listed in Table 14.2 were first scored by the first principal component of `transcan` transformed signs, denoted by PC_1. Knowing that the resulting weights may be too complex for clinical use, the primary reasons for analyzing the principal components were to see if some of the clusters could be removed from consideration so that the clinicians would not spend time developing scoring rules for them. Let us "peek" at Y to assist in scoring clusters at this point, but to do so in a very structured way that does not involve the examination of a large number of individual coefficients.

To judge any cluster scoring scheme, we must pick a tentative outcome model. For this purpose we chose the PO model. By using the 14 PC_1s corresponding to the 14 clusters, the fitted PO model had a likelihood ratio (LR) χ^2 of 1155 with 14 d.f., and the predictive discrimination of the clusters was quantified by a Somers' D_{xy} rank correlation between $X\hat{\beta}$ and Y of 0.596. The following clusters were not statistically important predictors and we assumed that the lack of importance of the PC_1s in predicting Y (adjusted for the other PC_1s) justified a conclusion that no sign within that cluster was clinically important in predicting Y: `hydration`, `hxprob`, `pustular`, `crying`, `fever.ill`, `stop.breath`, `labor`. This list was identified using a backward step-down procedure on the full model. The total Wald χ^2 for these seven PC_1s was 22.4 ($P = 0.002$). The reduced model had LR $\chi^2 = 1133$ with 7 d.f., $D_{xy} = 0.591$. The bootstrap validation in Section 14.11 is penalized for fitting the seven predictors.

TABLE 14.3: Clinician Combinations, Rankings, and Scorings of Signs

Cluster	Combined/Ranked Signs in Order of Severity	Weights
bul.conv	abb $\cup$ convul	0–1
drowsy	hcl, qcr>0, csd>0 $\cup$ slpm $\cup$ wake, aro>0, mvm>0	0–5
agitated	hcm, slpl, con=1, csa, con=2	0, 1, 2, 7, 8, 10
reffort	nfl>0, lcw>1, gru=1, gru=2, ccy	0–5
ausc	whz, coh, crs>0	0–3
feeding	hfa=1, hfa=2, hfa=3, absu=1 $\cup$ afe=1, absu=2 $\cup$ afe=2	0–5
abdominal	jau $\cup$ abd>0 $\cup$ omph	0–1

The clinicians were asked to rank the clinical severity of signs within each potentially important cluster. During this step, the clinicians also ranked severity levels of some of the component signs, and some cluster scores were simplified, especially when the signs within a cluster occurred infrequently. The clinicians also assessed whether the severity points or weights should be equally spaced, assigning unequally spaced weights for one cluster (agitated). The resulting rankings and sign combinations are shown in Table 14.3. The signs or sign combinations separated by a comma are treated as separate categories, whereas some signs were unioned ("or"–ed) when the clinicians deemed them equally important. As an example, if an additive cluster score was to be used for drowsy, the scorings would be 0 = none present, 1 = hcl, 2 = qcr>0, 3 = csd>0 or slpm or wake, 4 = aro>0, 5 = mvm>0 and the scores would be added.

This table reflects some data reduction already (unioning some signs and selection of levels of ordinal signs) but more reduction is needed. Even after signs are ranked within a cluster, there are various ways of assigning the cluster scores. We investigated six methods. We started with the purely statistical approach of using PC_1 to summarize each cluster. Second, all sign combinations within a cluster were unioned to represent a 0/1 cluster score. Third, only sign combinations thought by the clinicians to be severe were unioned, resulting in drowsy=aro>0 or mvm>0, agitated=csa or con=2, reffort=lcw>1 or gru>0 or ccy, ausc=crs>0, and feeding=absu>0 or afe>0. For clusters that are not scored 0/1 in Table 14.3, the fourth summarization method was a hierarchical one that used the weight of the worst applicable category as the cluster score. For example, if aro=1 but mvm=0, drowsy would be scored as 4. The fifth method counted the number of positive signs in the cluster. The sixth method summed the weights of all signs or sign combinations present. Finally, the worst sign combination present was again used as in the second method, but the points assigned to the category were data-driven ones obtained by using extra dummy variables. This provided an assessment of the adequacy of the clinician-specified weights. By comparing rows 4 and 7 in Table 14.4 we see that response data-driven sign weights have a slightly worse AIC, indicating that the number of extra β parameters estimated was not justified by the improvement in χ^2. The hierarchical method, using the clinicians' weights, performed quite well. The only cluster with inadequate clinician weights was ausc—see below. The PC_1 method, without any

TABLE 14.4: Predictive Information of Various Cluster Scoring Strategies

Scoring Method	LR χ^2	d.f.	AIC
PC_1 of each cluster	1133	7	1119
Union of all signs	1045	7	1031
Union of higher categories	1123	7	1109
Hierarchical (worst sign)	1194	7	1180
Additive, equal weights	1155	7	1141
Additive using clinician weights	1183	7	1169
Hierarchical, data-driven weights	1227	25	1177

guidance, performed well, as in [184]. The only reasons not to use it are that it requires a coefficient for every sign in the cluster and the coefficients are not translatable into simple scores such as $0, 1, \ldots$.

Representation of clusters by a simple union of selected signs or of all signs is inadequate, but otherwise the choice of methods is not very important in terms of explaining variation in Y. We chose the fourth method, a hierarchical severity point assignment (using weights that were prespecified by the clinicians), for its ease of use and of handling missing component variables (in most cases) and potential for speeding up the clinical exam (examining to detect more important signs first). Because of what was learned regarding the relationship between ausc and Y, we modified the ausc cluster score by redefining it as ausc=crs>0 (crepitations present). Note that neither the "tweaking" of ausc nor the examination of the seven scoring methods displayed in Table 14.4 are taken into account in the model validation.

14.4 Assessing Ordinality of Y for each X, and Unadjusted Checking of PO and CR Assumptions

Section 13.2 described a graphical method for assessing the ordinality assumption for Y separately with respect to each X, and for assessing PO and CR assumptions individually. Figure 14.2 is an example of such displays. For this dataset we expect strongly nonlinear effects for temp, rr, and hrat, so for those predictors we plot the mean absolute differences from suitable "normal" values as an approximate solution.

```
> par(mfrow=c(3,4))     # 3 x 4 matrix of plots
> plot.xmean.ordinaly(Y ~ age + abs(temp-37) + abs(rr-60) +
+                     abs(hrat-125) + waz + bul.conv +
+                     drowsy + agitated + reffort +
+                     ausc + feeding + abdominal, cr=T)
```

The plot is shown in Figure 14.2. Y does not seem to operate in an ordinal fashion with respect to age, $|rr-60|$, or ausc. For the other variables, ordinality holds, and

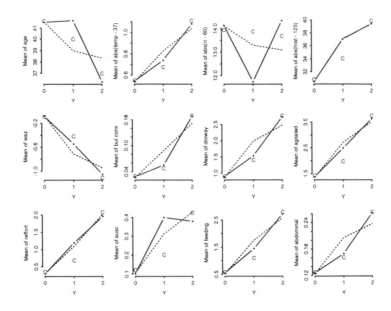

FIGURE 14.2: Examination of the ordinality of Y for each predictor by assessing how varying Y relate to the mean X, and whether the trend is monotonic. Solid lines connect the simple stratified means, and dashed lines connect the estimated expected value of $X|Y = j$ given that PO holds. Estimated expected values from the CR model are marked with Cs.

PO holds reasonably well for the other variables. For heart rate, the PO assumption appears to be satisfied perfectly. CR model assumptions appear to be more tenuous than PO assumptions, when one variable at a time is fitted.

14.5   A Tentative Full Proportional Odds Model

Based on what was determined in Section 14.3, the original list of 47 signs was reduced to seven predictors: two unions of signs (bul.conv, abdominal), one single sign (ausc), and four "worst category" point assignments (drowsy, agitated, reffort, feeding). Seven clusters were dropped for the time being because of weak associations with Y. Such a limited use of variable selection gets around the severe problems inherent with that technique.

At this point in model development add to the model age and vital signs: temp (temperature), rr (respiratory rate), hrat (heart rate), and waz, weight-for-age Z-score. Since age was expected to modify the interpretation of temp, rr, and hrat, and interactions between continuous variables would be difficult to use in the field, we categorized `age` into three intervals: 0–6 days ($n = 302$), 7–59 days ($n = 3042$), and 60–90 days ($n = 1208$).[a]

```
> ageg ← cut2(age, c(7,60))
```

The new variables `temp`, `rr`, `hrat`, `waz` were missing in, respectively, $n = 13, 11$, 147, and 20 infants. Since the three vital sign variables are somewhat correlated with each other, customized imputation models were developed to impute all the missing values without assuming linearity or even monotonicity of any of the regressions.

```
> vsign.trans ← transcan(∼ temp + hrat + rr, imputed=T)
> temp ← impute(vsign.trans, temp)
> hrat ← impute(vsign.trans, hrat)
> rr   ← impute(vsign.trans, rr)
```

After `transcan` estimated optimal restricted cubic spline transformations, `temp` could be predicted with adjusted $R^2 = 0.17$ from `hrat` and `rr`, `hrat` could be predicted with adjusted $R^2 = 0.14$ from `temp` and `rr`, and `rr` could be predicted with adjusted R^2 of only 0.06. The first two R^2, while not large, mean that customized imputations are more efficient than imputing with constants. Imputations on `rr` were closer to the median `rr` of 48/minute as compared with the other two vital signs whose imputations have more variation. In a similar manner, `waz` was imputed using `age`, birth weight, head circumference, body length, and prematurity (adjusted R^2 for predicting `waz` from the others was 0.74).

The continuous predictors `temp`, `hrat`, `rr` were not assumed to linearly relate to the log odds that $Y \geq j$. Restricted cubic spline functions with five knots for `temp`,`rr` and four knots for `hrat`,`waz` were used to model the effects of these variables:

```
> f1 ← lrm(Y ∼ ageg*(rcs(temp,5)+rcs(rr,5)+rcs(hrat,4)) +
+            rcs(waz,4) + bul.conv + drowsy + agitated +
+            reffort + ausc + feeding + abdominal,
+            x=T, y-T)   # x−T, y=T used by resid() below
```

This model has LR χ^2 of 1393 with 45 d.f. and $D_{xy} = 0.653$. Wald tests of nonlinearity and interaction are obtained using the statement `latex(anova(f1))`, whose output is shown in Table 14.5.

The bottom four lines of the table are the most important. First, there is strong evidence that some associations with Y exist (45 d.f. test) and very strong evidence of nonlinearity in one of the vital signs or in `waz` (26 d.f. test). There is moderately strong evidence for an interaction effect somewhere in the model (22 d.f. test). We see that the grouped age variable `ageg` is predictive of Y, but mainly as an effect modifier for `rr`, and `hrat`. `temp` is extremely nonlinear, and `rr` is moderately so. `hrat`, a difficult variable to measure reliably in young infants, is perhaps not important enough ($\chi^2 = 19.0, 9$ d.f.) to keep in the final model.

---

[a]These age intervals were also found to adequately capture most of the interaction effects.

TABLE 14.5: Wald Statistics for Y in the Proportional Odds Model

	χ^2	d.f.	P
ageg (Factor+Higher Order Factors)	41.49	24	0.0147
All Interactions	40.48	22	0.0095
temp (Factor+Higher Order Factors)	37.08	12	0.0002
All Interactions	6.77	8	0.5617
Nonlinear (Factor+Higher Order Factors)	31.08	9	0.0003
rr (Factor+Higher Order Factors)	81.16	12	< 0.0001
All Interactions	27.37	8	0.0006
Nonlinear (Factor+Higher Order Factors)	27.36	9	0.0012
hrat (Factor+Higher Order Factors)	19.00	9	0.0252
All Interactions	8.83	6	0.1836
Nonlinear (Factor+Higher Order Factors)	7.35	6	0.2901
waz	35.82	3	< 0.0001
Nonlinear	13.21	2	0.0014
bul.conv	12.16	1	0.0005
drowsy	17.79	1	< 0.0001
agitated	8.25	1	0.0041
reffort	63.39	1	< 0.0001
ausc	105.82	1	< 0.0001
feeding	30.38	1	< 0.0001
abdominal	0.74	1	0.3895
ageg × temp (Factor+Higher Order Factors)	6.77	8	0.5617
Nonlinear	6.40	6	0.3801
Nonlinear Interaction : f(A,B) vs. AB	6.40	6	0.3801
ageg × rr (Factor+Higher Order Factors)	27.37	8	0.0006
Nonlinear	14.85	6	0.0214
Nonlinear Interaction : f(A,B) vs. AB	14.85	6	0.0214
ageg × hrat (Factor+Higher Order Factors)	8.83	6	0.1836
Nonlinear	2.42	4	0.6587
Nonlinear Interaction : f(A,B) vs. AB	2.42	4	0.6587
TOTAL NONLINEAR	78.20	26	< 0.0001
TOTAL INTERACTION	40.48	22	0.0095
TOTAL NONLINEAR + INTERACTION	96.31	32	< 0.0001
TOTAL	1073.78	45	< 0.0001

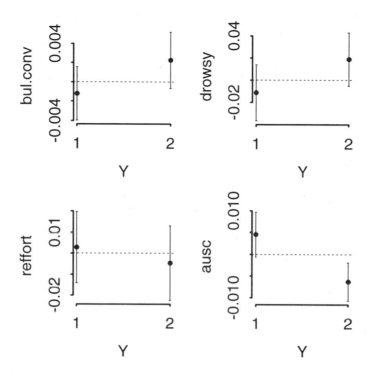

FIGURE 14.3: Binary logistic model score residuals for binary events derived from two cutoffs of the ordinal response Y. Note that the mean residuals, marked with closed circles, correspond closely to differences between solid and dashed lines at $Y = 1, 2$ in Figure 14.2. Score residual assessments for spline-expanded variables such as rr would have required one plot per d.f.

14.6   Residual Plots

Section 13.3.4 defined binary logistic score residuals for isolating the PO assumption in an ordinal model. For the tentative PO model, score residuals for four of the variables were plotted using

```
> par(mfrow=c(2,2) )
> resid(f1, 'score.binary', pl=T, which=c(17,18,20,21) )
```

The result is shown in Figure 14.3. We see strong evidence of non-PO for ausc and moderate evidence for drowsy and bul.conv, in agreement with Figure 14.2.

Partial residuals computed separately for each Y-cutoff (Section 13.3.4) are the most useful residuals for ordinal models as they simultaneously check linearity, find needed transformations, and check PO. In Figure 14.4, smoothed partial residual plots were obtained for all predictors, after first fitting a simple model in which every

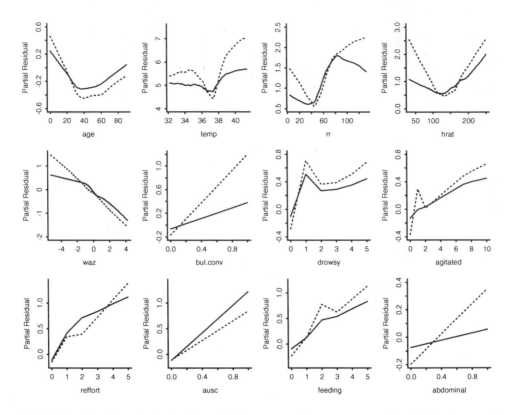

FIGURE 14.4: Smoothed partial residuals corresponding to two cutoffs of Y, from a model in which all predictors were assumed to operate linearly and additively. The smoothed curves estimate the actual predictor transformations needed. Solid lines denote $Y \geq 1$ while dashed lines denote $Y \geq 2$.

predictor was assumed to operate linearly. Interactions were temporarily ignored and age was used as a continuous variable.

```
> f2 ← lrm(Y ~ age + temp + rr + hrat + waz +
+              bul.conv + drowsy + agitated + reffort + ausc +
+              feeding + abdominal, x=T, y=T)
> par(mfrow=c(3,4))
> resid(f2, 'partial', pl=T)      # pl=T : plot
```

The degree of nonparallelism generally agreed with the degree of nonflatness in Figure 14.3 and with the other score residual plots that were not shown. The partial residuals show that temp is highly nonlinear and that it is much more useful in predicting $Y = 2$. For the cluster scores, the linearity assumption appears reasonable, except possibly for `drowsy`. Other nonlinear effects are taken into account using splines as before (except for `age`, which is categorized).

A model can have significant lack of fit with respect to some of the predictors and still yield quite accurate predictions. To see if that is the case for this PO model, we computed predicted probabilities of $Y = 2$ for all infants from the model and compared these with predictions from a customized binary logistic model derived to predict $\Pr(Y = 2)$. The mean absolute difference in predicted probabilities between the two models is only 0.02, but the 0.90 quantile of that difference is 0.059. For high-risk infants, discrepancies of 0.2 were common. Therefore we elected to consider a different model.

14.7   Graphical Assessment of Fit of CR Model

In order to take a first look at the fit of a CR model, let us consider the two binary events that need to be predicted, and assess linearity and parallelism over Y-cutoffs. Here we fit a sequence of binary fits and then use the `plot.lrm.partial` function, which assembles partial residuals for a sequence of fits and constructs one graph per predictor.

```
> cr0 <- lrm(Y==0 ~ age + temp + rr + hrat + waz +
+             bul.conv + drowsy + agitated + reffort + ausc +
+             feeding + abdominal, x=T, y=T)
# Use the update function to save repeating model right-hand side
# An indicator variable for Y=1 is the response variable below
> cr1 <- update(cr0, Y==1 ~ ., subset=Y>=1)
> plot.lrm.partial(cr0, cr1, center=T)
```

The output is in Figure 14.5. There is not much more parallelism here than in Figure 14.4. For the two most important predictors, `ausc` and `rr`, there are strongly differing effects for the different events being predicted (e.g., $Y = 0$ or $Y = 1|Y \geq 1$). As is often the case, there is no one constant β model that satisfies assumptions with respect to all predictors simultaneously, especially when there is evidence for nonordinality for `ausc` in Figure 14.2. The CR model will need to be generalized to adequately fit this dataset.

14.8   Extended Continuation Ratio Model

The CR model in its ordinary form has no advantage over the PO model for this dataset. But Section 13.4.6 discussed how the CR model can easily be extended to relax any of its assumptions. First we use the `cr.setup` function to set up the data for fitting a CR model using the binary logistic trick.

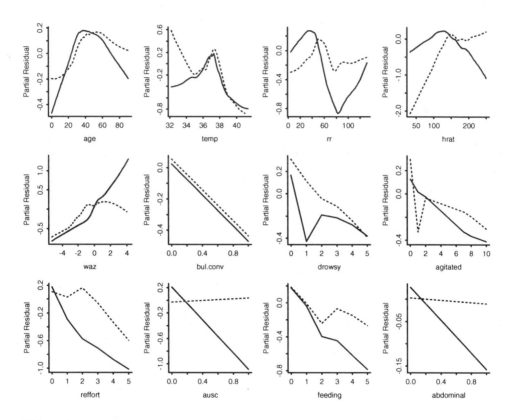

FIGURE 14.5: `loess` smoothed partial residual plots for binary models that are components of an ordinal continuation ratio model. Solid lines correspond to a model for $Y = 0$,
and dotted lines correspond to a model for $Y = 1|Y \geq 1$.

```
> u ← cr.setup(Y)
> attach(mydata[u$subs,])
> y        ← u$y
> cohort ← u$cohort
```

Here the `cohort` variable has values 'all', 'Y>=1' corresponding to the conditioning events in Equation 13.10. After the `attach` command runs, vectors such as `age` are lengthened (to 5553 records). Now we fit a fully extended CR model that makes no equal slopes assumptions; that is, the model *has* to fit Y assuming the covariables are linear and additive. At this point, we omit `hrat` but add back all variables that were deleted by examining their association with Y. Recall that most of these seven cluster scores were summarized using PC_1. Adding back "insignificant" variables will allow us to validate the model fairly using the bootstrap, as well as to obtain confidence intervals that are not falsely narrow.[11]

```
> full ← lrm(y ~ cohort*(ageg*(rcs(temp,5) + rcs(rr,5)) +
+      rcs(waz,4) + bul.conv + drowsy + agitated + reffort +
+      ausc + feeding + abdominal + hydration + hxprob +
+      pustular + crying + fever.ill + stop.breath + labor),
+                         x=T,y=T)
> # x=T, y=T is for pentrace, validate, calibrate below
> latex(anova(full))
```

This model has LR $\chi^2 = 1824$ with 87 d.f. Wald statistics produced by `latex(anova(full))` are in Table 14.6. For brevity tests of nonlinear effects and many tests with $P > 0.1$ are not shown. The global test of the constant slopes assumption in the CR model (test of all interactions involving `cohort`) has $\chi^2 = 172$ with 43 d.f., $P < 0.0001$. Consistent with Figure 14.5, the formal tests indicate that `ausc` is the biggest violator, followed by `waz` and `rr`.

14.9   Penalized Estimation

We know that the CR model must be extended to fit these data adequately. If the model is fully extended to allow for all `cohort` × predictor interactions, we have not gained any precision or power in using an ordinal model over using a polytomous logistic model. Therefore we seek some restrictions on the model's parameters. The `lrm` and `pentrace` functions allow for differing λ for shrinking different types of terms in the model. Here we want to do a grid search to determine the optimum penalty for simple main effect (noninteraction) terms and the penalty for interaction terms, most of which are terms interacting with `cohort` to allow for unequal slopes. The following code uses `pentrace` on the full extended CR model fit to find the optimum penalty factors. All combinations of the `simple` and `interaction` λs for which the interaction penalty $\geq$ the penalty for the simple parameters are examined.

TABLE 14.6: Wald Statistics for y in the Extended CR Model

	χ^2	d.f.	P
cohort	199.47	44	< 0.0001
All Interactions	172.12	43	< 0.0001
ageg	48.89	36	0.0742
temp	59.37	24	0.0001
rr	93.77	24	< 0.0001
waz	39.69	6	< 0.0001
bul.conv	10.80	2	0.0045
drowsy	15.19	2	0.0005
agitated	13.55	2	0.0011
reffort	51.85	2	< 0.0001
ausc	109.80	2	< 0.0001
feeding	27.47	2	< 0.0001
hxprob	6.62	2	0.0364
stop.breath	5.34	2	0.0693
labor	5.35	2	0.0690
ageg × temp	8.18	16	0.9432
ageg × rr	38.11	16	0.0015
cohort × rr	19.67	12	0.0736
cohort × waz	9.04	3	0.0288
cohort × ausc	38.11	1	< 0.0001
cohort × fever.ill	3.17	1	0.0749
cohort × stop.breath	2.99	1	0.0839
cohort × ageg × temp	2.22	8	0.9736
cohort × ageg × rr	10.22	8	0.2500
TOTAL NONLINEAR	93.36	40	< 0.0001
TOTAL INTERACTION	203.10	59	< 0.0001
TOTAL NONLINEAR + INTERACTION	257.70	67	< 0.0001
TOTAL	1211.73	87	< 0.0001

```
> pentrace(full, list(simple=c(0,.025,.05,.075,.1),
+                      interaction=c(0,10,50,100,125,150))))
```

Best penalty:

```
simple interaction    df    aic
  0.05            125 49.75 1672.6
```

```
simple interaction     df     aic     bic   aic.c
 0.000           0  87.000  1650.3  1074.2  1647.5
 0.000          10  60.628  1670.8  1269.4  1669.5
 0.025          10  60.110  1671.6  1273.5  1670.2
 0.050          10  59.797  1671.6  1275.6  1670.3
 0.075          10  59.581  1671.5  1276.9  1670.2
 0.100          10  59.421  1671.3  1277.8  1670.0
 0.000          50  54.640  1671.3  1309.5  1670.2
 0.025          50  54.135  1672.0  1313.5  1670.9
 0.050          50  53.829  1672.0  1315.5  1670.9
 0.075          50  53.619  1671.8  1316.8  1670.8
 0.100          50  53.463  1671.6  1317.6  1670.5
 0.000         100  51.613  1671.9  1330.1  1670.9
 0.025         100  51.113  1672.5  1334.1  1671.6
 0.050         100  50.809  1672.6  1336.1  1671.6
 0.075         100  50.600  1672.4  1337.3  1671.4
 0.100         100  50.445  1672.1  1338.1  1671.2
 0.000         125  50.553  1671.9  1337.2  1671.0
 0.025         125  50.054  1672.6  1341.1  1671.7
 0.050         125  49.750  1672.6  1343.2  1671.7
 0.075         125  49.542  1672.4  1344.4  1671.5
 0.100         125  49.387  1672.2  1345.1  1671.3
 0.000         150  49.653  1671.8  1343.0  1670.9
 0.025         150  49.155  1672.5  1347.0  1671.6
 0.050         150  48.852  1672.5  1349.0  1671.6
 0.075         150  48.643  1672.3  1350.2  1671.5
 0.100         150  48.489  1672.1  1351.0  1671.2
```

We see that shrinkage from 87 d.f. down to 49.8 effective d.f. results in an increase in AIC of 22.3. The optimum penalty factors were 0.05 for simple terms and 125 for interaction terms.

Let us now store a penalized version of the full fit, find where the effective d.f. were reduced, and compute χ^2 for each factor in the model. We take the effective d.f. for a collection of model parameters to be the sum of the diagonals of the matrix product defined underneath Gray's Equation 2.9[161] that correspond to those parameters.

```
> full.pen ← update(full,
+                    penalty=list(simple=.05, interaction=125))
> effective.df(full.pen)
```

Original and Effective Degrees of Freedom

	Original	Penalized
All	87	49.75
Simple Terms	20	19.98
Interaction or Nonlinear	67	29.77
Nonlinear	40	16.82
Interaction	59	22.57
Nonlinear Interaction	32	9.62

```
# Exclude interactions and cohort effects from plot
> plot(anova(full.pen), cex.labels=0.75, rm.ia=T,   # Figure 14.6
+      rm.other='cohort  (Factor+Higher Order Factors)')
> somers2(predict(full.pen)[cohort=='all'], y[cohort=='all'])
```

C	Dxy	n	Missing
0.836	0.672	4552	0

This will be the final model except for the model used in Section 14.10. The model has LR $\chi^2 = 1772$. The output of `effective.df` shows that noninteraction terms have barely been penalized, and coefficients of interaction terms have been shrunken from 59 d.f. to effectively 22.6 d.f. Predictive discrimination was assessed by computing the Somers' D_{xy} rank correlation between $X\hat{\beta}$ and whether $Y = 0$, in the subset of records for which $Y = 0$ is what was being predicted. Here $D_{xy} = 0.672$ and the ROC area is 0.836 (the unpenalized model had an apparent $D_{xy} = 0.676$ for the training sample). To summarize in another way the effectiveness of this model in screening infants for risks of any abnormality, the fraction of infants with predicted probabilities that $Y > 0$ being $< 0.05, > 0.25$, and > 0.5 are, respectively, 0.10, 0.28, and 0.14. `anova` output is plotted in Figure 14.6 to give a snapshot of the importance of the various predictors. The Wald statistics used here are computed on a variance–covariance matrix which is adjusted for penalization (using Gray Equation 2.6[161] before it was determined that the sandwich covariance estimator performs less well than the inverse of the penalized information matrix—see p. 209).

The full equation for the fitted model is obtained using the statement `latex(full.pen)`. Only the part of the equation used for predicting $\Pr(Y = 0)$ is shown.

$$\Pr\{y = 1\} = \frac{1}{1 + \exp(-X\beta)}, \quad \text{where}$$

$X\hat{\beta} =$

$\quad -5.543$

$\quad +0.1075\{ageg \in [\,7, 60)\} + 0.1971\{ageg \in [60, 90]\}$

$\quad +0.1979temp + 0.1092(temp - 36.2)^3_+ - 2.833(temp - 37)^3_+ + 5.071(temp - 37.3)^3_+$

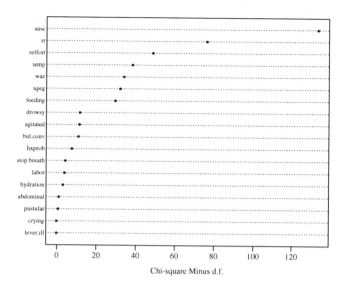

FIGURE 14.6: Importance of predictors in full penalized model, as judged by partial Wald χ^2 minus the predictor d.f. The Wald χ^2 values for each line in the dot plot include contributions from all higher-order effects. Interaction effects by themselves have been removed as has the cohort effect.

$$-2.508(\text{temp} - 37.7)^2_+ + 0.1606(\text{temp} - 39)^3_+$$
$$+0.02091\text{rr} - 6.337 \times 10^{-5}(\text{rr} - 32)^3_+ + 8.405 \times 10^{-5}(\text{rr} - 42)^3_+$$
$$+6.152 \times 10^{-5}(\text{rr} - 49)^3_+ - 0.0001018(\text{rr} - 59)^3_+ + 1.96 \times 10^{-5}(\text{rr} - 76)^3_+$$
$$-0.0759\text{waz} + 0.02509(\text{waz} + 2.9)^3_+ - 0.1185(\text{waz} + 0.75)^3_+ + 0.1226(\text{waz} - 0.28)^3_+$$
$$-0.02916(\text{waz} - 1.73)^3_+ - 0.4418\text{bul.conv} - 0.08185\text{drowsy} - 0.05327\text{agitated}$$
$$-0.2304\text{reffort} - 1.159\text{ausc} - 0.16\text{feeding} - 0.1609\text{abdominal}$$
$$-0.0541\text{hydration} + 0.08086\text{hxprob} + 0.00752\text{pustular} + 0.04712\text{crying}$$
$$+0.004299\text{fever.ill} - 0.3519\text{stop.breath} + 0.06864\text{labor}$$
$$+\{\text{ageg} \in [\,7, 60)\}[6.5 \times 10^{-5}\text{temp} - 0.0028(\text{temp} - 36.2)^3_+ - 0.008691(\text{temp} - 37)^3_+$$
$$-0.004988(\text{temp} - 37.3)^3_+ + 0.02592(\text{temp} - 37.7)^3_+ - 0.009445(\text{temp} - 39)^3_+]$$
$$+\{\text{ageg} \in [60, 90]\}[0.000132\text{temp} - 0.001826(\text{temp} - 36.2)^3_+ - 0.0164(\text{temp} - 37)^3_+$$
$$-0.0476(\text{temp} - 37.3)^3_+ + 0.09142(\text{temp} - 37.7)^3_+ - 0.02559(\text{temp} - 39)^3_+]$$
$$+\{\text{ageg} \in [\,7, 60)\}[-0.0009438\text{rr} - 1.045 \times 10^{-6}(\text{rr} - 32)^3_+ - 1.67 \times 10^{-6}(\text{rr} - 42)^3_+$$
$$-5.189 \times 10^{-6}(\text{rr} - 49)^3_+ + 1.429 \times 10^{-5}(\text{rr} - 59)^3_+ - 6.382 \times 10^{-6}(\text{rr} - 76)^3_+]$$
$$+\{\text{ageg} \in [60, 90]\}[-0.001921\text{rr} - 5.521 \times 10^{-6}(\text{rr} - 32)^3_+ - 8.628 \times 10^{-6}(\text{rr} - 42)^3_+$$
$$-4.147 \times 10^{-6}(\text{rr} - 49)^3_+ + 3.813 \times 10^{-5}(\text{rr} - 59)^3_+ - 1.984 \times 10^{-5}(\text{rr} - 76)^3_+]$$

and $\{c\} = 1$ if subject is in group c, 0 otherwise; $(x)_+ = x$ if $x > 0$, 0 otherwise.

Now consider displays of the shapes of effects of the predictors. For the continuous variables `temp` and `rr` that interact with age group, we show the effects for all three age groups separately for each Y cutoff. All effects have been centered so that the log odds at the median predictor value is zero when `cohort='all'`, so these plots actually show log odds relative to reference values. The patterns in Figure 14.7 are in agreement with those in Figure 14.5.

```
> par(mfrow=c(4,4))
> yl ← c(-2.5, 1)        # put all plots on common y-axis scale

# Plot predictors that interact with another predictor
# Vary ageg over all age groups, then vary temp over its
# default range (10th smallest to 10th largest values in data)
# Make a separate plot for each 'cohort'
# ref.zero centers effects using median x

> for(co in levels(cohort)) {
+    plot(full.pen, temp=NA, ageg=NA, cohort=co, ref.zero=T,
+         ylim=yl, conf.int=F)
+    text(37.5, 1.5, co)     # add title showing current cohort
+ }
> for(co in levels(cohort)) {
+    plot(full.pen, rr=NA,   ageg=NA, cohort=co, ref.zero=T,
+         ylim=yl, conf.int=F)
+    text(70, 1.5, co)
+ }

> # For each predictor that only interacts with cohort, show the
> # Differing effects of the predictor for predicting Pr(Y=0) and
> # Pr(Y=1 given Y exceeds 0) on the same graph

> plot(full.pen, waz     =NA, cohort=NA, ref.zero=T,
+      ylim=yl, conf.int=F)
> plot(full.pen, bul.conv=NA, cohort=NA, ref.zero=T,
+      ylim=yl, conf.int=F)
. . . .
> plot(full.pen, crying  =NA, cohort=NA, ref.zero=T,
+      ylim=yl, conf.int=F)
```

14.10 Using Approximations to Simplify the Model

Parsimonious models can be developed by approximating predictions from the model to any desired level of accuracy. Let $\hat{L} = X\hat{\beta}$ denote the predicted log odds

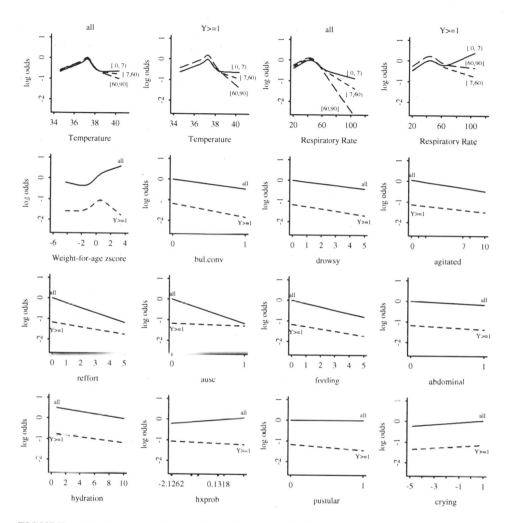

FIGURE 14.7: Centered effects of predictors on the log odds. The first four plots show interaction effects with the `age` intervals noted. For others, interaction with `cohort` are shown. For predictors having fewer than 10 unique values, x-axis tick marks appear only for values that occurred in the data. No plot was made for the `fever.ill, stop.breath,` or `labor` cluster scores. The title `all` refers to the prediction of $Y = 0 | Y \geq 0$, that is, $Y = 0$.

from the full penalized ordinal model, including multiple records for subjects with $Y > 0$. Then we can use a variety of techniques to approximate $\hat{L}$ from a subset of the predictors (in their raw form). With this approach one can immediately see what is lost over the full model by computing, for example, the mean absolute error in predicting $\hat{L}$. Another advantage to full model approximation is that shrinkage used in computing $\hat{L}$ is inherited by any model that predicts $\hat{L}$. In contrast, the usual stepwise methods result in $\hat{\beta}$ that are too large since the final coefficients are estimated as if the model structure were prespecified.   ☐1

CART would be particularly useful as a model approximator as it would result in a prediction tree that would be easy for health workers to use. Unfortunately, a 50-node CART was required to predict $\hat{L}$ with an $R^2 \geq 0.9$, and the mean absolute error in the predicted logit was still 0.4. This will happen when the model contains many important continuous variables.

Let's approximate the full model using its important components, by using a step-down technique predicting $\hat{L}$ from all of the component variables using ordinary least squares. In using step-down with the least squares function ols in Design there is a problem when the initial $R^2 = 1.0$ as in that case the estimate of $\sigma = 0$. This can be circumvented by specifying an arbitrary nonzero value of σ to ols (here 1.0), as we are not using the variance–covariance matrix from ols anyway. Since cohort interacts with the predictors, separate approximations can be developed for each level of Y. For this example we approximate the log odds that $Y = 0$ using the cohort of patients used for determining $Y = 0$, that is, $Y \geq 0$ or cohort='all'.

```
> plogit  ← predict(full.pen)
> f ← ols(plogit ∼ ageg*(rcs(temp,5) + rcs(rr,5)) +
+           rcs(waz,4) + bul.conv + drowsy + agitated + reffort +
+           ausc + feeding + abdominal + hydration + hxprob +
+           pustular + crying + fever.ill + stop.breath + labor,
+           subset=cohort='all', sigma=1)

> # Do fast backward stepdown
> fastbw(f, aics=1e10)
> # 1e10 causes all variables to eventually be
> # deleted so can see most important ones in order

> # Fit an approximation to the full penalized model using most
> # important variables
> full.approx ← ols(plogit ∼ rcs(temp,5) + ageg*rcs(rr,5) +
+                    rcs(waz,4) + bul.conv + drowsy + reffort +
+                    ausc + feeding,
+                    subset=cohort=='all')
```

The approximate model had R^2 against the full penalized model of 0.972, and the mean absolute error in predicting $\hat{L}$ was 0.17. The D_{xy} rank correlation between the approximate model's predicted logit and the binary event $Y = 0$ is 0.665 as compared with the full model's $D_{xy} = 0.672$. See Section 18.5 for an example of computing correct estimates of variance of the parameters in an approximate model.

Next turn to diagramming this model approximation so that all predicted values can be computed without the use of a computer. We draw a type of nomogram that converts each effect in the model to a 0 to 100 scale which is just proportional to the log odds. These points are added across predictors to derive the "Total Points," which are converted to $\hat{L}$ and then to predicted probabilities. For the interaction between rr and ageg, Design's nomogram function automatically constructs three rr axes—only one is added into the total point score for a given subject. Here we draw a nomogram for predicting the probability that $Y > 0$, which is $1 - \Pr(Y = 0)$. This probability is derived by negating $\hat{\beta}$ and $X\hat{\beta}$ in the model derived to predict $\Pr(Y = 0)$.

```
> f ← full.approx
> f$coefficients      ← -f$coefficients
> f$linear.predictors ← -f$linear.predictors

> nomogram(f,
+          temp=32:41, rr=seq(20,120,by=10),
+          waz=seq(-1.5,2,by=.5),
+          fun=plogis, funlabel='Pr(Y>0)',
+          fun.at=c(.02,.05,seq(.1,.9,by=.1),.95,.98))
```

The nomogram is shown in Figure 14.8. As an example in using the nomogram, a six-day-old infant gets approximately 9 points for having a respiration rate of 30/minute, 19 points for having a temperature of 39°C, 11 points for waz=0, 14 points for drowsy=5, and 15 points for reffort=2. Assuming that bul.conv=ausc=feeding=0, that infant gets 68 total points. This corresponds to $X\hat{\beta} = -0.6$ and a probability of 0.35. Values computed directly from the full.approx formula were $X\hat{\beta} = -0.68$ and a probability of 0.34.

2

14.11 Validating the Model

For the full CR model that was fitted using PMLE, we used 150 bootstrap replications to estimate and then to correct for optimism in various statistical indexes: D_{xy}, generalized R^2, intercept and slope of a linear recalibration equation for $X\hat{\beta}$, the maximum calibration error for $\Pr(Y = 0)$ based on the linear-logistic recalibration (Emax), and the Brier quadratic probability score B. PMLE is used at each of the 150 resamples. During the bootstrap simulations, we sample with replacement from the *patients* and not from the 5553 expanded *records*, hence the specification cluster=u$subs, where u$subs is the vector of sequential patient numbers computed from cr.setup above. To be able to assess predictive accuracy of a single predicted probability, the subset parameter is specified so that $\Pr(Y = 0)$ is being assessed

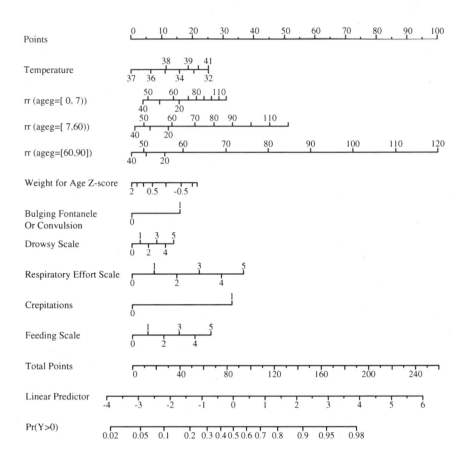

FIGURE 14.8: Nomogram for predicting $\Pr(Y > 0)$ from the penalized extended CR model, using an approximate model fitted using ordinary least squares ($R^2 = 0.972$ against the full model's predicted logits).

even though 5553 observations are used to develop each of the 150 models. The output and the S-PLUS statement used to obtain the output are shown below.

```
> validate(full.pen, B=150, cluster=u$subs, subset=cohort=='all')
```

	index.orig	training	test	optimism	index.corrected	n
Dxy	0.672	0.675	0.666	0.009	0.662	150
R2	0.376	0.383	0.370	0.013	0.363	150
Intercept	-0.031	-0.033	0.001	-0.034	0.003	150
Slope	1.029	1.031	1.002	0.029	1.000	150
Emax	0.000	0.000	0.001	0.001	0.001	150
B	0.120	0.119	0.121	-0.002	0.122	150

We see that for the apparent $D_{xy} = 0.672$ the optimism from overfitting was estimated to be 0.009 for the PMLE model, so the bias-corrected estimate of predictive discrimination is 0.662. The intercept and slope needed to recalibrate $X\hat{\beta}$ to a 45° line are very near (0, 1). The estimate of the maximum calibration error in predicting $\Pr(Y = 0)$ is 0.001 which is quite satisfactory. The corrected Brier score is 0.122.

The simple calibration statistics just listed do not address the issue of whether predicted values from the model are miscalibrated in a nonlinear way, so now we estimate an overfitting-corrected calibration curve nonparametrically.

```
> cal ← calibrate(full.pen, B=150, cluster=u$subs,
+                   subset=cohort=='all')
> plot(cal)
```

The results are shown in Figure 14.9. One can see a slightly nonlinear calibration function estimate, but the overfitting-corrected calibration is excellent everywhere, being only slightly worse than the apparent calibration. The estimated maximum calibration error is 0.043. The excellent validation for both predictive discrimination and calibration are a result of the large sample size, frequency distribution of Y, initial data reduction, and PMLE.

14.12 Summary

Clinically guided variable clustering and item weighting resulted in a great reduction in the number of candidate predictor degrees of freedom and hence increased the true predictive accuracy of the model. Scores summarizing clusters of clinical signs, along with temperature, respiration rate, and weight-for-age after suitable nonlinear transformation and allowance for interactions with age, are powerful predictors of the ordinal response. Graphical methods are effective for detecting lack of fit in the PO and CR models and for diagramming the final model. Model approximation allowed development of parsimonious clinical prediction tools. Approximate models

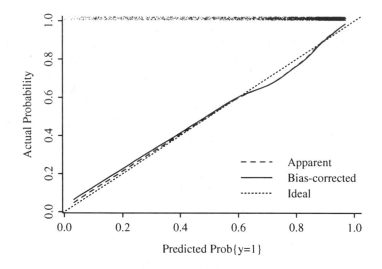

FIGURE 14.9: Bootstrap calibration curve for the full penalized extended CR model. 150 bootstrap repetitions were used in conjunction with the `loess` smoother.[76] Also shown is a "rug plot" to demonstrate how effective this model is in discriminating patients into low- and high-risk groups for $\Pr(Y = 0)$ (which corresponds with the derived variable value $y = 1$ when `cohort='all'`).

inherit the shrinkage from the full model. For the ordinal model developed here, substantial shrinkage of the full model was needed.

14.13 Further Reading

[1] The *lasso* method of Tibshirani[415, 416] also incorporates shrinkage into variable selection.

[2] To see how this compares with predictions using the full model, the extra clinical signs in that model that are not in the approximate model were predicted individually on the basis of $X\hat{\beta}$ from the reduced model along with the signs that are in that model, using ordinary linear regression. The signs not specified when evaluating the approximate model were then set to predicted values based on the values given for the 6-day-old infant above. The resulting $X\hat{\beta}$ for the full model is -0.81 and the predicted probability is 0.31, as compared with -0.68 and 0.34 quoted above.

14.14 Problems

Develop a proportional odds ordinal logistic model predicting the severity of functional disability (sfdm2) in SUPPORT. The highest level of this variable corresponds to patients dying before the two-month follow-up interviews. Consider this level as the most severe outcome. Consider the following predictors: age, sex, dzgroup, num.co, scoma, race (use all levels), meanbp, hrt, temp, pafi, alb, adlsc. The last variable is the baseline level of functional disability from the "activities of daily living scale."

1. For the variables adlsc, sex, age, meanbp, and others if you like, make plots of means of predictors stratified by levels of the response, to check for ordinality. On the same plot, show estimates of means assuming the proportional odds relationship between predictors and response holds. Comment on the evidence for ordinality and for proportional odds.

2. To allow for maximum adjustment of baseline functional status, treat this predictor as nominal (after rounding it to the nearest whole number; fractional values are the result of imputation) in remaining steps, so that all dummy variables will be generated. Make a single chart showing proportions of various outcomes stratified (individually) by adlsc, sex, age, meanbp. For continuous predictors use quartiles. You can pass the following function to the summary (summary.formula) function to obtain the proportions of patients having sfdm2 at or worse than each of its possible levels (other than the first level). An easy way to do this is to use the cumcategory function with the

Hmisc library's `summary.formula` function. Print estimates to only two significant digits of precision. Manually check the calculations for the `sex` variable using `table(sex, sfdm2)`. Then plot all estimates on a single graph using `plot(object, which=1:4)`, where `object` was created by `summary` (actually `summary.formula`). Note: for printing tables you may want to convert `sfdm2` to a 0–4 variable so that column headers are short and so that later calculations are simpler. You can use for example:

```
sfdm <- as.integer(sfdm2) - 1
```

3. Use an S-PLUS function such as the following to compute the *logits* of the cumulative proportions.

```
sf ← function(y)
  c('Y>=1'=qlogis(mean(y >= 1)), 'Y>=2'=qlogis(mean(y >= 2)),
    'Y>=3'=qlogis(mean(y >= 3)), 'Y>=4'=qlogis(mean(y >= 4)))
```

As the $Y = 3$ category is rare, it may be even better to omit the $Y \geq 4$ column above, as was done in Section 13.3.8 and Figure 13.1. For each predictor pick two rows of the `summary` table having reasonable sample sizes, and take the difference between the two rows. Comment on the validity of the proportional odds assumption by assessing how constant the row differences are across columns. Note: constant differences in log odds (logits) mean constant ratios of odds or constant relative effects of the predictor across outcome levels.

4. Make two plots nonparametrically relating `age` to all of the cumulative proportions or their logits. You can use commands such as the following (to use the S-PLUS `Hmisc` library). `plsmo`

```
for(i in 1:4) plsmo(age, sfdm >= i, add=i>1,
                    ylim=c(.2,.8), ylab='Proportion Y>=j')
for(i in 1:4) plsmo(age, sfdm >= i, add=i>1, fun=qlogis,
                    ylim=qlogis(c(.2,.8)), ylab='logit')
```

Comment on the linearity of the `age` effect (which of the two plots do you use?) and on the proportional odds assumption for `age`, by assessing parallelism in the second plot.

5. Impute `race` using the most frequent category and `pafi` and `alb` using "normal" values.

6. Fit a model to predict the ordinal response using all predictors. For continuous ones assume a smooth relationship but allow it to be nonlinear. Quantify the ability of the model to discriminate patients in the five outcomes. Do an overall likelihood ratio test for whether any variables are associated with the level of functional disability.

7. Compute partial tests of association for each predictor and a test of nonlinearity for continuous ones. Compute a global test of nonlinearity. Graphically display the ranking of importance of the predictors.

8. Display the shape of how each predictor relates to the log odds of exceeding any level of `sfdm2` you choose, setting other predictors to typical values (one value per predictor). By default, `plot.Design` will make predictions for the middle response category, which is a satisfactory choice here.

9. Use resampling to validate the Somers' D_{xy} rank correlation between predicted logit and the ordinal outcome. Also validate the generalized R^2, and slope shrinkage coefficient, all using a single S-PLUS statement. Comment on the quality (potential "exportability") of the model.

Chapter 15

Models Using Nonparametric Transformations of X and Y

15.1   Background

Fitting multiple regression models by the method of least squares is one of the most commonly used methods in statistics. There are a number of challenges to the use of least squares, even when it is only used for estimation and not inference, including the following.

1. How should continuous predictors be transformed so as to get a good fit?

2. Is it better to transform the response variable? How does one find a good transformation that simplifies the right-hand side of the equation?

3. What if Y needs to be transformed nonmonotonically (e.g., $|Y - 100|$ or $(Y - 120)^2$) before it will have any correlation with X?

When one is trying to draw an inference about population effects using confidence limits or hypothesis tests, the most common approach is to assume that the residuals have a normal distribution. This is equivalent to assuming that the conditional distribution of the response Y given the set of predictors X is normal with mean depending on X and variance that is (one hopes) a constant independent of X. The need for a distributional assumption to enable us to draw inferences creates a number of other challenges such as these.

1. If for the untransformed original scale of the response Y the distribution of the residuals is not normal with constant spread, ordinary methods will not yield correct inferences (e.g., confidence intervals will not have the desired coverage probability and the intervals will need to be asymmetric).

2. Quite often there is a transformation of Y that will yield well-behaving residuals. How do you find this transformation? Can you find a transformation for the Xs at the same time?

3. All classical statistical inferential methods assume that the full model was prespecified, that is, the model was not modified after examining the data. How does one correct confidence limits, for example, for data-based model and transformation selection?

15.2   Generalized Additive Models

Hastie and Tibshirani[191] have developed *generalized additive models* (GAMs) for a variety of distributions for Y. There are semiparametric GAMs, but most GAMs for continuous Y assume that the conditional distribution of Y is from a specific distribution family. GAMs nicely estimate the transformation each continuous X requires so as to optimize a fitting criterion such as sum of squared errors or log likelihood, subject to the degrees of freedom the analyst desires to spend on each predictor.

There is excellent software available for fitting a wide variety of GAMs, such as the powerful S-PLUS function, gam. gam automatically estimates the transformation each right-hand side variable should receive so as to optimize prediction of Y, and a number of distributions are allowed for Y. It is important to note, though, parametric GAMs assume that Y has already been transformed to fit the specified distribution family.

15.3   Nonparametric Estimation of Y-Transformation

When the model's left-hand side also needs transformation, either to improve R^2 or to achieve constant variance of the residuals (which increases the chances of satisfying a normality assumption), there are a few approaches available. One approach is Breiman and Friedman's *alternating conditional expectation* (ACE) method.[47] ACE simultaneously transforms both Y and each of the Xs so as to maximize the multiple R^2 between the transformed Y and the transformed Xs. The model is given by

$$g(Y) = f_1(X_1) + f_2(X_2) + \ldots + f_p(X_p). \tag{15.1}$$

ACE allows the analyst to impose restrictions on the transformations such as mono-tonicity. It allows for categorical predictors, whose categories will automatically be given numeric scores. The transformation for Y is allowed to be nonmonotonic. One feature of ACE is its ability to estimate the *maximal correlation* between an X and the response Y. Unlike the ordinary correlation coefficient (which assumes linear-ity) or Spearman's rank correlation (which assumes monotonicity), the maximal correlation has the property that it is zero if and only if X and Y are statistically independent. This property holds because ACE allows for nonmonotonic transfor-mations of all variables. The "super smoother" (see the S-PLUS `supsmu` function) is the basis for the nonparametric estimation of transformations for continuous Xs.

Tibshirani developed a different algorithm for nonparametric additive regression based on least squares, *additivity and variance stabilization* (AVAS).[414] Unlike ACE, AVAS forces $g(Y)$ to be monotonic. AVAS's fitting criteria is to maximize R^2 while forcing the transformation for Y to result in nearly constant variance of residuals. The model specification is the same as for ACE (Equation 15.3).

ACE and AVAS are powerful fitting algorithms, but they can result in overfit-ting (R^2 can be greatly inflated when one fits many predictors), and they provide no statistical inferential measures. As discussed earlier, the process of estimating transformations (especially those for Y) can result in significant variance under-estimation, especially for small sample sizes. The bootstrap can be used to correct the apparent R^2 resulting from these procedures for overfitting. As before, it es-timates the optimism (bias) in the apparent R^2, and this optimism is subtracted from the apparent R^2 to get a more trustworthy estimate. The bootstrap can also be used to compute confidence limits for all estimated transformations, and confidence limits for estimated predictor effects that take fully into account the uncertainty associated with the transformations. To do this, all steps involved in fitting the additive models must be repeated fresh for each resample.

Limited testing has shown that the sample size needs to exceed 100 for ACE and AVAS to provide stable estimates. In small sample sizes the bootstrap bias-corrected estimate of R^2 will be zero because the sample information did not support simultaneous estimation of all transformations.

15.4 Obtaining Estimates on the Original Scale

A common practice in least squares fitting is to attempt to rectify lack of fit by taking parametric transformations of Y before fitting; the logarithm is the most common transformation. If after transformation the model's residuals have a popu-lation median of zero, the inverse transformation of a predicted transformed value estimates the population median of Y given X. This is because unlike means, quan-tiles are transformation-preserving. Many analysts make the mistake of not reporting which population parameter is being estimated when inverse transforming $X\hat{\beta}$, and sometimes they even report that the mean is being estimated.

How would one go about estimating the population mean or other parameter on the untransformed scale? If the residuals are assumed to be normally distributed and if $\log(Y)$ is the transformation, the mean of the log-normal distribution, a function of both the mean and the variance of the residuals, can be used to derive the desired quantity. However, if the residuals are not normally distributed, this procedure will not result in the correct estimator. Duan[119] developed a "smearing" estimator for more nonparametrically obtaining estimates of parameters on the original scale. In the simple one-sample case without predictors in which one has computed $\hat{\theta} = \sum_{i=1}^{n} \log(Y_i)/n$, the residuals from this fitted value are given by $e_i = \log(Y_i) - \hat{\theta}$. The smearing estimator of the population mean is $\sum \exp[\hat{\theta} + e_i]/n$. In this simple case the result is the ordinary sample mean $\overline{Y}$.

The worth of Duan's smearing estimator is in regression modeling. Suppose that the regression was run on $g(Y)$ from which estimated values $\widehat{g(Y_i)} = X_i\hat{\beta}$ and residuals on the transformed scale $e_i = g(Y_i) - X_i\hat{\beta}$ were obtained. Instead of restricting ourselves to estimating the population mean, let $W(y_1, y_2, \ldots, y_n)$ denote any function of a vector of untransformed response values. To estimate the population mean in the homogeneous one-sample case, W is the simple average of all of its arguments. To estimate the population 0.25 quantile, W is the sample 0.25 quantile of $y_1, \ldots, y_n$. Then the smearing estimator of the population parameter estimated by W given X is $W(g^{-1}(a+e_1), g^{-1}(a+e_2), \ldots, g^{-1}(a+e_n))$, where g^{-1} is the inverse of the g transformation and $a = X\hat{\beta}$.

When using the AVAS algorithm, the monotonic transformation g is estimated from the data, and the predicted value of $\hat{g}(Y)$ is given by Equation 15.3. So we extend the smearing estimator as $W(\hat{g}^{-1}(a + e_1), \ldots, \hat{g}^{-1}(a + e_n))$, where a is the predicted transformed response given a. As $\hat{g}$ is nonparametric (i.e., a table look-up), the `areg.boot` function described below computes $\hat{g}^{-1}$ using reverse linear interpolation.

If residuals from $\hat{g}(Y)$ are assumed to be symmetrically distributed, their population median is zero and we can estimate the median on the untransformed scale by computing $\hat{g}^{-1}(X\hat{\beta})$. To be safe, `areg.boot` adds the median residual to $X\hat{\beta}$ when estimating the population median (the median residual can be ignored by specifying `statistic='fitted'` to functions that operate on objects created by `areg.boot`).

15.5   S-PLUS Functions

The S-PLUS `ace` function implements all the features of the ACE algorithm, and `avas` does likewise for AVAS. These functions are builtin to S-PLUS (see [307, pp. 236–242] for examples and a nice overview). The bootstrap and smearing capabilities mentioned above are offered for these estimation functions by the `areg.boot` ("additive regression using the bootstrap") function in the Hmisc library. Unlike the ace and avas functions, areg.boot uses the S-PLUS modeling language, making it easier for the analyst to specify the predictor variables and what is assumed about their relationships with the transformed Y. areg.boot also offers various estimation options with and without smearing. It can estimate the effect of changing one predictor, holding others constant, using the ordinary bootstrap to estimate the standard deviation of difference in two possibly transformed estimates (for two values of X), assuming normality of such differences. Normality is assumed to avoid generating a large number of bootstrap replications of time-consuming model fits. It would not be very difficult to add nonparametric bootstrap confidence limit capabilities to the software. areg.boot resamples every aspect of the modeling process it uses, just as Faraway[134] did for parametric least squares modeling.

areg.boot implements a variety of methods as shown in the simple example below. The monotone function restricts a variable's transformation to be monotonic, while the I function restricts it to be linear.

```
f ← areg.boot(Y ~ monotone(age) +
              sex + weight + I(blood.pressure))
```

```
plot(f)           # show transformations, CLs
Function(f)       # generate S-PLUS functions
                  # defining transformations
predict(f)        # get predictions,
                  # smearing estimates
summary(f)        # compute CLs on effects of
                  # each X
smearingEst()     # generalized smearing
                  # estimators
Mean(f)           # derive S-PLUS function to
                  # compute smearing mean Y
Quantile(f)       # derive S-PLUS function to
                  # compute smearing quantile
```

The methods are best described in a case study.

15.6 Case Study

As an example consider a dataset provided courtesy of Dr. John Schorling, Department of Medicine, University of Virginia School of Medicine, and found on the Web page for this text. The data consist of 19 variables on 403 subjects from 1046 subjects who were interviewed in a study to understand the prevalence of cardiovascular risk factors such as obesity and diabetes in central Virginia for African Americans.[456] Diabetes Mellitus Type II (adult onset diabetes) is associated most strongly with obesity. The waist/hip ratio may be a predictor of diabetes and heart disease. DM II is also associated with hypertension, as they may both be part of what has been labeled "Syndrome X." The 403 subjects were the ones who were actually screened for diabetes. A primary laboratory test for diabetes measured gylcosylated hemoglobin (GHb), also called glycated hemoglobin or hemoglobin A_{1c}. GHb has the advantage of reflecting average blood glucose for the preceding 60 to 90 days. GHb > 7.0 is usually taken as a positive diagnosis of diabetes.

At first glance some analysts might think that the best way to develop a model for diagnosing diabetes might be to fit a binary logistic model with GHb > 7 as the response variable. This is very wasteful of information, as it does not distinguish a GHb value of 2 from a 6.9, or a 7.1 from a 10. The waste of information will result in larger standard errors of $\hat{\beta}$, wider confidence bands, larger P-values, and lower power to detect risk factors. A better approach is to predict the continuous GHb value using a continuous response model such as ordinary multiple regression or using ordinal logistic regression. Then this model can be converted to predict the probability that GHb exceeds any cutoff of interest. For an ordinal logistic model having one intercept per possible value of GHb in the dataset (except for the lowest value), all probabilities are easy to compute. For ordinary regression this probability depends on the distribution of the residuals from the model.

Let us proceed with a least squares approach. An initial series of trial transformations for the response indicated that the reciprocal of GHb resulted in a model having residuals of nearly constant spread when plotted against predicted values. In addition, the residuals appeared well approximated by a normal distribution. On the other hand, a model developed on the original scale did not have constant spread of the residuals. It will be interesting to see if the nonparametric variance stabilizing function determined by `avas` will resemble the reciprocal of GHb.

Let's consider the following predictors: age, systolic blood pressure, total cholesterol, body frame (small, medium, large), weight, and hip circumference. Twelve subjects have missing body frame, and we should be able to impute this variable from other body size measurements. Let's do this using recursive partitioning with Atkinson and Therneau's `rpart` function. `rpart` will predict the probability that the polytomous response `frame` equals each of its three levels.

```
> library(rpart)
> r ← rpart(frame ~ gender + height + weight + waist + hip)
> plot(r); text(r)   # shows first split on waist, then
>                     # height,weight
> probs ← predict(r, diabetes)
> # Within each row of probs order from largest to smallest
> # Find column # of largest
> most.probable.category ← (t(apply(-probs, 1, order)))[,1]
> frame.pred ← levels(frame)[most.probable.category]
> table(frame, frame.pred)
```

```
       large medium small
 small     2     45    57
medium    10    158    16
 large    35     67     1
```

```
> frame ← impute(frame, frame.pred[is.na(frame)])
> describe(frame)
frame : Body Frame
   n missing imputed unique
 403       0      12      3

small (106, 26%), medium (193, 48%), large (104, 26%)

> table(frame[is.imputed(frame)])
 small medium large
     2      9     1
```

Other predictors are only missing on a handful of cases. Impute them with constants to avoid excluding any observations from the fit.

```
> bp.1s  ← impute(bp.1s)
> chol   ← impute(chol)
> weight ← impute(weight)
> hip    ← impute(hip)
```

Now fit the avas model. We used the default number of 100 bootstrap repetitions but only plot the first 20 estimates to see clearly how the bootstrap reestimates of transformations vary on the next plot. We use subject matter knowledge to restrict the transformations of age, weight, and hip to be monotonic. Had we wanted to restrict transformations to be linear, we would have specified the identity function, for example, I(weight).

```
> set.seed(721)            # so can reproduce bootstrap esimates
> f ← areg.boot(glyhb ∼ monotone(age) + bp.1s + chol + frame +
+                monotone(weight) + monotone(hip))
> options(digits=3)
> f


avas Additive Regression Model

areg.boot(x = glyhb ∼ monotone(age) + bp.1s + chol + frame +
          monotone(weight) + monotone(hip))

Categorical variables: frame
```

```
Frequencies of Missing Values Due to Each Variable
glyhb monotone(age) bp.1s chol frame monotone(weight) monotone(hip)
   13              0      0    0     0               0             0
```

```
n= 390   p= 6
```

```
Apparent R2 on transformed Y scale: 0.265
Bootstrap validated R2             : 0.201
```

```
Coefficients of standardized transformations:
```

```
 Intercept   age bp.1s  chol frame weight   hip
 -4.34e-009 1.06  1.51 0.953 0.708   1.26 0.653
```

Note that the coefficients above do not mean very much as the scale of the transformations is arbitrary. We see that the model was moderately overfitted (optimism in R^2 is 0.265 to 0.201).

Next we plot the transformations, 0.95 confidence bands, and a sample of the bootstrap estimates.

```
> plot(f, boot=20)
```

The plot is shown in Figure 15.1. Apparently, age and chol are the most important predictors.

Let's see how effective the transformation of glyhb was in stabilizing variance and making the residuals normally distributed.

```
> par(mfrow=c(2,2))            # Figure 15.2
> plot(fitted(f), resid(f))
> plot(predict(f), resid(f))
> qqnorm(resid(f)); abline(a=0, b=1)  # draws line of identity
```

We see from Figure 15.2 that the residuals have reasonably uniform spread and are distributed almost normally. A multiple regression run on untransformed variables did not fare nearly as well.

Now check whether the response transformation is close to the reciprocal of glyhb. First derive an S-PLUS representation of the fitted transformations. For nonparametric function estimates these are really table look-ups. Function creates a list of functions, named according to the variables in the model.

```
> funs ← Function(f)
> plot(1/glyhb, funs$glyhb(glyhb))    # Figure 15.3
```

Results are in Figure 15.3. An almost linear relationship is evidence that the reciprocal is a good transformation.[a]

---

[a]Beware that it may not help to know this, because if we redo the analysis using an ordinary linear model on 1/glyhb, standard errors would not take model selection into account.[134]

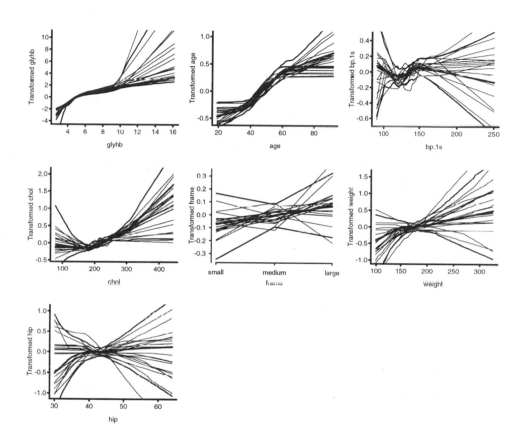

FIGURE 15.1: avas transformations: overall estimates, pointwise 0.95 confidence bands, and 20 bootstrap estimates (thinner lines).

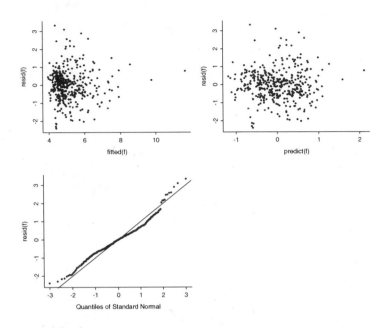

FIGURE 15.2: Distribution of residuals from the **avas** fit. The top left panel x-axis has $\hat{Y}$ on the original Y scale. The top right panel uses the transformed $\hat{Y}$ for the x-axis.

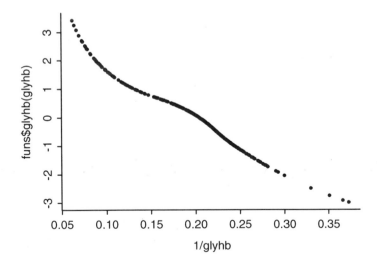

FIGURE 15.3: Agreement between the **avas** transformation for **glyhb** and the reciprocal of **glyhb**.

Now let us obtain approximate tests of effects of each predictor. summary does this by setting all other predictors to reference values (e.g., medians), and comparing predicted responses for a given level of the predictor X with predictions for the lowest setting of X. We use the three quartiles for continuous variables, but specify age settings manually. The default predicted response for summary is the median, which is used here. Therefore tests are for differences in median GHb.

```
> summary(f, values=list(age=c(20,30,40,50,60,70,80)))

Values to which predictors are set when estimating
effects of other predictors:

    glyhb age bp.1s chol frame weight hip
    4.84  50   136  204     2    173  42

Estimates of differences of effects on Median Y (from first X value),
and bootstrap standard errors of these differences.
Settings for X are shown as row headings.




Predictor: age
     Differences     S.E Lower 0.95 Upper 0.95     Z Pr(|Z|)
20      0.0000       NA         NA         NA NA       NA
30      0.0631 0.0456   -0.02632      0.153 1.38 0.166631
40      0.1824 0.0884    0.00906      0.356 2.06 0.039172
50      0.5250 0.1439    0.24302      0.807 3.65 0.000263
60      0.8674 0.2405    0.39598      1.339 3.61 0.000311
70      1.1213 0.3420    0.45104      1.792 3.28 0.001042
80      1.4240 0.6059    0.23659      2.611 2.35 0.018749


Predictor: bp.1s
      Differences     S.E Lower 0.95 Upper 0.95     Z Pr(|Z|)
122      0.0000       NA         NA         NA NA       NA
136      0.0851 0.0869    -0.0852      0.255 0.979 0.3274
148      0.2250 0.1276    -0.0251      0.475 1.763 0.0779


Predictor: chol
      Differences     S.E Lower 0.95 Upper 0.95     Z Pr(|Z|)
179      0.0000       NA         NA         NA NA       NA
204      0.0701 0.0614    -0.0503      0.190 1.14 0.2539
229      0.1875 0.1002    -0.0090      0.384 1.87 0.0615
```

```
Predictor: frame
        Differences    S.E Lower 0.95 Upper 0.95      Z Pr(|Z|)
  small     0.0000    NA         NA        NA   NA       NA
 medium     0.0505 0.116     -0.177     0.278 0.436    0.663
  large     0.1152 0.198     -0.274     0.504 0.581    0.562


Predictor: weight
        Differences    S.E Lower 0.95 Upper 0.95      Z Pr(|Z|)
   150     0.0000    NA         NA.       NA   NA       NA
   173     0.0216 0.113     -0.199     0.242 0.191    0.848
   200     0.1556 0.232     -0.298     0.609 0.672    0.501


Predictor: hip
        Differences    S.E Lower 0.95 Upper 0.95      Z Pr(|Z|)
    39    0.00000    NA         NA        NA   NA       NA
    42    0.00953 0.120     -0.226     0.245 0.0795   0.937
    46    0.02941 0.212     -0.385     0.444 0.1390   0.889
```

For example, when age increases from 20 to 70 we predict an increase in median GHb by 1.121 with standard error 0.342, when all other predictors are held to constants listed above. Setting them to other constants will yield different estimates of the age effect, as the transformation of glyhb is nonlinear. We see that only for age do some of the confidence intervals for effects exclude zero.

Next depict the fitted model by plotting predicted values, with age varying on the x-axis, and three curves corresponding to three values of chol. All other predictors are set to representative values. Figure 15.4 shows estimates of both the median and the mean GHb.

```
> newdat ← expand.grid(age=20:80,
+                       chol=quantile(chol,c(.25,.5,.75)),
+                       bp.1s=136, frame='medium',
+                       weight=173, hip=42),
+                       statistic=c('median','mean'))
> yhat ← c(predict(f, newdat[1:183,],   statistic='median'),
+           predict(f, newdat[184:366,], statistic='mean'))
> xYplot(yhat ~ age | statistic, groups=chol,    # in Hmisc
+         data=newdat, type='l', col=1,           # Figure 15.4
+         ylab='Glycosylated Hemoglobin',
+         label.curve=list(method='on top'))
```

The result is Figure 15.4. Note that none of the predictions is above 7.0. Determine the number of predicted transformed values in the entire dataset above 7.0.

```
> yhat.all ← fitted(f)
> sum(yhat.all > 7, na.rm=T)
[1] 25
```

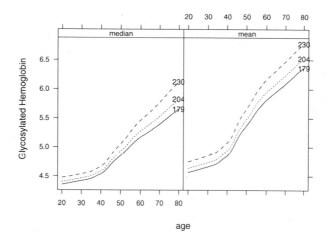

FIGURE 15.4: Predicted median (left panel) and mean (right panel) GHb as a function of age and chol.

So the model is not very useful for finding clinical levels of diabetes. To ascertain that a dedicated binary model would not do any better, we try GHb dichotomized at the diagnostic cutpoint.

```
> library(Design,T)
> h ← lrm(glyhb > 7 ~ rcs(age,4) + rcs(bp.1s,3) + rcs(chol,3) +
+          frame + rcs(weight,4) + rcs(hip,3))
> h


Logistic Regression Model

lrm(formula = glyhb > 7 ~ rcs(age, 4) + rcs(bp.1s, 3) +
    rcs(chol, 3) + frame + rcs(weight, 4) + rcs(hip, 3))



Frequencies of Responses
 FALSE TRUE
   330   60

Frequencies of Missing Values Due to Each Variable
 glyhb > 7 age bp.1s chol frame weight hip
    13      0    0     0    0     0     0

 Obs Max Deriv Model L.R. d.f. P     C   Dxy Gamma Tau-a   R2 Brier
 390   1e-007      71.3   14 0 0.819 0.637 0.639 0.166 0.29 0.105
```

	Coef	S.E.	Wald Z	P
Intercept	-16.804027	6.40143	-2.63	0.0087
age	0.023219	0.08806	0.26	0.7920
age'	0.266699	0.25501	1.05	0.2956
age''	-0.852166	0.63708	-1.34	0.1810
bp.1s	0.028259	0.02476	1.14	0.2537
bp.1s'	-0.025207	0.02404	-1.05	0.2944
chol	0.004649	0.01004	0.46	0.6432
chol'	0.003535	0.01046	0.34	0.7354
frame=medium	-0.246480	0.48146	-0.51	0.6087
frame=large	-0.266503	0.53384	-0.50	0.6176
weight	0.042962	0.03073	1.40	0.1621
weight'	-0.088281	0.09463	-0.93	0.3509
weight''	0.264845	0.29109	0.91	0.3629
hip	0.033904	0.12479	0.27	0.7859
hip'	-0.053349	0.13979	-0.38	0.7027

```
> anova(h)
            Wald Statistics          Response: glyhb > 7
```

Factor	Chi-Square	d.f.	P
age	23.85	3	0.0000
Nonlinear	6.82	2	0.0331
bp.1s	1.32	2	0.5178
Nonlinear	1.10	1	0.2944
chol	5.45	2	0.0657
Nonlinear	0.11	1	0.7354
frame	0.29	2	0.8630
weight	5.41	3	0.1443
Nonlinear	0.87	2	0.6457
hip	0.19	2	0.9111
Nonlinear	0.15	1	0.7027
TOTAL NONLINEAR	10.48	7	0.1630
TOTAL	45.65	14	0.0000

So far the results seem to be the same as using a continuous response. How many predicted probabilities of diabetes are in the "rule-in" range?

```
> p ← predict(h, type='fitted')
> sum(p > .9, na.rm=T)
[1] 0
```

Only one patient had a predicted probability > 0.8. So the risk factors are just not very strong although age does explain significant preclinical variation in GHb.

Chapter 16

Introduction to Survival Analysis

16.1   Background

Suppose that one wished to study the occurrence of some event in a population of subjects. If the time until the occurrence of the event were unimportant, the event could be analyzed as a binary outcome using the logistic regression model. For example, in analyzing mortality associated with open heart surgery, it may not matter whether a patient dies during the procedure or he dies after being in a coma for two months. For other outcomes, especially those concerned with chronic conditions, the time until the event is important. In a study of emphysema, death at eight years after onset of symptoms is different from death at six months. An analysis that simply counted the number of deaths would be discarding valuable information and sacrificing statistical power.

Survival analysis is used to analyze data in which the time until the event is of interest. The response variable is the time until that event and is often called a *failure time, survival time,* or *event time.* Examples of responses of interest include the time until cardiovascular death, time until death or myocardial infarction, time until failure of a light bulb, time until pregnancy, or time until occurrence of an ECG abnormality during exercise on a treadmill. Bull and Spiegelhalter[58] have an excellent overview of survival analysis.

The response, event time, is usually continuous, but survival analysis allows the response to be incompletely determined for some subjects. For example, suppose that after a five-year follow-up study of survival after myocardial infarction a patient is still alive. That patient's survival time is *censored* on the right at five years; that is, her survival time is known only to exceed five years. The response value to be used in the analysis is 5+. Censoring can also occur when a subject is lost to follow-up.   ②

If no responses are censored, standard regression models for continuous responses could be used to analyze the failure times by writing the expected failure time as a function of one or more predictors, assuming that the distribution of failure time is properly specified. However, there are still several reasons for studying failure time using the specialized methods of survival analysis.

1. Time to failure can have an unusual distribution. Failure time is restricted to be positive so it has a skewed distribution and will never be normally distributed.

2. The probability of surviving past a certain time is often more relevant than the expected survival time (and expected survival time may be difficult to estimate if the amount of censoring is large).

3. A function used in survival analysis, the hazard function, helps one to understand the mechanism of failure.[212]

Survival analysis is used often in industrial life-testing experiments, and it is heavily used in clinical and epidemiologic follow-up studies. Examples include a randomized trial comparing a new drug to placebo for its ability to maintain remission in patients with leukemia, and an observational study of prognostic factors in coronary heart disease. In the latter example subjects may well be followed for varying lengths of time, as they may enter the study over a period of many years.

When regression models are used for survival analysis, all the advantages of these models can be brought to bear in analyzing failure times. Multiple, independent prognostic factors can be analyzed simultaneously and treatment differences can be assessed while adjusting for heterogeneity and imbalances in baseline characteristics. Also, patterns in outcome over time can be predicted for individual subjects.

Even in a simple well-designed experiment, survival modeling can allow one to do the following in addition to making simple comparisons.

1. Test for and describe interactions with treatment. Subgroup analyses can easily generate spurious results and they do not consider interacting factors in a dose-response manner. Once interactions are modeled, relative treatment benefits can be estimated (e.g., hazard ratios), and analyses can be done to determine if some patients are too sick or too well to have even a relative benefit.

2. Understand prognostic factors (strength and shape).

3. Model absolute effect of treatment. First, a model for the probability of surviving past time t is developed. Then differences in survival probabilities for

patients on treatments A and B can be estimated. The differences will be due primarily to sickness (overall risk) of the patient and to treatment interactions.

4. Understand time course of treatment effect. The period of maximum effect or period of any substantial effect can be estimated from a plot of relative effects of treatment over time.

5. Gain power for testing treatment effects.

6. Adjust for imbalances in treatment allocation.

The last two advantages of survival analysis are relatively minor in a randomized clinical trial since randomization is expected to balance measured and unmeasured prognostic factors, and since adjustment for balanced predictors does not gain as much power as in ordinary least squares models.

16.2   Censoring, Delayed Entry, and Truncation

Responses may be left–censored and interval–censored besides being right–censored. *Interval–censoring* is present, for example, when a measuring device functions only for a certain range of the response; measurements outside that range are censored at an end of the scale of the device. Interval–censoring also occurs when the presence of a medical condition is assessed during periodic exams. When the condition is present, the time until the condition developed is only known to be between the current and the previous exam. *Left–censoring* means that an event is known to have occurred before a certain time. In addition, *left–truncation* and *delayed entry* are common. Nomenclature is confusing as many authors refer to delayed entry as left–truncation. Left–truncation really means that an unknown subset of subjects failed before a certain time and the subjects didn't get into the study. For example, one might study the survival patterns of patients who were admitted to a tertiary care hospital. Patients who didn't survive long enough to be referred to the hospital comprise the left-truncated group, and interesting questions such as the optimum timing of admission to the hospital cannot be answered from the data set.

Delayed entry occurs in follow-up studies when subjects are exposed to the risk of interest only after varying periods of survival. For example, in a study of occupational exposure to a toxic compound, researchers may be interested in comparing life length of employees with life expectancy in the general population. A subject must live until the beginning of employment before exposure is possible; that is, death cannot be observed before employment. The start of follow-up is delayed until the start of employment and it may be right–censored when follow-up ends. In some studies, a researcher may want to assume that for the purpose of modeling the shape of the hazard function, time zero is the day of diagnosis of disease, while patients enter the study at various times since diagnosis. Delayed entry occurs for patients who don't enter the study until some time after their diagnosis. Patients who die before study entry are left-truncated. Note that the choice of time origin is very important.[37, 58, 77, 93]

Heart transplant studies have been analyzed by considering time zero to be the time of enrollment in the study. Pretransplant survival is right–censored at the time of transplant. Transplant survival experience is based on delayed entry into the "risk set" to recognize that a transplant patient is not at risk of dying from transplant failure until after a donor heart is found. In other words, survival experience is not credited to transplant surgery until the day of transplant. Comparisons of transplant experience with medical treatment suffer from "waiting time bias" if transplant survival begins on the day of transplant instead of using delayed entry.[147, 302, 385]

There are several planned mechanisms by which a response is right–censored. *Fixed type I* censoring occurs when a study is planned to end after two years of follow-up, or when a measuring device will only measure responses up to a certain limit. There the responses are observed only if they fall below a fixed value C. In *type II censoring*, a study ends when there is a prespecified number of events. If, for example, 100 mice are followed until 50 die, the censoring time is not known in advance.

We are concerned primarily with *random type I right-censoring* in which each subject's event time is observed only if the event occurs before a certain time, but the censoring time can vary between subjects. Whatever the cause of censoring, we assume that the censoring is *noninformative* about the event; that is, the censoring is caused by something that is independent of the impending failure. Censoring is noninformative when it is caused by planned termination of follow-up or by a subject moving out of town for reasons unrelated to the risk of the event. If subjects are removed from follow-up because of a worsening condition, the *informative censoring* will result in biased estimates and inaccurate statistical inference about the survival experience. For example, if a patient's response is censored because of an adverse effect of a drug or noncompliance to the drug, a serious bias can result if patients with adverse experiences or noncompliance are also at higher risk of suffering the outcome. In such studies, efficacy can only be assessed fairly using the *intention to treat principle*: all events should be attributed to the treatment *assigned* even if the subject is later removed from that treatment.

4

16.3   Notation, Survival, and Hazard Functions

In survival analysis we use T to denote the response variable, as the response is usually the time until an event. Instead of defining the statistical model for the response T in terms of the expected failure time, it is advantageous to define it in terms of the *survival function*, $S(t)$, given by

$$S(t) = \text{Prob}\{T > t\} = 1 - F(t), \tag{16.1}$$

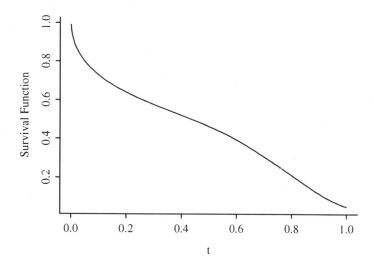

FIGURE 16.1: Survival function.

where $F(t)$ is the cumulative distribution function for T. If the event is death, $S(t)$ is the probability that death occurs after time t, that is, the probability that the subject will survive at least until time t. $S(t)$ is always 1 at $t = 0$; all subjects survive at least to time zero. The survival function must be nonincreasing as t increases. An example of a survival function is shown in Figure 16.1. In that example subjects are at very high risk of the event in the early period so that the $S(t)$ drops sharply. The risk is low for $0.1 \leq t \leq 0.6$, so $S(t)$ is somewhat flat. After $t = .6$ the risk again increases, so $S(t)$ drops more quickly.

Figure 16.2 depicts the *cumulative hazard function* corresponding to the survival function in Figure 16.1. This function is denoted by $\Lambda(t)$. It describes the accumulated risk up until time t, and as is shown later, is the negative of the log of the survival function. $\Lambda(t)$ is nondecreasing as t increases; that is, the accumulated risk increases or remains the same. Another important function is the *hazard function*, $\lambda(t)$, also called the *force of mortality*, or *instantaneous event (death, failure) rate*. The hazard at time t is related to the probability that the event will occur in a small interval around t, given that the event has not occurred before time t. By studying the event rate at a given time conditional on the event not having occurred by that time, one can learn about the mechanisms and forces of risk over time. Figure 16.3 depicts the hazard function corresponding to $S(t)$ in Figure 16.1. Notice that the hazard function allows one to more easily determine the phases of increased risk than looking for sudden drops in $S(t)$ or $\Lambda(t)$. The hazard function

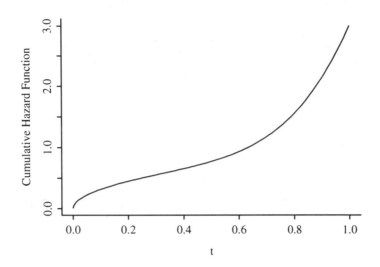

FIGURE 16.2: Cumulative hazard function.

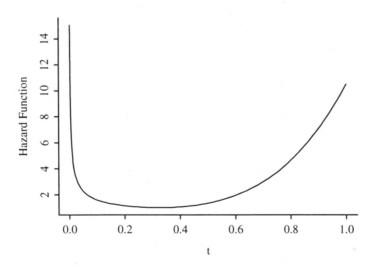

FIGURE 16.3: Hazard function.

is defined formally by

$$\lambda(t) = \lim_{u \to 0} \frac{\text{Prob}\{t < T \le t + u | T > t\}}{u}, \quad (16.2)$$

which using the law of conditional probability becomes

$$
\begin{aligned}
\lambda(t) &= \lim_{u \to 0} \frac{\text{Prob}\{t < T \le t + u\}/\text{Prob}\{T > t\}}{u} \\
&= \lim_{u \to 0} \frac{[F(t + u) - F(t)]/u}{S(t)} \\
&= \frac{\partial F(t)/\partial t}{S(t)} \quad (16.3) \\
&= \frac{f(t)}{S(t)},
\end{aligned}
$$

where $f(t)$ is the probability density function of T evaluated at t, the derivative or slope of the cumulative distribution function $1 - S(t)$. Since

$$\frac{\partial \log S(t)}{\partial t} = \frac{\partial S(t)/\partial t}{S(t)} = \frac{f(t)}{S(t)}, \quad (16.4)$$

the hazard function can also be expressed as

$$\lambda(t) = -\frac{\partial \log S(t)}{\partial t}, \quad (16.5)$$

the negative of the slope of the log of the survival function. Working backwards, the integral of $\lambda(t)$ is:

$$\int_0^t \lambda(v) dv = -\log S(t). \quad (16.6)$$

The integral or area under $\lambda(t)$ is defined to be $\Lambda(t)$, the cumulative hazard function. Therefore

$$\Lambda(t) = -\log S(t), \quad (16.7)$$

or

$$S(t) = \exp[-\Lambda(t)]. \quad (16.8)$$

So knowing any one of the functions $S(t)$, $\Lambda(t)$, or $\lambda(t)$ allows one to derive the other two functions. The three functions are different ways of describing the same distribution.

One property of $\Lambda(t)$ is that the expected value of $\Lambda(T)$ is unity, since if $T \sim S(t)$, the density of T is $\lambda(t)S(t)$ and

$$
\begin{aligned}
E[\Lambda(T)] &= \int_0^\infty \Lambda(t)\lambda(t)\exp(-\Lambda(t))dt \\
&= \int_0^\infty u\exp(-u)du \\
&= 1.
\end{aligned}
\tag{16.9}
$$

Now consider properties of the distribution of T. The population qth quantile (100qth percentile), T_q, is the time by which a fraction q of the subjects will fail. It is the value t such that $S(t) = 1 - q$; that is

$$
T_q = S^{-1}(1-q).
\tag{16.10}
$$

The median life length is the time by which half the subjects will fail, obtained by setting $S(t) = 0.5$:

$$
T_{0.5} = S^{-1}(0.5).
\tag{16.11}
$$

The qth quantile of T can also be computed by setting $\exp[-\Lambda(t)] = 1 - q$, giving

$$
\begin{aligned}
T_q &= \Lambda^{-1}[-\log(1-q)] \quad \text{and as a special case,} \\
T_{.5} &= \Lambda^{-1}(\log 2).
\end{aligned}
\tag{16.12}
$$

The mean or expected value of T (the expected failure time) is the area under the survival function for t ranging from 0 to ∞:

$$
\mu = \int_0^\infty S(v)dv.
\tag{16.13}
$$

Irwin has defined *mean restricted life* (see [229, 230]), which is the area under $S(t)$ up to a fixed time (usually chosen to be a point at which there is still adequate follow-up information).

The random variable T denotes a random failure time from the survival distribution $S(t)$. We need additional notation for the response and censoring information for the ith subject. Let T_i denote the response for the ith subject. This response is the time until the event of interest, and it may be censored if the subject is not followed long enough for the event to be observed. Let C_i denote the censoring time for the ith subject, and define the event indicator as

$$
\begin{aligned}
e_i &= 1 \quad \text{if the event was observed} \ (T_i \le C_i), \\
&= 0 \quad \text{if the response was censored} \ (T_i > C_i).
\end{aligned}
\tag{16.14}
$$

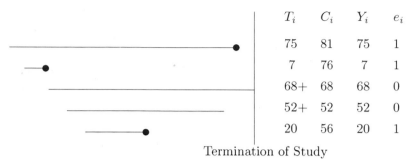

	T_i	C_i	Y_i	e_i
	75	81	75	1
	7	76	7	1
	68+	68	68	0
	52+	52	52	0
	20	56	20	1

Termination of Study

FIGURE 16.4: Some censored data. Circles denote events.

The observed response is

$$Y_i = \min(T_i, C_i), \tag{16.15}$$

which is the time that occurred first: the failure time or the censoring time. The pair of values (Y_i, e_i) contains all the response information for most purposes (i.e., the potential censoring time C_i is not usually of interest if the event occurred before C_i).

Figure 16.4 demonstrates this notation. The line segments start at study entry (survival time $t = 0$).

A useful property of the cumulative hazard function can be derived as follows. Let z be any cutoff time and consider the expected value of Λ evaluated at the earlier of the cutoff time or the actual failure time.

$$
\begin{aligned}
E[\Lambda(\min(T, z))] &= E[\Lambda(T)I(T \leq z) + \Lambda(z)I(T > z)] \\
&= E[\Lambda(T)I(T \leq z)] + \Lambda(z)S(z).
\end{aligned} \tag{16.16}
$$

Here $I(s)$ is the indicator function so that $I(s) = 1$ is s is true. The first term in the right–hand side is

$$
\begin{aligned}
&\int_0^\infty \Lambda(t)I(t \leq z)\lambda(t)\exp(-\Lambda(t))dt \\
&= \int_0^z \Lambda(t)\lambda(t)\exp(-\Lambda(t))dt \\
&= -[u\exp(-u) + \exp(-u)]\big|_0^{\Lambda(z)} \\
&= 1 - S(z)[\Lambda(z) + 1].
\end{aligned} \tag{16.17}
$$

Adding $\Lambda(z)S(z)$ results in

$$E[\Lambda(\min(T, z))] = 1 - S(z) = F(z). \tag{16.18}$$

It follows that $\sum_{i=1}^{n} \Lambda(\min(T_i, z))$ estimates the expected number of failures occurring before time z among the n subjects.

⑤

16.4   Homogeneous Failure Time Distributions

In this section we assume that each subject in the sample has the same distribution of the random variable T that represents the time until the event. In particular, there are no covariables that describe differences between subjects in the distribution of T. As before we use $S(t)$, $\lambda(t)$, and $\Lambda(t)$ to denote, respectively, the survival, hazard, and cumulative hazard functions.

The form of the true population survival distribution function $S(t)$ is almost always unknown, and many distributional forms have been used for describing failure time data. We consider first the two most popular parametric survival distributions: the exponential and Weibull distributions. The exponential distribution is a very simple one in which the hazard function is constant; that is, $\lambda(t) = \lambda$. The cumulative hazard and survival functions are then

$$
\begin{aligned}
\Lambda(t) &= \lambda t \quad \text{and} \\
S(t) &= \exp(-\Lambda(t)) = \exp(-\lambda t).
\end{aligned}
\tag{16.19}
$$

The median life length is $\Lambda^{-1}(\log 2)$ or

$$
T_{0.5} = \log(2)/\lambda.
\tag{16.20}
$$

The time by which $1/2$ of the subjects will have failed is then proportional to the reciprocal of the constant hazard rate λ . This is true also of the expected or mean life length, which is $1/\lambda$.

The exponential distribution is one of the few distributions for which a closed-form solution exists for the estimator of its parameter when censoring is present. This estimator is a function of the number of events and the total *person-years* of exposure. Methods based on person-years in fact implicitly assume an exponential distribution. The exponential distribution is often used to model events that occur "at random in time."[221] It has the property that the future lifetime of a subject is the same, no matter how "old" it is, or

$$
\text{Prob}\{T > t_0 + t | T > t_0\} = \text{Prob}\{T > t\}.
\tag{16.21}
$$

This "ageless" property also makes the exponential distribution a poor choice for modeling human survival except over short time periods.

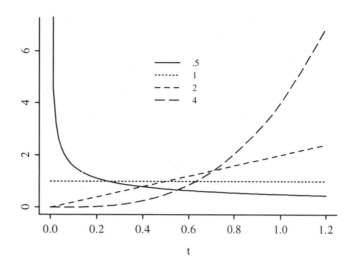

FIGURE 16.5: Some Weibull hazard functions with $\alpha = 1$ and various values of γ.

The Weibull distribution is a generalization of the exponential distribution. Its hazard, cumulative hazard, and survival functions are given by

$$
\begin{aligned}
\lambda(t) &= \alpha\gamma t^{\gamma-1} \\
\Lambda(t) &= \alpha t^{\gamma} \\
S(t) &= \exp(-\alpha t^{\gamma}).
\end{aligned}
\tag{16.22}
$$

The Weibull distribution with $\gamma = 1$ is an exponential distribution (with constant hazard). When $\gamma > 1$, its hazard is increasing with t, and when $\gamma < 1$ its hazard is decreasing. Figure 16.5 depicts some of the shapes of the hazard function that are possible. If T has a Weibull distribution, the median of T is

$$
T_{0.5} = [(\log 2)/\alpha]^{1/\gamma}.
\tag{16.23}
$$

There are many other traditional parametric survival distributions, some of which have hazards that are "bathtub shaped" as in Figure 16.3.[166, 221] The restricted cubic spline function described in Section 2.4.4 is an alternative basis for $\lambda(t)$.[196, 197] This function family allows for any shape of smooth $\lambda(t)$ since the number of knots can be increased as needed, subject to the number of events in the sample. Nonlinear terms in the spline function can be tested to assess linearity of hazard (Rayleighness) or constant hazard (exponentiality).

6

The restricted cubic spline hazard model with k knots is

$$\lambda_k(t) = a + bt + \sum_{j=1}^{k-2} \gamma_j w_j(t), \tag{16.24}$$

where the $w_j(t)$ are the restricted cubic spline terms of Equation 2.25. There terms are cubic terms in t. A set of knots $v_1, \ldots, v_k$ is selected from the quantiles of the uncensored failure times (see Section 2.4.4 and [196]).

The cumulative hazard function for this model is

$$\Lambda(t) = at + \frac{1}{2}t^2 + \frac{1}{4} \times \text{ quartic terms in t.} \tag{16.25}$$

Standard maximum likelihood theory is used to obtain estimates of the k unknown parameters to derive, for example, smooth estimates of $\lambda(t)$ with confidence bands. The flexible estimates of $S(t)$ using this method are as efficient as Kaplan–Meier estimates, but they are smooth and can be used as a basis for modeling predictor variables. The spline hazard model is particularly useful for fitting steeply falling and gently rising hazard functions that are characteristic of high-risk medical procedures.

16.5   Nonparametric Estimation of S and Λ

16.5.1   Kaplan–Meier Estimator

As the true form of the survival distribution is seldom known, it is useful to estimate the distribution without making any assumptions. For many analyses, this may be the last step, while in others this step helps one select a statistical model for more in-depth analyses. When no event times are censored, a nonparametric estimator of $S(t)$ is $1 - F_n(t)$ where $F_n(t)$ is the usual empirical cumulative distribution function based on the observed failure times $T_1, \ldots, T_n$. Let $S_n(t)$ denote this empirical survival function. $S_n(t)$ is given by the fraction of observed failure times that exceed t:

$$S_n(t) = [\text{number of } T_i > t]/n. \tag{16.26}$$

When censoring is present, $S(t)$ can be estimated (at least for t up until the end of follow-up) by the Kaplan–Meier[228] product-limit estimator. This method is based on conditional probabilities. For example, suppose that every subject has been followed for 39 days or has died within 39 days so that the proportion of subjects surviving at least 39 days can be computed. After 39 days, some subjects may be lost to follow-up besides those removed from follow-up because of death within 39 days. The proportion of those still followed 39 days who survive day 40 is computed. The probability of surviving 40 days from study entry equals the probability of surviving day 40 after living 39 days, multiplied by the chance of surviving 39 days.

TABLE 16.1

Day	No. Subjects At Risk	Deaths	Censored	Cumulative Survival
12	100	1	0	$99/100 = .99$
30	99	2	1	$97/99 \times 99/100 = .97$
60	96	0	3	$96/96 \times .97 = .97$
72	93	3	0	$90/93 \times .97 = .94$
.	.	.	.	.
.	.	.	.	.

The life table in Table 16.1 demonstrates the method in more detail. We suppose that 100 subjects enter the study and none die or are lost before day 12.

Times in a life table should be measured as precisely as possible. If the event being analyzed is death, the failure time should usually be specified to the nearest day. We assume that deaths occur on the day indicated and that being censored on a certain day implies the subject survived through the end of that day. The data used in computing Kaplan–Meier estimates consist of $(Y_i, e_i), i = 1, 2, \ldots, n$ using notation defined previously. Primary data collected to derive (Y_i, e_i) usually consist of entry date, event date (if subject failed), and censoring date (if subject did not fail). Instead, the entry date, date of event/censoring, and event/censoring indicator e_i may be specified.

The Kaplan–Meier estimator is called the product-limit estimator because it is the limiting case of actuarial survival estimates as the time periods shrink so that an entry is made for each failure time. An entry need not be in the table for censoring times (when no failures occur at that time) as long as the number of subjects censored is subtracted from the next number at risk. Kaplan–Meier estimates are preferred to actuarial estimates because they provide more resolution and make fewer assumptions. In constructing a yearly actuarial life table, for example, it is traditionally assumed that subjects censored between two years were followed 0.5 years.

The product-limit estimator is a nonparametric maximum likelihood estimator [226, pp. 10–13]. The formula for the Kaplan–Meier product-limit estimator of $S(t)$ is as follows. Let k denote the number of failures in the sample and let $t_1, t_2, \ldots, t_k$ denote the unique event times (ordered for ease of calculation). Let d_i denote the number of failures at t_i and n_i be the number of subjects *at risk* at time t_i; that is, n_i = number of failure/censoring times $> t_i$. The estimator is then

$$S_{\mathrm{KM}}(t) = \prod_{i:t_i < t} (1 - d_i/n_i). \tag{16.27}$$

TABLE 16.2

i	t_i	n_i	d_i	$(n_i - d_i)/n_i$
1	1	7	1	6/7
2	3	6	2	4/6
3	9	2	1	1/2

The Kaplan–Meier estimator of $\Lambda(t)$ is $\Lambda_{\mathrm{KM}}(t) = -\log S_{\mathrm{KM}}(t)$. An estimate of quantile q of failure time is $S_{\mathrm{KM}}^{-1}(1 - q)$, if follow-up is long enough so that $S_{\mathrm{KM}}(t)$ drops as low as $1 - q$. If the last subject followed failed so that $S_{\mathrm{KM}}(t)$ drops to zero, the expected failure time can be estimated by computing the area under the Kaplan–Meier curve.

To demonstrate computation of $S_{\mathrm{KM}}(t)$, imagine a sample of failure times given by

$$1 \quad 3 \quad 3 \quad 6^+ \quad 8^+ \quad 9 \quad 10^+,$$

where + denotes a censored time. The quantities needed to compute S_{KM} are in Table 16.2. Thus

$$
\begin{aligned}
S_{\mathrm{KM}}(t) &= 1, \quad 0 \le t < 1 \\
&= 6/7 = .85, \quad 1 \le t < 3 \\
&= (6/7)(4/6) = .57, \quad 3 \le t < 9 \\
&= (6/7)(4/6)(1/2) = .29, \quad 9 \le t < 10.
\end{aligned}
\tag{16.28}
$$

Note that the estimate of $S(t)$ is undefined for $t > 10$ since not all subjects have failed by $t = 10$ but no follow-up extends beyond $t = 10$. A graph of the Kaplan–Meier estimate is found in Figure 16.6.

The variance of $S_{\mathrm{KM}}(t)$ can be estimated using Greenwood's formula [226, p. 14], and using normality of $S_{\mathrm{KM}}(t)$ in large samples this variance can be used to derive a confidence interval for $S(t)$. A better method is to derive an asymmetric confidence interval for $S(t)$ based on a symmetric interval for $\log \Lambda(t)$. This latter method ensures that a confidence limit does not exceed one or fall below zero, and is more accurate since $\log \Lambda_{\mathrm{KM}}(t)$ is more normally distributed than $S_{\mathrm{KM}}(t)$. Once a confidence interval, say $[a, b]$ is determined for $\log \Lambda(t)$, the confidence interval for $S(t)$ is computed by $[\exp\{-\exp(b)\}, \exp\{-\exp(a)\}]$. The formula for an estimate of the variance of interest is [226, p. 15]:

$$
\mathrm{Var}\{\log \Lambda_{\mathrm{KM}}(t)\} = \frac{\sum_{i:t_i < t} d_i/[n_i(n_i - d_i)]}{\{\sum_{i:t_i < t} \log[(n_i - d_i)/n_i]\}^2}.
\tag{16.29}
$$

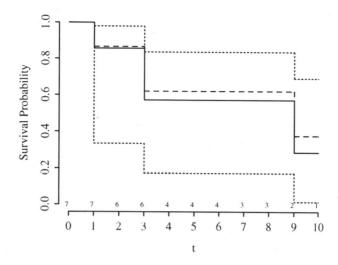

FIGURE 16.6:   Kaplan–Meier product-limit estimator with 0.95 confidence bands. The Altschuler–Nelson–Aalen–Fleming–Harrington estimator is depicted with the dashed lines.

Letting s denote the square root of this variance estimate, an approximate $1 - \alpha$ confidence interval for $\log \Lambda(t)$ is given by $\log \Lambda_{\mathrm{KM}}(t) \pm zs$, where z is the $1 - \alpha/2$ standard normal critical value. After simplification, the confidence interval for $S(t)$ becomes

$$S_{\mathrm{KM}}(t)^{\exp(\pm zs)}. \tag{16.30}$$

Note that confidence limits constructed in this manner are not defined for $t >$ last failure/censoring time if the last time represents a failure (i.e., if S_{KM} drops to zero).

Miller[316] showed that if the parametric form of $S(t)$ is known to be Weibull with known shape parameter, the Kaplan–Meier estimator is very inefficient (i.e., has high variance) when compared to the parametric maximum likelihood estimator.

16.5.2   Altschuler–Nelson Estimator

Altschuler[14], Nelson[323], Aalen[1] and Fleming and Harrington[140] proposed estimators of $\Lambda(t)$ or of $S(t)$ based on an estimator of $\Lambda(t)$:

$$\hat{\Lambda}(t) = \sum_{i:t_i < t} \frac{d_i}{n_i}$$
$$S_\Lambda(t) = \exp(-\hat{\Lambda}(t)). \tag{16.31}$$

$S_\Lambda(t)$ has advantages over $S_{\mathrm{KM}}(t)$. First, $\sum_{i=1}^{n} \hat{\Lambda}(Y_i) = \sum_{i=1}^{n} e_i$ [412, Appendix 3]. In other words, the estimator gives the correct expected number of events. Second, there is a wealth of asymptotic theory based on the Altschuler–Nelson estimator.[140]

See Figure 16.6 for an example of the $S_\Lambda(t)$ estimator. This estimator has the same variance as $S_{\mathrm{KM}}(t)$ for large enough samples.   9

16.6   Analysis of Multiple Endpoints

Clinical studies frequently assess multiple endpoints. A cancer clinical trial may, for example, involve recurrence of disease and death, whereas a cardiovascular trial may involve nonfatal myocardial infarction and death. Endpoints may be combined, and the new event (e.g., time until infarction or death) may be analyzed with any of the tools of survival analysis because only the usual censoring mechanism is used. Sometimes the various endpoints may need separate study, however, because they may have different risk factors.

When the multiple endpoints represent multiple causes of a terminating event (e.g., death), Prentice et al. have developed standard methods for analyzing cause-specific hazards[344] [226, pp. 163–178]. Their methods allow each cause of failure to be analyzed separately, censoring on the other causes. They do not assume any mechanism for cause removal nor make any assumptions regarding the interrelation among causes of failure. However, analyses of competing events using data where some causes of failure are removed in a different way from the original dataset will give rise to different inferences.

When the multiple endpoints represent a mixture of fatal and nonfatal outcomes, the analysis may be more complex. The same is true when one wishes to jointly study an event-time endpoint and a repeated measurement.   10

16.6.1   Competing Risks

When events are independent, each event may also be analyzed separately by censoring on all other events as well as censoring on loss to follow-up. This will yield an unbiased estimate of an easily interpreted cause-specific $\lambda(t)$ or $S(t)$ because censoring is noninformative [226, pp. 168–169]. One minus $S_{\mathrm{KM}}(t)$ computed in this manner will correctly estimate the probability of failing from the event in the absence of other events. Even when the competing events are not independent, the cause-specific hazard model may lead to valid results, but the resulting model does not allow one to estimate risks conditional on removal of one or more causes of the event. See Kay[233] for a nice example of competing risks analysis when a treatment reduces the risk of death from one cause but increases the risk of death from another cause.   11

Larson and Dinse[258] have an interesting approach that jointly models the time until (any) failure and the failure type. For r failure types, they use an r-category polytomous logistic model to predict the probability of failing from each cause. They assume that censoring is unrelated to cause of event.

16.6.2 Competing Dependent Risks

In many medical and epidemiologic studies one is interested in analyzing multiple causes of death. If the goal is to estimate cause-specific failure probabilities, treating subjects dying from extraneous causes as censored and then computing the ordinary Kaplan–Meier estimate results in biased (high) survival estimates[148, 154]. If cause m is of interest, the cause-specific hazard function is defined as

$$\lambda_m(t) = \lim_{u \to 0} \frac{\Pr\{\text{fail from cause } m \text{ in } [t, t+u) | \text{alive at } t\}}{u}. \tag{16.32}$$

The *cumulative incidence function* or probability of failure from cause m by time t is given by

$$F_m(t) = \int_0^t \lambda_m(u) S(u) du, \tag{16.33}$$

where $S(u)$ is the probability of surviving (ignoring cause of death), which equals $\exp[-\int_0^u (\sum \lambda_m(x)) dx]$ [148]; [306, Chapter 10]; [71, 281]. As previously mentioned, $1 - F_m(t) = \exp[-\int_0^t \lambda_m(u) du]$ only if failures due to other causes are eliminated and if the cause-specific hazard of interest remains unchanged in doing so.[148]

Again letting $t_1, t_2, \ldots, t_k$ denote the unique ordered failure times, a nonparametric estimate of $F_m(t)$ is given by

$$\hat{F}_m(t) = \sum_{i: t_i \le t} \frac{d_{mi}}{n_i} S_{\text{KM}}(t_{i-1}), \tag{16.34}$$

where d_{mi} is the number of failures of type m at time t_i and n_i is the number of subjects at risk of failure at t_i.

Pepe and others[330, 332, 333] showed how to use a combination of Kaplan–Meier estimators to derive an estimator of the probability of being free of event 1 by time t given event 2 has not occurred by time t (see also [238]). Let T_1 and T_2 denote, respectively, the times until events 1 and 2. Let $S_1(t)$ and $S_2(t)$ denote, respectively, the two survival functions. Let us suppose that event 1 is not a terminating event (e.g., is not death) and that even after event 1 subjects are followed to ascertain occurrences of event 2. The probability that $T_1 > t$ given $T_2 > t$ is

$$\begin{aligned} \Pr\{T_1 > t | T_2 > t\} &= \frac{\Pr\{T_1 > t \text{ and } T_2 > t\}}{\Pr\{T_2 > t\}} \\ &= \frac{S_{12}(t)}{S_2(t)}, \end{aligned} \tag{16.35}$$

where $S_{12}(t)$ is the survival function for $\min(T_1, T_2)$, the earlier of the two events. Since $S_{12}(t)$ does not involve any informative censoring (assuming as always that loss to follow-up is noninformative), S_{12} may be estimated by the Kaplan–Meier estimator $S_{\mathrm{KM}_{12}}$ (or by S_Λ). For the type of event 1 we have discussed above, S_2 can also be estimated without bias by S_{KM_2}. Thus we estimate, for example, the probability that a subject still alive at time t will be free of myocardial infarction as of time t by $S_{\mathrm{KM}_{12}}/S_{\mathrm{KM}_2}$.

Another quantity that can easily be computed from ordinary survival estimates is $S_2(t) - S_{12}(t) = [1 - S_{12}(t)] - [1 - S_2(t)]$, which is the probability that event 1 occurs by time t and that event 2 has not occurred by time t.

The ratio estimate above is used to estimate the survival function for one event given that another has not occurred. Another function of interest is the *crude survival function* which is a *marginal* distribution; that is, it is the probability that $T_1 > t$ whether or not event 2 occurs:[245]

$$
\begin{aligned}
S_c(t) &= 1 - F_1(t) \\
F_1(t) &= \mathrm{Prob}\{T_1 \le t\},
\end{aligned}
\tag{16.36}
$$

where $F_1(t)$ is the *crude incidence function* defined previously. Note that the $T_1 \le t$ implies that the occurrence of event 1 is part of the probability being computed. If event 2 is a terminating event so that some subjects can never suffer event 1, the crude survival function for T_1 will never drop to zero. The crude survival function can be interpreted as the survival distribution of W where $W = T_1$ if $T_1 < T_2$ and $W = \infty$ otherwise.[245]

16.6.3 State Transitions and Multiple Types of Nonfatal Events

In many studies there is one final, absorbing state (death, all causes) and multiple live states. The live states may represent different health states or phases of a disease. For example, subjects may be completely free of cancer, have an isolated tumor, metastasize to a distant organ, and die. Unlike this example, the live states need not have a definite ordering. One may be interested in estimating *transition probabilities*, for example, the probability $\pi_{ij}(t_1, t_2)$ that an individual in state i at time t_1 is in state j after an additional time t_2. Strauss and Shavelle[404] have developed an extended Kaplan–Meier estimator for this situation. Let $S^i_{KM}(t|t_1)$ denote the ordinary Kaplan–Meier estimate of the probability of not dying before time t (ignoring distinctions between multiple live states) for a cohort of subjects beginning follow-up at time t_1 in state i. This is an estimate of the probability of surviving an additional t time units (in any live state) given that the subject was alive and in state i at time t_1. Strauss and Shavelle's estimator is given by

$$
\pi_{ij}(t_1, t_2) = \frac{n_{ij}(t_1, t_2)}{n_i(t_1, t_2)} S^i_{KM}(t_2|t_1),
\tag{16.37}
$$

where $n_i(t_1, t_2)$ is the number of subjects in live state i at time t_1 who are alive and uncensored t_2 time units later, and $n_{ij}(t_1, t_2)$ is the number of such subjects in state j t_2 time units beyond t_1.

12

16.6.4 Joint Analysis of Time and Severity of an Event

In some studies, an endpoint is given more weight if it occurs earlier or if it is more severe clinically, or both. For example, the event of interest may be myocardial infarction, which may be of any severity from minimal damage to the left ventricle to a fatal infarction. Berridge and Whitehead[36] have provided a promising model for the analysis of such endpoints. Their method assumes that the severity of endpoints which do occur is measured on an ordinal categorical scale and that severity is assessed at the time of the event. Berridge and Whitehead's example was time until first headache, with severity of headaches graded on an ordinal scale. They proposed a joint hazard of an individual who responds with ordered category j:

$$\lambda_j(t) - \lambda(t)\pi_j(t), \qquad (16.38)$$

where $\lambda(t)$ is the hazard for the failure time and $\pi_j(t)$ is the probability of an individual having event severity j given she fails at time t. Note that a shift in the distribution of response severity is allowed as the time until the event increases.

13

16.6.5 Analysis of Multiple Events

It is common to choose as an endpoint in a clinical trial an event that can recur. Examples include myocardial infarction, gastric ulcer, pregnancy, and infection. Using only the time until the first event can result in a loss of statistical information and power.[a] There are specialized multivariate survival models (whose assumptions are extremely difficult to verify) for handling this setup, but in many cases a simpler approach will be efficient.

The simpler approach involves modeling the marginal distribution of the time until each event.[280, 331] Here one forms one record per subject per event, and the survival time is the time to the first event for the first record, or is the time from the previous event to the next event for all later records. This approach yields consistent estimates of distribution parameters as long as the marginal distributions are correctly specified.[447] One can allow the number of previous events to influence the hazard function of another event by modeling this count as a covariable.

The multiple events within subject are not independent, so variance estimates must be corrected for intracluster correlation. The clustered sandwich covariance

---

[a]An exception to this is the case in which once an event occurs for the first time, that event is likely to recur multiple times for any patient. Then the latter occurrences are redundant.

matrix estimator described in Section 9.5 and in [280] will provide consistent estimates of variances and covariances even if the events are dependent. Lin[280] also discussed how this method can easily be used to model multiple events of differing types.

14

16.7   S-Plus Functions

The `event.chart` function of Lee et al.[275] will draw a variety of charts for displaying raw survival time data, for both single and multiple events per subject. Relationships with covariables can also be displayed. This function is in the `Hmisc` library.

The analyses described in this chapter can be viewed as special cases of the Cox proportional hazards model.[92] The programs for Cox model analyses described in Section 19.12 can be used to obtain the results described here, as long as there is at least one stratification factor in the model. There are, however, several S-Plus functions that are pertinent to the homogeneous or stratified case. The S-Plus function `survfit`, and its particular renditions of the print, plot, lines, and points generic functions (all part of the `survival` library written by Terry Therneau) will compute, print, and plot Kaplan–Meier and Nelson survival estimates. Confidence intervals for $S(t)$ may be based on S, Λ, or $\log \Lambda$. `survfit` and other functions described in later chapters use Therneau's `Surv` function to combine the response variable and event indicator into a single S-Plus "survival time" object. In its simplest form, use `Surv(y, event)`, where `y` is the failure/right–censoring time and `event` is the event/censoring indicator, usually coded `T/F`, $0 =$ censored $1 =$ event or $1 =$ censored $2 =$ event. If the event status variable has other coding (e.g., 3 means death), use `Surv(y, s==3)`. To handle interval time-dependent covariables, or to use Andersen and Gill's *counting process* formulation of the Cox model,[16] use the notation `Surv(tstart, tstop, status)`. The counting process notation allows subjects to enter and leave risk sets at random. For each time interval for each subject, the interval is made up of `tstart`$< t \leq$`tstop`. For time-dependent stratification, there is an optional `origin` argument to `Surv` that indicates the hazard shape time origin at the time of crossover to a new stratum. A `type` argument is used to handle left– and interval–censoring, especially for parametric survival models. Possible values of `type` are `"left"`,`"right"`,`"counting"`,`"interval"`,`"interval2"`.

The `Surv` expression will usually be used inside another function, but it is fine to save the result of `Surv` in another object and to use this object in the particular fitting function.

`survfit` is invoked by the following, with default parameter settings indicated.

```
units(y) <- "Month"
# Default is "Day" - used for axis labels, etc.
survfit(Surv(y, event) ~ svar1 + svar2 + ... , data, subset,
        na.action=na.delete,
```

```
        type=c("kaplan-meier","fleming-harrington"),
        error=c("greenwood","tsiatis"), se.fit=T,
        conf.int=.95,
        conf.type=c("log-log","log","plain","none"))
```

If there are no stratification variables (svar1, ...), omit them. To print a table of estimates, use

```
    f ← survfit(. . .)
    print(f)      # print brief summary of f
    summary(f, times, censored=F, digits=3)
```

For failure times stored in days, use

```
    f ← survfit(Surv(futime, event) ∼ sex)
    summary(f, seq(30,180,by=30))
```

to print monthly estimates.

To plot the object returned by survfit, use

```
    plot(f, conf.int=T, mark.time=T, mark=3, col=1, lty=1,
        lwd=1, cex=1, log=F, yscale=1, xscale=1,
        xlab="", ylab="", xaxs="i", ...)
```

This invokes plot.survfit. You can also use survplot (here, actually survplot.-survfit) for other options that include automatic curve labeling and showing the number of subjects at risk at selected times. Figure 16.6 was drawn with the statements

```
    tt ← c(1,3,3,6,8,9,10)
    stat ← c(1,1,1,0,0,1,0)
    S ← Surv(tt, stat)
    survplot(survfit(S),conf="bands",n.risk=T,xlab="t")
    survplot(survfit(S, type="fleming-harrington", conf.int=F),
        add=T, lty=3)
```

Stratified estimates, with four treatments distinguished by line type and curve labels, could be drawn by

```
    units(y) <- "Year"
    f ← survfit(Surv(y, stat) ∼ treatment)
    survplot(f, ylab="Fraction Pain-Free")
```

The groupkm in Design computes and optionally plots $S_{KM}(u)$ or $\log \Lambda_{KM}(u)$ (if loglog=T) for fixed u with automatic stratification on a continuous predictor x. As in cut2 (Section 6.2) you can specify the number of subjects per interval (default is m=50), the number of quantile groups (g), or the actual cutpoints (cuts). groupkm plots the survival or log–log survival estimate against mean x in each x interval.

The `bootkm` function in the `Hmisc` library bootstraps Kaplan–Meier survival estimates or Kaplan–Meier estimates of quantiles of the survival time distribution. It is easy to use `bootkm` to compute, for example, a nonparametric confidence interval for the ratio of median survival times for two groups.

See the Web site for a list of functions from other users for nonparametric estimation of $S(t)$ with left–, right–, and interval–censored data. The adaptive linear spline log-hazard fitting function `heft`[244] is in `StatLib`.

16.8   Further Reading

[1] Some excellent general references for survival analysis are [40, 58, 80, 93, 141, 195, 212, 226, 239, 264, 273, 306, 327, 388, 411].

[2] See Goldman,[151] Bull and Spiegelhalter,[58] and Lee et al.[275] for ways to construct descriptive graphs depicting right–censored data.

[3] Some useful references for left–truncation are [58, 77, 167, 351].

[4] See [266, p. 164] for some ideas for detecting informative censoring. Bilker and Wang[38] discuss *right–truncation* and contrast it with right–censoring.

[5] Arjas[22] has applications based on properties of the cumulative hazard function.

[6] Kooperberg et al.[244, 402] have an adaptive method for fitting hazard functions using linear splines in the log hazard. Mudholkar et al.[319] presented a generalized Weibull model allowing for a variety of hazard shapes.

[7] Hollander et al.[207] provide a nonparametric *simultaneous* confidence band for $S(t)$, surprisingly using likelihood ratio methods.

[8] See [454] for a discussion of how the efficiency of Kaplan–Meier estimators can be improved by interpolation as opposed to piecewise flat step functions. That paper also discusses a variety of other estimators, some of which are significantly more efficient than Kaplan–Meier.

[9] See [77, 167, 302, 385, 420, 423] for methods of estimating S or Λ in the presence of left–truncation. See Turnbull[422] for nonparametric estimation of $S(t)$ with left–, right–, and interval–censoring, and Kooperberg and Clarkson[243] for a flexible parametric approach to modeling that allows for interval–censoring. Lindsey and Ryan[285] have a nice tutorial on the analysis of interval–censored data.

[10] Hogan and Laird[205, 206] developed methods for dealing with mixtures of fatal and nonfatal outcomes, including some ideas for handling outcome-related dropouts on the repeated measurements. See also Finkelstein and Schoenfeld.[138] The 30 April 1997 issue of *Statistics in Medicine* (Vol. 16) is devoted to methods for analyzing multiple endpoints as well as designing multiple endpoint studies. The papers in that issue are invaluable, as is Therneau and Hamilton[413] and Therneau and Grambsch.[411]

[11] See Lunn and McNeil[296] and Marubini and Valsecchi [306, Chapter 10] for practical approaches to analyzing competing risks using ordinary Cox proportional hazards models. A nice overview of competing risks with comparisons of various approaches is found in Tai et al..[407]

12   Shen and Thall[384] have developed a flexible parametric approach to multistate survival analysis.

13   Lancar et al.[255] developed a method for analyzing repeated events of varying severities.

14   Lawless and Nadeau[266] have a very good description of models dealing with recurrent events. They use the notion of the *cumulative mean function*, which is the expected number of events experienced by a subject by a certain time. Lawless[265] contrasts this approach with other approaches. See Aalen et al.[3] for a nice example in which multivariate failure times (time to failure of fillings in multiple teeth per subject) are analyzed. Francis and Fuller[144] developed a graphical device for depicting complex event history data. Therneau and Hamilton[413] have very informative comparisons of various methods for modeling multiple events, showing the importance of whether the analyst starts the clock over after each event. Kelly and Lim[235] have another very useful paper comparing various methods for analzing recurrent events. Wang and Chang[442] demonstrated the difficulty of using Kaplan–Meier estimates for recurrence time data.

16.9 Problems

1. Make a rough drawing of a hazard function from birth for a man who develops significant coronary artery disease at age 50 and undergoes coronary artery bypass surgery at age 55.

2. Define in words the relationship between the hazard function and the survival function.

3. In a study of the life expectancy of light bulbs as a function of the bulb's wattage, 100 bulbs of various wattage ratings were tested until each had failed. What is wrong with using the product-moment linear correlation test to test whether wattage is associated with life length concerning (a) distributional assumptions and (b) other assumptions?

4. A placebo-controlled study is undertaken to ascertain whether a new drug decreases mortality. During the study, some subjects are withdrawn because of moderate to severe side effects. Assessment of side effects and withdrawal of patients is done on a blinded basis. What statistical technique can be used to obtain an unbiased treatment comparison of survival times? State at least one efficacy endpoint that can be analyzed unbiasedly.

5. Consider long-term follow-up of patients in the support dataset. What proportion of the patients have censored survival times? Does this imply that one cannot make accurate estimates of chances of survival? Make a histogram or empirical distribution function estimate of the *censored* follow-up times. What is the typical follow-up duration for a patient in the study who has survived so

far? What is the typical survival time for patients who have died? Taking censoring into account, what is the median survival time from the Kaplan–Meier estimate of the overall survival function? Estimate the median graphically or using any other sensible method.

6. Plot Kaplan–Meier survival function estimates stratified by `dzclass`. Estimate the median survival time and the first quartile of time until death for each of the four disease classes.

7. Repeat Problem 6 except for tertiles of `meanbp`.

8. The commonly used log-rank test for comparing survival times between groups of patients is a special case of the test of association between the grouping variable and survival time in a Cox proportional hazards regression model. Depending on how one handles tied failure times, the log-rank χ^2 statistic exactly equals the score χ^2 statistic from the Cox model, and the likelihood ratio and Wald χ^2 test statistics are also appropriate. To obtain global score or LR χ^2 tests and P-values you can use a statement[b] such as

   ```
   cph(Survobject ~ predictor)
   ```

   where `Survobject` is a survival time object created by the `Surv` function. Obtain the log-rank (score) χ^2 statistic, degrees of freedom, and P-value for testing for differences in survival time between levels of `dzclass`. Interpret this test, referring to the graph you produced in Problem 6 if needed.

9. Do preliminary analyses of survival time using the Mayo Clinic primary biliary cirrhosis dataset described in Section 8.12. Make graphs of Altschuler–Nelson or Kaplan–Meier survival estimates stratified separately by a few categorical predictors and by categorized versions of one or two continuous predictors. Estimate median failure time for the various strata. You may want to suppress confidence bands when showing multiple strata on one graph. See [244] for parametric fits to the survival and hazard function for this dataset.

---

[b] `cph` is in the **Design** library. It is similar to the built-in **coxph** function.

Chapter 17

Parametric Survival Models

17.1 Homogeneous Models (No Predictors)

The nonparametric estimator of $S(t)$ is a very good descriptive statistic for displaying survival data. For many purposes, however, one may want to make more assumptions to allow the data to be modeled in more detail. By specifying a functional form for $S(t)$ and estimating any unknown parameters in this function, one can

1. easily compute selected quantiles of the survival distribution;

2. estimate (usually by extrapolation) the expected failure time;

3. derive a concise equation and smooth function for estimating $S(t)$, $\Lambda(t)$, and $\lambda(t)$; and

4. estimate $S(t)$ more precisely than $S_{\text{KM}}(t)$ or $S_\Lambda(t)$ if the parametric form is correctly specified.

17.1.1 Specific Models

Parametric modeling requires choosing one or more distributions. The Weibull and exponential distributions were discussed in Chapter 17. Other commonly used survival distributions are obtained by transforming T and using a standard distribution. The log transformation is most commonly employed. The *log-normal* distribution specifies that $\log(T)$ has a normal distribution with mean μ and variance σ^2. Stated another way, $\log(T) \sim \mu + \sigma\epsilon$, where ϵ has a standard normal distribution. Then

$S(t) = 1 - \Phi((\log(t) - \mu)/\sigma)$, where Φ is the standard normal cumulative distribution function. The *log-logistic* distribution is given by $S(t) = [1 + \exp(-(\log(t) - \mu)/\sigma)]^{-1}$. Here $\log(T) \sim \mu + \sigma\epsilon$ where ϵ follows a logistic distribution $[1 + \exp(-u)]^{-1}$. The *log extreme value* distribution is given by $S(t) = \exp[-\exp((\log(t) - \mu)/\sigma)]$, and $\log(T) \sim \mu + \sigma\epsilon$, where $\epsilon \sim 1 - \exp[-\exp(u)]$.

17.1.2   Estimation

Maximum likelihood (ML) estimation is used to estimate the unknown parameters of $S(t)$. The general method presented in Chapter 9 must be augmented, however, to allow for censored failure times. The basic idea is as follows. Again let T be a random variable representing time until the event, T_i be the (possibly censored) failure time for the ith observation, and Y_i denote the observed failure or censoring time $\min(T_i, C_i)$, where C_i is the censoring time. If Y_i is uncensored, observation i contributes a factor to the likelihood equal to the density function for T evaluated at Y_i, $f(Y_i)$. If Y_i instead represents a censored time so that $T_i = Y_i^+$, it is only known that T_i exceeds Y_i. The contribution to the likelihood function is the probability that $T_i > C_i$ (equal to $\text{Prob}\{T_i > Y_i\}$). This probability is $S(Y_i)$. The joint likelihood over all observations $i = 1, 2, \ldots, n$ is

$$L = \prod_{i:Y_i \text{ uncensored}}^{n} f(Y_i) \prod_{i:Y_i \text{ censored}}^{n} S(Y_i). \tag{17.1}$$

There is one more component to L: the distribution of censoring times if these are not fixed in advance. Recall that we assume that censoring is noninformative, that is, it is independent of the risk of the event. This independence implies that the likelihood component of the censoring distribution simply multiplies L and that the censoring distribution contains little information about the survival distribution. In addition, the censoring distribution may be very difficult to specify. For these reasons we can maximize L separately to estimate parameters of $S(t)$ and ignore the censoring distribution.

Recalling that $f(t) = \lambda(t)S(t)$ and $\Lambda(t) = -\log S(t)$, the log likelihood can be written as

$$\log L = \sum_{i:Y_i \text{ uncensored}}^{n} \log \lambda(Y_i) - \sum_{i=1}^{n} \Lambda(Y_i). \tag{17.2}$$

All observations then contribute an amount to the log likelihood equal to the negative of the cumulative hazard evaluated at the failure/censoring time. In addition, uncensored observations contribute an amount equal to the log of the hazard function evaluated at the time of failure. Once L or $\log L$ is specified, the general ML methods outlined earlier can be used without change in most situations. The principal difference is that censored observations contribute less information to the statistical inference than uncensored observations. For distributions such as the log-normal that are written only in terms of $S(t)$, it may be easier to write the likelihood in terms of $S(t)$ and $f(t)$.

As an example, we turn to the exponential distribution, for which log L has a simple form that can be maximized explicitly. Recall that for this distribution $\lambda(t) = \lambda$ and $\Lambda(t) = \lambda t$. Therefore,

$$\log L = \sum_{i:Y_i \text{ uncensored}}^{n} \log \lambda - \sum_{i=1}^{n} \lambda Y_i. \tag{17.3}$$

Letting n_u denote the number of uncensored event times,

$$\log L = n_u \log \lambda - \sum_{i=1}^{n} \lambda Y_i. \tag{17.4}$$

Letting w denote the sum of all failure/censoring times ("person years of exposure"):

$$w = \sum_{i=1}^{n} Y_i, \tag{17.5}$$

the derivatives of $\log L$ are given by

$$\frac{\partial \log L}{\partial \lambda} = n_u/\lambda - w$$
$$\frac{\partial^2 \log L}{\partial \lambda^2} = -n_u/\lambda^2. \tag{17.6}$$

Equating the derivative of $\log L$ to zero implies that the MLE of λ is

$$\hat{\lambda} = n_u/w \tag{17.7}$$

or the number of failures per person-years of exposure. By inserting the MLE of λ into the formula for the second derivative we obtain the observed estimated information, w^2/n_u. The estimated variance of $\hat{\lambda}$ is thus n_u/w^2 and the standard error is $n_u^{1/2}/w$. The precision of the estimate depends primarily on n_u.

Recall that the expected life length μ is $1/\lambda$ for the exponential distribution. The MLE of μ is w/n_u and its estimated variance is w^2/n_u^3. The MLE of $S(t)$, $\hat{S}(t)$, is $\exp(-\hat{\lambda}t)$, and the estimated variance of $\log(\hat{\Lambda}(t))$ is simply $1/n_u$.

As an example, consider the sample listed previously,

$$1 \quad 3 \quad 3 \quad 6^+ \quad 8^+ \quad 9 \quad 10^+.$$

Here $n_u = 4$ and $w = 40$, so the MLE of λ is 0.1 failure per person-period. The estimated standard error is $2/40 = 0.05$. Estimated expected life length is 10 units with a standard error of 5 units. Estimated median failure time is $\log(2)/0.1 = 6.931$. The estimated survival function is $\exp(-0.1t)$, which at $t = 1, 3, 9, 10$ yields $0.90, 0.74, 0.41$, and 0.37, which can be compared to the product limit estimates listed earlier $(0.85, 0.57, 0.29, 0.29)$.

Now consider the Weibull distribution. The log likelihood function is

$$\log L = \sum_{i:Y_i \text{ uncensored}} \log[\alpha\gamma Y_i^{\gamma-1}] - \sum_{i=1}^{n} \alpha Y_i^{\gamma}. \tag{17.8}$$

Although $\log L$ can be simplified somewhat, it cannot be solved explicitly for α and γ. An iterative method such as the Newton–Raphson method is used to compute the MLEs of α and γ. Once these estimates are obtained, the estimated variance–covariance matrix and other derived quantities such as $\hat{S}(t)$ can be obtained in the usual manner.

For the dataset used in the exponential fit, the Weibull fit follows.

$$
\begin{aligned}
\hat{\alpha} &= 0.0728 \\
\hat{\gamma} &= 1.164 \\
\hat{S}(t) &= \exp(-0.0728t^{1.164}) \\
\hat{S}^{-1}(0.5) &= [(\log 2)/\hat{\alpha}]^{1/\hat{\gamma}} = 6.935 \text{ (estimated median)}.
\end{aligned} \tag{17.9}
$$

This fit is very close to the exponential fit since $\hat{\gamma}$ is near 1.0. Note that the two medians are almost equal. The predicted survival probabilities for the Weibull model for $t = 1, 3, 9, 10$ are, respectively, $0.93, 0.77, 0.39, 0.35$.

Sometimes a formal test can be made to assess the fit of the proposed parametric survival distribution. For the data just analyzed, a formal test of exponentiality versus a Weibull alternative is obtained by testing $H_0 : \gamma = 1$ in the Weibull model. A score test yielded $\chi^2 = 0.14$ with 1 d.f., $p = 0.7$, showing little evidence for nonexponentiality (note that the sample size is too small for this test to have any power).

17.1.3 Assessment of Model Fit

The fit of the hypothesized survival distribution can often be checked easily using graphical methods. Nonparametric estimates of $S(t)$ and $\Lambda(t)$ are primary tools for this purpose. For example, the Weibull distribution $S(t) = \exp(-\alpha t^{\gamma})$ can be rewritten by taking logarithms twice:

$$\log[-\log S(t)] = \log \Lambda(t) = \log \alpha + \gamma(\log t). \tag{17.10}$$

The fit of a Weibull model can be assessed by plotting $\log \hat{\Lambda}(t)$ versus $\log t$ and checking whether the curve is approximately linear. Also, the plotted curve provides approximate estimates of α (the antilog of the intercept) and γ (the slope). Since an exponential distribution is a special case of a Weibull distribution when $\gamma = 1$, exponentially distributed data will tend to have a graph that is linear with a slope of 1.

For any assumed distribution $S(t)$, a graphical assessment of goodness of fit can be made by plotting $S^{-1}[S_\Lambda(t)]$ or $S^{-1}[S_{\text{KM}}(t)]$ against t and checking for linearity. For log distributions, S specifies the distribution of $\log(T)$, so we plot against $\log t$. For a log-normal distribution we thus plot $\Phi^{-1}[S_\Lambda(t)]$ against $\log t$, where Φ^{-1} is the inverse of the standard normal cumulative distribution function. For a log-logistic distribution we plot $\text{logit}[S_\Lambda(t)]$ versus $\log t$. For an extreme value distribution we use $\log - \log$ plots as with the Weibull distribution. Parametric model fits can also be checked by plotting the fitted $\hat{S}(t)$ and $S_\Lambda(t)$ against t on the same graph.

17.2   Parametric Proportional Hazards Models

In this section we present one way to generalize the survival model to a survival regression model. In other words, we allow the sample to be heterogeneous by adding predictor variables $X = \{X_1, X_2, \ldots, X_k\}$. As with other regression models, X can represent a mixture of binary, polytomous, continuous, spline-expanded, and even ordinal predictors (if the categories are scored to satisfy the linearity assumption). Before discussing ways in which the regression part of a survival model might be specified, first recall how regression effects have been modeled in other settings. In multiple linear regression, the regression effect $X\beta = \beta_0 + \beta_1 X_1 + \beta_2 X_2 + \ldots + \beta_k X_k$ can be thought of as an increment in the expected value of the response Y. In binary logistic regression, $X\beta$ specifies the log odds that $Y = 1$, or $\exp(X\beta)$ multiplies the odds that $Y = 1$.

17.2.1   Model

The most widely used survival regression specification is to allow the hazard function $\lambda(t)$ to be multiplied by $\exp(X\beta)$. The survival model is thus generalized from a hazard function $\lambda(t)$ for the failure time T to a hazard function $\lambda(t)\exp(X\beta)$ for the failure time given the predictors X:

$$\lambda(t|X) = \lambda(t)\exp(X\beta). \tag{17.11}$$

This regression formulation is called the *proportional hazards (PH)* model. The $\lambda(t)$ part of $\lambda(t|X)$ is sometimes called an *underlying hazard function* or a *hazard function for a standard subject*, which is a subject with $X\beta = 0$. Any parametric hazard function can be used for $\lambda(t)$, and as we show later, $\lambda(t)$ can be left completely unspecified without sacrificing the ability to estimate β, by the use of Cox's semi-parametric PH model.[92] Depending on whether the underlying hazard function $\lambda(t)$

has a constant scale parameter, $X\beta$ may or may not include an intercept β_0. The term $\exp(X\beta)$ can be called a *relative hazard function* and in many cases it is the function of primary interest as it describes the (relative) effects of the predictors.

The PH model can also be written in terms of the cumulative hazard and survival functions:

$$
\begin{aligned}
\Lambda(t|X) &= \Lambda(t)\exp(X\beta) \\
S(t|X) &= \exp[-\Lambda(t)\exp(X\beta)] = \exp[-\Lambda(t)]^{\exp(X\beta)}.
\end{aligned} \tag{17.12}
$$

$\Lambda(t)$ is an "underlying" cumulative hazard function. $S(t|X)$, the probability of surviving past time t given the values of the predictors X, can also be written as

$$
S(t|X) = S(t)^{\exp(X\beta)}, \tag{17.13}
$$

where $S(t)$ is the "underlying" survival distribution, $\exp(-\Lambda(t))$. The effect of the predictors is to multiply the hazard and cumulative hazard functions by a factor $\exp(X\beta)$, or equivalently to raise the survival function to a power equal to $\exp(X\beta)$.

17.2.2 Model Assumptions and Interpretation of Parameters

In the general regression notation of Section 2.2, the log hazard or log cumulative hazard can be used as the property of the response T evaluated at time t that allows distributional and regression parts to be isolated and checked. The PH model can be linearized with respect to $X\beta$ using the following identities.

$$
\begin{aligned}
\log \lambda(t|X) &= \log \lambda(t) + X\beta \\
\log \Lambda(t|X) &= \log \Lambda(t) + X\beta.
\end{aligned} \tag{17.14}
$$

No matter which of the three model statements are used, there are certain assumptions in a parametric PH survival model. These assumptions are listed below.

1. The true form of the underlying functions (λ, Λ, and S) should be specified correctly.

2. The relationship between the predictors and log hazard or log cumulative hazard should be linear in its simplest form. In the absence of interaction terms, the predictors should also operate additively.

3. The way in which the predictors affect the distribution of the response should be by multiplying the hazard or cumulative hazard by $\exp(X\beta)$ or equivalently by adding $X\beta$ to the log hazard or log cumulative hazard at each t. The effect of the predictors is assumed to be the same at all values of t since $\log \lambda(t)$ can be separated from $X\beta$. In other words, the PH assumption implies no t by predictor interaction.

The regression coefficient for X_j, β_j, is the increase in log hazard or log cumulative hazard at any fixed point in time if X_j is increased by one unit and all other predictors are held constant. This can be written formally as

$$\beta_j = \log \lambda(t|X_1, X_2, \ldots, X_j + 1, X_{j+1}, \ldots, X_k) - \log \lambda(t|X_1, \ldots, X_j, \ldots, X_k),$$
(17.15)

which is equivalent to the log of the ratio of the hazards at time t. The regression coefficient can just as easily be written in terms of a ratio of hazards at time t. The ratio of hazards at $X_j + d$ versus X_j, all other factors held constant, is $\exp(\beta_j d)$. Thus the effect of increasing X_j by d is to increase the hazard of the event by a factor of $\exp(\beta_j d)$ at all points in time, assuming X_j is linearly related to $\log \lambda(t)$. In general, the ratio of hazards for an individual with predictor variable values X^* compared to an individual with predictors X is

$$
\begin{aligned}
X^* : X \text{ hazard ratio} &= [\lambda(t)\exp(X^*\beta)]/[\lambda(t)\exp(X\beta)] \\
&= \exp(X^*\beta)/\exp(X\beta) = \exp[(X^* - X)\beta].
\end{aligned}
$$
(17.16)

If there is only one predictor X_1 and that predictor is binary, the PH model can be written

$$
\begin{aligned}
\lambda(t|X_1 = 0) &= \lambda(t) \\
\lambda(t|X_1 = 1) &= \lambda(t)\exp(\beta_1).
\end{aligned}
$$
(17.17)

Here $\exp(\beta_1)$ is the $X_1 = 1 : X_1 = 0$ hazard ratio. This simple case has no regression assumption but assumes PH and a form for $\lambda(t)$. If the single predictor X_1 is continuous, the model becomes

$$\lambda(t|X_1) = \lambda(t)\exp(\beta_1 X).$$
(17.18)

Without further modification (such as taking a transformation of the predictor), the model assumes a straight line in the log hazard or that for all t, an increase in X by one unit increases the hazard by a factor of $\exp(\beta_1)$.

As in logistic regression, much more general regression specifications can be made, including interaction effects. Unlike logistic regression, however, a model containing, say age, sex, and age $\times$ sex interaction is not equivalent to fitting two separate models. This is because even though males and females are allowed to have unequal age slopes, both sexes are assumed to have the underlying hazard function proportional to $\lambda(t)$ (i.e., the PH assumption holds for sex in addition to age).

17.2.3 Hazard Ratio, Risk Ratio, and Risk Difference

Other ways of modeling predictors can also be specified besides a multiplicative effect on the hazard. For example, one could postulate that the effect of a predictor

TABLE 17.1

Subject	5-Year Survival		Difference	Mortality Ratio (T/C)
	C	T		
1	0.98	0.99	0.01	$0.01/0.02 = 0.5$
2	0.80	0.89	0.09	$0.11/0.2 = 0.55$
3	0.25	0.50	0.25	$0.5/0.75 = 0.67$

is to add to the hazard of failure instead of to multiply it by a factor. The effect of a predictor could also be described in terms of a mortality ratio (relative risk), risk difference, odds ratio, or increase in expected failure time. However, just as an odds ratio is a natural way to describe an effect on a binary response, a hazard ratio is often a natural way to describe an effect on survival time. One reason is that a hazard ratio *can* be constant.

Table 17.1 provides treated (T) to control (C) survival (mortality) differences and mortality ratios for three hypothetical types of subjects. We suppose that subjects 1, 2, and 3 have increasingly worse prognostic factors. For example, the age at baseline of the subjects might be 30, 50, and 70 years, respectively. We assume that the treatment affects the hazard by a constant multiple of 0.5 (i.e., PH is in effect and the constant hazard ratio is 0.5). Note that $S_T = S_C^{0.5}$. Notice that the mortality difference and ratio depend on the survival of the control subject. A control subject having "good" predictor values will leave little room for an improved prognosis from the treatment.

The hazard ratio is a basis for describing the mechanism of an effect. In the above example, it is reasonable that the treatment affect each subject by lowering her hazard of death by a factor of 2, even though less sick subjects have a low mortality difference. Hazard ratios also lead to good statistical tests for differences in survival patterns and to predictive models. Once the model is developed, however, survival differences may better capture the impact of a risk factor. Absolute survival differences rather than relative differences (hazard ratios) also relate more closely to statistical power. For example, even if the effect of a treatment is to halve the hazard rate, a population where the control survival is 0.99 will require a much larger sample than will a population where the control survival is 0.3.

Figure 17.1 depicts the relationship between survival $S(t)$ of a control subject at any time t, relative reduction in hazard (h), and difference in survival $S(t) - S(t)^h$. This figure demonstrates that absolute clinical benefit is primarily a function of the baseline risk of a subject. Clinical benefit will also be a function of factors that interact with treatment, that is, factors that modify the relative benefit of treatment. Once a model is developed for estimating $S(t|X)$, this model can be used to estimate absolute benefit as a function of baseline risk factors as well as factors that interact with a treatment. Let X_1 be a binary treatment indicator and

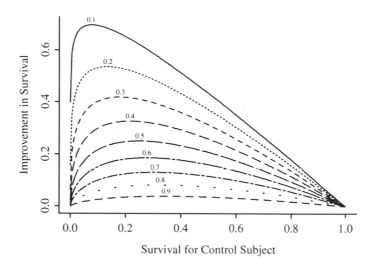

FIGURE 17.1: Absolute clinical benefit as a function of survival in a control subject and the relative benefit (hazard ratio). The hazard ratios are given for each curve.

let $A = \{X_2, \ldots, X_p\}$ be the other factors (which for convenience we assume do not interact with X_1). Then the estimate of $S(t|X_1 = 0, A) - S(t|X_1 = 1, A)$ can be plotted against $S(t|X_1 = 0)$ or against levels of variables in A to display absolute benefit versus overall risk or specific subject characteristics.

17.2.4 Specific Models

Let $X\beta$ denote the linear combination of predictors excluding an intercept term. Using the PH formulation, an exponential survival regression model[150] can be stated as

$$
\begin{aligned}
\lambda(t|X) &= \lambda \exp(X\beta) \\
S(t|X) &= \exp[-\lambda t \exp(X\beta)] = \exp(-\lambda t)^{\exp(X\beta)}.
\end{aligned} \tag{17.19}
$$

The parameter λ can be thought of as the antilog of an intercept term since the model could be written $\lambda(t|X) = \exp[(\log \lambda) + X\beta]$. The effect of X on the expected or median failure time is as follows.

$$
\begin{aligned}
E\{T|X\} &= 1/[\lambda \exp(X\beta)] \\
T_{0.5}|X &= (\log 2)/[\lambda \exp(X\beta)].
\end{aligned} \tag{17.20}
$$

The exponential regression model can be written in another form that is more numerically stable by replacing the λ parameter with an intercept term in $X\beta$, specifically $\lambda = \exp(\beta_0)$. After redefining $X\beta$ to include β_0, λ can be dropped in all the above formulas.

The Weibull regression model is defined by one of the following functions (assuming that $X\beta$ does not contain an intercept).

$$
\begin{aligned}
\lambda(t|X) &= \alpha\gamma t^{\gamma-1}\exp(X\beta) \\
\Lambda(t|X) &= \alpha t^\gamma \exp(X\beta) \\
S(t|X) &= \exp[-\alpha t^\gamma \exp(X\beta)] \\
&= [\exp(-\alpha t^\gamma)]^{\exp(X\beta)}.
\end{aligned}
\tag{17.21}
$$

Note that the parameter α in the homogeneous Weibull model has been replaced with $\alpha\exp(X\beta)$. The median survival time is given by

$$
T_{0.5}|X = \{\log 2/[\alpha\exp(X\beta)]\}^{1/\gamma}.
\tag{17.22}
$$

As with the exponential model, the parameter α could be dropped (and replaced with $\exp(\beta_0)$) if an intercept β_0 is added to $X\beta$.

For numerical reasons it is sometimes advantageous to write the Weibull PH model as

$$
S(t|X) = \exp(-\Lambda(t|X)),
\tag{17.23}
$$

where

$$
\Lambda(t|X) = \exp(\gamma\log t + X\beta).
\tag{17.24}
$$

17.2.5 Estimation

The parameters in λ and β are estimated by maximizing a log likelihood function constructed in the same manner as described in Section 17.1. The only difference is the insertion of $\exp(X_i\beta)$ in the likelihood function:

$$
\log L = \sum_{i:Y_i\ \text{uncensored}} \log[\lambda(Y_i)\exp(X_i\beta)] - \sum_{i=1}^{n}\Lambda(Y_i)\exp(X_i\beta).
\tag{17.25}
$$

Once $\hat\beta$, the MLE of β, is computed along with the large-sample standard error estimates, hazard ratio estimates and their confidence intervals can readily be computed. Letting s denote the estimated standard error of $\hat\beta_j$, a $1-\alpha$ confidence interval for the $X_j + 1 : X_j$ hazard ratio is given by $\exp[\hat\beta_j \pm zs]$, where z is the $1-\alpha/2$ critical value for the standard normal distribution.

Once the parameters of the underlying hazard function are estimated, the MLE of $\lambda(t)$, $\hat\lambda(t)$, can be derived. The MLE of $\lambda(t|X)$, the hazard as a function of t and X, is given by

$$
\hat\lambda(t|X) = \hat\lambda(t)\exp(X\hat\beta).
\tag{17.26}
$$

The MLE of $\Lambda(t)$, $\hat{\Lambda}(t)$, can be derived from the integral of $\hat{\lambda}(t)$ with respect to t. Then the MLE of $S(t|X)$ can be derived:

$$\hat{S}(t|X) = \exp[-\hat{\Lambda}(t)\exp(X\hat{\beta})]. \tag{17.27}$$

For the Weibull model, we denote the MLEs of the hazard parameters α and γ by $\hat{\alpha}$ and $\hat{\gamma}$. The MLE of $\lambda(t|X)$, $\Lambda(t|X)$, and $S(t|X)$ for this model are

$$\begin{aligned}
\hat{\lambda}(t|X) &= \hat{\alpha}\hat{\gamma}t^{\hat{\gamma}-1}\exp(X\hat{\beta}) \\
\hat{\Lambda}(t|X) &= \hat{\alpha}t^{\hat{\gamma}}\exp(X\hat{\beta}) \\
\hat{S}(t|X) &= \exp[-\hat{\Lambda}(t|X)].
\end{aligned} \tag{17.28}$$

Confidence intervals for $S(t|X)$ are best derived using general matrix notation to derive an estimate s of the standard error of $\log[\hat{\lambda}(t|X)]$ from the estimated information matrix of all hazard and regression parameters. A confidence interval for $\hat{S}$ will be of the form

$$\hat{S}(t|X)^{\exp(\pm zs)}. \tag{17.29}$$

The MLEs of β and of the hazard shape parameters lead directly to MLEs of the expected and median life length. For the Weibull model the MLE of the median life length given X is

$$\hat{T}_{0.5}|X = \{\log 2/[\hat{\alpha}\exp(X\hat{\beta})]\}^{1/\hat{\gamma}}. \tag{17.30}$$

For the exponential model, the MLE of the expected life length for a subject having predictor values X is given by

$$\hat{E}(T|X) = [\hat{\lambda}\exp(X\hat{\beta})]^{-1}, \tag{17.31}$$

where $\hat{\lambda}$ is the MLE of λ.

17.2.6 Assessment of Model Fit

Three assumptions of the parametric PH model were listed in Section 17.2.2. We now lay out in more detail what relationships need to be satisfied. We first assume a PH model with a single binary predictor X_1. For a general underlying hazard function $\lambda(t)$, all assumptions of the model are displayed in Figure 17.2. In this case, the assumptions are PH and a shape for $\lambda(t)$.

If $\lambda(t)$ is Weibull, the two curves will be linear if $\log t$ is plotted instead of t on the x-axis. Note also that if there is no association between X and survival ($\beta_1 = 0$), estimates of the two curves will be close and will intertwine due to random variability. In this case, PH is not an issue.

If the single predictor is continuous, the relationships in Figures 17.3 and 17.4 must hold. Here linearity is assumed (unless otherwise specified) besides PH and the form of $\lambda(t)$. In Figure 17.3, the curves must be parallel for any choices of

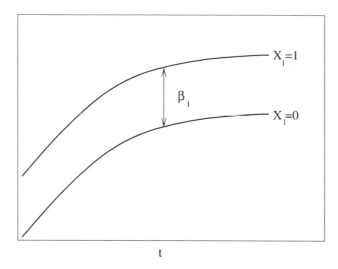

FIGURE 17.2: PH model with one binary predictor. Y-axis is $\log \lambda(t)$ or $\log \Lambda(t)$. For $\log \Lambda(t)$, the curves must be nondecreasing. For $\log \lambda(t)$, they may be any shape.

times t_1 and t_2 as well as each individual curve being linear. Also, the difference between ordinates needs to conform to the assumed distribution. This difference is $\log[\lambda(t_2)/\lambda(t_1)]$ or $\log[\Lambda(t_2)/\Lambda(t_1)]$.

Figure 17.4 highlights the PH assumption. The relationship between the two curves must hold for any two values c and d of X_1. The shape of the function for a given value of X_1 must conform to the assumed $\lambda(t)$. For a Weibull model, the functions should each be linear in $\log t$.

When there are multiple predictors, the PH assumption can be displayed in a way similar to Figures 17.2 and 17.4 but with the population additionally cross-classified by levels of the other predictors besides X_1. If there is one binary predictor X_1 and one continuous predictor X_2, the relationship in Figure 17.5 must hold at each time t if linearity is assumed for X_2 and there is no interaction between X_1 and X_2. Methods for verifying the regression assumptions (e.g., splines and residuals) and the PH assumption are covered in detail under the Cox PH model in Chapter 19.

The method for verifying the assumed shape of $S(t)$ in Section 17.1.3 is also useful when there are a limited number of categorical predictors. To validate a Weibull PH model one can stratify on X and plot $\log \Lambda_{\mathrm{KM}}(t|X \text{ stratum})$ against $\log t$. This graph simultaneously assesses PH in addition to shape assumptions— all curves should be parallel as well as straight. Straight but nonparallel (non-PH) curves indicate that a series of Weibull models with differing γ parameters will fit.

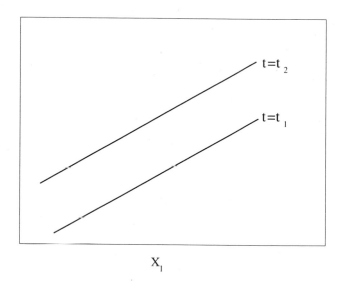

FIGURE 17.3: PH model with one continuous predictor. Y-axis is $\log \lambda(t)$ or $\log \Lambda(t)$; for $\log \Lambda(t)$, drawn for $t_2 > t_1$. The slope of each line is β_1.

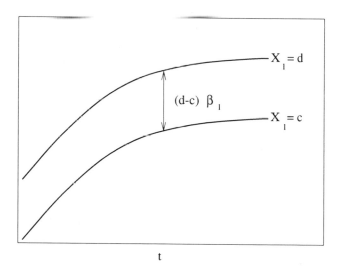

FIGURE 17.4: PH model with one continuous predictor. Y-axis is $\log \lambda(t)$ or $\log \Lambda(t)$. For $\log \lambda$, the functions need not be monotonic.

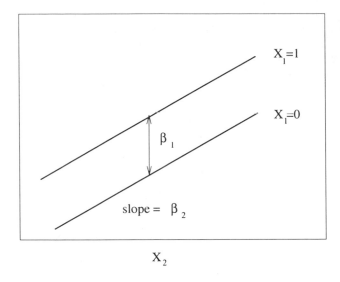

FIGURE 17.5: Regression assumptions, linear additive PH or AFT model with two predictors. For PH, Y-axis is $\log \lambda(t)$ or $\log \Lambda(t)$ for a fixed t. For AFT, Y-axis is $\log(T)$.

17.3   Accelerated Failure Time Models

17.3.1   Model

Besides modeling the effect of predictors by a multiplicative effect on the hazard function, other regression effects can be specified. The *accelerated failure time (AFT) model* is commonly used; it specifies that the predictors act multiplicatively on the failure time or additively on the log failure time. The effect of a predictor is to alter the rate at which a subject proceeds along the time axis (i.e., to accelerate the time to failure [226, pp. 33–35]). The model is   2

$$S(t|X) = \psi((\log(t) - X\beta)/\sigma), \qquad (17.32)$$

where ψ is any standardized survival distribution function. The parameter σ is called the *scale parameter*. The model can also be stated as $(\log(T) - X\beta)/\sigma \sim \psi$ or $\log(T) = X\beta + \sigma\epsilon$, where ϵ is a random variable from the distribution ψ. Sometimes the untransformed T is used in place of $\log(T)$. When the log form is used, the models are said to be log-normal, log-logistic, and so on.

The exponential and Weibull are the only two distributions that can describe either a PH or an AFT model.   3

17.3.2 Model Assumptions and Interpretation of Parameters

The $\log \lambda$ or $\log \Lambda$ transformation of the PH model has the following equivalent for AFT models.

$$\psi^{-1}[S(t|X)] = (\log(t) - X\beta)/\sigma. \tag{17.33}$$

Letting as before ϵ denote a random variable from the distribution S, the model is also

$$\log(T) = X\beta + \sigma\epsilon. \tag{17.34}$$

So the property of the response T of interest for regression modeling is $\log(T)$. In the absence of censoring, we could check the model by plotting an X against $\log T$ and checking that the residuals $\log(T) - X\hat{\beta}$ are distributed as ψ to within a scale factor.

The assumptions of the AFT model are thus the following.

  1. The true form of ψ (the distributional family) is correctly specified.

  2. In the absence of nonlinear and interaction terms, each X_j affects $\log(T)$ or $\psi^{-1}[S(t|X)]$ linearly.

  3. Implicit in these assumptions is that σ is a constant independent of X.

A one-unit change in X_j is then most simply understood as a β_j change in the log of the failure time. The one-unit change in X_j increases the failure time by a factor of $\exp(\beta_j)$.

The median survival time is obtained by solving $\psi((\log(t) - X\beta)/\sigma) = 0.5$ giving

$$T_{0.5}|X = \exp[X\beta + \sigma\psi^{-1}(0.5)] \tag{17.35}$$

17.3.3 Specific Models

Common choices for the distribution function ψ in Equation 17.32 are the extreme value distribution $\psi(u) = \exp(-\exp(u))$, the logistic distribution $\psi(u) = [1 + \exp(u)]^{-1}$, and the normal distribution $\psi(u) = 1 - \Phi(u)$. The AFT model equivalent of the Weibull model is obtained by using the extreme value distribution, negating β, and replacing γ with $1/\sigma$ in Equation 17.24:

$$\begin{aligned} S(t|X) &= \exp[-\exp((\log(t) - X\beta)/\sigma)] \\ T_{0.5}|X &= [\log(2)]^\sigma \exp(X\beta). \end{aligned} \tag{17.36}$$

The exponential model is obtained by restricting $\sigma = 1$ in the extreme value distribution.

The log-normal regression model is

$$S(t|X) = 1 - \Phi((\log(t) - X\beta)/\sigma), \tag{17.37}$$

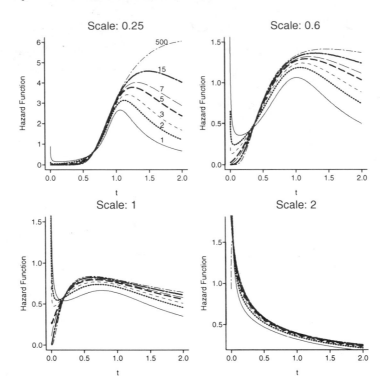

FIGURE 17.6:   Log t distribution for $\sigma = 0.25, 0.6, 1, 2$ and for degrees of freedom $1, 2, 3, 5, 7, 15, 500$ (almost log-normal). The top left plot has degrees of freedom written in the plot.

and the log-logistic model is

$$S(t|X) = [1 + \exp((\log(t) - X\beta)/\sigma)]^{-1}. \tag{17.38}$$

The t distribution allows for more flexibility by varying the degrees of freedom. Figure 17.6 depicts possible hazard functions for varying σ and degrees of freedom. However, the log t distribution does not have a late increasing hazard phase typical of human survival.

All three of these parametric survival models have median survival time $T_{0.5}|X = \exp(X\beta)$.

17.3.4   Estimation

Maximum likelihood estimation is used much the same as in Section 17.2.5. Care must be taken in the choice of initial values; iterative methods are especially prone to problems in choosing the initial $\hat{\sigma}$. Estimation works better if σ is parameterized as $\exp(\delta)$. Once β and σ $(\exp(\delta))$ are estimated, MLEs of secondary parameters such as survival probabilities and medians can readily be obtained:

$$
\begin{aligned}
\hat{S}(t|X) &= \psi((\log(t) - X\hat{\beta})/\hat{\sigma}) \\
\hat{T}_{0.5}|X &= \exp[X\hat{\beta} + \hat{\sigma}\psi^{-1}(0.5)].
\end{aligned}
\tag{17.39}
$$

For normal and logistic distributions, $\hat{T}_{0.5}|X = \exp(X\hat{\beta})$. The MLE of the effect on $\log(T)$ of increasing X_j by d units is $\hat{\beta}_j d$ if X_j is linear and additive.

The delta (statistical differential) method can be used to compute an estimate of the variance of $f = [\log(t) - X\hat{\beta}]/\hat{\sigma}$. Let $(\hat{\beta}, \hat{\delta})$ denote the estimated parameters, and let $\hat{V}$ denote the estimated covariance matrix for these parameter estimates. Let F denote the vector of derivatives of f with respect to $(\beta_0, \beta_1, \ldots, \beta_p, \delta)$; that is, $F = [-1, -X_1, -X_2, \ldots, -X_p, -(\log(t) - X\hat{\beta})]/\hat{\sigma}$. The variance of f is then approximately

$$
\operatorname{Var}(f) = F\hat{V}F'.
\tag{17.40}
$$

Letting s be the square root of the variance estimate and $z_{1-\alpha/2}$ be the normal critical value, a $1 - \alpha$ confidence limit for $S(t|X)$ is

$$
\psi((\log(t) - X\hat{\beta})/\hat{\sigma} \pm z_{1-\alpha/2} \times s).
\tag{17.41}
$$

17.3.5 Residuals

For an AFT model, standardized residuals are simply

$$
r = (\log(T) - X\hat{\beta})/\sigma.
\tag{17.42}
$$

When T is right-censored, r is right-censored. Censoring must be taken into account, for example, by displaying Kaplan–Meier estimates based on groups of residuals rather than showing individual residuals. The residuals can be used to check for lack of fit as described in the next section. Note that examining individual uncensored residuals is not appropriate, as their distribution is conditional on $T_i < C_i$, where C_i is the censoring time.

Cox and Snell[94] proposed a type of general residuals that also work for censored data. Using their method on the cumulative probability scale results in the probability integral transformation. If the probability of failure before time t given X is $S(t|X)$, $F(T|X) = 1 - S(T|X)$ has a uniform $[0, 1]$ distribution, where T is a subject's actual failure time. When T is right-censored, so is $1 - S(T|X)$. Substituting $\hat{S}$ for S results in an approximate uniform $[0, 1]$ distribution for any value of X. One minus the Kaplan–Meier estimate of $1 - \hat{S}(T|X)$ (using combined data for all X) is compared against a $45°$ line to check for goodness of fit. A more stringent assessment is obtained by repeating this process while stratifying on X.

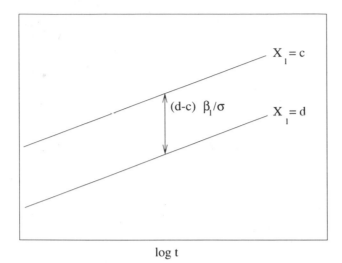

FIGURE 17.7: AFT model with one predictor. Y-axis is $\psi^{-1}[S(t|X)] = (\log(t) - X\beta)/\sigma$. Drawn for $d > c$. The slope of the lines is σ^{-1}.

17.3.6   Assessment of Model Fit

For a single binary predictor, all assumptions of the AFT model are depicted in Figure 17.7. That figure also shows the assumptions for any two values of a single continuous predictor that behaves linearly. For a single continuous predictor, the relationships in Figure 17.8 must hold for any two follow-up times. The regression assumptions are isolated in Figure 17.5.

To verify the fit of a log-logistic model with age as the only predictor, one could stratify by quartiles of age and check for linearity and parallelism of the four logit $S_\Lambda(t)$ or $S_{\mathrm{KM}}(t)$ curves over increasing t as in Figure 17.7, which stresses the distributional assumption (no T by X interaction and linearity vs. $\log(t)$). To stress the linear regression assumption while checking for absence of time interactions (part of the distributional assumptions), one could make a plot like Figure 17.8. For each decile of age, the logit transformation of the 1-, 3-, and 5-year survival estimates for that decile would be plotted against the mean age in the decile. This checks for linearity and constancy of the age effect over time. Regression splines will be a more effective method for checking linearity and determining transformations. This is demonstrated in Chapter 19 with the Cox model, but identical methods apply here.

As an example, consider data from Kalbfleisch and Prentice [226, pp. 1-2], who present data from Pike[341] on the time from exposure to the carcinogen DMBA to mortality from vaginal cancer in rats. The rats are divided into two groups on the basis of a pretreatment regime. Survival times in days (with censored times marked [+]) are found in Table 17.2. The top left plot in Figure 17.9 displays non-

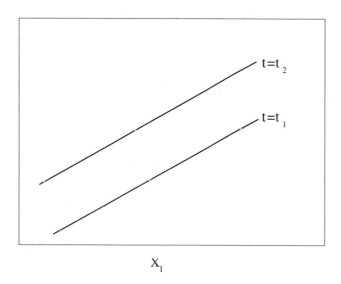

FIGURE 17.8:   AFT model with one continuous predictor. Y-axis is $\psi^{-1}[S(t|X)] = (\log(t) - X\beta)/\sigma$. Drawn for $t_2 > t_1$. The slope of each line is β_1/σ and the difference between the lines is $\log(t_2/t_1)/\sigma$.

TABLE 17.2

Group 1	143	164	188	188	190	192	206	209	213	216
	220	227	230	234	246	265	304	216+	244+	
Group 2	142	156	163	198	205	232	232	233	233	233
	233	239	240	261	280	280	296	296	323	204+
	344+									

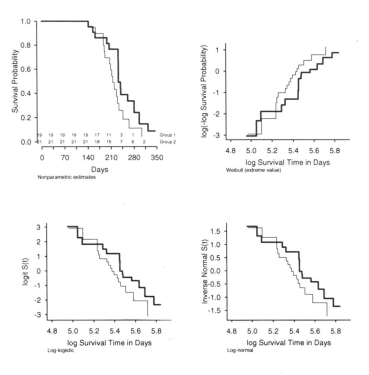

FIGURE 17.9: Altschuler–Nelson–Fleming–Harrington nonparametric survival estimates for rats treated with DMBA,[341] along with various transformations of the estimates for checking distributional assumptions of three parametric survival models. Thick lines correspond to Group 2.

parametric survival estimates for the two groups, with the number of rats "at risk" at each 30-day mark written above the x-axis. The remaining three plots are for checking assumptions of three models. None of the parametric models presented will completely allow for such a long period with no deaths. Neither will any allow for the early crossing of survival curves. Log-normal and log-logistic models yield very similar results due to the similarity in shapes between $\Phi(z)$ and $[1 + \exp(-z)]^{-1}$ for nonextreme z. All three transformations show good parallelism after the early crossing. The log-logistic and log-normal transformations are slightly more linear. The fitted models are:

$$S_{\text{extreme}}(t) = \exp[-\exp(\frac{\log(t) - 5.45 - 0.132\{\text{Group 2}\}}{0.183})]$$

$$S_{\text{log-logistic}}(t) = [1 + \exp(\frac{\log(t) - 5.38 - 0.105\{\text{Group 2}\}}{0.116})]^{-1} \quad (17.43)$$

TABLE 17.3

Model	Group 2:1 Failure Time Ratio	Median Survival Time	
		Group 1	Group 2
Extreme Value (Weibull)	1.14	217	248
Log-logistic	1.11	217	241
Log-normal	1.10	217	238

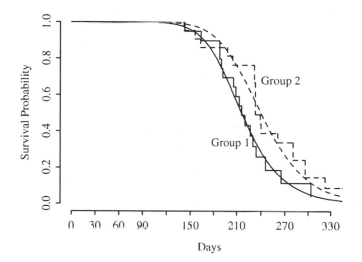

FIGURE 17.10: Agreement between fitted log-logistic model and nonparametric survival estimates for rat vaginal cancer data.

$$S_{\text{log-normal}}(t) = 1 - \Phi\left(\frac{\log(t) - 5.38 - 0.0931\{\text{Group } 2\}}{0.210}\right).$$

The estimated failure time ratios and median failure times for the two groups are given in Table 17.3. For example, the effect of going from Group 1 to Group 2 is to increase log failure time by 0.132 for the extreme value model, giving a Group 2:1 failure time ratio of $\exp(0.132) = 1.14$. This ratio is also the ratio of median survival times.

We choose the log-logistic model for its simpler form. The fitted survival curves are plotted with the nonparametric estimates in Figure 17.10. Excellent agreement is seen, except for 150 to 180 days for Group 2. The standard error of the regression coefficient for group in the log-logistic model is 0.0636 giving a Wald χ^2 for group differences of $(.105/.0636)^2 = 2.73, P = 0.1$.

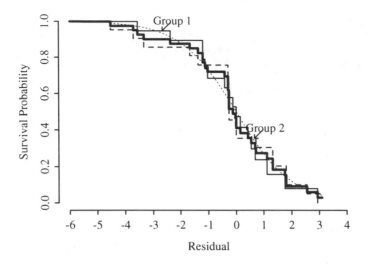

FIGURE 17.11: Kaplan–Meier estimates of distribution of standardized censored residuals from the log-logistic model, along with the assumed standard log-logistic distribution (dashed curve). Thick step function is the estimated distribution of all residuals, and other step functions are the estimated distributions of residuals stratified by group, as indicated.

The Weibull PH form of the fitted extreme value model, using Equation 17.24, is

$$S(t|X) = \exp[-\exp(5.46\log(t) - 29.781 - 0.721\{\text{Group 2}\})] \qquad (17.44)$$

A sensitive graphical verification of the distributional assumptions of the AFT model is obtained by plotting the estimated survival distribution of standardized residuals (Equation 17.3.5), censored identically to the way T is censored. This distribution is plotted along with the theoretical distribution ψ. The assessment may be made more stringent by stratifying the residuals by important subject characteristics and plotting separate survival function estimates; they should all have the same standardized distribution (e.g., same σ).

As an example, Figure 17.11 shows the Kaplan–Meier estimate of the distribution of residuals, Kaplan–Meier estimates stratified by group, and the assumed log-logistic distribution.

Section 18.2 has a more in-depth example of this approach.

5

17.3.7   Validating the Fitted Model

AFT models may be validated for both calibration and discrimination accuracy using the same methods that are presented for the Cox model in Section 19.10.

The method discussed there for checking calibration is based on choosing a single follow-up time and constructing rather arbitrary intervals of predicted probabilities. Checking the distributional assumptions of the model is also a check of calibration accuracy in a sense. Another indirect calibration assessment may be obtained from a set of Cox–Snell residuals (Section 17.3.5) or by using ordinary residuals as just described. A higher resolution indirect calibration assessment based on plotting individual uncensored failure times is available when the theoretical censoring times for those observations are known. Let C denote a subject's censoring time and F the cumulative distribution of a failure time T. The expected value of $F(T|X)$ is 0.5 when T is an actual failure time random variable. The expected value for an event time that is observed *because it is uncensored* is the expected value of $F(T|T \leq C, X) = 0.5F(C|X)$. A smooth plot (using, say, loess) of $F(T|X) - 0.5F(C|X)$ against $X\hat{\beta}$ should be a flat line through $y = 0$ if the model is well calibrated. A smooth plot of $2F(T|X)/F(C|X)$ against $X\hat{\beta}$ (or anything else) should be a flat line through $y = 1$. This method assumes that the model is calibrated well enough that we can substitute $1 - \hat{S}(C|X)$ for $F(C|X)$.

17.4   Buckley–James Regression Model

Buckley and James[56] developed a method for estimating regression coefficients using least squares after imputing censored residuals. Their method does not assume a distribution for survival time or the residuals, but is aimed at estimating expected survival time or expected log survival time given predictor variables. This method has been generalized to allow for smooth nonlinear effects and interactions in the S-PLUS bj function in the Design library, written by Janez Stare and Frank Harrell.

17.5   Design Formulations

Various designs can be formulated with survival regression models just as with other regression models. By constructing the proper dummy variables, ANOVA and ANOCOVA models can easily be specified for testing differences in survival time between multiple treatments. Interactions and complex nonlinear effects may also be modeled.

17.6   Test Statistics

As discussed previously, likelihood ratio, score, and Wald statistics can be derived from the maximum likelihood analysis, and the choice of test statistic depends on the circumstance and on computational convenience.

17.7   Quantifying Predictive Ability

See Section 19.9 for a generalized measure of concordance between predicted and observed survival time (or probability of survival) for right-censored data.

17.8   S-PLUS Functions

Therneau's `survreg` function (part of his `survival` library) can fit regression models in the AFT family with left–, right–, or interval–censoring. The time variable can be untransformed or log-transformed (the default). Distributions supported are extreme value (Weibull and exponential), normal, logistic, and Student-t. The version of `survreg` in `Design` that fits parametric survival models in the same framework as `lrm`, `ols`, and `cph` is called `psm`. The same AFT notation is used as SAS `PROC LIFEREG`. `psm` works with `print`, `coef`, `formula`, `specs`, `summary`, `anova`, `plot`, `predict`, `fastbw`, `latex`, `nomogram`, `validate`, `calibrate`, `survest`, and `survplot` functions for obtaining and plotting predicted survival probabilities. The `dist` argument to `psm` can be `"extreme"`, `"logistic"`, `"gaussian"`, `"exponential"`, `"t"` or any abbreviation of those names to fit, respectively, extreme value, logistic, normal, and exponential (extreme value with scale fixed at one) models. The scale can be fixed at any value, and `link` specifies the transformation of T: `"log"` or `"identity"`. To fit a model with no covariables, use the command `psm(Surv(d.time, event) ∼ 1)`. To restate a Weibull or exponential model in PH form, use the `pphsm` function. An example of how many of the functions are used is found below.

```
> units(d.time) ← "Year"
> f ← psm(Surv(d.time,cdeath) ∼ lsp(age,65)*sex)
> # default is extreme value (Weibull)
> anova(f)
> summary(f)              # summarize effects with delta log T
> latex(f)                # typeset mathematical form of fitted model
> survest(f, times=1)   # 1y survival estimates for all subjects
> survest(f, expand.grid(sex="female", age=30:80), times=1:2)
> # 1y, 2y survival estimates vs. age, for females
> survest(f, data.frame(sex="female",age=50))
> # survival curve for an individual subject
> survplot(f, sex=NA, age=50, n.risk=T)
> # survival curves for each sex, adjusting age to 50
> f.ph ← pphsm(f)       # convert from AFT to PH
> summary(f.ph)           # summarize with hazard ratios
>                         # instead of changes in log(T)
```

Figure 17.9 was produced with

```
> group ← c(rep("Group 1",19),rep("Group 2",21))
```

```
> group ← factor(group)
> days ← c(143,164,188,188,190,192,206,209,213,216,220,227,230,
+             234,246,265,304,216,244,142,156,163,198,205,232,232,
+             233,233,233,233,239,240,261,280,280,296,296,323,204,344)
> death ← rep(1,40)
> death[c(18,19,39,40)] ← 0
> units(days) ← "Day"
> S ← Surv(days,death)

> f ← survfit(S ~ group, type="fleming")
> par(mfrow=c(2,2))
> survplot(f, n.risk=T, label.curves=F,
+           dots=F, conf="none", lwd=c(1,3.5), lty=1)
> title(sub="Nonparametric estimates",adj=0,cex=.7)
> par(mar=c(5,4,4,2)+.1)
> # undo special rt margin used by n.risk

> # Check fits of Weibull, log-logistic, log-normal
> xl ← c(4.8, 5.9)
> survplot(f, loglog=T, logt=T, conf="none", xlim=xl,
+           label.curves=F, lwd=c(1,3.5), lty=1)
> title(sub="Weibull (extreme value)",adj=0,cex=.7)
> survplot(f, fun=function(y)log(y/(1-y)),
+           ylab="logit S(t)", logt=T,
+           conf="none", xlim=xl,
+           label.curves=F, lwd=c(1,3.5), lty=1)
> title(sub="Log-logistic",adj=0,cex=.7)
> survplot(f, fun=qnorm, ylab="Inverse Normal S(t)",
+           logt=T, conf="none", xlim=xl,
+           label.curves=F, lwd=c(1,3.5), lty=1)
> title(sub="Log-normal",adj=0,cex=.7)
```

Figure 17.10 was produced with the following, with f denoting the nonparametric survival estimates from survfit above. Output from psm and other functions is shown also.

```
> g ← psm(S ~ group, dist="logistic", y=T)
> # y=T is for resid(g) below
> g
```

Parametric Survival Model: Logistic Distribution

```
 Obs Events Model L.R. d.f.      P    R2
  40     36       2.71    1 0.0997 0.09
```

Call:

```
sm(formula = S ~ group, dist = "logistic")
Deviance Residuals:
    Min    1Q Median    3Q  Max
  -2.51 -0.721 -0.057 0.805 2.51

Coefficients:
               Value Std. Error z value       p
  (Intercept)  5.376     0.0448  119.90 0.00e+00
group=Group 2  0.105     0.0636    1.65 9.87e-02
  Log(scale) -2.154     0.1412  -15.26 1.35e-52


      Null Deviance: 53.6 on 39 degrees of freedom
  Residual Deviance: 50.9 on 37 degrees of freedom  (LL= 0.871 2.226 )
  Number of Newton-Raphson Iterations: 3

> summary(g)


            Effects               Response : S


                    Factor Low High Diff. Effect S.E. Lower 0.95 Upper 0.95
  group - Group 2:Group 1 1    2    NA    0.11  0.06     -0.02       0.23
        T ratio          1    2    NA    1.11    NA      0.98       1.26


> survplot(g, group=NA)
> survplot(f, add=T, label.curves=F, conf="none")
```

Figure 17.11 was produced by:

```
> r ← resid(g, 'cens')
> survplot(survfit(r ~ group), conf='none', xlab='Residual')
> # survfit computed Kaplan-Meier esimates of distribution of censored r
> par(lwd=4)
> survplot(survfit(r), conf='none', add=T)
> lines(r, lwd=1)       # draws theoretical distribution
```

Special functions work with objects created by psm to create S functions that contain the analytic form for predicted survival probabilities (Survival), hazard functions (Hazard), quantiles of survival time (Quantile), and mean or expected survival time (Mean). Once the S functions are constructed, they can be used in a variety of contexts. The survplot and survest functions have a special argument for psm fits: what. The default is what="survival" to estimate or plot survival probabilities. Specifying what="hazard" will plot hazard functions. plot.Design also has a special argument for psm fits: time. Specifying a single value for time results in survival probability for that time being plotted instead of $X\hat{\beta}$. Examples of many of the functions appear below, with the output of the survplot command shown in Figure 17.12.

```
> med    ← Quantile(g)
> meant  ← Mean(g)
> haz    ← Hazard(g)
> surv   ← Survival(g)
> surv

function(times, lp,
    parms = structure(.Data = -2.15437786646329,
                      .Names = "Log(scale)"),
    transform = structure(.Data = "log", .Names = "link")) {
    t.trans ← glm.links["link", transform]$link(times)
    structure(1/(1 + exp((t.trans - lp)/exp(parms))),
              names = NULL)
}


> # Compute median survival time
> med(lp=range(g$linear.predictors))
[1] 216.09 240.03


> # Another way:
> xbeta ← predict(g, data.frame(group=c("Group 1","Group 2")))
> xbeta


      1      2
 5.3757 5.4808

> med(lp=xbeta)        # use meant(xbeta) to get mean survival time
[1] 216.09 240.03


> # Still another: (shows APPROXIMATE c.l.)
> plot(g, group=NA, fun=function(x)med(lp=x),
    ylab="Median Survival Time")


> # Compute survival probability at 210 days
> surv(210, xbeta)
[1] 0.56127 0.75998


> # Plot estimated hazard functions and add median
> # survival times to graph
> survplot(g, group=NA, what="hazard")
> m ← format(med(lp=xbeta))
> text(60, .02, paste("Group 1 median: ", m[1],"\n",
+      "Group 2 median: ", m[2], sep=""))
> # Another way:
> plot(1:330, haz(1:330, g$coef[1]))
> lines(1:330, haz(1:330, g$coef[1]+g$coef[2]))
```

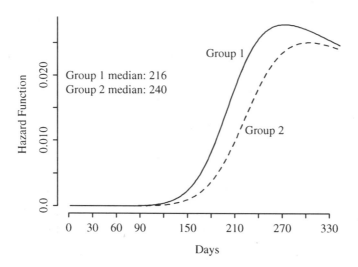

FIGURE 17.12: Estimated hazard functions for log-logistic fit to rat vaginal cancer data, along with median survival times.

The S object called `survreg.distributions` of Therneau has detailed information for extreme-value, logistic, normal, and t distributions. For each distribution, components include the deviance function, an algorithm for obtaining starting parameter estimates, a LaTeX representation of the survival function, and S functions defining the survival, hazard, quantile functions, and basic survival inverse function (which could have been used in Figure 17.9). Figure 17.6 was produced by the following program.

```
> # Retrieve analytic hazard function for t-distribution
> haz ← survreg.distributions$t$hazard
> # also look at t$survival.inverse, $quantile, $survival
> par(mfrow=c(2,2))
> times ← c(seq(0,.25,length=100),seq(.26,2,length=150))
> i ← 0
> high ← c(6,1.5,1.5,1.75)
> low  ← c(0,0,0,.25)
> dfs ← c(1,2,3,5,7,15,500)
> for(scale in c(.25,.6,1,2)) {
+    i ← i+1
+    plot(0,0,xlim=c(0,2),ylim=c(low[i],high[i]),
+        xlab="t",ylab="Hazard Function",type="n")
+    col ← 1.09
+    for(df in dfs) {
+      col ← col-.09
+      lines(times, haz(times, 0, c(log(scale), df), "log"),
```

```
+           col=col)
+      if(i==1) text(1.7, haz(1.7,0,c(log(scale),df),"log"),
+                   format(df))
+   }
+ title(paste("Scale:",format(scale)))
+ }
```

Design's `val.surv` function is useful for indirect external validation of parametric models using Cox–Snell residuals and other approaches of Section 17.3.7. The `plot` method for an object created by `val.surv` makes it easy to stratify all computations by a variable of interest to more stringently validate the fit with respect to that variable.

Design's `bj` function fits the Buckley–James model for right-censored responses.

Kooperberg et al.'s adaptive linear spline log-hazard model[243, 244, 402] has been implemented in the S function `hare` in StatLib. Their procedure searches for second-order interactions involving predictors (and linear splines of them) and linear splines in follow-up time (allowing for nonproportional hazards).

17.9 Further Reading

[1] Wellek[449] developed a test statistic for a specified maximum survival difference after relating this difference to a hazard ratio.

[2] Hougaard[217] compared accelerated failure time models with proportional hazard models.

[3] Gore et al.[155] discuss how an AFT model (the log-logistic model) gives rise to varying hazard ratios.

[4] See Hillis[201] for other types of residuals and plots that use them.

[5] See Gore et al.[155] and Lawless[264] for other methods of checking assumptions for AFT models. Lawless is an excellent text for in-depth discussion of parametric survival modeling.

17.10 Problems

1. For the failure times (in days)

$$1 \quad 3 \quad 3^+ \quad 6^+ \quad 7^+$$

compute MLEs of the following parameters of an exponential distribution by hand: λ, μ, $T_{0.5}$, and $S(3 \text{ days})$. Compute 0.95 confidence limits for λ and $S(3)$, basing the latter on $\log[\Lambda(t)]$.

2. For the same data in Problem 1, compute MLEs of parameters of a Weibull distribution. Also compute the MLEs of $S(3)$ and $T_{0.5}$.

Chapter 18

Case Study in Parametric Survival Modeling and Model Approximation

Consider the random sample of 1000 patients from the SUPPORT study,[241] described in Section 3.10. In this case study we develop a parametric survival time model (accelerated failure time model) for time until death for the acute disease subset of SUPPORT (acute respiratory failure, multiple organ system failure, coma). We eliminate the chronic disease categories because the shapes of the survival curves are different between acute and chronic disease categories. To fit both acute and chronic disease classes would require a log-normal model with σ parameter that is disease-specific.

Patients had to survive until day 3 of the study to qualify. The baseline physiologic variables were measured during day 3.

18.1 Descriptive Statistics

First we create a variable `acute` to flag the categories of interest, and print univariable descriptive statistics for the data subset.

```
> library(Hmisc,T); library(Design,T)
> acute ← support$dzclass %in% c('ARF/MOSF','Coma')
> describe(support[acute,])    # actually used latex(describe)
```

support[acute,]
35 Variables   537 Observations

---

age : Age

n	missing	unique	Mean	.05	.10	.25	.50	.75	.90	.95
537	0	529	60.7	28.49	35.22	47.93	63.67	74.49	81.54	85.56

lowest : 18.04 18.41 19.76 20.30 20.31
highest: 91.62 91.82 91.93 92.74 95.51

---

death : Death at any time up to NDI date:31DEC94

n	missing	unique	Sum	Mean
537	0	2	356	0.6629

---

sex

n	missing	unique
537	0	2

female (251, 47%), male (286, 53%)

---

hospdead : Death in Hospital

n	missing	unique	Sum	Mean
537	0	2	201	0.3743

---

slos : Days from Study Entry to Discharge

n	missing	unique	Mean	.05	.10	.25	.50	.75	.90	.95
537	0	85	23.44	4.0	5.0	9.0	15.0	27.0	47.4	68.2

lowest :   3   4   5   6   7, highest: 145 164 202 236 241

---

d.time : Days of Follow-Up

n	missing	unique	Mean	.05	.10	.25	.50	.75	.90	.95
537	0	340	446.1	4	6	16	182	724	1421	1742

lowest :   3   4   5   6   7, highest: 1977 1979 1982 2011 2022

---

dzgroup : Disease Group

n	missing	unique
537	0	3

ARF/MOSF w/Sepsis (391, 73%), Coma (60, 11%), MOSF w/Malig (86, 16%)

---

dzclass : Disease Class

n	missing	unique
537	0	2

ARF/MOSF (477, 89%), Coma (60, 11%)

---

num.co : number of comorbidities

n	missing	unique	Mean
537	0	7	1.525

	0	1	2	3	4	5	6
Frequency	111	196	133	51	31	10	5
%	21	36	25	9	6	2	1

edu : Years of Education

.... | . . . .

	n	missing	unique	Mean	.05	.10	.25	.50	.75	.90	.95
	411	126	22	12.03	7	8	10	12	14	16	17

lowest : 0 1 2 3 4, highest: 17 18 19 20 22

---

income

	n	missing	unique
	335	202	4

under \$11k (158, 47%), \$11-\$25k (79, 24%), \$25-\$50k (63, 19%)
>\$50k (35, 10%)

---

scoma : SUPPORT Coma Score based on Glasgow D3

	n	missing	unique	Mean	.05	.10	.25	.50	.75	.90	.95
	537	0	11	19.24	0	0	0	0	37	55	100

	0	9	26	37	41	44	55	61	89	94	100
Frequency	301	50	44	19	17	43	11	6	8	6	32
%	56	9	8	4	3	8	2	1	1	1	6

---

charges : Hospital Charges

	n	missing	unique	Mean	.05	.10	.25	.50	.75	.90	.95
	517	20	516	86652	11075	15180	27389	51079	100904	205562	283411

lowest :   3448   4432   4574   5555   5849
highest: 504660 538323 543761 706577 740010

---

totcst : Total RCC cost

	n	missing	unique	Mean	.05	.10	.25	.50	.75	.90	.95
	471	66	471	46360	6359	8449	15412	29308	57028	108927	141569

lowest :   0   2071   2522   3191   3325
highest: 269057 269131 338955 357919 390460

---

totmcst : Total micro-cost

	n	missing	unique	Mean	.05	.10	.25	.50	.75	.90	.95
	331	206	328	39022	6131	8283	14415	26323	54102	87495	111920

lowest :   0   1562   2478   2626   3421
highest: 144234 154709 198047 234876 271467

---

avtisst : Average TISS, Days 3-25

	n	missing	unique	Mean	.05	.10	.25	.50	.75	.90	.95
	536	1	205	29.83	12.46	14.50	19.62	28.00	39.00	47.17	50.37

lowest :   4.000   5.667   8.000   9.000   9.500
highest: 58.500 59.000 60.000 61.000 64.000

---

race : Race

	n	missing	unique
	535	2	5

	white	black	asian	other	hispanic
Frequency	417	84	4	8	22
%	78	16	1	1	4

meanbp : Mean Arterial Blood Pressure Day 3

n	missing	unique	Mean	.05	.10	.25	.50	.75	.90	.95
537	0	109	83.28	41.8	49.0	59.0	73.0	111.0	124.4	135.0

lowest :   0 20 27 30 32, highest: 155 158 161 162 180

wblc : White Blood Cell Count Day 3

n	missing	unique	Mean	.05	.10	.25	.50	.75	.90
532	5	241	14.1	0.8999	4.5000	7.9749	12.3984	18.1992	25.1891

.95
30.1873

lowest :   0.05000   0.06999   0.09999   0.14999   0.19998
highest: 51.39844 58.19531 61.19531 79.39062 100.00000

hrt : Heart Rate Day 3

n	missing	unique	Mean	.05	.10	.25	.50	.75	.90	.95
537	0	111	105	51	60	75	111	126	140	155

lowest :   0 11 30 36 40, highest: 189 193 199 232 300

resp : Respiration Rate Day 3

n	missing	unique	Mean	.05	.10	.25	.50	.75	.90	.95
537	0	45	23.72	8	10	12	24	32	39	40

lowest :   0   4   6   7   8, highest: 48 49 52 60 64

temp : Temperature (celcius) Day 3

n	missing	unique	Mean	.05	.10	.25	.50	.75	.90	.95
537	0	61	37.52	35.50	35.80	36.40	37.80	38.50	39.09	39.50

lowest : 32.50 34.00 34.09 34.90 35.00
highest: 40.20 40.59 40.90 41.00 41.20

pafi : PaO2/(.01*FiO2) Day 3

n	missing	unique	Mean	.05	.10	.25	.50	.75	.90	.95
500	37	357	227.2	86.99	105.08	137.88	202.56	290.00	390.49	433.31

lowest : 45.00 48.00 53.33 54.00 55.00
highest: 574.00 595.12 640.00 680.00 869.38

alb : Serum Albumin Day 3

n	missing	unique	Mean	.05	.10	.25	.50	.75	.90	.95
346	191	34	2.668	1.700	1.900	2.225	2.600	3.100	3.400	3.800

lowest : 1.100 1.200 1.300 1.400 1.500
highest: 4.100 4.199 4.500 4.699 4.800

bili : Bilirubin Day 3

n	missing	unique	Mean	.05	.10	.25	.50	.75	.90
386	151	88	2.678	0.3000	0.4000	0.6000	0.8999	2.0000	6.5996

.95
13.1743

lowest :   0.09999   0.19998   0.29999   0.39996   0.50000
highest: 22.59766 30.00000 31.50000 35.00000 39.29688

crea : Serum creatinine Day 3

n	missing	unique	Mean	.05	.10	.25	.50	.75	.90	.95
537	0	84	2.232	0.6000	0.7000	0.8999	1.3999	2.5996	5.2395	7.3197

lowest :   0.3   0.4   0.5   0.6   0.7, highest: 10.4 10.6 11.2 11.6 11.8

sod : Serum sodium Day 3

n	missing	unique	Mean	.05	.10	.25	.50	.75	.90	.95
537	0	38	138.1	129	131	134	137	142	147	150

lowest : 118 120 121 126 127, highest: 156 157 158 168 175

ph : Serum pH (arterial) Day 3

n	missing	unique	Mean	.05	.10	.25	.50	.75	.90	.95
500	37	49	7.416	7.270	7.319	7.380	7.420	7.470	7.510	7.529

lowest : 6.960 6.989 7.069 7.119 7.130
highest: 7.560 7.569 7.590 7.600 7.659

glucose : Glucose Day 3

n	missing	unique	Mean	.05	.10	.25	.50	.75	.90	.95
297	240	179	167.7	76.0	89.0	106.0	141.0	200.0	292.4	347.2

lowest :   30   42   52   55   68, highest: 446 468 492 576 598

bun : BUN Day 3

n	missing	unique	Mean	.05	.10	.25	.50	.75	.90	.95
304	233	100	38.91	8.00	11.00	16.75	30.00	56.00	79.70	100.70

lowest :   1   3   4   5   6, highest: 123 124 125 128 146

urine : Urine Output Day 3

n	missing	unique	Mean	.05	.10	.25	.50	.75	.90	.95
303	234	262	2095	20.3	364.0	1156.5	1870.0	2795.0	4008.6	4817.5

lowest :   0   5   8   15   20, highest: 6865 6920 7360 7560 7750

adlp : ADL Patient Day 3

n	missing	unique	Mean
104	433	8	1.577

	0	1	2	3	4	5	6	7
Frequency	51	19	7	6	4	7	8	2
%	49	18	7	6	4	7	8	2

adls : ADL Surrogate Day 3

n	missing	unique	Mean
392	145	8	1.86

	0	1	2	3	4	5	6	7
Frequency	185	68	22	18	17	20	39	23
%	47	17	6	5	4	5	10	6

sfdm2 : Severe Functional Disability Month 2

```
  n missing unique
468      69      5
```

```
no(M2 and SIP pres) (134, 29%), adl>=4 (>=5 if sur) (78, 17%)
SIP>=30 (30, 6%), Coma or Intub (5, 1%), <2 mo. follow-up (221, 47%)
```

adlsc : Imputed ADL Calibrated to Surrogate

```
  n missing unique  Mean   .05    .10    .25    .50    .75    .90    .95
537 0          144   2.119 0.000 0.000 0.000 1.839 3.375 6.000 6.000
```

```
lowest : 0.0000 0.4948 0.4948 1.0000 1.1667
highest: 5.7832 6.0000 6.3398 6.4658 7.0000
```

Next, distributions of continuous predictors, stratified by coma versus acute respiratory failure/multiple organ system failure, are plotted. Then patterns of missing data are displayed.

```
> ecdf(support[acute,c(1,12,14,18,19:31,35)],
+       group=support$dzclass, lty=1:2,
+       label.curves=F, subtitles=F)          # Figure 18.1
> # Show patterns of missing data
> plot(naclus(support[acute,]), hang=.05) # Figure 18.2
```

The `Hmisc` `varclus` function is used to quantify and depict associations between predictors, allowing for general nonmonotonic relationships. This is done by using Hoeffding's D as a similarity measure for all possible pairs of predictors instead of the default similarity, Spearman's ρ.

```
> attach(support[acute,])
> vc ← varclus(~ age+sex+dzgroup+num.co+edu+income+scoma+race+
+               meanbp+wblc+hrt+resp+temp+pafi+alb+bili+crea+sod+
+               ph+glucose+bun+urine+adlsc, sim='hoeffding')
> plot(vc)                                  # Figure 18.3
```

18.2 Checking Adequacy of Log-Normal Accelerated Failure Time Model

Let us check whether a parametric survival time model will fit the data, with respect to the key prognostic factors. First, Kaplan–Meier estimates stratified by disease group are computed, and plotted after inverse normal transformation, against $\log t$. Parallelism and linearity indicate goodness of fit to the log normal distribution for disease group. Then a more stringent assessment is made by fitting an initial model and computing right-censored residuals. These residuals, after dividing by $\hat{\sigma}$, should all have a normal distribution if the model holds. We compute Kaplan–Meier estimates of the distribution of the residuals and overlay the estimated survival

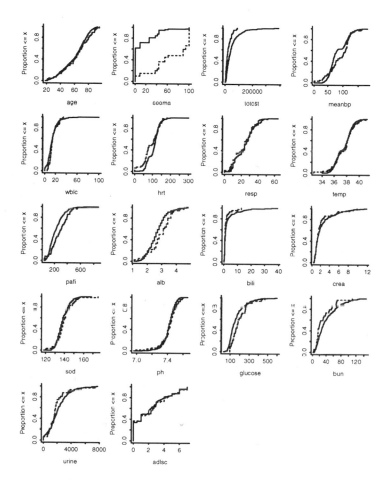

FIGURE 18.1: Empirical cumulative distribution functions for selected continuous variables, stratified by disease class. ARF/MOSF is shown with a solid line, and Coma with a dotted line.

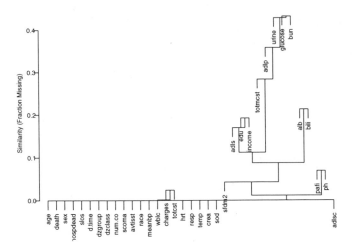

FIGURE 18.2: Cluster analysis showing which predictors tend to be missing on the same patients.

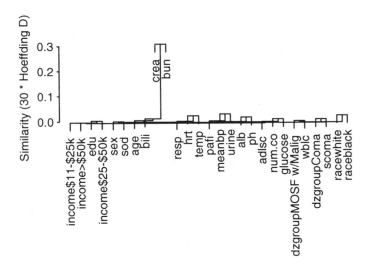

FIGURE 18.3: Hierarchical clustering of potential predictors using Hoeffding D as a similarity measure. Categorical predictors are automatically expanded into dummy variables.

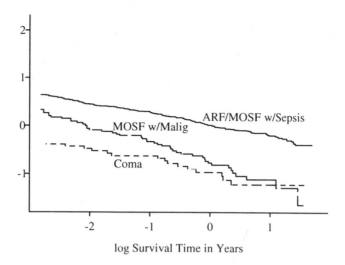

FIGURE 18.4: $\Phi^{-1}(S_{KM}(t))$ stratified by dzgroup. Linearity and semiparallelism indicate a reasonable fit to the log-normal accelerated failure time model with respect to one predictor.

distribution with the theoretical Gaussian one. This is done overall, and then to get more stringent assessments of fit, residuals are stratified by key predictors and plots are produced that contain multiple Kaplan–Meier curves along with a single theoretical normal curve. All curves should hover about the normal distribution. To gauge the natural variability of stratified residual distribution estimates, the residuals are also stratified by a random number that has no bearing on the goodness of fit.

```
> dd ← datadist(support[acute,])
> # describe distributions of variables to Design
> options(datadist='dd')

> # Generate right-censored survival time variable
> years ← d.time/365.25
> units(years) ← 'Year'
> S ← Surv(years, death)

> # Show normal inverse Kaplan-Meier estimates stratified by dzgroup
> survplot(survfit(S ∼ dzgroup), conf='none',
+          fun=qnorm,logt=T)    # Figure 18.4

> f ← psm(S ∼ dzgroup + rcs(age,5) + rcs(meanbp,5),
+          dist='gaussian', y=T)
```

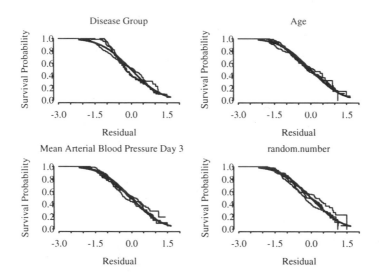

FIGURE 18.5: Kaplan–Meier estimates of distributions of normalized, right-censored residuals from the fitted log-normal survival model. Residuals are stratified by important variables in the model (by quartiles of continuous variables), plus a random variable to depict the natural variability. Theoretical standard Gaussian distributions of residuals are shown with a thick solid line.

```
> r ← resid(f)

> par(mfrow=c(2,2))
> survplot(r, dzgroup, label.curve=F)
> survplot(r, age,     label.curve=F)
> survplot(r, meanbp,  label.curve=F)
> random.number ← runif(length(age))
> survplot(r, random.number, label.curve=F)     # Figure 18.5
```

The fit for dzgroup is not great but overall fit is good.

Now remove from consideration predictors that are missing in more than 0.2 of patients. Many of these were collected only for the second half of SUPPORT. Of those continuous variables to be included in the model, find which ones have enough potential predictive power to justify allowing for nonlinear relationships, which spend more d.f. For each variable compute Spearman ρ^2 based on multiple linear regression of rank(x), rank(x)^2, and the survival time, truncating survival time at the shortest follow-up for survivors (356 days; see Section 4.1). Remaining missing values are imputed using the "most normal" values, a procedure found to work adequately for this particular study. Race is imputed using the modal category.

```
> shortest.follow.up ← min(d.time[death==0], na.rm=T)
```

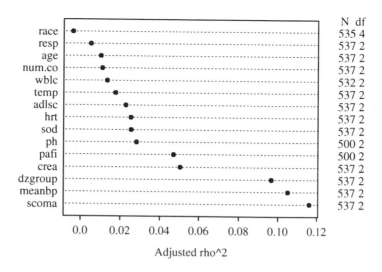

FIGURE 18.6: Generalized Spearman ρ^2 rank correlation between predictors and truncated survival time.

```
> d.timet ← pmin(d.time, shortest.follow.up)

> w ← spearman2(d.timet ∼ age + num.co + scoma + meanbp +
+               hrt + resp + temp + crea + sod + adlsc +
+               wblc + pafi + ph + dzgroup + race, p=2)
> plot(w)          # Figure 18.6


> # Compute number of missing values per variable
> sapply(llist(age,num.co,scoma,meanbp,hrt,resp,temp,crea,sod,adlsc,
+               wblc,pafi,ph), function(x) sum(is.na(x)))
> # Can also do naplot(naclus(support[acute,]))
```

age	num.co	scoma	meanbp	hrt	resp	temp	crea	sod	adlsc	wblc	pafi	ph
0	0	0	0	0	0	0	0	0	0	5	37	37

```
> # Can also use the Hmisc naclus and naplot functions to do this

> # Impute missing values with normal or modal values
> wblc.i ← impute(wblc.i, 9)
> pafi.i ← impute(pafi.i, 333.3)
> ph.i   ← impute(ph.i, 7.4)
> race2  ← race
> levels(race2) ← list(white='white',other=levels(race)[-1])
> race2[is.na(race2)] ← 'white'
> dd ← datadist(dd, wblc.i, pafi.i, ph.i, race2)
```

Now a log-normal survival model is fitted, with number of parameters corresponding to nonlinear effects determined from Spearman ρ^2 analysis.

```
> # Singular information matrix when included ph.i
> f ← psm(S ∼ rcs(age,3)+sex+dzgroup+pol(num.co,2)+
+                pol(scoma,2)+pol(adlsc,2)+race2+rcs(meanbp,5)+
+                rcs(hrt,3)+resp+rcs(temp,3)+
+                rcs(crea,5)+sod+rcs(wblc.i,3)+rcs(pafi.i,3),
+           dist='gaussian')
> f
```

```
Parametric Survival Model: Gaussian Distribution

 Obs Events Model L.R. d.f. P   R2
 537    356      271.06  30 0 0.49
```

```
.   .   .   .   .   .   .   .
```

18.3   Summarizing the Fitted Model

First let's plot the shape of the effect of each predictor on log survival time. All effects are centered so that they can be placed on a common scale. This allows the relative strength of various predictors to be judged. Then Wald χ^2 statistics, penalized for d.f., are plotted in descending order. Next, relative effects of varying predictors over reasonable ranges (survival time ratios varying continuous predictors from the first to the third quartile) are charted.

```
> par(mfrow=c(3,5))
> plot(f, ref.zero=T, ylim=c(-3,2), lwd.conf=.6,
+      vnames='names', abbrev=T)        # Figure 18.7
> plot(anova(f))                        # Figure 18.8
> anova(f)                              # Table 18.1
> options(digits=3)
> plot(summary(f), log=T)               # Figure 18.9
```

18.4   Internal Validation of the Fitted Model Using the Bootstrap

Let us decide whether there was significant overfitting during the development of this model, using the bootstrap.

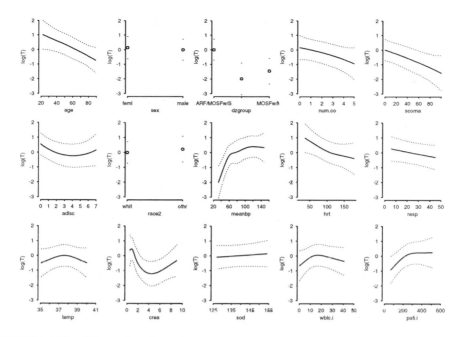

FIGURE 18.7: Effect of each predictor on log survival time. Predicted values have been centered so that predictions at predictor reference values are zero. Pointwise 0.95 confidence bands are also shown. As all Y-axes have the same scale, it is easy to see which predictors are strongest.

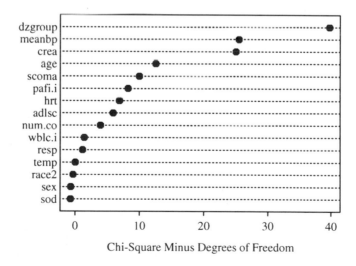

FIGURE 18.8: Contribution of variables in predicting survival time in log-normal model.

TABLE 18.1: Wald Statistics for S

	χ^2	d.f.	P
age	14.55	2	0.0007
Nonlinear	0.04	1	0.8367
sex	0.34	1	0.5603
dzgroup	41.78	2	< 0.0001
num.co	5.99	2	0.0501
Nonlinear	0.14	1	0.7106
scoma	11.98	2	0.0025
Nonlinear	0.06	1	0.8019
adlsc	7.94	2	0.0188
Nonlinear	3.67	1	0.0553
race2	0.69	1	0.4069
meanbp	29.49	4	< 0.0001
Nonlinear	11.81	3	0.0081
hrt	8.91	2	0.0116
Nonlinear	0.58	1	0.4463
resp	2.19	1	0.1392
temp	2.06	2	0.3562
Nonlinear	1.97	1	0.1600
crea	28.99	4	< 0.0001
Nonlinear	18.95	3	0.0003
sod	0.31	1	0.5752
wblc.i	3.48	2	0.1756
Nonlinear	3.47	1	0.0624
pafi.i	10.25	2	0.0059
Nonlinear	2.72	1	0.0994
TOTAL NONLINEAR	50.83	14	< 0.0001
TOTAL	251.19	30	< 0.0001

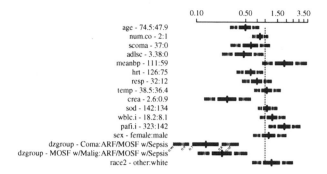

FIGURE 18.9: Estimated survival time ratios for default settings of predictors. For example, when age changes from its lower quartile to the upper quartile (47.9y to 74.5y), median survival time decreases by half. Different shaded areas of bars indicate different confidence levels, ranging from 0.7 to 0.99.

```
> # First add data to model fit so bootstrap can resample from the data
> g ← update(f, x=T, y=T)
> validate(g, B=50, dxy=T)
```

```
Divergence or singularity in 7 samples
          index.orig training   test optimism index.corrected  n
Dxy           0.4763   0.4986 0.4511    0.048          0.4287 43
R2            0.4877   0.5319 0.4433    0.089          0.3991 43
Intercept     0.0000   0.0000 0.4588   -0.459          0.4588 43
Slope         1.0000   1.0000 0.9225    0.077          0.9225 43
D             0.3002   0.3311 0.2703    0.061          0.2394 43
U            -0.0022  -0.0021 0.0049   -0.007          0.0048 43
Q             0.3025   0.3333 0.2654    0.068          0.2346 43
```

Judging from D_{xy} and R^2 there is a moderate amount of overfitting. The slope shrinkage factor (0.92) is not troublesome, however. An almost unbiased estimate of future predictive discrimination on similar patients is given by the corrected D_{xy} of 0.43. This index equals the difference between the probability of concordance and the probability of discordance of pairs of predicted survival times and pairs of observed survival times, accounting for censoring.

Next, a bootstrap overfitting-corrected calibration curve is estimated. Patients are stratified by the predicted probability of surviving one year, such that there are at least 60 patients in each group.

```
> cal ← calibrate(g, u=1, m=60)
> plot(cal)                # Figure 18.10
> rm(g)                    # remove large object
```

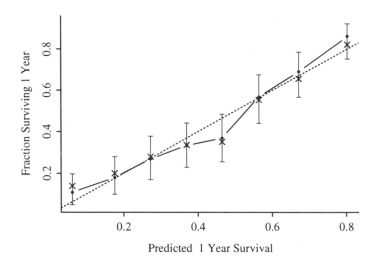

FIGURE 18.10: Bootstrap validation of calibration curve. Dots represent apparent calibration accuracy; ×s represent bootstrap estimates corrected for overfitting.

Of the eight prognostic groups, the leftmost one having the worst average prognosis did not validate very well, consistent with indexes of overfitting listed above. The remaining prognostic spectrum appears to validate well.

18.5   Approximating the Full Model

The fitted log-normal model is perhaps too complex for routine use and for routine data collection. Let us develop a simplified model that can predict the predicted values of the full model with high accuracy ($R^2 = 0.967$). The simplification is done using a fast backward step-down against the full model predicted values.

```
> Z ← predict(f)      # X*beta hat
> a ← ols(Z ~ rcs(age,3)+sex+dzgroup+pol(num.co,2)+
+               pol(scoma,2)+pol(adlsc,2)+race2+
+               rcs(meanbp,5)+rcs(hrt,3)+resp+
+               rcs(temp,3)+rcs(crea,5)+sod+rcs(wblc.i,3)+
+               rcs(pafi.i,3), sigma=1)
> # sigma=1 is used to prevent sigma hat from being zero when R2=1.0
> # since we start out by approximating Z with all component variables
> fastbw(a, aics=10000)      # fast backward step-down
```

Deleted	Chi-Sq	d.f.	P	Residual	d.f.	P	AIC	R2
sex	2.05	1	0.1518	2.05	1	0.1518	0.05	0.999
sod	2.29	1	0.1302	4.35	2	0.1139	0.35	0.997
race2	4.41	1	0.0357	8.76	3	0.0327	2.76	0.994
temp	8.00	2	0.0183	16.75	5	0.0050	6.75	0.989
resp	14.76	1	0.0001	31.51	6	0.0000	19.51	0.980
wblc.i	19.88	2	0.0000	51.39	8	0.0000	35.39	0.967
num.co	35.80	2	0.0000	87.19	10	0.0000	67.19	0.944
adlsc	51.31	2	0.0000	138.51	12	0.0000	114.51	0.912
pafi.i	50.05	2	0.0000	188.56	14	0.0000	160.56	0.880
hrt	77.06	2	0.0000	265.62	16	0.0000	233.62	0.831
age	64.25	2	0.0000	329.87	18	0.0000	293.87	0.790
scoma	76.20	2	0.0000	406.07	20	0.0000	366.07	0.741
crea	320.25	4	0.0000	726.32	24	0.0000	678.32	0.538
meanbp	403.08	4	0.0000	1129.40	28	0.0000	1073.40	0.281
dzgroup	441.14	2	0.0000	1570.54	30	0.0000	1510.54	0.000

```
> f.approx ← ols(Z ~ dzgroup + rcs(meanbp,5) +
+                    rcs(crea,5) + pol(scoma,2) + rcs(age,3) +
+                    rcs(hrt,3) + rcs(pafi.i,3) + pol(adlsc,2)+
+                    pol(num.co,2), x=T)    # x=T to get variances
> f.approx$stats
```

```
    n Model L.R. d.f.    R2 Sigma
  537        1836   22 0.967 0.316
```

We can estimate the variance–covariance matrix of the coefficients of the reduced model using Equation 5.2 in Section 5.4.2. The computations below result in a covariance matrix that does not include elements related to the scale parameter. In the code x is the matrix T in Section 5.4.2. The Varcov function is in Design.

```
> V ← Varcov(f,regcoef.only=T)           # var(full model)
> X ← g$x                                # full model design
> x ← f.approx$x                         # approx. model design
> w ← solve(t(x) %*% x, t(x)) %*% X      # contrast matrix
> v ← w %*% V %*% t(w)
```

Let's compare the variance estimates (diagonals of v) with variance estimates from a reduced model that is fitted against the actual outcomes.

```
> f.sub ← psm(S ~ dzgroup + rcs(meanbp,5) + rcs(crea,5) +
+               pol(scoma,2) + rcs(age,3) + rcs(hrt,3) +
+               rcs(pafi.i,3) + pol(adlsc,2) +
+               pol(num.co,2), dist='gaussian')

> diag(v)/diag(Varcov(f.sub,regcoef.only=T))
```

The ratios ranged from 0.979 to 0.984, so the estimated variances from the reduced model are actually slightly smaller than those that would have been obtained from stepwise variable selection in this case, had variable selection used a stopping rule that resulted in the same set of variables being selected. Now let us compute Wald statistics for the reduced model.

```
> f.approx$var ← v
> anova(f.approx, test='Chisq', ss=F)
```

The results are shown in Table 18.2. Note the similarity of the statistics to those found in the table for the full model. This would not be the case had deleted variables been very collinear with retained variables.

TABLE 18.2: Wald Statistics for Z

	χ^2	d.f.	P
dzgroup	54.60	2	< 0.0001
meanbp	30.50	4	< 0.0001
Nonlinear	10.80	3	0.0128
crea	32.10	4	< 0.0001
Nonlinear	22.10	3	0.0001
scoma	11.60	2	0.0030
Nonlinear	0.11	1	0.7369
age	13.40	2	0.0012
Nonlinear	0.10	1	0.7477
hrt	10.80	2	0.0045
Nonlinear	0.34	1	0.5626
pafi.i	10.10	2	0.0063
Nonlinear	2.43	1	0.1193
adlsc	6.62	2	0.0364
Nonlinear	2.93	1	0.0872
num.co	6.37	2	0.0414
Nonlinear	0.06	1	0.8051
TOTAL NONLINEAR	45.50	12	< 0.0001
TOTAL	242.00	22	< 0.0001

The equation for the simplified model follows. The model is also depicted graphically in Figure 18.11. The nomogram allows one to calculate mean and median survival time. Survival probabilities could have easily been added as additional axes.

```
> # Typeset mathematical form of approximate model
> w ← latex(f.approx)
```

$$E(Z) = X\beta,$$

where

$X\hat{\beta} =$

-1.43

$-1.99\{\text{Coma}\} - 1.74\{\text{MOSF w/Malig}\}$

$+0.0693 \text{ meanbp} - 0.0000302(\text{meanbp} - 41.8)_+^3 + 0.0000761(\text{meanbp} - 61)_+^3$

$-0.0000469(\text{meanbp} - 73)_+^3 + 3.25 \times 10^{-06}(\text{meanbp} - 109)_+^3$

$-2.32 \times 10^{-06}(\text{meanbp} - 135)_+^3$

$+0.161 \text{ crea} - 1.93(\text{crea} - 0.6)_+^3 + 3.31(\text{crea} - 0.9)_+^3 - 1.44(\text{crea} - 1.4)_+^3$

$+0.0451(\text{crea} - 2.4)_+^3 + 0.0115(\text{crea} - 7.32)_+^3 - 0.011413 \text{ scoma} - 0.000041\text{scoma}^2$

$-0.0197 \text{ age} - 2.27 \times 10^{-06}(\text{age} - 35.2)_+^3 + 5.89 \times 10^{-06}(\text{age} - 63.7)_+^3$

$-3.62 \times 10^{-06}(\text{age} - 81.5)_+^3$

$-0.0137 \text{ hrt} + 5.64 \times 10^{-07}(\text{hrt} - 60)_+^3 - 1.55 \times 10^{-06}(\text{hrt} - 111)_+^3$

$+9.91 \times 10^{-07}(\text{hrt} - 140)_+^3$

$+0.00646 \text{ pafi.i} - 6.85 \times 10^{-08}(\text{pafi.i} - 108)_+^3 + 1.13 \times 10^{-07}(\text{pafi.i} - 218)_+^3$

$-4.47 \times 10^{-08}(\text{pafi.i} - 385)_+^3 - 0.3418 \text{ adlsc} + 0.0416\text{adlsc}^2$

$-0.1624 \text{ num.co} - 0.0117\text{num.co}^2$

and $\{c\} = 1$ if subject is in group c, 0 otherwise; $(x)_+ = x$ if $x > 0$, 0 otherwise.

```
> # Derive S-PLUS functions that express mean and quantiles
> # of survival time for specific linear predictors analytically
> expected.surv <  Mean(f)
> quantile.surv <- Quantile(f)
> expected.surv

function(lp, parms = structure(.Data = 0.812110283722707,
          .Names = "Log(scale)"),
transform = structure(.Data = "log", .Names = "link"))
{
names(parms) <- NULL
switch(transform,
        identity = lp,
        log = exp(lp + exp(2 * parms)/2),
        stop(paste(transform, "not implemented")))
}
```

```
> quantile.surv

function(q = 0.5, lp,
          parms = structure(.Data = 0.812110283722707,
          .Names = "Log(scale)"),
          transform = structure(.Data = "log",
                                      .Names = "link"))
{
names(parms) ← NULL
inv ← glm.links["inverse", transform]$inverse
f ← function(lp, q, parms)
lp + exp(parms) * qnorm(q)
names(q) ← format(q)
drop(inv(outer(lp, q, FUN = f, parms = parms)))
}

> median.surv   ← function(x) quantile.surv(lp=x)


> # Improve variable labels for the nomogram
> f.approx ← Newlabels(f.approx,
+              c('Disease Group','Mean Arterial BP',
+                'Creatinine','SUPPORT Coma Score','Age',
+                'Heart Rate', 'PaO2/(.01*FiO2)','ADL',
+                '# Comorbidities'))

> nomogram(f.approx,
+          fun=list('Median Survival Time'=median.surv,
+                   'Mean Survival Time'  =expected.surv),
+          fun.at=c(.1,.25,.5,1,2,5,10,20,40),
+          cex.var=1,cex.axis=.75)
> # Figure 18.11
```

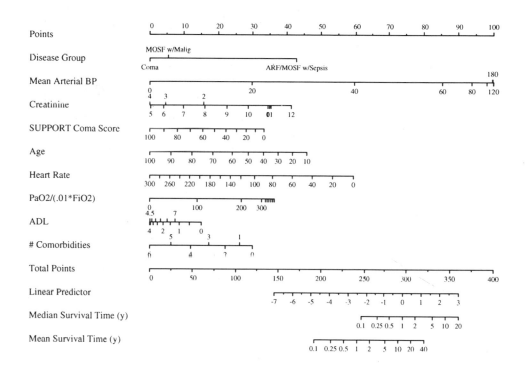

FIGURE 18.11:   Nomogram for predicting median and mean survival time, based on approximation of full model.

18.6   Problems

Analyze the Mayo Clinic PBC dataset.

1. Graphically assess whether Weibull (extreme value), exponential, log-logistic, or log-normal distributions will fit the data, using a few apparently important stratification factors.

2. For the best fitting parametric model from among the four examined, fit a model containing several sensible covariables, both categorical and continuous. Do a Wald test for whether each factor in the model has an association with survival time, and a likelihood ratio test for the simultaneous contribution of all predictors. For classification factors having more than two levels, be sure that the Wald test has the appropriate degrees of freedom. For continuous factors, verify or relax linearity assumptions. If using a Weibull model, test whether a simpler exponential model would be appropriate. Interpret all estimated coefficients in the model. Write the full survival model in mathematical form. Generate a predicted survival curve for a patient with a given set of characteristics.

See [244] for an analysis of this dataset using linear splines in time and in the covariables.

Chapter 19

Cox Proportional Hazards Regression Model

19.1 Model

19.1.1 Preliminaries

The Cox proportional hazards model[92] is the most popular model for the analysis of survival data. It is a semiparametric model; it makes a parametric assumption concerning the effect of the predictors on the hazard function, but makes no assumption regarding the nature of the hazard function $\lambda(t)$ itself. The Cox PH model assumes that predictors act multiplicatively on the hazard function but does not assume that the hazard function is constant (i.e., exponential model), Weibull, or any other particular form. The regression portion of the model is fully parametric; that is, the regressors are linearly related to log hazard or log cumulative hazard. In many situations, either the form of the true hazard function is unknown or it is complex, so the Cox model has definite advantages. Also, one is usually more interested in the effects of the predictors than in the shape of $\lambda(t)$, and the Cox approach allows the analyst to essentially ignore $\lambda(t)$, which is often not of primary interest.

   The Cox PH model uses only the rank ordering of the failure and censoring times and thus is less affected by outliers in the failure times than fully parametric methods. The model contains as a special case the popular log-rank test for comparing survival between two groups. For estimating and testing regression coefficients, the Cox model is as efficient as parametric models (e.g., Weibull model with PH) even when all assumptions of the parametric model are satisfied.[123]

When a parametric model's assumptions are not true (e.g., when a Weibull model is used and the population is not from a Weibull survival distribution so that the choice of model is incorrect), the Cox analysis is more efficient than the parametric analysis. As shown below, diagnostics for checking Cox model assumptions are very well developed.

19.1.2   Model Definition

The Cox PH model is most often stated in terms of the hazard function:

$$\lambda(t|X) = \lambda(t)\exp(X\beta). \tag{19.1}$$

We do not include an intercept parameter in $X\beta$ here. Note that this is identical to the parametric PH model stated earlier. There is an important difference, however, in that now we do not assume any specific shape for $\lambda(t)$. For the moment, we are not even interested in estimating $\lambda(t)$. The reason for this departure from the fully parametric approach is due to an ingenious conditional argument by Cox.[92] Cox argued that when the PH model holds, information about $\lambda(t)$ is not very useful in estimating the parameters of primary interest, β. By special conditioning in formulating the log likelihood function, Cox showed how to derive a valid estimate of β that does not require estimation of $\lambda(t)$ as $\lambda(t)$ dropped out of the new likelihood function. Cox's derivation focuses on using the information in the data that relates to the relative hazard function $\exp(X\beta)$.

19.1.3   Estimation of β

Cox's derivation of an estimator of β can be loosely described as follows. Let $t_1 < t_2 < \ldots < t_k$ represent the unique ordered failure times in the sample of n subjects; assume for now that there are no tied failure times (tied censoring times are allowed) so that $k = n$. Consider the set of individuals at risk of failing an instant before failure time t_i. This set of individuals is called the *risk set* at time t_i, and we use R_i to denote this risk set. R_i is the set of subjects j such that the subject had not failed or been censored by time t_i; that is, the risk set R_i includes subjects with failure/censoring time $Y_j \geq t_i$.

The conditional probability that individual i is the one that failed at t_i, given that the subjects in the set R_i are at risk of failing, and given further that exactly one failure occurs at t_i, is

$$\text{Prob}\{\text{subject } i \text{ fails at } t_i | R_i \text{ and one failure at } t_i\} \;=\; \frac{\text{Prob}\{\text{subject } i \text{ fails at } t_i | R_i\}}{\text{Prob}\{\text{ one failure at } t_i | R_i\}} \tag{19.2}$$

using the rules of conditional probability. This conditional probability equals

$$\frac{\lambda(t_i)\exp(X_i\beta)}{\sum_{j\in R_i}\lambda(t_i)\exp(X_j\beta)} = \frac{\exp(X_i\beta)}{\sum_{j\in R_i}\exp(X_j\beta)} = \frac{\exp(X_i\beta)}{\sum_{Y_j\geq t_i}\exp(X_j\beta)} \qquad (19.3)$$

independent of $\lambda(t)$. To understand this likelihood, consider a special case where the predictors have no effect; that is, $\beta = 0$ [64, pp. 48–49]. Then $\exp(X_i\beta) = \exp(X_j\beta) = 1$ and Prob{subject i is the subject that failed at $t_i|R_i$ and one failure occurred at t_i} is $1/n_i$ where n_i is the number of subjects at risk at time t_i.

By arguing that these conditional probabilities are themselves conditionally independent across the different failure times, a total likelihood can be computed by multiplying these individual likelihoods over all failure times. Cox termed this a *partial likelihood* for β:

$$L(\beta) = \prod_{Y_i \text{ uncensored}} \frac{\exp(X_i\beta)}{\sum_{Y_j\geq Y_i}\exp(X_j\beta)}. \qquad (19.4)$$

The log partial likelihood is

$$\log L(\beta) = \sum_{Y_i \text{ uncensored}} \{X_i\beta - \log[\sum_{Y_j\geq Y_i}\exp(X_j\beta)]\}. \qquad (19.5)$$

Cox and others have shown that this partial log likelihood can be treated as an ordinary log likelihood to derive valid (partial) MLEs of β. Note that this log likelihood is unaffected by the addition of a constant to any or all of the Xs. This is consistent with the fact that an intercept term is unnecessary and cannot be estimated since the Cox model is a model for the relative hazard and does not directly estimate the underlying hazard $\lambda(t)$.

When there are tied failure times in the sample, the true partial log likelihood function involves permutations so it can be time-consuming to compute. When the number of ties is not large, Breslow[49] has derived a satisfactory approximate log likelihood function. The formula given above, when applied without modification to samples containing ties, actually uses Breslow's approximation. If there are ties so that $k < n$ and $t_1,\ldots,t_k$ denote the unique failure times as we originally intended, Breslow's approximation is written as

$$\log L(\beta) = \sum_{i=1}^{k}\{S_i\beta - d_i\log[\sum_{Y_j\geq t_i}\exp(X_j\beta)]\}, \qquad (19.6)$$

where $S_i = \sum_{j\in D_i}X_j$, D_i is the set of indexes j for subjects failing at time t_i, and d_i is the number of failures at t_i.

Efron[123] derived another approximation to the true likelihood that is significantly more accurate than the Breslow approximation and often yields estimates that are very close to those from the more cumbersome permutation likelihood:[198]

$$\log L(\beta) = \sum_{i=1}^{k} \{ S_i \beta - \sum_{j=1}^{d_i} \log[\sum_{Y_j \geq t_i} \exp(X_j \beta) $$

$$- \frac{j-1}{d_i} \sum_{l \in \mathcal{D}_i} \exp(X_l \beta)] \}. \tag{19.7}$$

In the special case when all tied failure times are from subjects with identical $X_i\beta$, the Efron approximation yields the exact (permutation) marginal likelihood (Therneau, personal communication, 1993).

Kalbfleisch and Prentice[225] showed that Cox's partial likelihood, in the absence of predictors that are functions of time, is a marginal distribution of the *ranks* of the failure/censoring times.

19.1.4   Model Assumptions and Interpretation of Parameters

The Cox PH regression model has the same assumptions as the parametric PH model except that no assumption is made regarding the shape of the underlying hazard or survival functions $\lambda(t)$ and $S(t)$. The Cox PH model assumes, in its most basic form, linearity and additivity of the predictors with respect to log hazard or log cumulative hazard. It also assumes the PH assumption of no time by predictor interactions; that is, the predictors have the same effect on the hazard function at all values of t. The relative hazard function $\exp(X\beta)$ is constant through time and the survival functions for subjects with different values of X are powers of each other. If, for example, the hazard of death at time t for treated patients is half that of control patients at time t, this same hazard ratio is in effect at any other time point. In other words, treated patients have a consistently better hazard of death over all follow-up time.

The regression parameters are interpreted the same as in the parametric PH model. The only difference is the absence of hazard shape parameters in the model, since the hazard shape is not estimated in the Cox partial likelihood procedure.

19.1.5   Example

Consider again the rat vaginal cancer data from Section 17.3.6. Figure 19.1 displays the nonparametric survival estimates for the two groups along with estimates derived from the Cox model (by a method discussed later). The predicted survival curves from the fitted Cox model are in good agreement with the nonparametric estimates, again verifying the PH assumption for these data. The estimates of the group effect from a Cox model (using the exact likelihood since there are ties, along with both Efron's and Breslow's approximations) as well as from a Weibull model and an exponential model are shown in Table 19.1. The exponential model, with its

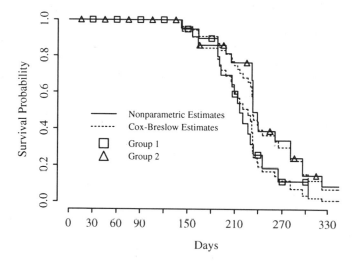

FIGURE 19.1: Altschuler–Nelson–Fleming–Harrington nonparametric survival estimates and Cox-Breslow estimates for rat data[341]

constant hazard, cannot accommodate the long early period with no failures. The group predictor was coded as $X_1 = 0$ and $X_1 - 1$ for Groups 1 and 2, respectively. For this example, the Breslow likelihood approximation resulted in $\hat{\beta}$ closer to that from maximizing the exact likelihood. Note how the group effect (47% reduction in hazard of death by the exact Cox model) is underestimated by the exponential model (9% reduction in hazard). The hazard ratio from the Weibull fit agrees with the Cox fit.

TABLE 19.1

Model	Group Regression Coefficient	S.E.	Wald P-Value	Group 2:1 Hazard Ratio
Cox (Exact)	−0.629	0.361	0.08	0.533
Cox (Efron)	−0.569	0.347	0.10	0.566
Cox (Breslow)	−0.596	0.348	0.09	0.551
Exponential	−0.093	0.334	0.78	0.911
Weibull (AFT)	0.132	0.061	0.03	–
Weibull (PH)	−0.721	–	–	0.486

19.1.6   Design Formulations

Designs are no different for the Cox PH model than for other models except for one minor distinction. Since the Cox model does not have an intercept parameter, the group omitted from X in an ANOVA model will go into the underlying hazard function. As an example, consider a three-group model for treatments A, B, and C. We use the two dummy variables

$$X_1 \;=\; 1 \quad \text{if treatment is A, 0 otherwise, and}$$
$$X_2 \;=\; 1 \quad \text{if treatment is B, 0 otherwise.}$$

The parameter β_1 is the A : C log hazard ratio or difference in hazards at any time t between treatment A and treatment C. β_2 is the B : C log hazard ratio ($\exp(\beta_2)$ is the B : C hazard ratio, etc.). Since there is no intercept parameter, there is no direct estimate of the hazard function for treatment C or any other treatment; only relative hazards are modeled.

As with all regression models, a Wald, score, or likelihood ratio test for differences between any treatments is conducted by testing $H_0 : \beta_1 = \beta_2 = 0$ with 2 d.f.

19.1.7   Extending the Model by Stratification

A unique feature of the Cox PH model is its ability to adjust for factors that are not modeled. Such factors usually take the form of polytomous stratification factors that are either too difficult to model or do not satisfy the PH assumption. For example, a subject's occupation or clinical study site may take on dozens of levels and the sample size may not be large enough to model this nominal variable with dozens of dummy variables. Also, one may know that a certain predictor (either a polytomous one or a continuous one that is grouped) may not satisfy PH and it may be too complex to model the hazard ratio for that predictor as a function of time.

The idea behind the *stratified* Cox PH model is to allow the form of the underlying hazard function to vary across levels of the stratification factors. A stratified Cox analysis ranks the failure times separately within strata. Suppose that there are b strata indexed by $j = 1, 2, \ldots, b$. Let C denote the stratum identification. For example, $C = 1$ or 2 may stand for the female and male strata, respectively. The stratified PH model is

$$\lambda(t|X, C = j) \;=\; \lambda_j(t)\exp(X\beta), \quad \text{or}$$
$$S(t|X, C = j) \;=\; S_j(t)^{\exp(X\beta)}. \tag{19.8}$$

Here $\lambda_j(t)$ and $S_j(t)$ are, respectively, the underlying hazard and survival functions for the jth stratum. The model does not assume any connection between the shapes of these functions for different strata.

In this stratified analysis, the data are stratified by C but, by default, a common vector of regression coefficients is fitted across strata. These common regression coefficients can be thought of as "pooled" estimates. For example, a Cox model with age as a (modeled) predictor and sex as a stratification variable essentially estimates the common slope of age by pooling information about the age effect over the two sexes. The effect of age is adjusted by sex differences, but no assumption is made about how sex affects survival. There is no PH assumption for sex. Levels of the stratification factor C can represent multiple stratification factors that are cross-classified. Since these factors are not modeled, no assumption is made regarding interactions among them.

At first glance it appears that stratification causes a loss of efficiency. However, in most cases the loss is small as long as the number of strata is not too large with regard to the total number of events. A stratum that contains no events contributes no information to the analysis, so such a situation should be avoided if possible.

The stratified or "pooled" Cox model is fitted by formulating a separate log likelihood function for each stratum, but with each log likelihood having a common β vector. If different strata are made up of independent subjects, the strata are independent and the likelihood functions are multiplied together to form a joint likelihood over strata. Log likelihood functions are thus added over strata. This total log likelihood function is maximized once to derive a pooled or stratified estimate of β and to make an inference about β. No inference can be made about the stratification factors. They are merely "adjusted for."

Stratification is useful for checking the PH and linearity assumptions for one or more predictors. Predicted Cox survival curves (Section 19.2) can be derived by modeling the predictors in the usual way, and then stratified survival curves can be estimated by using those predictors as stratification factors. Other factors for which PH is assumed can be modeled in both instances. By comparing the modeled versus stratified survival estimates, a graphical check of the assumptions can be made. Figure 19.1 demonstrates this method although there are no other factors being adjusted for and stratified Cox estimates are KM estimates. The stratified survival estimates are derived by stratifying the dataset to obtain a separate underlying survival curve for each stratum, while pooling information across strata to estimate coefficients of factors that are modeled.

Besides allowing a factor to be adjusted for without modeling its effect, a stratified Cox PH model can also allow a modeled factor to interact with strata.[103, 132, 410] For the age–sex example, consider the following model with X_1 denoting age and $C = 1, 2$ denoting females and males, respectively.

$$\begin{aligned}
\lambda(t|X_1, C = 1) &= \lambda_1(t)\exp(\beta_1 X_1) \\
\lambda(t|X_1, C = 2) &= \lambda_2(t)\exp(\beta_1 X_1 + \beta_2 X_1).
\end{aligned} \qquad (19.9)$$

This model can be simplified to

$$\lambda(t|X_1, C = j) = \lambda_j(t) \exp(\beta_1 X_1 + \beta_2 X_2) \qquad (19.10)$$

if X_2 is a product interaction term equal to 0 for females and X_1 for males. The β_2 parameter quantifies the interaction between age and sex: it is the difference in the age slope between males and females. Thus the interaction between age and sex can be quantified and tested, even though the effect of sex is not modeled!

The stratified Cox model is commonly used to adjust for hospital differences in a multicenter randomized trial. With this method, one can allow for differences in outcome between q hospitals without estimating $q - 1$ parameters. Treatment $\times$ hospital interactions can be tested efficiently without computational problems by estimating only the treatment main effect, after stratifying on hospital. The score statistic (with $q - 1$ d.f.) for testing $q - 1$ treatment $\times$ hospital interaction terms is then computed ("residual χ^2" in a stepwise procedure with treatment $\times$ hospital terms as candidate predictors).

The stratified Cox model turns out to be a generalization of the conditional logistic model for analyzing matched set (e.g., case-control) data.[50] Each stratum represents a set, and the number of "failures" in the set is the number of "cases" in that set. For $r : 1$ matching (r may vary across sets), the Breslow[49] likelihood may be used to fit the conditional logistic model exactly. For $r : m$ matching, an exact Cox likelihood must be computed.

19.2   Estimation of Survival Probability and Secondary Parameters

As discussed above, once a partial log likelihood function is derived, it is used as if it were an ordinary log likelihood function to estimate β, estimate standard errors of β, obtain confidence limits, and make statistical tests. Point and interval estimates of hazard ratios are obtained in the same fashion as with parametric PH models discussed earlier.

The Cox model and parametric survival models differ markedly in how one estimates $S(t|X)$. Since the Cox model does not depend on a choice of the underlying survival function $S(t)$, fitting a Cox model does not result directly in an estimate of $S(t|X)$. However, several authors have derived secondary estimates of $S(t|X)$. One method is the *discrete hazard model* of Kalbfleisch and Prentice [226, pp. 36–37, 84–87]. Their estimator has two advantages: it is an extension of the Kaplan–Meier estimator and is identical to S_{KM} if the estimated value of β happened to be zero or there are no covariables being modeled; and it is not affected by the choice of what constitutes a "standard" subject having the underlying survival function $S(t)$. In other words, it would not matter whether the standard subject is one having age equal to the mean age in the sample or the median age in the sample; the estimate of $S(t|X)$ as a function of X = age would be the same (this is also true of another estimator which follows).

Let $t_1, t_2, \ldots, t_k$ denote the unique failure times in the sample. The discrete hazard model assumes that the probability of failure is greater than zero only at observed failure times. The probability of failure at time t_j given that the subject has not failed before that time is also the hazard of failure at time t_j since the model is discrete. The hazard at t_j for the standard subject is written λ_j. Letting $\alpha_j = 1 - \lambda_j$, the underlying survival function can be written

$$S(t_i) = \prod_{j=0}^{i-1} \alpha_j, i = 1, 2, \ldots, k \quad (\alpha_0 = 1). \tag{19.11}$$

A separate equation can be solved using the Newton–Raphson method to estimate each α_j. If there is only one failure at time t_i, there is a closed-form solution for the maximum likelihood estimate of α_i, a_i, letting j denote the subject who failed at t_i. $\hat{\beta}$ denotes the partial MLE of β.

$$\hat{\alpha}_i = [1 - \exp(X_j\hat{\beta})/ \sum_{Y_m \geq Y_j} \exp(X_m\hat{\beta})]^{\exp(-X_j\hat{\beta})}. \tag{19.12}$$

If $\hat{\beta} = 0$, this formula reduces to a conditional probability component of the product-limit estimator, 1 - (1/number at risk).

The estimator of the underlying survival function is

$$\hat{S}(t) = \prod_{j:t_j < t} \hat{\alpha}_j, \tag{19.13}$$

and the estimate of the probability of survival past time t for a subject with predictor values X is

$$\hat{S}(t|X) = \hat{S}(t)^{\exp(X\hat{\beta})}. \tag{19.14}$$

When the model is stratified, estimation of the α_j and S is carried out separately within each stratum once $\hat{\beta}$ is obtained by pooling over strata. The stratified survival function estimates can be thought of as stratified Kaplan–Meier estimates adjusted for X, with the adjustment made by assuming PH and linearity. As mentioned previously, these stratified adjusted survival estimates are useful for checking model assumptions and for providing a simple way to incorporate factors that violate PH.

The stratified estimates are also useful in themselves as descriptive statistics without making assumptions about a major factor. For example, in a study from Califf et al. [61] to compare medical therapy to coronary artery bypass grafting (CABG), the model was stratified by treatment but adjusted for a variety of baseline characteristics by modeling. These adjusted survival estimates do not assume a form for the effect of surgery. Figure 19.2 displays unadjusted (Kaplan–Meier) and adjusted survival curves, with baseline predictors adjusted to their mean levels in the combined sample. Notice that valid adjusted survival estimates are obtained even though the curves cross (i.e., PH is violated for the treatment variable). These curves are essentially product limit estimates with respect to treatment and Cox PH estimates with respect to the baseline descriptor variables.

The Kalbfleisch–Prentice discrete underlying hazard model estimates of the α_j are one minus estimates of the hazard function at the discrete failure times. However, these estimated hazard functions are usually too "noisy" to be useful unless the sample size is very large or the failure times have been grouped (say by rounding).

Just as Kalbfleisch and Prentice have generalized the Kaplan–Meier estimator to allow for covariables, Breslow[49] has generalized the Altschuler– Nelson–Aalen– Fleming–Harrington estimator to allow for covariables. Using the notation in Section 19.1.3, Breslow's estimate is derived through an estimate of the cumulative hazard function:

$$\hat{\Lambda}(t) = \sum_{i:t_i < t} \frac{d_i}{\sum_{Y_i \geq t_i} \exp(X_i \hat{\beta})}. \tag{19.15}$$

For any X, the estimates of Λ and S are

$$\begin{aligned} \hat{\Lambda}(t|X) &= \hat{\Lambda}(t) \exp(X\hat{\beta}) \\ \hat{S}(t|X) &= \exp[-\hat{\Lambda}(t) \exp(X\hat{\beta})]. \end{aligned} \tag{19.16}$$

More asymptotic theory has been derived from the Breslow estimator than for the Kalbfleisch–Prentice estimator. Another advantage of the Breslow estimator is that it does not require iterative computations for $d_i > 1$. Lawless [264, p. 362] states that the two survival function estimators differ little except in the right-hand tail when all d_is are unity. Like the Kalbfleisch–Prentice estimator, the Breslow estimator is invariant under different choices of "standard subjects" for the underlying survival $S(t)$.

Somewhat complex formulas are available for computing confidence limits of $\hat{S}(t|X)$.[421]

19.3   Test Statistics

Wald, score, and likelihood ratio statistics are useful and valid for drawing inferences about β in the Cox model. The score test deserves special mention here. If there is a single binary predictor in the model that describes two groups, the score test for assessing the importance of the binary predictor is virtually identical to the Mantel–Haenszel log-rank test for comparing the two groups. If the analysis is stratified for other (nonmodeled) factors, the score test from a stratified Cox model is equivalent to the corresponding stratified log-rank test. Of course, the likelihood ratio or Wald

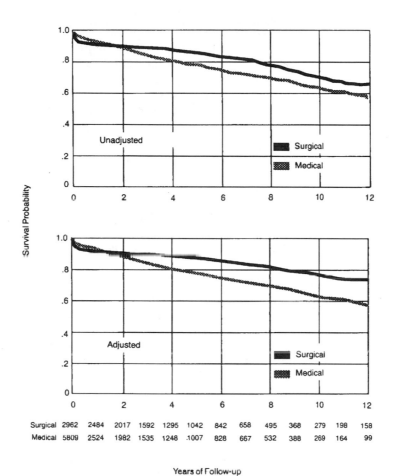

FIGURE 19.2: Unadjusted (Kaplan–Meier) and adjusted (Cox–Kalbfleisch–Prentice) estimates of survival. Top, Kaplan–Meier estimates for patients treated medically and surgically at Duke University Medical Center from November 1969 through December 1984.
These survival curves are not adjusted for baseline prognostic factors. Numbers of patients alive at each follow-up interval for each group are given at the bottom of the figure.
Bottom, survival curves for patients treated medically or surgically after adjusting for all
known important baseline prognostic characteristics.[61] Reprinted by permission, American
Medical Association.

TABLE 19.2

Residual	Purposes
Martingale	Assessing adequacy of a hypothesized predictor transformation. Graphing an estimate of a predictor transformation (Section 19.5.1).
Score	Detecting overly influential observations (Section 19.8). Robust estimate of covariance matrix of $\hat{\beta}$ (Section 9.5).[283]
Schoenfeld	Testing PH assumption (Section 19.5.2). Graphing estimate of hazard ratio function (Section 19.5.2).

tests could also be used in this situation, and in fact the likelihood ratio test may be better than the score test (i.e., type I errors by treating the likelihood ratio test statistic as having a χ^2 distribution may be more accurate than using the log-rank statistic).

The Cox model can be thought of as a generalization of the log-rank procedure since it allows one to test continuous predictors, perform simultaneous tests of various predictors, and adjust for other continuous factors without grouping them. Although a stratified log-rank test does not make assumptions regarding the effect of the adjustment (stratifying) factors, it makes the same assumption (i.e., PH) as the Cox model regarding the treatment effect for the statistical test of no difference in survival between groups.

19.4   Residuals

Therneau et al.[412] discussed four types of residuals from the Cox model: martingale, score, Schoenfeld, and deviance. The first three have been proven to be very useful, as indicated in Table 19.2.

4

19.5   Assessment of Model Fit

As stated before, the Cox model makes the same assumptions as the parametric PH model except that it does not assume a given shape for $\lambda(t)$ or $S(t)$. Because the Cox PH model is so widely used, methods of assessing its fit are dealt with in more detail than was done with the parametric PH models.

19.5.1 Regression Assumptions

Regression assumptions (linearity, additivity) for the PH model are displayed in Figures 17.3 and 17.5. As mentioned earlier, the regression assumptions can be verified by stratifying by X and examining $\log \hat{\Lambda}(t|X)$ or $\log[\Lambda_{KM}(t|X)]$ estimates as a function of X at fixed time t. However, as was pointed out in logistic regression, the stratification method is prone to problems of high variability of estimates. The sample size must be moderately large before estimates are precise enough to observe trends through the "noise." If one wished to divide the sample by quintiles of age and 15 events were thought to be needed in each stratum to derive a reliable estimate of $\log[\Lambda_{KM}(2 \text{ years})]$, there would need to be 75 events in the entire sample. If the Kaplan–Meier estimates were needed to be adjusted for another factor that was binary, twice as many events would be needed to allow the sample to be stratified by that factor.

Figure 19.3 displays Kaplan–Meier three-year log cumulative hazard estimates stratified by sex and decile of age. The simulated sample consists of 2000 hypothetical subjects (368 of whom had events), with 1196 males (142 deaths) and 804 females (226 deaths). The sample was drawn from a population with a known survival distribution that is exponential with hazard function

$$\lambda(t|X_1, X_2) = .02 \exp[.8X_1 + .04(X_2 - 50)], \qquad (19.17)$$

where X_1 represents the sex group (0 = male, 1 = female) and X_2 age in years, and censoring is uniform. Thus for this population PH, linearity, and additivity hold. Notice the amount of variability and wide confidence limits in the stratified nonparametric survival estimates.

As with the logistic model and other regression models, the restricted cubic spline function is an excellent tool for modeling the regression relationship with very few assumptions. A four-knot spline Cox PH model in two variables (X_1, X_2) that assumes linearity in X_1 and no $X_1 \times X_2$ interaction is given by

$$\begin{aligned} \lambda(t|X) &= \lambda(t) \exp(\beta_1 X_1 + \beta_2 X_2 + \beta_3 X_2' + \beta_4 X_2''), \\ &= \lambda(t) \exp(\beta_1 X_1 + f(X_2)), \end{aligned} \qquad (19.18)$$

where X_2' and X_2'' are spline component variables as described earlier and $f(X_2)$ is the spline function or spline transformation of X_2 given by

$$f(X_2) = \beta_2 X_2 + \beta_3 X_2' + \beta_4 X_2''. \qquad (19.19)$$

In linear form the Cox model without assuming linearity in X_2 is

$$\log \lambda(t|X) = \log \lambda(t) + \beta_1 X_1 + f(X_2). \qquad (19.20)$$

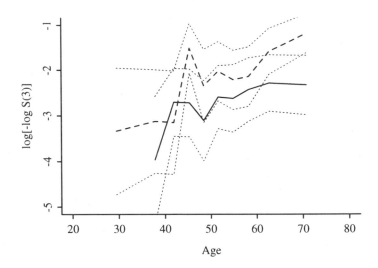

FIGURE 19.3: Kaplan–Meier log Λ estimates by sex and deciles of age, with 0.95 confidence limits. Solid line is for males, dashed line for females.

By computing partial MLEs of β_2, β_3, and β_4, one obtains the estimated transformation of X_2 that yields linearity in log hazard or log cumulative hazard.

A similar model that does not assume PH in X_1 is the Cox model stratified on X_1. Letting the stratification factor be $C = X_1$, this model is

$$
\begin{aligned}
\log \lambda(t | X_2, C = j) &= \log \lambda_j(t) + \beta_1 X_2 + \beta_2 X_2' + \beta_3 X_2'' \\
&= \log \lambda_j(t) + f(X_2).
\end{aligned}
\tag{19.21}
$$

This model does assume no $X_1 \times X_2$ interaction.

Figure 19.4 displays the estimated spline function relating age and sex to $\log[\Lambda(3)]$ in the simulated dataset, using the additive model stratified on sex. The fitted equation, after simplifying the restricted cubic spline to simpler (unrestricted) form, is $X\hat{\beta} = -3.54 + 7.50 \times 10^{-2}\text{age} - 1.48 \times 10^{-5}(\text{age} - 30.7)_+^3 - 1.03 \times 10^{-5}(\text{age} - 45.4)_+^3 + 5.59 \times 10^{-5}(\text{age} - 54.8)_+^3 - 3.07 \times 10^{-5}(\text{age} - 69.6)_+^3$. Notice that the spline estimates are closer to the true linear relationships than were the Kaplan–Meier estimates, and the confidence limits are much tighter. The spline estimates impose a smoothness on the relationship and also use more information from the data by treating age as a continuous ordered variable. Also, unlike the stratified Kaplan–Meier estimates, the modeled estimates can make the assumption of no age $\times$ sex interaction. When this assumption is true, modeling effectively boosts the sample size in estimating a common function for age across both sex groups. Of course, this assumption can be tested and interactions can be modeled if necessary.

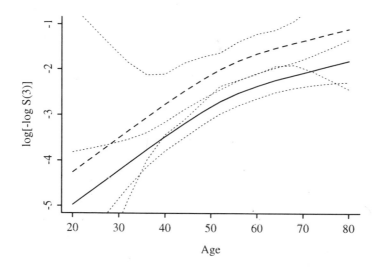

FIGURE 19.4: Cox PH model stratified on sex, using spline function for age, no interaction. 0.95 confidence limits also shown. Soline line is for males, dashed line is for females.

A formal test of the linearity assumption of the Cox PH model in the above example is obtained by testing $H_0 : \beta_2 = \beta_3 = 0$. The χ^2 statistic with 2 d.f. is 4.04, $P = 0.09$.

A Cox model that still does not assume PH for $X_1 = C$ but which allows for an $X_1 \times X_2$ interaction is

$$
\begin{aligned}
\log \lambda(t|X_2, C = j) = \log \lambda_j(t) \quad &+ \quad \beta_1 X_2 + \beta_2 X_2' + \beta_3 X_2'' \\
&+ \quad \beta_4 X_1 X_2 + \beta_5 X_1 X_2' \\
&+ \quad \beta_6 X_1 X_2''.
\end{aligned}
\tag{19.22}
$$

This model allows the relationship between X_2 and log hazard to be a smooth nonlinear function and the shape of the X_2 effect to be completely different for each level of X_1 if X_1 is dichotomous. Figure 19.5 displays a fit of this model at $t = 3$ years for the simulated dataset. The fitted equation is $X\hat{\beta} = -3.93 + 9.86 \times 10^{-2}\text{age} - 2.91 \times 10^{-5}(\text{age} - 30.7)_+^3 + 8.72 \times 10^{-6}(\text{age} - 45.4)_+^3 + 6.22 \times 10^{-5}(\text{age} - 54.8)_+^3 - 4.19 \times 10^{-5}(\text{age} - 69.6)_+^3 + \{\text{Female}\}[-3.50 \times 10^{-2}\text{age} + 1.90 \times 10^{-5}(\text{age} - 30.7)_+^3 - 1.76 \times 10^{-5}(\text{age} - 45.4)_+^3 - 2.10 \times 10^{-5}(\text{age} - 54.8)_+^3 + 1.97 \times 10^{-5}(\text{age} - 69.6)_+^3]$. The test for interaction yielded $\chi^2 = 1.25$ with 3 d.f., $P = 0.74$. The simultaneous test for linearity and additivity yielded $\chi^2 = 5.81$ with 5 d.f., $P = 0.33$. Note that allowing the model to be very flexible (not assuming linearity in age, additivity between age and sex, and PH for sex) still resulted in estimated regression functions that

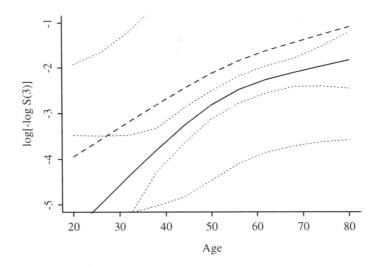

FIGURE 19.5: Cox PH model stratified on sex, with interaction between age spline and sex. 0.95 confidence limits are also shown. Solid line is for males, dashed line for females.

are very close to the true functions. However, confidence limits in this unrestricted model are much wider.

Figure 19.6 displays the estimated relationship between left ventricular ejection fraction (LVEF) and log hazard ratio for cardiovascular death in a sample of patients with significant coronary artery disease. The relationship is estimated using three knots placed at quantiles 0.05, 0.5, and 0.95 of LVEF. Here there is significant non-linearity (Wald $\chi^2 = 9.6$ with 1 d.f.). The graphs lead directly to a transformation of LVEF that satisfies the linearity assumption:

$$
\begin{aligned}
\text{LVEF}' &= \text{LVEF} & \text{if } \text{LVEF} \le 0.5, \\
&= 0.5 & \text{if } \text{LVEF} > 0.5, \quad (19.23)
\end{aligned}
$$

that is, the transformation min(LVEF,0.5). This transformation has the best log likelihood "for the money" as judged by the Akaike information criterion (AIC = $-2 \log$ L.R. $-2\times$ no. parameters = 127). The AICs for 3, 4, 5, and 6-knot spline fits were, respectively, 126, 124, 122, and 120. Had the suggested transformation been more complicated than a truncation, a tentative transformation could have been checked for adequacy by expanding the new transformed variable into a new spline function and testing it for linearity.

Other methods based on smoothed residual plots are also valuable tools for selecting predictor transformations. Therneau et al.[412] describe residuals based on martingale theory that can estimate transformations of any number of predictors omitted from a Cox model fit, after adjusting for other variables included in the

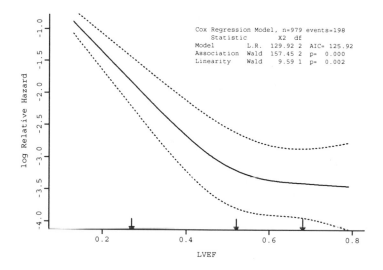

FIGURE 19.6: Restricted cubic spline estimate of relationship between LVEF and relative log hazard from a sample of 979 patients and 198 cardiovascular deaths. Data from the Duke Cardiovascular Disease Databank.

fit. Figure 19.7 used various smoothing methods on the points (LVEF, residual). First, the S-PLUS loess function[65] was used to obtain a smoothed scatterplot fit and approximate 0.95 confidence bars. Second, an ordinary least squares model, representing LVEF as a restricted cubic spline with five default knots, was fitted. Ideally, both fits should have used weighted regression as the residuals do not have equal variance. Predicted values from this fit along with 0.95 confidence limits are shown. The loess and spline-linear regression agree extremely well. Third, Cleveland's lowess scatterplot smoother[76] was used on the martingale residuals against LVEF. The suggested transformation from all three is very similar to that of Figure 19.6. For smaller sample sizes, the raw residuals should also be displayed. There is one vector of martingale residuals that is plotted against all of the predictors. When correlations among predictors are mild, plots of estimated predictor transformations without adjustment for other predictors (i.e., marginal transformations) may be useful. Martingale residuals may be obtained quickly by fixing $\hat{\beta} = 0$ for all predictors. Then smoothed plots of predictor against residual may be made for all predictors. Table 19.3 summarizes some of the ways martingale residuals may be used. See section 10.5 for more information on checking the regression assumptions. The methods for examining interaction surfaces described there apply without modification to the Cox model (except that the nonparametric regression surface does not apply because of censoring).

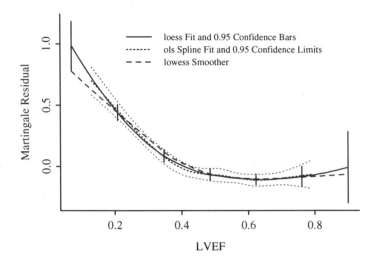

FIGURE 19.7: Three smoothed estimates relating martingale residuals[412] to LVEF.

TABLE 19.3

Purpose	Method
Estimate transformation for a single variable	Force $\hat{\beta}_1 = 0$ and compute residuals from the null regression
Check linearity assumption for a single variable	Compute $\hat{\beta}_1$ and compute residuals from the linear regression
Estimate marginal transformations for p variables	Force $\hat{\beta}_1, \ldots, \hat{\beta}_p = 0$ and compute residuals from the global null model
Estimate transformation for variable i adjusted for other $p - 1$ variables	Estimate $p - 1$ βs, forcing $\hat{\beta}_i = 0$ Compute residuals from mixed global/null model

19.5.2   Proportional Hazards Assumption

Even though assessment of fit of the regression part of the Cox PH model corresponds with other regression models such as the logistic model, the Cox model has its own distributional assumption in need of validation. Here, of course, the distributional assumption is not as stringent as with other survival models, but we do need to validate how the survival or hazard functions for various subjects are connected. There are many graphical and analytical methods of verifying the PH assumption. Two of the methods have already been discussed: a graphical examination of parallelism of $\log \Lambda$ plots, and a comparison of stratified and unstratified models (as in Figure 19.1). Muenz[320] suggested a simple modification that will make nonproportional hazards more apparent: plot $\Lambda_{\mathrm{KM}_1}(t)/\Lambda_{\mathrm{KM}_2}(t)$ against t and check for flatness. The points on this curve can be passed through a smoother. One can also plot differences in $\log(-\log S(t))$ against t.[103] Arjas[22] developed a graphical method based on plotting the estimated cumulative hazard versus the cumulative number of events in a stratum as t progresses.

There are other methods for assessing whether PH holds that may be more direct. Gore et al.,[155] Harrell and Lee,[182] and Kay[233] (see also Anderson and Senthilselvan[20]) describe a method for allowing the log hazard ratio (Cox regression coefficient) for a predictor to be a function of time by fitting specially stratified Cox models. Their method assumes that the predictor being examined for PH already satisfies the linear regression assumption. Follow-up time is stratified into intervals and a separate model is fitted to compute the regression coefficient within each interval, assuming that the effect of the predictor is constant only within that small interval. It is recommended that intervals be constructed so that there is roughly an equal number of events in each. The number of intervals should allow at least 10 or 20 events per interval.

The interval-specific log hazard ratio is estimated by excluding all subjects with event/censoring time before the start of the interval and censoring all events that occur after the end of the interval. This process is repeated for all desired time intervals. By plotting the log hazard ratio and its confidence limits versus the interval, one can assess the importance of a predictor as a function of follow-up time and learn how to model non-PH using more complicated models containing predictor by time interactions. If the hazard ratio is approximately constant within broad time intervals, the time stratification method can be used for fitting and testing the predictor $\times$ time interaction [182, p. 827]; [67].

Consider as an example the rat vaginal cancer data used in Figures 17.9, 17.10, and 19.1. Recall that the PH assumption appeared to be satisfied for the two groups although Figure 17.9 demonstrated some non-Weibullness. Figure 19.8 contains a Λ ratio plot.[320] You can see that the ratio is not stable from 160 to 190 days, but is mostly flat thereafter. Interval-specific estimates of the group 2 : group 1 log hazard ratios are shown in Table 19.4 with intervals specified to yield equal numbers of deaths. The Efron likelihood was used. The number of observations is declining

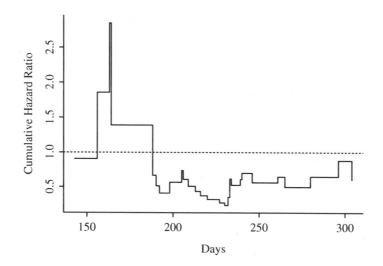

FIGURE 19.8:   Estimate of Λ_2/Λ_1 based on $-\log$ of Altschuler–Nelson–Fleming–Harrington nonparametric survival estimates.

TABLE 19.4

Time Interval	Observations	Deaths	Log Hazard Ratio	Standard Error
$[0, 209)$	40	12	-0.47	0.59
$[209, 234)$	27	12	-0.72	0.58
$234 +$	14	12	-0.50	0.64

TABLE 19.5

Time Interval	Observations	Deaths	Log Hazard Ratio	Standard Error
[0, 21)	110	26	−0.46	0.47
[21, 52)	84	26	−0.90	0.50
[52, 118)	59	26	−1.35	0.50
118 +	28	26	−1.04	0.45

TABLE 19.6

Time Interval	Observations	Deaths	Log Hazard Ratio	Standard Error
[0, 19]	137	27	−0.053	0.010
[19, 49)	112	26	−0.047	0.009
[49, 99]	85	27	−0.036	0.012
99 +	28	26	−0.012	0.014

over time because computations in each interval were based on animals followed at least to the start of that interval. The overall Cox regression coefficient was −0.57 with a standard error of 0.35. There does not appear to be any trend in the hazard ratio over time, indicating a constant hazard ratio or proportional hazards.

Now consider the Veterans Administration Lung Cancer dataset [226, pp. 60, 223–4]. Log Λ plots indicated that the four cell types did not satisfy PH. To simplify the problem, omit patients with "large" cell type and let the binary predictor be 1 if the cell type is "squamous" and 0 if it is "small" or "adeno." We are assessing whether survival patterns for the two groups "squamous" versus "small" or "adeno" have PH. Interval-specific estimates of the squamous : small,adeno log hazard ratios (using Efron's likelihood) are found in Table 19.5. Times are in days. There is evidence of a trend of a decreasing hazard ratio over time which is consistent with the observation that squamous cell patients had equal or worse survival in the early period but decidedly better survival in the late phase.

From the same dataset now examine the PH assumption for Karnofsky performance status using data from all subjects, if the linearity assumption is satisfied. Interval-specific regression coefficients for this predictor are given in Table 19.6. There is good evidence that the importance of performance status is decreasing over time and that it is not a prognostic factor after roughly 99 days. In other words, once a patient survives 99 days, the performance status does not contain much information concerning whether the patient will survive 120 days. This non-PH would be more difficult to detect from Kaplan–Meier plots stratified on performance status unless performance status was stratified carefully.

7

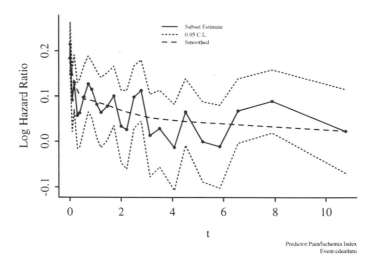

FIGURE 19.9: Stratified hazard ratios for pain/ischemia index over time. Data from the Duke Cardiovascular Disease Databank.

Figure 19.9 displays a log hazard ratio plot for a larger dataset in which more time strata can be formed. In 3299 patients with coronary artery disease, 827 suffered cardiovascular death or nonfatal myocardial infarction. Time was stratified into intervals containing approximately 30 events, and within each interval the Cox regression coefficient for an index of anginal pain and ischemia was estimated. The pain/ischemia index, one component of which is unstable angina, is seen to have a strong effect for only six months. After that, survivors have stabilized and knowledge of the angina status in the previous six months is not informative.

Another method for graphically assessing the log hazard ratio over time is based on Schoenfeld's *partial residuals*[336, 377] with respect to each predictor in the fitted model. The residual is the contribution of the first derivative of the log likelihood function with respect to the predictor's regression coefficient, computed separately at each risk set or unique failure time. In Figure 19.10 the "loess-smoothed"[65] (with approximate 0.95 confidence bars) and "super-smoothed"[146] relationship between the residual and unique failure time is shown for the same data as Figure 19.9. For smaller n, the raw residuals should also be displayed to convey the proper sense of variability. The agreement with the pattern in Figure 19.9 is evident.

Pettitt and Bin Daud[336] suggest scaling the partial residuals by the information matrix components. They also propose a score test for PH based on the Schoenfeld residuals. Grambsch and Therneau[157] found that the Pettitt–Bin Daud standardization is sometimes misleading in that non-PH in one variable may cause the residual plot for another variable to display non-PH. The Grambsch–Therneau weighted

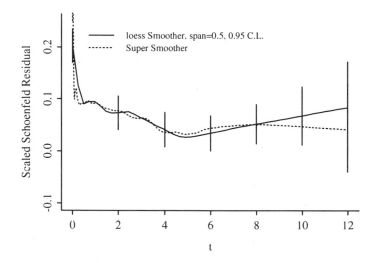

FIGURE 19.10: Smoothed weighted[157] Schoenfeld[377] residuals for the same data in Figure 19.9. Test for PH based on the correlation (ρ) between the individual weighted Schoenfeld residuals and the rank of failure time yielded $\rho = -0.23, z = -6.73, P = 2 \times 10^{-11}$.

residual solves this problem and also yields a residual that is on the same scale as the log relative hazard ratio. Their residual is

$$\hat{\beta} + dR\hat{V}, \tag{19.24}$$

where d is the total number of events, R is the $n \times p$ matrix of Schoenfeld residuals, and $\hat{V}$ is the estimated covariance matrix for $\hat{\beta}$. This new residual can also be the basis for tests for PH, by correlating a user-specified function of unique failure times with the weighted residuals.

The residual plot is computationally very attractive since the score residual components are byproducts of Cox maximum likelihood estimation. Another attractive feature is the lack of need to categorize the time axis. Unless approximate confidence intervals are derived from smoothing techniques, a lack of confidence intervals from most software is one disadvantage of the method.

Formal tests for PH can be based on time-stratified Cox regression estimates.[20, 182] Alternatively, more complex (and probably more efficient) formal tests for PH can be derived by specifying a form for the time by predictor interaction (using what is called a time-dependent covariable in the Cox model) and testing coefficients of such interactions for significance. The obsolete Version 5 SAS PHGLM procedure used a computationally fast procedure based on an approximate score statistic that tests for linear correlation between the rank order of the failure times in the sample and Schoenfeld's partial residuals.[175, 182] This test is available in S-PLUS (for both

TABLE 19.7

t	log Hazard Ratio
10	−0.36
36	−0.64
83.5	−0.83
200	−1.02

weighted and unweighted residuals) using Therneau's `cox.zph` function that is built into S-PLUS. For the results in Figure 19.10, the test for PH is highly significant (correlation coefficient $= -0.23$, normal deviate $z = -6.73$). Since there is only one regression parameter, the weighted residuals are a constant multiple of the unweighted ones, and have the same correlation coefficient.

[10]

Another method for checking the PH assumption which is especially applicable to a polytomous predictor involves taking ratios of parametrically estimated hazard functions estimated separately for each level of the predictor. For example, suppose that a risk factor X is either present ($X = 1$) or absent ($X = 0$), and suppose that separate Weibull distributions adequately fit the survival pattern of each group. If there are no other predictors to adjust for, define the hazard function for $X = 0$ as $\alpha\gamma t^{\gamma-1}$ and the hazard for $X = 1$ as $\delta\theta t^{\theta-1}$. The $X = 1 : X = 0$ hazard ratio is

$$\frac{\alpha\gamma t^{\gamma-1}}{\delta\theta t^{\theta-1}} = \frac{\alpha\gamma}{\delta\theta} t^{\gamma-\theta}. \tag{19.25}$$

The hazard ratio is constant if the two Weibull shape parameters (γ and θ) are equal. These Weibull parameters can be estimated separately and a Wald test statistic of $H_0 : \gamma = \theta$ can be computed by dividing the square of their difference by the sum of the squares of their estimated standard errors, or better by a likelihood ratio test. A plot of the estimate of the hazard ratio above as a function of t may also be informative.

[11]

In the VA lung cancer data, the MLEs of the Weibull shape parameters for squamous cell cancer was 0.77 and for the combined small + adeno was 0.99. SAS **PROC LIFEREG** provided estimates of the reciprocals of these parameters of 1.293 and 1.012 with respective standard errors of 0.183 and 0.0912. A Wald test for differences in these reciprocals provides a rough test for a difference in the shape estimates. The Wald χ^2 is 1.89 with 1 d.f. indicating slight evidence for non-PH.

The fitted Weibull hazard function for squamous cell cancer is $.0167t^{0.23}$ and for adeno + small is $0.0144t^{-0.01}$. The estimated hazard ratio is then $1.16t^{-0.22}$ and the log hazard ratio is $0.148 - 0.22 \log t$. By evaluating this Weibull log hazard ratio at interval midpoints (arbitrarily using $t = 200$ for the last (open) interval) we obtain log hazard ratios that are in good agreement with those obtained by time-stratifying the Cox model as shown in Table 19.7.

There are many methods of assessing PH using time-dependent covariables in the Cox model.[155, 398] Gray[161, 162] mentions a flexible and efficient method of estimating the hazard ratio function using time-dependent covariables that are $X \times$ spline term interactions. Gray's method uses B-splines and requires one to maximize a *penalized* log-likelihood function. Verweij and van Houwelingen[438] developed a more nonparametric version of this approach. Hess[199] uses simple restricted cubic splines to model the time-dependent covariable effects (see also [4, 197]). Suppose that $k = 4$ knots are used and that a covariable X is already transformed correctly. The model is

$$\log \lambda(t|X) = \log \lambda(t) + \beta_1 X + \beta_2 Xt + \beta_3 Xt' + \beta_4 Xt'', \qquad (19.26)$$

where t', t'' are constructed spline variables (Equation 2.25). The $X + 1 : X$ log hazard ratio function is estimated by

$$\hat{\beta}_1 + \hat{\beta}_2 t + \hat{\beta}_3 t' + \hat{\beta}_4 t''. \qquad (19.27)$$

This method can be generalized to allow for simultaneous estimation of the shape of the X effect and $X \times t$ interaction using spline surfaces in (X, t) instead of (X_1, X_2) (Section 2.7.2).

Table 19.8 summarizes many facets of verifying assumptions for PH models. The trade-offs of the various methods for assessing proportional hazards are given in Table 19.9.

12

13

19.6   What to Do When PH Fails

When a factor violates the PH assumption and a test of association is not needed, the factor can be adjusted for through stratification as mentioned earlier. This is especially attractive if the factor is categorical. For continuous predictors, one may want to stratify into quantile groups. The continuous version of the predictor can still be adjusted for as a covariable to account for any residual linearity within strata.

When a test of significance is needed and the P-value is impressive, the "principle of conservatism" could be invoked, as the P-value would likely have been more impressive had the factor been modeled correctly. Predicted survival probabilities using this approach will be erroneous in certain time intervals.

An efficient test of association can be done using time-dependent covariables [306, pp. 208–217]. For example, in the model

$$\lambda(t|X) = \lambda_0(t) \exp(\beta_1 X + \beta_2 X \times \log(t + 1)) \qquad (19.28)$$

TABLE 19.8: Assumptions of the Proportional Hazards Model

Variables	Assumptions	Verification
Response Variable T Time Until Event	Shape of $\lambda(t\|X)$ for fixed X as $t \uparrow$ Cox: none Weibull: t^θ	Shape of $S_{\text{KM}}(t)$
Interaction Between X and T	Proportional hazards— effect of X does not depend on T (e.g., treatment effect is constant over time)	<ul><li>Categorical X: check parallelism of stratified $\log[-\log S(t)]$ plots as $t \uparrow$</li><li>Muenz[320] cum. hazard ratio plots</li><li>Arjas[22] cum. hazard plots</li><li>Check agreement of stratified and modeled estimates</li><li>Hazard ratio plots</li><li>Smoothed Schoenfeld residual plots and correlation test (time vs. residual)</li><li>Test time-dependent covariable such as $X \times \log(t+1)$</li><li>Ratio of parametrically estimated $\lambda(t)$</li></ul>
Individual Predictors X	Shape of $\lambda(t\|X)$ for fixed t as $X \uparrow$ Linear: $\log \lambda(t\|X) = \log \lambda(t) + \beta X$ Nonlinear: $\log \lambda(t\|X) = \log \lambda(t) + f(X)$	<ul><li>k-level ordinal X : linear term $+ k - 2$ dummy variables</li><li>Continuous X: polynomials, spline functions, smoothed martingale residual plots</li></ul>
Interaction Between X_1 and X_2	Additive effects: effect of X_1 on $\log \lambda$ is independent of X_2 and vice versa	Test nonadditive terms (e.g., products)

TABLE 19.9

Method	Requires Grouping X	Requires Grouping t	Computa-tional Efficiency	Yields Formal Test	Yields Estimate of $\lambda_2(t)/\lambda_1(t)$	Requires Fitting 2 Models	Must Choose Smoothing Parameter
log[− log], Muenz, Arjas plots	x		x			x	
Dabrowska log $\hat{\Lambda}$ difference plots	x		x	x		x	
Stratified vs. Modeled Estimates	x		x			x	
Hazard ratio plot		x		?	x	x	?
Schoenfeld residual plot			x		x		x
Schoenfeld residual correlation test			x	x			
Fit time-dependent covariables				x	x		
Ratio of parametric estimates of $\lambda(t)$	x		x	x	x	x	

one tests $H_0 : \beta_1 = \beta_2 = 0$ with 2 d.f. This is similar to the approach used by [51]. Stratification on time intervals can also be used:[20, 155, 182]

$$\lambda(t|X) = \lambda_0(t)\exp[\beta_1 X + \beta_2 X \times I(t > c)], \qquad (19.29)$$

where $I(t > c) = 1$ when $t > c$. If this step-function model holds, and if a sufficient number of subjects have late follow-up, you can also fit a model for early outcomes and a separate one for late outcomes using interval-specific censoring as discussed in Section 19.5.2. The dual model approach provides easy to interpret models, assuming that proportional hazards is satisfied within each interval.

Kronborg and Aaby[251] and Dabrowska et al.[103] provide tests for differences in $\Lambda(t)$ at specific t based on stratified PH models. These can also be used to test for treatment effects when PH is violated for treatment but not for adjustment variables. Differences in mean restricted life length (differences in areas under survival curves up to a fixed finite time) can also be useful for comparing therapies when PH fails.[230]

Parametric models that assume an effect other than PH, for example, the log-logistic model,[155] can be used to allow a predictor to have a constantly increasing or decreasing effect over time. If one predictor satisfies PH but another does not, this approach will not work.

[14]

19.7   Collinearity

See Section 4.6 for the general approach using variance inflation factors.

19.8 Overly Influential Observations

Therneau et al.[412] describe the use of *score residuals* for assessing influence in Cox and related regression models. They show that the *infinitesimal jackknife* estimate of the influence of observation i on β equals $V s'$, where V is the estimated variance–covariance matrix of the p regression estimates b and $s = (s_{i1}, s_{i2}, \ldots, s_{ip})$ is the vector of score residuals for the p regression coefficients for the ith observation. Let $S_{n \times p}$ denote the matrix of score residuals over all observations. Then an approximation to the unstandardized change in b (DFBETA) is SV. Standardizing by the standard errors of b found from the diagonals of V, $e = (V_{11}, V_{22}, \ldots, V_{pp})^{1/2}$, yields

$$\text{DFBETAS} = SV \, \text{Diag}(e)^{-1}, \tag{19.30}$$

where $\text{Diag}(e)$ is a diagonal matrix containing the estimated standard errors.

As discussed in Section 6.2, identification of overly influential observations is facilitated by printing, for each predictor, the list of observations containing DFBETAS $> u$ for any parameter associated with that predictor. The choice of cutoff u depends on the sample size among other things. A typical choice might be $u = 0.2$ indicating a change in a regression coefficient of 0.2 standard errors.

19.9 Quantifying Predictive Ability

To obtain a unitless measure of predictive ability for a Cox PH model we can use the R index described Section 9.8.3, which is the square root of the fraction of log likelihood explained by the model of the log likelihood that could be explained by a perfect model, penalized for the complexity of the model. The lowest (best) possible -2 log likelihood for the Cox model is zero, which occurs when the predictors can perfectly rank order the survival times. Therefore, as was the case with the logistic model, the quantity L^* from Section 9.8.3 is zero and an R index that is penalized for the number of parameters in the model is given by

$$R^2 = (\text{LR} - 2p)/L^0, \tag{19.31}$$

where p is the number of parameters estimated and L^0 is the -2 log likelihood when β is restricted to be zero (i.e., there are no predictors in the model). R will be near one for a perfectly predictive model and near zero for a model that does not discriminate between short and long survival times. The R index does not take into account any stratification factors. If stratification factors are present, R will be near one if survival times can be perfectly ranked within strata even though there is overlap between strata.

Schemper[368] and Korn and Simon[248] have reported that R^2 is too sensitive to the distribution of censoring times and have suggested alternatives based on the distance between estimated Cox survival probabilities (using predictors) and Kaplan–Meier estimates (ignoring predictors). Kent and O'Quigley[236] also report problems with R^2 and suggest a more complex measure. Schemper[370] investigated the Maddala–Magee[297, 298] index R^2_{LR} described in Section 9.8.3, applied to Cox regression:

$$
\begin{aligned}
R^2_{\text{LR}} &= 1 - \exp(-\text{LR}/n) \\
&= 1 - \omega^{2/n},
\end{aligned}
\tag{19.32}
$$

where ω is the null model likelihood divided by the fitted model likelihood.

For many situations, R^2_{LR} performed as well as Schemper's more complex measure[368, 371] and hence it is preferred because of its ease of calculation (assuming that PH holds). Ironically, Schemper[370] demonstrated that the n in the formula for this index is the total number of observations, not the number of events. To make the R^2 index have a maximum value of 1.0, we use the Nagelkerke[322] R^2_{N} discussed in Section 9.8.3.

An easily interpretable index of discrimination for survival models is derived from Kendall's τ and Somers' D_{xy} rank correlation,[393] the Gehan–Wilcoxon statistic for comparing two samples for survival differences, and the Brown–Hollander–Korwar nonparametric test of association for censored data.[178, 184] This index, c, is a generalization of the area under the ROC curve discussed under the logistic model, in that it applies to a continuous response variable that can be censored. The c index is the proportion of all pairs of subjects whose survival time can be ordered such that the subject with the higher predicted survival is the one who survived longer. Two subjects' survival times cannot be ordered if both subjects are censored or if one has failed and the follow-up time of the other is less than the failure time of the first. The c index is a probability of concordance between predicted and observed survival, with $c = 0.5$ for random predictions and $c = 1$ for a perfectly discriminating model. The c index is relatively unaffected by the amount of censoring. D_{xy} is obtained from $2(c - 0.5)$.

19.10   Validating the Fitted Model

Separate bootstrap or cross-validation assessments can be made for calibration and discrimination of Cox model survival and log relative hazard estimates.

19.10.1   Validation of Model Calibration

One approach to validation of the calibration of predictions is to obtain unbiased estimates of the difference between Cox predicted and Kaplan–Meier survival estimates at a fixed time u. Here is one sequence of steps.

1. Obtain cutpoints (e.g., deciles) of predicted survival at time u so as to have a given number of subjects (e.g., 50) in each interval of predicted survival. These cutpoints are based on the distribution of $\hat{S}(u|X)$ in the whole sample for the "final" model (for data-splitting, instead use the model developed in the training sample). Let k denote the number of intervals used.

2. Compute the average $\hat{S}(u|X)$ in each interval.

3. Compare this with the Kaplan–Meier survival estimates at time u, stratified by intervals of $\hat{S}(u|X)$. Let the differences be denoted by $d = (d_1, \ldots, d_k)$.

4. Use bootstrapping or cross-validation to estimate the overoptimism in d and then to correct d to get a more fair assessment of these differences. For each repetition, repeat any stepwise variable selection or stagewise significance testing using the same stopping rules as were used to derive the "final" model. No more than $B = 200$ replications are needed to obtain accurate estimates.

5. If desired, the bias-correct d can be added to the original stratified Kaplan–Meier estimates to obtain a bias-corrected calibration curve.

As an example, consider a dataset of 20 random uniformly distributed predictors for a sample of size 200. Let the failure time be another random uniform variable that is independent of *all* the predictors, and censor half of the failure times at random. Divide the observations into quintiles of predicted 0.5-year survival, so that there are 40 observations per stratum. Due to fitting 20 predictors to 100 events, there will apparently be fair agreement between predicted and Kaplan–Meier survival over all strata (the dots in Figure 19.11). However, the bias-corrected calibrations (the Xs in the figure) give a more truthful answer: examining the Xs across levels of predicted survival demonstrate that predicted and observed survival are actually unrelated, in agreement with how the data were generated.

19.10.2   Validation of Discrimination and Other Statistical Indexes

Here bootstrapping and cross-validation are used as for logistic models (Section 10.9). We can obtain bootstrap bias-corrected estimates of c or equivalently D_{xy}. To instead obtain a measure of relative calibration or slope shrinkage, we can bootstrap the apparent estimate of $\gamma = 1$ in the model

$$\lambda(t|X) = \lambda(t)\exp(\gamma Xb). \tag{19.33}$$

Besides being a measure of calibration in itself, the bootstrap estimate of γ also leads to an unreliability index U which measures how far the model maximum log likelihood (which allows for an overall slope correction) is from the log likelihood

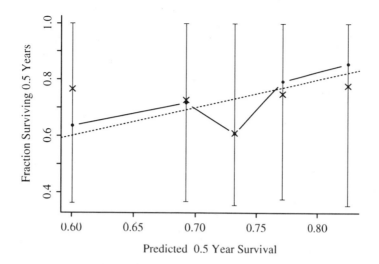

FIGURE 19.11: Calibration of random predictions using Efron's bootstrap with $B = 50$ resamples and 40 patients per interval. Dataset has $n = 200$, 100 uncensored observations, 20 random predictors, $\chi^2_{20} = 9.87$. •: apparent calibration; ×: bias-corrected calibration.

evaluated at "frozen" regression coefficients ($\gamma \doteq 1$) (see [183] and Section 10.9).

$$U = \frac{\text{LR}(\hat{\gamma}Xb) - \text{LR}(Xb)}{L^0}, \tag{19.34}$$

where L^0 is the -2 log likelihood for the null model (Section 9.8.3). Similarly, a discrimination index D^{183} can be derived from the -2 log likelihood at the shrunken linear predictor, penalized for estimating one parameter (γ) (see also [433, p. 1318] and [85]):

$$D = \frac{\text{LR}(\hat{\gamma}Xb) - 1}{L^0}. \tag{19.35}$$

D is the same as R^2 discussed above when $p = 1$ (indicating only one reestimated parameter, γ), the penalized proportion of explainable log likelihood that was explained by the model. Because of the remark of Schemper,[368] all of these indexes may unfortunately be functions of the censoring pattern.

An index of overall quality that penalizes discrimination for unreliability is

$$Q = D - U = \frac{\text{LR}(Xb) - 1}{L^0}. \tag{19.36}$$

Q is a normalized and penalized -2 log likelihood that is evaluated at the uncorrected linear predictor.

TABLE 19.10

Index	Original Sample	Training Sample	Test Sample	Optimism	Corrected Index
D_{xy}	−0.16	−0.31	−0.09	−0.22	0.06
R_N^2	0.05	0.15	0.00	0.15	−0.10
Slope	1.00	1.00	0.25	0.75	0.25
D	0.01	0.04	0.00	0.04	−0.02
U	0.00	0.00	0.00	0.00	0.00
Q	0.01	0.04	0.00	0.04	−0.02

For the random predictions used in Figure 19.11, the bootstrap estimates with $B = 50$ resamples are found in Table 19.10. It can be seen that the apparent correlation ($D_{xy} = -0.16$) does not hold up after correcting for overfitting ($D_{xy} = 0.06$). Also, the extreme slope shrinkage (0.25) indicates extreme overfitting.

See [433, Section 6] and [437] and Section 17.3.7 for still more useful methods for validating the Cox model.

19.11   Describing the Fitted Model

As with logistic modeling, once a Cox PH model has been fitted and all its assumptions verified, the final model needs to be presented and interpreted. The fastest way to describe the model is to interpret each effect in it. For each predictor the change in log hazard per desired units of change in the predictor value may be computed, or the antilog of this quantity, $\exp(\beta_j \times$ change in $X_j)$, may be used to estimate the hazard ratio holding all other factors constant. When X_j is a nonlinear factor, changes in predicted $X\beta$ for sensible values of X_j such as quartiles can be used as described in Section 10.10. Of course for nonmodeled stratification factors, this method is of no help. Figure 19.12 depicts a way to display estimated surgical : medical hazard ratios in the presence of a significant treatment by disease severity interaction and a secular trend in the benefit of surgical therapy (treatment by year of diagnosis interaction).

Often, the use of predicted survival probabilities may make the model more interpretable. If the effect of only one factor is being displayed and that factor is polytomous or predictions are made for specific levels, survival curves (with or without adjustment for other factors not shown) can be drawn for each level of the predictor of interest, with follow-up time on the x-axis. Figure 19.2 demonstrated this for a factor which was a stratification factor. Figure 19.13 extends this by displaying survival estimates stratified by treatment but adjusted to various levels of two modeled factors, one of which, year of diagnosis, interacted with treatment.

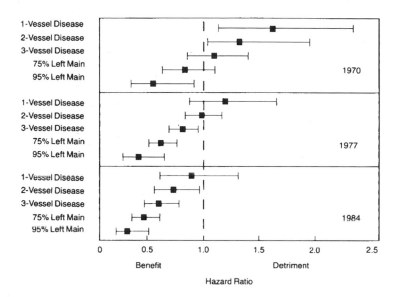

FIGURE 19.12: A display of an interaction between treatment and extent of disease, and between treatment and calendar year of start of treatment. Comparison of medical and surgical average hazard ratios for patients treated in 1970, 1977, and 1984 according to coronary anatomy. Closed squares represent point estimates; bars represent 0.95 confidence limits of average hazard ratios.[61] Reprinted by permission, American Medical Association.

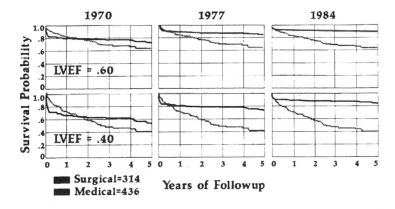

FIGURE 19.13: Cox–Kalbfleisch–Prentice survival estimates stratifying on treatment and adjusting for several predictors. Estimates are for patients with left main disease and normal or impaired ventricular function.[347] Reprinted by permission, Mosby, Inc. / Harcourt Health Sciences.

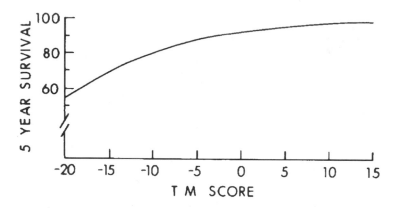

FIGURE 19.14: Cox model predictions with respect to a continuous variable. X-axis shows the range of the treadmill score seen in clinical practice and Y-axis shows the corresponding five-year survival probability predicted by the Cox regression model for the 2842 study patients.[304] Reprinted by permission, American College of Physicians—American Society of Internal Medicine.

When a continuous predictor is of interest, it is usually more informative to display that factor on the x-axis with estimated survival at one or more time points on the y-axis. When the model contains only one predictor, even if that predictor is represented by multiple terms such as a spline expansion, one may simply plot that factor against the predicted survival. Figure 19.14 depicts the relationship between treadmill exercise score, which is a weighted linear combination of several predictors in a Cox model, and the probability of surviving five years.

When displaying the effect of a single factor after adjusting for multiple predictors which are not displayed, care only need be taken for the values to which the predictors are adjusted (e.g., grand means). When instead the desire is to display the effect of multiple predictors simultaneously, an important continuous predictor can be displayed on the x-axis while separate curves or graphs are made for levels of other factors. Figure 19.15, which corresponds to the $\log \Lambda$ plots in Figure 19.5, displays the joint effects of age and sex on the three-year survival probability. Age is modeled with a cubic spline function, and the model includes terms for an age $\times$ sex interaction.

Besides making graphs of survival probabilities estimated for given levels of the predictors, nomograms have some utility in specifying a fitted Cox model. A nomogram can be used to compute $X\hat{\beta}$, the estimated log hazard for a subject with a set of predictor values X relative to the "standard" subject. The central line in the nomogram will be on this linear scale unlike the logistic model nomograms given in Section 10.10 which further transformed $X\hat{\beta}$ into $[1 + \exp(-X\hat{\beta})]^{-1}$. Alternatively, the central line could be on the nonlinear $\exp(X\hat{\beta})$ hazard ratio scale or survival at fixed t.

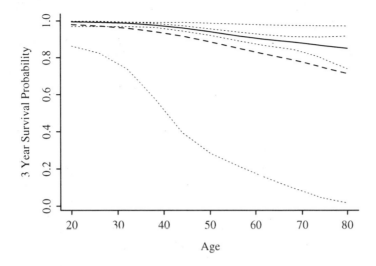

FIGURE 19.15: Survival estimates for model stratified on sex, with interaction.

A graph of the estimated underlying survival function $\hat{S}(t)$ as a function of t can be coupled with the nomogram used to compute $X\hat{\beta}$. The survival for a specific subject, $\hat{S}(t|X)$ is obtained from $\hat{S}(t)^{\exp(X\hat{\beta})}$. Alternatively, one could graph $\hat{S}(t)^{\exp(X\hat{\beta})}$ for various values of $X\hat{\beta}$ (e.g., $X\hat{\beta} = -2, -1, 0, 1, 2$) so that the desired survival curve could be read directly, at least to the nearest tabulated $X\hat{\beta}$. For estimating survival at a fixed time, say two years, one only need to provide the constant $\hat{S}(t)$. The nomogram could even be adapted to include a nonlinear scale $\hat{S}(2)^{\exp(X\hat{\beta})}$ to allow direct computation of two-year survival.

19.12 S-Plus Functions

Harrell's cpower, spower, and ciapower (in the Hmisc library) perform power calculations for Cox tests in follow-up studies. cpower computes power for a two-sample Cox (log-rank) test with random patient entry over a fixed duration and a given length of minimum follow-up. The expected number of events in each group is estimated by assuming exponential survival. cpower uses a slight modification of the method of Schoenfeld[378] (see [334]). Separate specification of noncompliance in the active treatment arm and "drop-in" from the control arm into the active arm are allowed, using the method of Lachin and Foulkes.[253] The ciapower function computes power of the Cox interaction test in a 2×2 setup using the method of Peterson and George.[334] It does not take noncompliance into account. The spower function simulates power for two-sample tests (the log-rank test by default) allowing for very complex conditions such as continuously varying treatment effect and noncompliance probabilities.

The S-PLUS function `cph` written by Harrell is a slight modification of the `coxph` function written by Terry Therneau (in his `survival` library in StatLib) to work in the `Design` framework. `cph` computes MLEs of Cox and stratified Cox PH models, overall score and likelihood ratio χ^2 statistics for the model, martingale residuals, the linear predictor ($X\hat{\beta}$ centered to have mean 0), and collinearity diagnostics. Efron, Breslow, and exact partial likelihoods are supported (although the exact likelihood is very computationally intensive if ties are frequent). The function also fits the Andersen–Gill[16] generalization of the Cox PH model. This model allows for predictor values to change over time in the form of step functions as well as allowing time-dependent stratification (subjects can jump to different hazard function shapes). The Andersen–Gill formulation allows multiple events per subject and permits subjects to move in and out of risk at any desired time points. The latter feature allows time zero to have a more general definition. (See Section 9.5 for methods of adjusting the variance–covariance matrix of $\hat{\beta}$ for dependence in the events per subject.) The printing function corresponding to `cph` prints the Nagelkerke index R_N^2 described in Section 19.9. `cph` works in conjunction with the generic functions such as `specs`, `predict`, `summary`, `anova`, `fastbw`, `which.influence`, `latex`, `residuals`, `coef`, `nomogram`, and `plot` described in Section 6.2, the same as the logistic regression function `lrm` does. For the purpose of plotting predicted survival at a single time, `plot` has an additional argument `time` for plotting `cph` fits. It also has an argument `loglog` which if `T` causes instead log -log survival to be plotted on the y-axis. `cph` has all the arguments described in Section 6.2 and some that are specific to it.

Similar to `Survival.psm`, there are `Survival.cph`, `Quantile.cph`, and `Mean.cph` functions which create other S-PLUS functions to evaluate survival probabilities and perform other calculations, based on a `cph` fit with `surv=T`. These functions, unlike all the others, allow polygon (linear interpolation) estimation of survival probabilities, quantiles, and mean survival time as an option. `Quantile.cph` is the only automatic way for obtaining survival quantiles with `cph`. Quantile estimates will be missing when the survival curve does not extend long enough. Likewise, survival estimates will be missing for $t >$ maximum follow-up time, when the last event time is censored. `Mean.cph` computes the mean survival time if the last failure time in each stratum is uncensored. Otherwise, `Mean.cph` may be used to compute restricted mean lifetime using a user-specified truncation point.[229] `Quantile` and `Mean` are especially useful with `plot` and `nomogram`. `Survival` is useful with `nomogram` (`plot` automatically handles `Survival` for ordinary step-function estimates):

```
f ← cph(..., surv=T)
med ← Quantile(f)
nomogram(f, fun=function(x) med(lp=x),
        funlabel='Median Survival Time')
# fun tranforms the linear predictors
srv ← Survival(f)
```

```
rmean ← Mean(f, tmax=3, method='approx')
nomogram(f, fun=list(function(x) srv(3, x), rmean),
        funlabel=c('3-Year Survival Prob.','Restricted Mean'))
# med, srv, expected are more complicated if strata are present
```

Figures 19.3, 19.4, 19.5 and 19.15 were produced by

```
n ← 2000
.Random.seed ← c(49,39,17,36,23,0,43,51,6,54,50,1)
# to be able to regenerate same data
age ← 50 + 12*rnorm(n)
label(age) ← "Age"
sex <- sample(c('Male','Female'), n, rep=T, prob=c(.6, .4))
cens ← 15*runif(n)
h ← .02*exp(.04*(age-50)+.8*(sex=='Female'))
t ← -log(runif(n))/h
e ← ifelse(t<=cens,1,0)
t ← pmin(t, cens)
units(t) ← "Year"
age.dec ← cut2(age, g=10, levels.mean=T)
Srv ← Surv(t,e)
f ← cph(Srv ~ strat(age.dec)+strat(sex), surv=T)
# surv=T speeds up computations, and confidence limits
# when there are no covariables are still accurate.
plot(f, age.dec=NA, sex=NA, time=3, loglog=T,
     val.lev=T, ylim=c(-5,-1))


f ← cph(Srv ~ rcs(age,4)+strat(sex), x=T, y=T)
# Get accurate C.L. for any age
# Note: for evaluating shape of regression, we would not
#   ordinarily bother to get 3-year survival probabilities -
#   would just use X * beta. We do so here to use same scale
#   as nonparametric estimates
f
anova(f)
ages ← seq(20, 80, by=4)
# Evaluate at fewer points. Default is 100
# Take much RAM if we use the exact C.L. formula with n=100
plot(f, age=ages, sex=NA, time=3, loglog=T, ylim=c(-5,-1))


f ← cph(Srv ~ rcs(age,4)*strat(sex), x=T, y=T)
anova(f)
ages ← seq(20, 80, by=6)
# Still fewer points - more parameters in model
plot(f, age=ages, sex=NA, time=3, loglog=T, ylim=c(-5,-1))
plot(f, age=ages, sex=NA, time=3)
# Having x=T, y=T in fit also allows computation of
#   influence statistics
```

```
resid(f, "dfbetas")
which.influence(f)
```

The S-PLUS program below demonstrates how several cph-related functions work well with the nomogram function to display this last fit. Here predicted three-year survival probabilities and median survival time (when defined) are displayed against age and sex. The fact that a nonlinear effect interacts with a stratified factor is taken into account.

```
srv ← Survival(f)   # use an f that used surv=T
# Define functions to compute 3-year estimates as a function
#  of the linear predictors (X*Beta)
surv.f ← function(lp) srv(3, lp, stratum="sex=Female")
surv.m ← function(lp) srv(3, lp, stratum="sex=Male")
quant ← Quantile(f)
# Define functions to compute median survival time
med.f ← function(lp) quant(.5, lp, stratum="sex=Female")
med.m ← function(lp) quant(.5, lp, stratum="sex=Male")
nomogram(f, fun=list(surv.m, surv.f, med.m, med.f),
         funlabel=c("S(3 | Male)","S(3 | Female)",
                    "Median (Male)","Median (Female)"),
         fun.at=list(c(.8,.9,.95,.98,.99),
                     c(.1,.3,.5,.7,.8,.9,.95,.98),
                     c(8,12),c(1,2,4,8,12)))
```

The standard errors of log–log survival probabilities computed by cph and the confidence intervals derived by the associated functions survest and survplot are only proper when the model contains only stratification factors or when predictions are made at the means of all covariables, unless you store in the fit object the data used in fitting the model using the options x=T, y=T. The survfit.cph and survest functions are modifications of Therneau's survfit.coxph function that can obtain predicted survival probabilities and confidence intervals for any setting of predictors. survfit.cph and survest are called as needed when you request plots.

The survest function is used to obtain predicted survival curves or survival at a given vector of times, for a desired set of predictor values and a fit produced by cph. Confidence limits may be obtained also, as can the standard error of the log–log survival.

The survplot function is similar in some ways to the plot function, but it plots follow-up time on the x-axis. It plots step-function survival curves with confidence bands or confidence bars for Cox models. Figure 19.1 was produced by the following S-PLUS program.

```
units(days) ← "Day"
S ← Surv(days,death)
f.mod ← cph(S ~ group, surv=T, x=T,y=T)
f.strat ← cph(S ~ strat(group), surv=T)
```

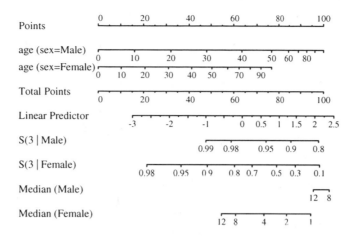

FIGURE 19.16: Nomogram from a fitted stratified Cox model that allowed for interaction between age and sex, and nonlinearity in age. The axis for median survival time is truncated on the left where the median is beyond the last follow-up time.

```
survplot(f.strat, group=NA, lty=c(1,1),
         label.curves=list(keys=c(0,2), key.inc=30,
                           keyloc='none'))
survplot(f.mod, group=NA, lty=c(2,2), add=T, label.curves=F)
legend(c(13,160),c(.38,.54),
       c("Nonparametric Estimates","Cox-Breslow Estimates"),
       lty=1:2, bty="n")
legend(c(13,160),c(.22,.38),
       c("Group 1","Group 2"), marks=c(0,2), cex=.75, bty="n")
```

The cumulative hazard ratio plot in Figure 19.8 was produced by:

```
f ← cph(S ~ strat(group), surv=T)
# For both strata, evaluate S(t) at combined set of death times
times ← sort(unique(days[death==1]))
est   ← survest(f, data.frame(group=levels(group)),
                times=times, conf.type="none")$surv
cumhaz ← -log(est)
plot(times, cumhaz[2,]/cumhaz[1,], xlab="Days",
     ylab="Cumulative Hazard Ratio", type="s")
abline(h=1, lty=2)
```

The `rcspline.plot` function described in Section 10.11 can fit a spline-expanded Cox PH model and plot the estimated spline function and confidence limits. Figure 19.6 was produced using

```
rcspline.plot(lvef, d.time, event=cdeath, nk=3)
```

The corresponding smoothed martingale residual plot for LVEF in Figure 19.7 was created with

```
cox ← cph(Surv(d.time,cdeath) ~ lvef, iter.max=0)
res ← resid(cox)
g ← loess(res ~ lvef)
plot(g, coverage=0.95, confidence=7, xlab="LVEF",
     ylab="Martingale Residual")
g ← ols(res ~ rcs(lvef,5))
plot(g, lvef=NA, add=T, lty=2)
lines(lowess(lvef, res, iter=0), lty=3)
legend(.3,1.15,c("loess Fit and 0.95 Confidence Bars",
                 "ols Spline Fit and 0.95 Confidence Limits",
                 "lowess Smoother"), lty=1:3, bty="n")
```

Because we desired residuals with respect to the omitted predictor LVEF, the parameter iter.max=0 had to be given to make cph stop the estimation process at the starting parameter estimates (default of zero). The effect of this is to ignore the predictors when computing the residuals; that is, to compute residuals from a flat line rather than the usual residuals from a fitted straight line.

The residuals.cph function is a slight modification of Therneau's residuals.-coxph function to obtain martingale, Schoenfeld, score, deviance residuals, or approximate DFBETA or DFBETAS. Since martingale residuals are always stored by cph (assuming there are covariables present), residuals.cph merely has to pick them off the fit object and reinsert rows that were deleted due to missing values. For other residuals, you must have stored the design matrix and Surv object with the fit by using ..., x=T, y=T. Storing the design matrix with x=T ensures that the same transformation parameters (e.g., knots) are used in evaluating the model as were used in fitting it. To use residuals.cph you can use the abbreviation resid. See the help file for residuals.cph for an example of how martingale residuals may be used to quickly plot univariable (unadjusted) relationships for several predictors.

Figure 19.10, which used smoothed scaled Schoenfeld partial residuals[377] to estimate the form of a predictor's log hazard ratio over time, was made with

```
Srv ← Surv(dm.time,cdeathmi)
cox ← cph(Srv ~ pi, x=T, y=T)
cox.zph(cox, "rank")      # Test for PH for each column of X
res ← resid(cox, "scaledsch")
time ← as.numeric(names(res))
# Use dimnames(res)[[1]] if more than one predictor
f ← loess(res ~ time, span=0.50)
plot(f, coverage=0.95, confidence=7, xlab="t",
     ylab="Scaled Schoenfeld Residual", ylim=c(-.1,.25))
lines(supsmu(time, res),lty=2)
```

```
legend(1.1,.21,c("loess Smoother with span=0.50 and 0.95 C.L.",
                 "Super Smoother"), lty=1:2, bty="n")
```

The computation and plotting of scaled Schoenfeld residuals could have been done automatically in this case by using the single command `plot(cox.zph(cox))`, although `cox.zph` defaults to plotting against the Kaplan–Meier transformation of follow-up time.

The `hazard.ratio.plot` function in **Design** repeatedly estimates Cox regression coefficients and confidence limits within time intervals. The log hazard ratios are plotted against the mean failure/censoring time within the interval. Figure 19.9 was created with

```
hazard.ratio.plot(pi, Srv)        # Srv was Surv(dm.time, ...)
```

If you have multiple degree of freedom factors, you may want to score them into linear predictors before using `hazard.ratio.plot`. The `predict` function with argument `type="terms"` will produce a matrix with one column per factor to do this (Section 6.2).

Therneau's `cox.zph` function implements Harrell's Schoenfeld residual correlation test for PH. This function also stores results that can easily be passed to a plotting method for `cox.zph` to automatically plot smoothed residuals that estimate the effect of each predictor over time.

Therneau has also written an S-PLUS function `survdiff` that compares two or more survival curves using the $G - \rho$ family of rank tests (Harrington and Fleming[189]).

The `rcorr.cens` function in the **Hmisc** library computes the c index and the corresponding generalization of Somers' D_{xy} rank correlation for a censored response variable. `rcorr.cens` also works for uncensored and binary responses (see ROC area in Section 10.8), although its use of all possible pairings makes it slow for this purpose.

The `calibrate` function for `cph` constructs a bootstrap or cross-validation optimism-corrected calibration curve by resampling the differences between average Cox predicted survival and Kaplan–Meier estimates at a single time point (see Section 19.10.1). Figure 19.11 was produced by

```
n  ← 200
p  ← 20
xx ← matrix(rnorm(n*p),nrow=n,ncol=p)
y  ← runif(n)
units(y) ← "Year"
e  ← c(rep(0,n/2),rep(1,n/2))
f.rand ← cph(Surv(y,e) ~ xx, x=T, y=T, time.inc=.5, surv=T)
cal <- calibrate(f.rand, u=.5, m=40, method="boot", B=50)
plot(cal, subtitles=F)
```

The `validate` function for `cph` fits validates several statistics describing Cox model fits—slope shrinkage, R_N^2, D, U, Q, and D_{xy}. The `val.surv` function can also be of use in externally validating a Cox model using the methods presented in Section 17.3.7.

19.13   Further Reading

[1]   Good general texts for the Cox PH model include Cox and Oakes,[93] Kalbfleisch and Prentice,[226] Lawless,[264] Collett,[80] Marubini and Valsecchi,[306] and Klein and Moeschberger.[239] Therneau and Grambsch[411] describe the many ways the standard Cox model may be extended.

[2]   Cupples et al.[101] and Marubini and Valsecchi [306, pp. 201–206] present good description of various methods of computing "adjusted survival curves."

[3]   See Altman and Andersen[10] for simpler approximate formulas. Cheng et al.[72] derived methods for obtaining pointwise and simultaneous confidence bands for $S(t)$ for future subjects, and Henderson[195] has a comprehensive discussion of the use of Cox models to estimate survival time for individual subjects.

[4]   Aalen[2] and Valsecchi et al.[429] discuss other residuals useful in graphically checking survival model assumptions.

[5]   [284] has other methods for generating confidence intervals for martingale residual plots.

[6]   Lin et al.[284] describe other methods of checking transformations using *cumulative* martingale residuals.

[7]   A parametric analysis of the VA dataset using linear splines and incorporating $X \times t$ interactions is found in [244].

[8]   See [157, 336] for some methods for obtaining confidence bands for Schoenfeld residual plots.

[9]   [324, 348] compared the power of the test for PH based on the correlation between failure time and Schoenfeld residuals with the power of several other tests.

[10]   See Lin et al.[284] for another approach to deriving a formal test of PH using residuals. Other graphical methods for examining the PH assumption are due to Gray,[160] who used hazard smoothing to estimate hazard ratios as a function of time, and Thaler,[409] who developed a nonparametric estimator of the hazard ratio over time for time-dependent covariables. See Valsecchi et al.[429] for other useful graphical assessments of PH.

[11]   A related test of constancy of hazard ratios may be found in [348]. Also, see Schemper[369] for related methods.

[12]   See [369] for a variation of the standard Cox likelihood to allow for non-PH.

[13]   An excellent review of graphical methods for assessing PH may be found in Hess.[200]

[14]   Schemper[369] provides a way to determine the effect of falsely assuming PH by comparing the Cox regression coefficient to a well-described average log hazard ratio. Zucker[466] shows how dependent a weighted log-rank test is on the true hazard ratio

function, when the weights are derived from a hypothesized hazard ratio function. Valsecchi et al.[429] proposed a method that is robust to non-PH that occurs in the late follow-up period. Their method uses down-weighting of certain types of "outliers." See Herndon and Harrell[197] for a flexible parametric PH model with time-dependent covariables, which uses the restricted cubic spline function to specify $\lambda(t)$.

15   See van Houwelingen and le Cessie [433, Eq. 61] and Verweij and van Houwelingen[437] for an interesting index of cross-validated predictive accuracy. Schemper and Henderson[373] relate explained variation to predictive accuracy in Cox models.

16   See similar indexes in Schemper[366] and a related idea in [433, Eq. 63]. See Korn and Simon,[248] Schemper and Stare,[375] and Henderson[195] for nice comparisons of various measures.

17   Altman and Royston[13] have a good discussion of validation of prognostic models and present several examples of validation using a simple discrimination index.

Chapter 20

Case Study in Cox Regression

20.1 Choosing the Number of Parameters and Fitting the Model

Consider the randomized trial of estrogen for treatment of prostate cancer[60] described in Chapter 8. Let us now develop a model for time until death (of any cause). There are 354 deaths among the 502 patients. If we only wanted to test for a drug effect on survival time, a simple rank-based analysis would suffice. To be able to test for differential treatment effect or to estimate prognosis or expected absolute treatment benefit for individual patients, however, we need a multivariable survival model.

In this case study we do not make use of data reductions obtained in Chapter 8 but show simpler (partial) approaches to data reduction. We do use the `transcan` results for imputation.[a]

First let's assess the wisdom of fitting a full additive model that does not assume linearity of effect for any predictor. Categorical predictors are expanded using dummy variables. For `pf` we could lump the last two categories as before since the last category has only two patients. Likewise, we could combine the last two levels of `ekg`. Continuous predictors are expanded by fitting four-knot restricted cubic spline

---

[a]This case study used an older version of `transcan` that computed different imputed values for `ekg` than those shown in Section 8.5. The ordering of levels of `ekg` is also different here.

TABLE 20.1

Predictor	Name	d.f.	Original Levels
Dose of estrogen	rx	3	placebo, 0.2, 1.0, 5.0 mg estrogen
Age in years	age	3	
Weight index: wt(kg)−ht(cm)+200	wt	3	
Performance rating	pf	2	normal, in bed < 50% of time, in bed > 50%, in bed always
History of cardiovascular disease	hx	1	present/absent
Systolic blood pressure/10	sbp	3	
Diastolic blood pressure/10	dbp	3	
Electrocardiogram code	ekg	5	normal, benign, rhythm disturb., block, strain, old myocardial infarction, new MI
Serum hemoglobin (g/100ml)	hg	3	
Tumor size (cm^2)	sz	3	
Stage/histologic grade combination	sg	3	
Serum prostatic acid phosphatase	ap	3	
Bone metastasis	bm	1	present/absent

functions, which contain two nonlinear terms and thus have a total of three d.f. Table 20.1 defines the candidate predictors and lists their d.f. The variable stage is not listed as it can be predicted with high accuracy from sz,sg,ap,bm (stage could have been used as a predictor for imputing missing values on sz, sg). There are a total of 36 candidate d.f. that should not be artificially reduced by "univariable screening" or graphical assessments of association with death. This is about 1/10 as many predictor d.f. as there are deaths, so there is some hope that a fitted model may validate. Let us also examine this issue by estimating the amount of shrinkage using Equation 4.1. We first use the previous transcan output to impute missing data.

```
> '%nin%' ← function(a,b) match(a, b, nomatch=0) == 0
> # tells which elements of a are not in b

> levels(ekg)[levels(ekg) %in% c('old MI','recent MI')] ← 'MI'
> # combines last 2 levels and uses a new name, MI

> pf.coded ← as.integer(pf)      # save original pf, recode to 1-4
> levels(pf)   ← c(levels(pf)[1:3], levels(pf)[3])
> # combine last 2 levels

> w ← prostate.transcan      # just to save typing for next 5 lines
```

```
> sz  ← impute(w, sz)
> sg  ← impute(w, sg)
> age ← impute(w, age)
> wt  ← impute(w, wt)
> ekg ← impute(w, ekg)

> dd ← datadist(rx, age, wt, pf, pf.coded, heart, map, hg,
+               sz, sg, ap, bm)
> options(datadist='dd')

> units(dtime) ← 'Month'
> S ← Surv(dtime, status!-'alive')

> f ← cph(S ~ rx + rcs(age,4) + rcs(wt,4) + pf + hx +
+             rcs(sbp,4) + rcs(dbp,4) + ekg + rcs(hg,4) +
+             rcs(sg,4) + rcs(sz,4) + rcs(ap,4) + bm)
```

The likelihood ratio χ^2 statistic is 140 with 36 d.f. This test is highly significant so some modeling is warranted. The AIC value (on the χ^2 scale) is $140-2\times36 = 68$. The rough shrinkage estimate is 0.743 (104/140) so we estimate that 26% of the model fitting will be noise, especially with regard to calibration accuracy. The approach of Spiegelhalter[397] is to fit this full model and to shrink predicted values. We instead try to do data reduction (blinded to individual χ^2 statistics from the above model fit) to see if a reliable model can be obtained without shrinkage. A good approach at this point might be to do a variable clustering analysis followed by single degree of freedom scoring for individual predictors or for clusters of predictors. Instead we do an informal data reduction. The strategy is listed in Table 20.2. For ap, more exploration is desired to be able to model the shape of effect with such a highly skewed distribution. Since we expect the tumor variables to be strong prognostic factors we retain them as separate variables. No assumption is made for the dose-response shape for estrogen, as there is reason to expect a nonmonotonic effect due to competing risks for cardiovascular death.

```
> heart ← hx + ekg %in% c('normal','benign')
> label(heart) ← 'Heart Disease Code'
> map    ← (2*dbp + sbp)/3
> label(map) ← 'Mean Arterial Pressure/10'

> f ← cph(S ~ rx + rcs(age,4) + rcs(wt,3) + pf.coded +
+             heart + rcs(map,3) + rcs(hg,4) +
+             rcs(sg,3) + rcs(sz,3) + rcs(log(ap),6) + bm,
+             x=T, y=T, surv=T, time.inc=5*12)
> # x, y for predict, validate, calibrate;
> # surv, time.inc for calibrate
```

The total savings is thus 11 d.f. The likelihood ratio χ^2 is 126 with 25 d.f., with a slightly improved AIC of 76. The rough shrinkage estimate is slightly better at

TABLE 20.2

Variables	Reductions	d.f. Saved
wt	Assume variable not important enough for 4 knots; use 3 knots	1
pf	Assume linearity	1
hx,ekg	Make new 0,1,2 variable and assume linearity: 2 = hx and ekg not normal or benign, 1 = either, 0 = none	5
sbp,dbp	Combine into mean arterial bp and use 3 knots: map = (2 dbp + sbp)/3	4
sg	Use 3 knots	1
sz	Use 3 knots	1
ap	Look at shape of effect of ap in detail, and take log before expanding as spline to achieve numerical stability: add 2 knots	−2

0.80, but still worrisome. A further data reduction could be done, such as using the transcan transformations determined from selfconsistency of predictors, but we stop here and use this model.

Now examine this model in more detail by examining coefficients and summarizing multiple parameters within predictors using Wald statistics.

```
> f

Cox Proportional Hazards Model

cph(formula = S ~ rx + rcs(age, 4) + rcs(wt, 3) +
        pf.coded + heart + rcs(map, 3) + rcs(hg, 4) +
        rcs(sz, 3) + rcs(sg, 3) + rcs(log(ap), 6) + bm,
        x=T, y=T, surv=T, time.inc=5*12)

Obs Events Model L.R. d.f. P Score Score P    R2
502    354         126   25 0   135      0 0.221


                       coef se(coef)      z       p
rx=0.2 mg estrogen  3.74e-03 1.50e-01  0.0250 9.80e-01
rx=1.0 mg estrogen -4.21e-01 1.66e-01 -2.5427 1.10e-02
rx=5.0 mg estrogen -9.73e-02 1.58e-01 -0.6176 5.37e-01
              age -1.17e-02 2.35e-02 -0.4995 6.17e-01
             age' 2.00e-02 3.86e-02  0.5190 6.04e-01
            age'' 2.71e-01 4.95e-01  0.5482 5.84e-01
               wt -2.46e-02 9.39e-03 -2.6175 8.86e-03
```

```
       wt'   1.84e-02 1.12e-02   1.6379 1.01e-01
  pf.coded   2.25e-01 1.21e-01   1.8625 6.25e-02
     heart   4.18e-01 8.08e-02   5.1723 2.31e-07
       map   3.24e-02 8.49e-02   0.3817 7.03e-01
      map'  -4.57e-02 9.41e-02  -0.4857 6.27e-01
        hg  -1.56e-01 7.68e-02  -2.0343 4.19e-02
       hg'   7.42e-02 2.10e-01   0.3530 7.24e-01
      hg''   5.08e-01 1.27e+00   0.4014 6.88e-01
        sz   1.00e-02 1.44e-02   0.6955 4.87e-01
       sz'   8.79e-03 2.37e-02   0.3715 7.10e-01
        sg   7.19e-02 7.86e-02   0.9138 3.61e-01
       sg'  -7.04e-03 9.83e-02  -0.0716 9.43e-01
        ap  -7.96e-01 3.11e-01  -2.5584 1.05e-02
       ap'   4.89e+01 2.18e+01   2.2482 2.46e-02
      ap''  -3.64e+02 1.59e+02  -2.2909 2.20e-02
     ap'''   4.04e+02 1.75e+02   2.3057 2.11e-02
    ap''''  -9.69e+01 4.16e+01  -2.3311 1.97e-02
        bm   3.25e-02 1.81e-01   0.1790 8.58e-01
```

```
> # The dose effect is apparently nonlinear.

> latex(anova(f))          # Table 20.3
```

There are 12 parameters associated with nonlinear effects, and the overall test of linearity indicates the strong presences of nonlinearity for at least one of the variables age,wt,map,hg,sz,sg,ap. There is a difference in survival time between at least two of the doses of estrogen.

20.2 Checking Proportional Hazards

Now that we have a tentative model, let us examine the model's distributional assumptions using smoothed scaled Schoenfeld residuals. A messy detail is how to handle multiple regression coefficients per predictor. Here we do an approximate analysis in which each predictor is scored by adding up all the terms in the model to transform that predictor to optimally relate to the log hazard (at least if the *shape* of the effect does not change with time). In doing this we are temporarily ignoring the fact that the individual regression coefficients were estimated from the data. For dose of estrogen, for example, we code the effect as 0 (placebo), 0.0037 (0.2 mg), -0.421 (1.0 mg), and -0.0972 (5.0 mg), and age is transformed as $-.0117$ age $+ 0.02$ age' $+0.271$ age'', which in the most simple form is

$$-1.17 \times 10^{-2} \text{age} + 3.48 \times 10^{-5} (\text{age} - 56)_+^3 + 4.71 \times 10^{-4} (\text{age} - 71)_+^3$$
$$-1.01 \times 10^{-3} (\text{age} - 75)_+^3 + 5.09 \times 10^{-4} (\text{age} - 80)_+^3.$$

TABLE 20.3: Wald Statistics for S

	χ^2	d.f.	P
rx	8.38	3	0.0387
age	12.85	3	0.0050
Nonlinear	8.18	2	0.0168
wt	8.87	2	0.0118
Nonlinear	2.68	1	0.1014
pf.coded	3.47	1	0.0625
heart	26.75	1	< 0.0001
map	0.25	2	0.8803
Nonlinear	0.24	1	0.6272
hg	11.85	3	0.0079
Nonlinear	6.92	2	0.0314
sz	10.60	2	0.0050
Nonlinear	0.14	1	0.7102
sg	3.14	2	0.2082
Nonlinear	0.01	1	0.9429
ap	13.17	5	0.0218
Nonlinear	12.93	4	0.0116
bm	0.03	1	0.8579
TOTAL NONLINEAR	30.28	12	0.0025
TOTAL	128.08	25	< 0.0001

In S-PLUS the `predict` function easily summarizes multiple terms and produces a matrix (here, `z`) containing the total effects for each predictor. Matrix factors can easily be included in model formulas.

```
> z ← predict(f, type='terms')
> # required x=T above to store design matrix
> f.short ← cph(S ~ z, x=T, y=T)
# store raw x, y so can get residuals
```

The fit `f.short` based on the matrix of single d.f. predictors `z` has the same LR χ^2 of 126 as the fit `f`, but with a falsely low 11 d.f. All regression coefficients are unity.

Now we compute scaled Schoenfeld residuals separately for each predictor and test the PH assumption using the "correlation with time" test. Also plot smoothed trends in the residuals. The `plot` method for `cox.zph` objects uses restricted cubic splines to smooth the relationship.

```
> phtest ← cox.zph(f.short, transform='identity')
> phtest
```

	rho	chisq	p
rx	0.12965	6.5451	0.0105
age	-0.08911	2.8518	0.0913
wt	-0.00878	0.0269	0.8697
pf.coded	-0.06238	1.4278	0.2321
heart	0.01017	0.0451	0.8319
map	0.03928	0.4998	0.4796
hg	-0.06678	1.7368	0.1876
sz	-0.05262	0.9834	0.3214
sg	-0.04276	0.6474	0.4210
ap	0.01237	0.0558	0.8133
bm	0.04891	0.9241	0.3364
GLOBAL	NA	15.3776	0.1659

Only the drug effect significantly changes over time ($P = 0.01$ for testing the correlation rho between the scaled Schoenfeld residual and time), but when a global test of PH is done penalizing for 11 d.f., the P value is 0.17. A graphical examination of the trends doesn't find anything interesting for the last 10 variables. A residual plot is drawn for `rx` alone and is shown in Figure 20.1.

```
> plot(phtest, var='rx')
```

We ignore the possible increase in effect of estrogen over time. If this non-PH is real, a more accurate model might be obtained by stratifying on `rx` or by using a time $\times$ `rx` interaction as a time-dependent covariable.

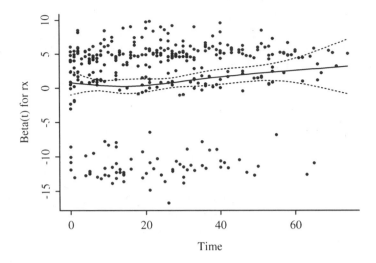

FIGURE 20.1: Raw and spline-smoothed scaled Schoenfeld residuals for dose of estrogen, nonlinearly coded from the Cox model fit, with ± 2 standard errors.

20.3   Testing Interactions

Note that the model has several insignificant predictors. These are not deleted, as that would not improve predictive accuracy and it would make accurate confidence intervals hard to obtain. At this point it would be reasonable to test prespecified interactions. Here we test all interactions with dose. Since the multiple terms for many of the predictors (and for **rx**) make for a great number of d.f. for testing interaction (and a loss of power), we do approximate tests on the data-driven codings of predictors. *P*-values for these tests are likely to be somewhat anticonservative.

```
> z.dose ← z[,"rx"]    # same as saying z[,1] - get first column
> z.other ← z[,-1]      # all but the first column of z
> f.ia ← cph(S ~ z.dose * z.other)
> anova(f.ia)
```

Factor	Chi-Square	d.f.	P
z.dose (Factor+Higher Order Factors)	18.9	11	0.062
All Interactions	12.2	10	0.273
z.other (Factor+Higher Order Factors)	134.3	20	0.000
All Interactions	12.2	10	0.273
z.dose * z.other (Factor+Higher Order Factors)	12.2	10	0.273
TOTAL	137.3	21	0.000

The global test of additivity has $P = 0.27$, so we ignore the interactions (and also forget to penalize for having looked for them below!).

20.4   Describing Predictor Effects

Let us plot how each predictor is related to the log hazard of death, including 0.95 confidence bands. Note that due to a peculiarity of the Cox model the standard error of the predicted $X\hat\beta$ is zero at the reference values (medians here, for continuous predictors).

```
> par(mfrow=c(3,4))      # 4 x 3 matrix of graphs, Figure 20.2
> r <- c(-1,1)           # use common y-axis range for all
> plot(f, rx=NA,         ylim=r)
> plot(f, age=NA,        ylim=r)
> scat1d(age)
> plot(f, wt=NA,         ylim=r)
  . . .
```

20.5   Validating the Model

We first validate this model for Somers' D_{xy} rank correlation between predicted log hazard and observed survival time, and for slope shrinkage. The bootstrap is used (with 200 resamples) to penalize for possible overfitting, as discussed in Section 5.2.

```
> validate(f, B=200, dxy=T, pr=T)
```

	index.orig	training	test	optimism	index.corrected	n
Dxy	-0.337377	-0.364644	-0.30976	-0.05488	-0.28250	200
R2	0.221444	0.261369	0.18445	0.07691	0.14453	200
Slope	1.000000	1.000000	0.78464	0.21536	0.78464	200

Here "training" refers to accuracy when evaluated on the bootstrap sample used to fit the model, and "test" refers to the accuracy when this model is applied without modification to the original sample. The apparent D_{xy} is -0.34, but a better estimate of how well the model will discriminate prognoses in the future is $D_{xy} = -0.28$. The bootstrap estimate of slope shrinkage is 0.78, surprisingly close to the simple heuristic estimate. The shrinkage coefficient could easily be used to shrink predictions to yield better calibration.

Finally, we validate the model (without using the shrinkage coefficient) for calibration accuracy in predicting the probability of surviving five years. The bootstrap is used to estimate the optimism in how well predicted five-year survival from the final Cox model tracks Kaplan–Meier five-year estimates, stratifying by grouping patients in subsets with about 70 patients per interval of predicted five-year survival.

```
> cal <- calibrate(f, B=200, u=5*12, m=70)
> cal              # same as print(cal)
```

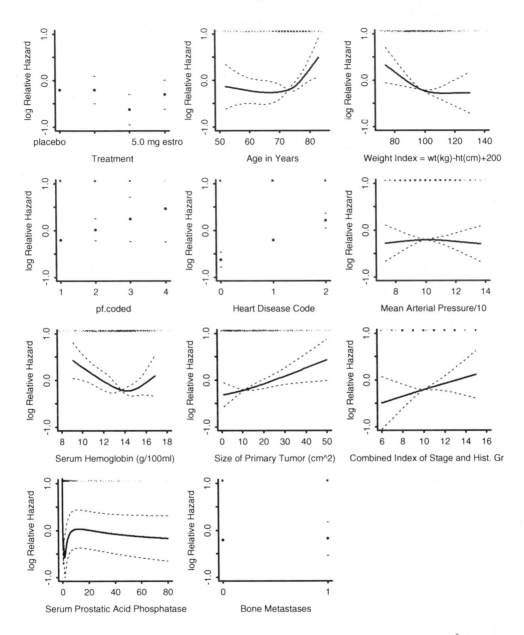

FIGURE 20.2: Shape of each predictor on log hazard of death. Y-axis shows $X\hat{\beta}$, but the predictors not plotted are set to reference values. "Rug plots" on the top of each graph show the data density of the predictor. Note the highly nonmonotonic relationship with ap, and the increased slope after age 70 which has been found in outcome models for various diseases.

```
calibrate.cph(fit = f, u = 5 * 12, m = 70, B = 200)
```

	index.orig	training	test	mean.optimism	mean.corrected	n
[1,]	-0.00749	0.01663	0.0577	-0.037003	0.02951	185
[2,]	0.01729	-0.00567	0.0109	-0.029964	0.04725	199
[3,]	-0.04261	-0.00367	0.0219	-0.020202	-0.02240	200
[4,]	-0.00965	-0.04743	-0.0320	0.000298	-0.00995	200
[5,]	-0.02419	-0.01553	-0.0264	0.008957	-0.03314	200
[6,]	0.02834	0.04143	-0.0169	0.032414	-0.00407	200
[7,]	0.02784	0.01456	-0.0254	0.047881	-0.02004	200

	mean.predicted	KM	KM.corrected	std.err
[1,]	0.0357	0.0282	0.0652	0.240
[2,]	0.1346	0.1519	0.1819	0.157
[3,]	0.2221	0.1795	0.1997	0.147
[4,]	0.3048	0.2952	0.2949	0.153
[5,]	0.3910	0.3668	0.3579	0.157
[6,]	0.4860	0.5143	0.4819	0.178
[7,]	0.6277	0.6556	0.6077	0.208

```
> plot(cal)
```

The estimated calibration curves are shown in Figure 20.3. Bootstrap calibration is very good except for the two groups with extremely bad prognosis—their survival is slightly better than predicted, consistent with regression to the mean. Even there, the absolute error is low despite a large relative error.

20.6 Presenting the Model

To present point and interval estimates of predictor effects we draw a hazard ratio chart (Figure 20.4), and to make a final presentation of the model we draw a nomogram having multiple "predicted value" axes. Since the ap relationship is so nonmonotonic, use a 20 : 1 hazard ratio for this variable.

```
> plot(summary(f, ap=c(1,20)), log=T)
```

The ultimate graphical display for this model will be a nomogram relating the predictors to $X\beta$, estimated three- and five-year survival probabilities and median survival time. It is easy to add as many "output" axes as desired to a nomogram.

```
> surv  ← Survival(f)
> surv3 ← function(x) surv(3*12,lp=x)
> surv5 ← function(x) surv(5*12,lp=x)
> quan  ← Quantile(f)
> med   ← function(x) quan(lp=x)/12
```

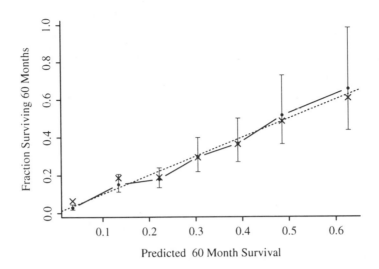

FIGURE 20.3: Bootstrap estimate of calibration accuracy for five-year estimates from the final Cox model. Dots correspond to apparent predictive accuracy. X marks the bootstrap-corrected estimates.

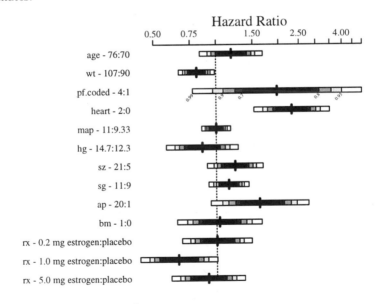

FIGURE 20.4: Hazard ratios and multilevel confidence bars for effects of predictors in model, using default ranges except for ap.

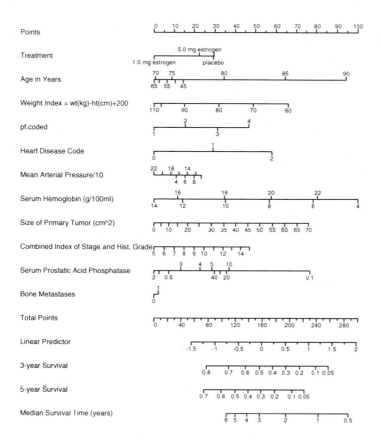

FIGURE 20.5: Nomogram for predicting survival probabilities and median survival time.

```
> ss     ← c(.05,.1,.2,.3,.4,.5,.6,.7,.8,.9,.95)

> nomogram(f, ap=c(.1,.5,1,2,3,4,5,10,20,30,40),
+          fun=list(surv3, surv5, med),
+          funlabel=c('3-year Survival','5-year Survival',
+                   'Median Survival Time (years)'),
+          fun.at=list(ss, ss, c(.5,1:6)), xfrac=.65)
```

20.7   Problems

Perform Cox regression analyses of survival time using the Mayo Clinic PBC dataset described in Section 8.12. Provide model descriptions, parameter estimates, and conclusions on a page that is separate from computer printouts.

1. Assess the nature of the association of several predictors of your choice. For polytomous predictors, perform a log-rank-type score test (or k-sample ANOVA extension if there are more than two levels). For continuous predictors, plot a smooth curve that estimates the relationship between the predictor and the log hazard or log–log survival. Use both parametric and nonparametric (using martingale residuals) approaches. Make a test of H_0 : predictor is not associated with outcome versus H_a : predictor is associated (by a smooth function). The test should have more than 1 d.f. If there is no evidence that the predictor is associated with outcome, omit that predictor from consideration for now. Make a formal test of linearity of each remaining continuous predictor. Use restricted cubic spline functions with four knots. Decide whether or how each predictor should be transformed or whether a spline function should be retained. If you feel that you can't narrow down the number of candidate predictors without examining the outcomes, and the number is too great to be able to derive a reliable model, use a data reduction technique and combine many of the variables into a summary index.

2. For factors that remain, assess the PH assumption using at least two methods, after ensuring that continuous predictors are transformed to be as linear as possible. In addition, for polytomous predictors, derive log cumulative hazard estimates adjusted for continuous predictors that do not assume anything about the relationship between the polytomous factor and survival.

3. Derive a final Cox PH model. Stratify on polytomous factors that do not satisfy the PH assumption. Decide whether to categorize and stratify on continuous factors that may strongly violate PH. Remember that in this case you can still model the continuous factor to account for any residual regression after adjusting for strata intervals. Test for and include clearly important two-way interactions, including interactions between a modeled factor and a stratification factor. Interpret the parameters in the final model. Also interpret the final model by providing some predicted survival curves in which an important continuous predictor is on the x-axis, predicted survival is on the y-axis, separate curves are drawn for levels of another factor, and any other factors in the model are adjusted to specified constants or to the grand mean. The estimated survival probabilities should be computed at $t = 100$ days.

4. Verify, in an unbiased fashion, your "final" model, for either calibration or discrimination. Validate intermediate steps, not just the final parameter estimates.

Appendix

Datasets, R Packages and S-Plus Libraries, and Internet Resources

Central Web Site and Datasets

The Web site for information related to this book is `biostat.mc.vanderbilt.edu/rms`. This site contains links to several other Web sites and it holds most of the datasets mentioned in the text for downloading. These datasets are in fully annotated R `save` and S-Plus transport format (`.sdd` files); some of these are also available in other formats. The datasets were selected because of the variety of types of response and predictor variables, sample size, and numbers of missing values. These files may be imported using the `File ... Import` menus under S-Plus, or using the `data.restore` function. In R they may be read using the `load` function, `load(url())` to read directly from the Web, or by using the `Hmisc` package's `getHdata` function to do the same. From the Web site there are links to other useful dataset sources. Links to presentations and technical reports related to the text are also found on this site, as is information for instructors for obtaining quizzes and answer sheets, extra problems, and solutions to these and to many of the problems in the text. Details about one semester courses and short courses based on the text are also found there.

R Packages and S-Plus Libraries

The `Design` package written by the author, so named because it maintains detailed information about a model's design matrix so that many analyses using the model fit are automated, is a large library of R and S-Plus functions. Most of these functions analyze model fits, validate them, or make presentation graphics from them, but the `Design` library also contains special model–fitting functions for binary and ordinal logistic regression (optionally using penalized maximum likelihood), penalized and unpenalized least squares, and parametric and semiparametric survival models. `Design` pays special attention to computing predicted values in that design matrix attributes (e.g., knots for splines, categories for categorical predictors) are "remembered" so that predictors are properly transformed while predictions are being generated. This library of functions makes extensive use of a wealth of survival analysis software written by Terry Therneau of the Mayo Foundation. This `survival` library is now a standard part of S-Plus and is available for R.

The author's `Hmisc` package contains other miscellaneous functions used in the text. These are functions that do not operate on model fits that used the enhanced design attributes stored by the `Design` package. Functions in `Hmisc` include facilities for data reduction, imputation, power and sample size calculation, advanced table making, recoding variables, translating SAS datasets into R or S-Plus data frames while preserving all data attributes (including variable and value labels and special missing values), drawing and annotating plots, and converting certain R or S-Plus objects to LaTeX[254] typeset form. The latter capability, provided by a family of `latex` functions, completes the conversion to LaTeX of many of the objects created by the `Design` package. `Design` contains several LaTeX methods that create LaTeX code for typesetting model fits in algebraic notation, for printing ANOVA and regression effect (e.g., odds ratio) tables, and other applications. `Design`'s LaTeX methods were used extensively in the text, especially for writing restricted cubic spline function fits in simplest notation.

The latest versions of the packages are available from the main Web site or from `CRAN` (see below). It is necessary to install the `Hmisc` package in order to use the `Design` package. `Hmisc` and `Design` come already installed with S-Plus on Windows. The Web site also contains more in-depth overviews of the libraries.

The add-on packages run on UNIX, Linux, and Microsoft Windows systems. For R, the packages also run on Mac OS X. For most systems, the packages may be automatically downloaded and installed using R's `install.packages` function or using menus under R on Windows. Current information about the availability of the libraries on various platforms is found on the Web site.

R-help, S-news *and* CRAN

To subscribe to the highly informative and helpful `R-help` or `S-news` group, see the Web site. `R-help` and `S-news` are appropriate for asking general questions about R and S-Plus including those about finding or writing functions to do specific analyses (for questions specific to a package, contact the author of that package). For R, another resource is the `CRAN` repository at `www.r-project.org`.

Multiple Imputation

The `Impute` E-mail list maintained by Robert Harris of the University of Texas Southwestern is an invaluable source of information regarding missing data problems. To subscribe to this list, see the Web site. Other excellent sources of online information are Joseph Schafer's "Multiple Imputation Frequently Asked Questions" site and Stef van Buuren and Karin Oudshoorn's "Multiple Imputation Online" site, for which links exist on the main Web site.

Introductory R *and S-Plus and Add-on Package Text*

Readers can download "An Introduction to S and to the `Hmisc` and `Design` Libraries" by C. F. Alzola and F. E. Harrell from the Web site. This text has a good deal of information about importing and preparing data for analysis, creating derived variables, exploratory graphics, table making, imputation, simulation, sample size and power calculations, annotating plots, reproducible analysis, and many other methods. The `www.r-project.org` site also has many useful documents.

Bibliography

An extensive annotated bibliography containing all the references in this text as well as other references concerning predictive methods, survival analysis, logistic regression, prognosis, diagnosis, modeling strategies, model validation, practical Bayesian methods, clinical trials, graphical methods, papers for teaching statistical methods, the bootstrap, and many other areas may be found on the main Web site.

SAS

SAS macros for fitting restricted cubic splines and for other basic operations are freely available from the main Web site. The Web site also has notes on SAS usage for some of the methods presented in the text.

References

Numbers in brackets [ ] following entries are page references to citations.

[1] O. O. Aalen. Nonparametric inference in connection with multiple decrement models. *Scandanavian Journal of Statistics*, 3:15–27, 1976. [403]

[2] O. O. Aalen. Further results on the non-parametric linear regression model in survival analysis. *Statistics in Medicine*, 12:1569–1588, 1993. [506]

[3] O. O. Aalen, E. Bjertness, and T. Sønju. Analysis of dependent survival data applied to lifetimes of amalgam fillings. *Statistics in Medicine*, 14:1819–1829, 1995. [411]

[4] M. Abrahamowicz, T. MacKenzie, and J. M. Esdaile. Time-dependent hazard ratio: Modeling and hypothesis testing with applications in lupus nephritis. *Journal of the American Medical Association*, 91:1432–1439, 1996. [489]

[5] A. Agresti. A survey of models for repeated ordered categorical response data. *Statistics in Medicine*, 8:1209–1224, 1989. [342]

[6] H. Ahn and W. Loh. Tree-structured proportional hazards regression modeling. *Biometrics*, 50:471–485, 1994. [37, 176]

[7] K. Akazawa, T. Nakamura, and Y. Palesch. Power of logrank test and Cox regression model in clinical trials with heterogeneous samples. *Statistics in Medicine*, 16:583–597, 1997. [4]

[8] J. M. Alho. On the computation of likelihood ratio and score test based confidence intervals in generalized linear models. *Statistics in Medicine*, 11:923–930, 1992. [211]

[9] D. G. Altman. Categorising continuous covariates (letter to the editor). *British Journal of Cancer*, 64:975, 1991. [8]

[10] D. G. Altman and P. K. Andersen. A note on the uncertainty of a survival probability estimated from Cox's regression model. *Biometrika*, 73:722–724, 1986. [9, 506]

[11] D. G. Altman and P. K. Andersen. Bootstrap investigation of the stability of a Cox regression model. *Statistics in Medicine*, 8:771–783, 1989. [57, 59, 359]

[12] D. G. Altman, B. Lausen, W. Sauerbrei, and M. Schumacher. Dangers of using 'optimal' cutpoints in the evaluation of prognostic factors. *Journal of the National Cancer Institute*, 86:829–835, 1994. [8]

[13] D. G. Altman and P. Royston. What do we mean by validating a prognostic model? *Statistics in Medicine*, 19:453–473, 2000. [4, 101, 507]

[14] B. Altschuler. Theory for the measurement of competing risks in animal experiments. *Mathematical Biosciences*, 6:1–11, 1970. [403]

[15] C. F. Alzola and F. E. Harrell. An Introduction to S-Plus and the Hmisc and Design Libraries. Available from **hesweb1.med.virginia.edu/biostat/s.**, 2001. Electronic book, 299 pages. [x, 107]

[16] P. K. Andersen and R. D. Gill. Cox's regression model for counting processes: A large sample study. *Annals of Statistics*, 10:1100–1120, 1982. [408, 500]

[17] G. L. Anderson and T. R. Fleming. Model misspecification in proportional hazards regression. *Biometrika*, 82:527–541, 1995. [4]

[18] J. A. Anderson. Regression and ordered categorical variables. *Journal of the Royal Statistical Society B*, 46:1–30, 1984. [342]

[19] J. A. Anderson and P. R. Philips. Regression, discrimination and measurement models for ordered categorical variables. *Applied Statistics*, 30:22–31, 1981. [342]

[20] J. A. Anderson and A. Senthilselvan. A two-step regression model for hazard functions. *Applied Statistics*, 31:44–51, 1982. [483, 487, 491]

[21] D. F. Andrews and A. M. Herzberg. *Data*. Springer-Verlag, New York, 1985. [147]

[22] E. Arjas. A graphical method for assessing goodness of fit in Cox's proportional hazards model. *Journal of the American Statistical Association*, 83:204–212, 1988. [410, 483, 490]

[23] H. R. Arkes, N. V. Dawson, T. Speroff, F. E. Harrell, C. Alzola, R. Phillips, N. Desbiens, R. K. Oye, W. Knaus, A. F. Connors, and the SUPPORT Investigators. The covariance decomposition of the probability score and its use in evaluating prognostic estimates. *Medical Decision Making*, 15:120–131, 1995. [247]

[24] B. G. Armstrong and M. Sloan. Ordinal regression models for epidemiologic data. *American Journal of Epidemiology*, 129:191–204, 1989. [338, 339, 340, 342]

[25] D. Ashby, C. R. West, and D. Ames. The ordered logistic regression model in psychiatry: Rising prevalence of dementia in old people's homes. *Statistics in Medicine*, 8:1317–1326, 1989. [342]

[26] A. C. Atkinson. A note on the generalized information criterion for choice of a model. *Biometrika*, 67:413–418, 1980. [58, 202]

[27] D. Bamber. The area above the ordinal dominance graph and the area below the receiver operating characteristic graph. *Journal of Mathematical Psychology*, 12:387–415, 1975. [247]

[28] J. Banks. Nomograms. In S. Kotz and N. L. Johnson, editors, *Encyclopedia of Statistical Sciences*, Volume 6. Wiley, New York, 1985. [98, 256]

[29] J. Barnard and D. B. Rubin. Small-sample degrees of freedom with multiple imputation. *Biometrika*, 86:948–955, 1999. [50]

[30] R. A. Becker, J. M. Chambers, and A. R. Wilks. *The New S Language*. Wadsworth and Brooks/Cole, Pacific Grove, CA, 1988. [105]

[31] H. Belcher. The concept of residual confounding in regression models and some applications. *Statistics in Medicine*, 11:1747–1758, 1992. [8]

[32] D. A. Belsley. *Conditioning Diagnostics: Collinearity and Weak Data in Regression*. Wiley, New York, 1991. [84]

[33] D. A. Belsley, E. Kuh, and R. E. Welsch. *Regression Diagnostics: Identifying Influential Data and Sources of Collinearity*. Wiley, New York, 1980. [76]

[34] J. K. Benedetti, P. Liu, H. N. Sather, J. Seinfeld, and M. A. Epton. Effective sample size for tests of censored survival data. *Biometrika*, 69:343–349, 1982. [61]

[35] K. N. Berk and D. E. Booth. Seeing a curve in multiple regression. *Technometrics*, 37:385–398, 1995. [265]

[36] D. M. Berridge and J. Whitehead. Analysis of failure time data with ordinal categories of response. *Statistics in Medicine*, 10:1703–1710, 1991. [338, 339, 342, 407]

[37] C. Berzuini and D. Clayton. Bayesian analysis of survival on multiple time scales. *Statistics in Medicine*, 13:823–838, 1994. [392]

[38] W. B. Bilker and M. Wang. A semiparametric extension of the Mann-Whitney test for randomly truncated data. *Biometrics*, 52:10–20, 1996. [410]

[39] D. A. Binder. Fitting Cox's proportional hazards models from survey data. *Biometrika*, 79:139–147, 1992. [211]

[40] E. H. Blackstone. Analysis of death (survival analysis) and other time-related events. In F. J. Macartney, editor, *Current Status of Clinical Cardiology*, pages 55–101. MTP Press Limited, Lancaster, UK, 1986. [410]

[41] M. Blettner and W. Sauerbrei. Influence of model-building strategies on the results of a case-control study. *Statistics in Medicine*, 12:1325–1338, 1993. [103]

[42] D. D. Boos. On generalized score tests. *American Statistician*, 46:327–333, 1992. [210]

[43] J. G. Booth and S. Sarkar. Monte Carlo approximation of bootstrap variances. *American Statistician*, 52:354–357, 1998. [101]

[44] R. Brant. Assessing proportionality in the proportional odds model for ordinal logistic regression. *Biometrics*, 46:1171–1178, 1990. [342]

[45] S. R. Brazer, F. S. Pancotto, T. T. Long III, F. E. Harrell, K. L. Lee, M. P. Tyor, and D. B. Pryor. Using ordinal logistic regression to estimate the likelihood of colorectal neoplasia. *Journal of Clinical Epidemiology*, 44:1263–1270, 1991. [342]

[46] L. Breiman. The little bootstrap and other methods for dimensionality selection in regression: X-fixed prediction error. *Journal of the American Statistical Association*, 87:738–754, 1992. [58, 84, 92, 94, 102, 103, 202]

[47] L. Breiman and J. H. Friedman. Estimating optimal transformations for multiple regression and correlation (with discussion). *Journal of the American Statistical Association*, 80:580–619, 1985. [68, 170, 376]

[48] L. Breiman, J. H. Friedman, R. A. Olshen, and C. J. Stone. *Classification and Regression Trees*. Wadsworth and Brooks/Cole, Pacific Grove, CA, 1984. [26, 37, 119]

[49] N. E. Breslow. Covariance analysis of censored survival data. *Biometrics*, 30:89–99, 1974. [467, 472, 474]

[50] N. E. Breslow, N. E. Day, K. T. Halvorsen, R. L. Prentice, and C. Sabai. Estimation of multiple relative risk functions in matched case-control studies. *American Journal of Epidemiology*, 108:299–307, 1978. [472]

[51] N. E. Breslow, L. Edler, and J. Berger. A two-sample censored-data rank test for acceleration. *Biometrics*, 40:1049–1062, 1984. [491]

[52] G. W. Brier. Verification of forecasts expressed in terms of probability. *Monthly Weather Review*, 75:1–3, 1950. [247]

[53] D. Brownstone. Regression strategies. In *Proceedings of the 20th Symposium on the Interface between Computer Science and Statistics*, pages 74–79, Washington, DC, 1988. American Statistical Association. [96]

[54] S. F. Buck. A method of estimation of missing values in multivariate data suitable for use with an electronic computer. *Journal of the Royal Statistical Society B*, 22:302–307, 1960. [47]

[55] S. T. Buckland, K. P. Burnham, and N. H. Augustin. Model selection: An integral part of inference. *Biometrics*, 53:603–618, 1997. [8, 9, 202]

[56] J. Buckley and I. James. Linear regression with censored data. *Biometrika*, 66:429–36, 1979. [435]

[57] P. Buettner, C. Garbe, and I. Guggenmoos-Holzmann. Problems in defining cutoff points of continuous prognostic factors: Example of tumor thickness in primary cutaneous melanoma. *Journal of Clinical Epidemiology*, 50:1201–1210, 1997. [8]

[58] K. Bull and D. Spiegelhalter. Survival analysis in observational studies. *Statistics in Medicine*, 16:1041–1074, 1997. [389, 392, 410]

[59] M. Buyse. R^2: A useful measure of model performance when predicting a dichotomous outcome. *Statistics in Medicine*, 19:271–274, 2000. Letter to the Editor regarding *Statistics in Medicine* 18:375–384; 1999. [265]

[60] D. P. Byar and S. B. Green. The choice of treatment for cancer patients based on covariate information: Application to prostate cancer. *Bulletin Cancer, Paris*, 67:477–488, 1980. [147, 269, 509]

[61] R. M. Califf, F. E. Harrell, K. L. Lee, J. S. Rankin, et al. The evolution of medical and surgical therapy for coronary artery disease. *Journal of the American Medical Association*, 261:2077–2086, 1989. [473, 475, 497]

[62] R. M. Califf, H. R. Phillips, et al. Prognostic value of a coronary artery jeopardy score. *Journal of the American College of Cardiology*, 5:1055–1063, 1985. [205]

[63] J. Carpenter and J. Bithell. Bootstrap confidence intervals: when, which, what? A practical guide for medical statisticians. *Statistics in Medicine*, 19:1141–1164, 2000. [101, 211]

[64] W. H. Carter, G. L. Wampler, and D. M. Stablein. *Regression Analysis of Survival Data in Cancer Chemotherapy*. Marcel Dekker, New York, 1983. [467]

[65] J. M. Chambers and T. J. Hastie, editors. *Statistical Models in S*. Wadsworth and Brooks/Cole, Pacific Grove, CA, 1992. [x, 25, 37, 106, 119, 238, 239, 257, 481, 486]

[66] L. E. Chambless and K. E. Boyle. Maximum likelihood methods for complex sample data: Logistic regression and discrete proportional hazards models. *Communications in Statistics A*, 14:1377–1392, 1985. [211]

[67] R. Chappell. A note on linear rank tests and Gill and Schumacher's tests of proportionality. *Biometrika*, 79:199–201, 1992. [483]

[68] C. Chatfield. Avoiding statistical pitfalls (with discussion). *Statistical Science*, 6:240–268, 1991. [76]

[69] C. Chatfield. Model uncertainty, data mining and statistical inference (with discussion). *Journal of the Royal Statistical Society A*, 158:419–466, 1995. [vii, 6, 7, 8, 9, 57, 84, 103, 202]

[70] S. Chatterjee and B. Price. *Regression Analysis by Example*. Wiley, New York, second edition, 1991. [65, 84]

[71] S. C. Cheng, J. P. Fine, and L. J. Wei. Prediction of cumulative incidence function under the proportional hazards model. *Biometrics*, 54:219–228, 1998. [405]

[72] S. C. Cheng, L. J. Wei, and Z. Ying. Predicting survival probabilities with semiparametric transformation models. *Journal of the American Statistical Association*, 92:227–235, 1997. [506]

[73] A. Ciampi, A. Negassa, and Z. Lou. Tree-structured prediction for censored survival data and the Cox model. *Journal of Clinical Epidemiology*, 48:675–689, 1995. [37]

[74] A. Ciampi, J. Thiffault, J.-P. Nakache, and B. Asselain. Stratification by stepwise regression, correspondence analysis and recursive partition. *Computational Statistics and Data Analysis*, 1986:185–204, 1986. [37, 67]

[75] L. A. Clark and D. Pregibon. Tree-based models. In J. M. Chambers and T. J. Hastie, editors, *Statistical Models in S*, Chapter 9, pages 377–419. Wadsworth and Brooks/Cole, Pacific Grove, CA, 1992. [37]

[76] W. S. Cleveland. Robust locally weighted regression and smoothing scatterplots. *Journal of the American Statistical Association*, 74:829–836, 1979. [24, 119, 233, 334, 370, 481]

[77] A. Cnaan and L. Ryan. Survival analysis in natural history studies of disease. *Statistics in Medicine*, 8:1255–1268, 1989. [392, 410]

[78] T. J. Cole, C. J. Morley, A. J. Thornton, M. A. Fowler, and P. H. Hewson. A scoring system to quantify illness in babies under 6 months of age. *Journal of the Royal Statistical Society A*, 154:287–304, 1991. [342]

[79] D. Collett. *Modelling Binary Data.* Chapman and Hall, London, 1991. [210, 265, 334]

[80] D. Collett. *Modelling Survival Data in Medical Research.* Chapman and Hall, London, 1994. [410, 506]

[81] A. F. Connors, T. Speroff, N. V. Dawson, C. Thomas, F. E. Harrell, D. Wagner, N. Desbiens, L. Goldman, A. W. Wu, R. M. Califf, W. J. Fulkerson, H. Vidaillet, S. Broste, P. Bellamy, J. Lynn, W. A. Knaus, and The SUPPORT Investigators. The effectiveness of right heart catheterization in the initial care of critically ill patients. *Journal of the American Medical Association*, 276:889–897, 1996. [3]

[82] E. F. Cook and L. Goldman. Asymmetric stratification: An outline for an efficient method for controlling confounding in cohort studies. *American Journal of Epidemiology*, 127:626–639, 1988. [27, 227]

[83] J. Copas. The effectiveness of risk scores: The logit rank plot. *Applied Statistics*, 48:165–183, 1999. [265]

[84] J. B. Copas. Regression, prediction and shrinkage (with discussion). *Journal of the Royal Statistical Society B*, 45:311–354, 1983. [84]

[85] J. B. Copas. Cross-validation shrinkage of regression predictors. *Journal of the Royal Statistical Society B*, 49:175–183, 1987. [95, 102, 265, 495]

[86] J. B. Copas. Unweighted sum of squares tests for proportions. *Applied Statistics*, 38:71–80, 1989. [231]

[87] J. B. Copas and T. Long. Estimating the residual variance in orthogonal regression with variable selection. *The Statistician*, 40:51–59, 1991. [57]

[88] C. Cox. Location-scale cumulative odds models for ordinal data: A generalized non-linear model approach. *Statistics in Medicine*, 14:1191–1203, 1995. [342]

[89] D. R. Cox. The regression analysis of binary sequences (with discussion). *Journal of the Royal Statistical Society B*, 20:215–242, 1958. [12, 216]

[90] D. R. Cox. Two further applications of a model for binary regression. *Biometrika*, 45:562–565, 1958. [249, 250]

[91] D. R. Cox. Further results on tests of separate families of hypotheses. *Journal of the Royal Statistical Society B*, 24:406–424, 1962. [203]

[92] D. R. Cox. Regression models and life-tables (with discussion). *Journal of the Royal Statistical Society B*, 34:187–220, 1972. [35, 37, 161, 205, 211, 334, 408, 417, 465, 466]

[93] D. R. Cox and D. Oakes. *Analysis of Survival Data*. Chapman and Hall, London, 1984. [392, 410, 506]

[94] D. R. Cox and E. J. Snell. A general definition of residuals (with discussion). *Journal of the Royal Statistical Society B*, 30:248–275, 1968. [429]

[95] D. R. Cox and E. J. Snell. *The Analysis of Binary Data*. Chapman and Hall, London, second edition, 1989. [204]

[96] D. R. Cox and N. Wermuth. A comment on the coefficient of determination for binary responses. *American Statistician*, 46:1–4, 1992. [204, 247]

[97] J. G. Cragg and R. Uhler. The demand for automobiles. *Canadian Journal of Economics*, 3:386–406, 1970. [205, 247]

[98] S. L. Crawford, S. L. Tennstedt, and J. B. McKinlay. A comparison of analytic methods for non-random missingness of outcome data. *Journal of Clinical Epidemiology*, 48:209–219, 1995. [50]

[99] N. J. Crichton and J. P. Hinde. Correspondence analysis as a screening method for indicants for clinical diagnosis. *Statistics in Medicine*, 8:1351–1362, 1989. [67]

[100] N. J. Crichton, J. P. Hinde, and J. Marchini. Models for diagnosing chest pain: Is CART useful? *Statistics in Medicine*, 16:717–727, 1997. [37]

[101] L. A. Cupples, D. R. Gagnon, R. Ramaswamy, and R. B. D'Agostino. Age-adjusted survival curves with application in the Framingham Study. *Statistics in Medicine*, 14:1731–1744, 1995. [506]

[102] E. E. Cureton and R. B. D'Agostino. *Factor Analysis, An Applied Approach*. Erlbaum, Hillsdale, NJ, 1983. [66, 72, 84, 85]

[103] D. M. Dabrowska, K. A. Doksum, N. J. Feduska, R. Husing, and P. Neville. Methods for comparing cumulative hazard functions in a semi-proportional hazard model. *Statistics in Medicine*, 11:1465–1476, 1992. [471, 483, 491]

[104] R. B. D'Agostino, A. J. Belanger, E. W. Markson, M. Kelly-Hayes, and P. A. Wolf. Development of health risk appraisal functions in the presence of multiple indicators: The Framingham Study nursing home institutionalization model. *Statistics in Medicine*, 14:1757–1770, 1995. [66, 84, 85]

[105] R. B. D'Agostino, Jr. and D. B. Rubin. Estimating and using propensity scores with partially missing data. *Journal of the American Statistical Association*, 95:749–759, 2000. [50]

[106] C. E. Davis, J. E. Hyde, S. I. Bangdiwala, and J. J. Nelson. An example of dependencies among variables in a conditional logistic regression. In S. Moolgavkar and R. Prentice, editors, *Modern Statistical Methods in Chronic Disease Epidemiology*, pages 140–147. Wiley, New York, 1986. [65, 116, 244]

[107] R. B. Davis and J. R. Anderson. Exponential survival trees. *Statistics in Medicine*, 8:947–961, 1989. [37]

[108] A. C. Davison and D. V. Hinkley. *Bootstrap Methods and Their Application*. Cambridge University Press, Cambridge, 1997. [58, 87, 90, 101]

[109] R. J. M. Dawson. The 'unusual episode' data revisited. *Journal of Statistics Education*, 3(3), 1995. Online journal at `www.amstat.org/publications/jse/v3n3/-datasets.dawson.html`. [299]

[110] C. de Boor. *A Practical Guide to Splines*. Springer-Verlag, New York, 1978. [20, 36]

[111] S. Derksen and H. J. Keselman. Backward, forward and stepwise automated subset selection algorithms: Frequency of obtaining authentic and noise variables. *British Journal of Mathematical and Statistical Psychology*, 45:265–282, 1992. [57]

[112] T. F. Devlin and B. J. Weeks. Spline functions for logistic regression modeling. In *Proceedings of the Eleventh Annual SAS Users Group International Conference*, pages 646–651, Cary, NC, 1986. SAS Institute, Inc. [18, 20]

[113] T. DiCiccio and B. Efron. More accurate confidence intervals in exponential families. *Biometrika*, 79:231–245, 1992. [211]

[114] E. Dickson, P. M. Grambsch, T. R. Fleming, L. D. Fisher, and A. Langworthy. Prognosis in primary biliary cirrhosis: Model for decision making. *Hepatology*, 10:1–7, 1989. [176]

[115] N. Doganaksoy and J. Schmee. Comparisons of approximate confidence intervals for distributions used in life-data analysis. *Technometrics*, 35:175–184, 1993. [195, 211]

[116] A. Donner. The relative effectiveness of procedures commonly used in multiple regression analysis for dealing with missing values. *American Statistician*, 36:378–381, 1982. [43, 47]

[117] D. Draper. Assessment and propagation of model uncertainty (with discussion). *Journal of the Royal Statistical Society B*, 57:45–97, 1995. [8, 9]

[118] M. Drum and P. McCullagh. Comment on Regression models for discrete longitudinal responses by G. M. Fitzmaurice, N. M. Laird, and A. G. Rotnitzky. *Statistical Science*, 8:300–301, 1993. [193]

[119] N. Duan. Smearing estimate: A nonparametric retransformation method. *Journal of the American Statistical Association*, 78:605–610, 1983. [378]

[120] R. Dudley, F. E. Harrell, L. Smith, D. B. Mark, R. M. Califf, D. B. Pryor, D. Glower, J. Lipscomb, and M. Hlatky. Comparison of analytic models for estimating the effect of clinical factors on the cost of coronary artery bypass graft surgery. *Journal of Clinical Epidemiology*, 46:261–271, 1993. [x]

[121] S. Durrleman and R. Simon. Flexible regression models with cubic splines. *Statistics in Medicine*, 8:551–561, 1989. [36]

[122] J. P. Eaton and C. A. Haas. *Titanic: Triumph and Tragedy*. W. W. Norton, New York, second edition, 1995. [299]

[123] B. Efron. The efficiency of Cox's likelihood function for censored data. *Journal of the American Statistical Association*, 72:557–565, 1977. [465, 467]

[124] B. Efron. Estimating the error rate of a prediction rule: Improvement on cross-validation. *Journal of the American Statistical Association*, 78:316–331, 1983. [58, 93, 94, 95, 96, 102, 249]

[125] B. Efron. How biased is the apparent error rate of a prediction rule? *Journal of the American Statistical Association*, 81:461–470, 1986. [84, 94]

[126] B. Efron. Missing data, imputation, and the bootstrap (with discussion). *Journal of the American Statistical Association*, 89:463–479, 1994. [47, 48]

[127] B. Efron and G. Gong. A leisurely look at the bootstrap, the jackknife, and cross-validation. *American Statistician*, 37:36–48, 1983. [94]

[128] B. Efron and C. Morris. Stein's paradox in statistics. *Scientific American*, 236:119–127, 1977. [63]

[129] B. Efron and R. Tibshirani. Bootstrap methods for standard errors, confidence intervals, and other measures of statistical accuracy. *Statistical Science*, 1:54–77, 1986. [58, 87, 94, 194]

[130] B. Efron and R. Tibshirani. *An Introduction to the Bootstrap*. Chapman and Hall, New York, 1993. [58, 87, 94, 95, 101, 194, 196]

[131] B. Efron and R. Tibshirani. Improvements on cross-validation: The .632+ bootstrap method. *Journal of the American Statistical Association*, 92:548–560, 1997. [102]

[132] G. E. Eide, E. Omenaas, and A. Gulsvik. The semi-proportional hazards model revisited: Practical reparameterizations. *Statistics in Medicine*, 15:1771–1777, 1996. [471]

[133] D. Faraggi and R. Simon. A simulation study of cross-validation for selecting an optimal cutpoint in univariate survival analysis. *Statistics in Medicine*, 15:2203–2213, 1996. [8]

[134] J. J. Faraway. The cost of data analysis. *Journal of Computational and Graphical Statistics*, 1:213–229, 1992. [8, 9, 81, 84, 95, 96, 340, 379, 382]

[135] S. E. Feinberg. *The Analysis of Cross-Classified Data*. MIT Press, Cambridge, MA, second edition, 1980. [331, 338]

[136] Z. Feng, D. McLerran, and J. Grizzle. A comparison of statistical methods for clustered data analysis with Gaussian error. *Statistics in Medicine*, 15:1793–1806, 1996. [194, 211]

[137] L. Ferré. Determining the dimension in sliced inverse regression and related methods. *Journal of the American Statistical Association*, 93:132–149, 1998. [84]

[138] D. M. Finkelstein and D. A. Schoenfeld. Combining mortality and longitudinal measures in clinical trials. *Statistics in Medicine*, 18:1341–1354, 1999. [410]

[139] G. M. Fitzmaurice. A caveat concerning independence estimating equations with multivariate binary data. *Biometrics*, 51:309–317, 1995. [211]

[140] T. R. Fleming and D. P. Harrington. Nonparametric estimation of the survival distribution in censored data. *Communications in Statistics*, 13(20):2469–2486, 1984. [403, 404]

[141] T. R. Fleming and D. P. Harrington. *Counting Processes & Survival Analysis*. Wiley, New York, 1991. [176, 410]

[142] I. Ford, J. Norrie, and S. Ahmadi. Model inconsistency, illustrated by the Cox proportional hazards model. *Statistics in Medicine*, 14:735–746, 1995. [4]

[143] E. B. Fowlkes. Some diagnostics for binary logistic regression via smoothing. *Biometrika*, 74:503–515, 1987. [265]

[144] B. Francis and M. Fuller. Visualization of event histories. *Journal of the Royal Statistical Society A*, 159:301–308, 1996. [411]

[145] D. Freedman, W. Navidi, and S. Peters. *On the Impact of Variable Selection in Fitting Regression Equations*, pages 1–16. Lecture Notes in Economics and Mathematical Systems. Springer-Verlag, New York, 1988. [95]

[146] J. H. Friedman. A variable span smoother. Technical Report 5, Laboratory for Computational Statistics, Department of Statistics, Stanford University, 1984. [25, 68, 119, 208, 260, 486]

[147] M. H. Gail. Does cardiac transplantation prolong life? A reassessment. *Annals of Internal Medicine*, 76:815–817, 1972. [392]

[148] J. J. Gaynor, E. J. Feuer, C. C. Tan, D. H. Wu, C. R. Little, D. J. Straus, D. D. Clarkson, and M. F. Brennan. On the use of cause-specific failure and conditional failure probabilities: Examples from clinical oncology data. *Journal of the American Statistical Association*, 88:400–409, 1993. [405]

[149] S. A. Glantz and B. K. Slinker. *Primer of Applied Regression and Analysis of Variance*. McGraw-Hill, New York, 1990. [64]

[150] M. Glasser. Exponential survival with covariance. *Journal of the American Statistical Association*, 62:561–568, 1967. [421]

[151] A. I. Goldman. EVENTCHARTS: Visualizing survival and other timed-events data. *American Statistician*, 46:13–18, 1992. [410]

[152] R. Goldstein. The comparison of models in discrimination cases. *Jurimetrics Journal*, 34:215–234, 1994. [211]

[153] G. Gong. Cross-validation, the jackknife, and the bootstrap: Excess error estimation in forward logistic regression. *Journal of the American Statistical Association*, 81:108–113, 1986. [94]

[154] T. A. Gooley, W. Leisenring, J. Crowley, and B. E. Storer. Estimation of failure probabilities in the presence of competing risks: New representations of old estimators. *Statistics in Medicine*, 18:695–706, 1999. [405]

[155] S. M. Gore, S. J. Pocock, and G. R. Kerr. Regression models and non-proportional hazards in the analysis of breast cancer survival. *Applied Statistics*, 33:176–195, 1984. [441, 483, 489, 491]

[156] W. Gould. Confidence intervals in logit and probit models. *Stata Technical Bulletin*, STB-14:26–28, July 1993. [184]

[157] P. Grambsch and T. Therneau. Proportional hazards tests and diagnostics based on weighted residuals. *Biometrika*, 81:515–526, 1994. Amendment and corrections in 82: 668 (1995). [334, 486, 487, 506]

[158] P. M. Grambsch and P. C. O'Brien. The effects of transformations and preliminary tests for non-linearity in regression. *Statistics in Medicine*, 10:697–709, 1991. [28, 32, 56]

[159] B. I. Graubard and E. L. Korn. Regression analysis with clustered data. *Statistics in Medicine*, 13:509–522, 1994. [211]

[160] R. J. Gray. Some diagnostic methods for Cox regression models through hazard smoothing. *Biometrics*, 46:93–102, 1990. [506]

[161] R. J. Gray. Flexible methods for analyzing survival data using splines, with applications to breast cancer prognosis. *Journal of the American Statistical Association*, 87:942–951, 1992. [25, 36, 37, 64, 207, 208, 361, 362, 489]

[162] R. J. Gray. Spline-based tests in survival analysis. *Biometrics*, 50:640–652, 1994. [25, 36, 37, 489]

[163] M. J. Greenacre. Correspondence analysis of multivariate categorical data by weighted least-squares. *Biometrika*, 75:457–467, 1988. [67]

[164] S. Greenland. Alternative models for ordinal logistic regression. *Statistics in Medicine*, 13:1665–1677, 1994. [342]

[165] S. Greenland and W. D. Finkle. A critical look at methods for handling missing covariates in epidemiologic regression analyses. *American Journal of Epidemiology*, 142:1255–1264, 1995. [42, 51]

[166] A. J. Gross and V. A. Clark. *Survival Distributions: Reliability Applications in the Biomedical Sciences.* Wiley, New York, 1975. [399]

[167] S. T. Gross and T. L. Lai. Nonparametric estimation and regression analysis with left-truncated and right-censored data. *Journal of the American Statistical Association*, 91:1166–1180, 1996. [410]

[168] A. Guisan and F. E. Harrell. Ordinal response regression models in ecology. *Journal of Vegetation Science*, 11:617–626, 2000. [342]

[169] P. Gustafson. Bayesian regression modeling with interactions and smooth effects. *Journal of the American Statistical Association*, 95:795–806, 2000. [37]

[170] M. Halperin, W. C. Blackwelder, and J. I. Verter. Estimation of the multivariate logistic risk function: A comparison of the discriminant function and maximum likelihood approaches. *Journal of Chronic Diseases*, 24:125–158, 1971. [217]

[171] D. J. Hand. *Construction and Assessment of Classification Rules.* Wiley, Chichester, 1997. [265]

[172] T. L. Hankins. Blood, dirt, and nomograms. *Chance*, 13:26–37, 2000. [98, 103, 256]

[173] J. A. Hanley and B. J. McNeil. The meaning and use of the area under a receiver operating characteristic (ROC) curve. *Radiology*, 143:29–36, 1982. [247]

[174] F. E. Harrell. The LOGIST Procedure. In *SUGI Supplemental Library Users Guide*, pages 269–293. SAS Institute, Inc., Cary, NC, Version 5 edition, 1986. [58]

[175] F. E. Harrell. The PHGLM Procedure. In *SUGI Supplemental Library Users Guide*, pages 437–466. SAS Institute, Inc., Cary, NC, Version 5 edition, 1986. [487]

[176] F. E. Harrell. Comparison of strategies for validating binary logistic regression models. Unpublished manuscript, 1991. [95, 249]

[177] F. E. Harrell. Semiparametric modeling of health care cost and resource utilization. Available from `hesweb1.med.virginia.edu/biostat/presentations`, 1999. [x]

[178] F. E. Harrell, R. M. Califf, D. B. Pryor, K. L. Lee, and R. A. Rosati. Evaluating the yield of medical tests. *Journal of the American Medical Association*, 247:2543–2546, 1982. [493]

[179] F. E. Harrell and R. Goldstein. A survey of microcomputer survival analysis software: The need for an integrated framework. *American Statistician*, 51:360–373, 1997. [120]

[180] F. E. Harrell and K. L. Lee. A comparison of the *discrimination* of discriminant analysis and logistic regression under multivariate normality. In P. K. Sen, editor, *Biostatistics: Statistics in Biomedical, Public Health, and Environmental Sciences. The Bernard G. Greenberg Volume*, pages 333–343. North-Holland, Amsterdam, 1985. [203, 205, 217, 248]

[181] F. E. Harrell and K. L. Lee. The practical value of logistic regression. In *Proceedings of the Tenth Annual SAS Users Group International Conference*, pages 1031–1036, 1985. [231]

[182] F. E. Harrell and K. L. Lee. Verifying assumptions of the Cox proportional hazards model. In *Proceedings of the Eleventh Annual SAS Users Group International Conference*, pages 823–828, Cary, NC, 1986. SAS Institute, Inc. [483, 487, 491]

[183] F. E. Harrell and K. L. Lee. Using logistic model calibration to assess the quality of probability predictions. Unpublished manuscript, 1991. [249, 250, 261, 495]

[184] F. E. Harrell, K. L. Lee, R. M. Califf, D. B. Pryor, and R. A. Rosati. Regression modeling strategies for improved prognostic prediction. *Statistics in Medicine*, 3:143–152, 1984. [61, 85, 351, 493]

[185] F. E. Harrell, K. L. Lee, and D. B. Mark. Multivariable prognostic models: Issues in developing models, evaluating assumptions and adequacy, and measuring and reducing errors. *Statistics in Medicine*, 15:361–387, 1996. [xi, 84]

[186] F. E. Harrell, K. L. Lee, D. B. Matchar, and T. A. Reichert. Regression models for prognostic prediction: Advantages, problems, and suggested solutions. *Cancer Treatment Reports*, 60:1071–1077, 1985. [37, 61]

[187] F. E. Harrell, K. L. Lee, and B. G. Pollock. Regression models in clinical studies: Determining relationships between predictors and response. *Journal of the National Cancer Institute*, 80:1198–1202, 1988. [26, 36]

[188] F. E. Harrell, P. A. Margolis, S. Gove, K. E. Mason, E. K. Mulholland, D. Lehmann, L. Muhe, S. Gatchalian, and H. F. Eichenwald. Development of a clinical prediction model for an ordinal outcome: The World Health Organization ARI Multicentre Study of clinical signs and etiologic agents of pneumonia, sepsis, and meningitis in young infants. *Statistics in Medicine*, 17:909–944, 1998. [xi, 64, 80, 345]

[189] D. P. Harrington and T. R. Fleming. A class of rank test procedures for censored survival data. *Biometrika*, 69:553–566, 1982. [505]

[190] T. Hastie. Discussion of "The use of polynomial splines and their tensor products in multivariate function estimation" by C. J. Stone. *Applied Statistics*, 22:177–179, 1994. [33]

[191] T. Hastie and R. Tibshirani. *Generalized Additive Models*. Chapman and Hall, London, 1990. [25, 36, 119, 376]

[192] T. J. Hastie, J. L. Botha, and C. M. Schnitzler. Regression with an ordered categorical response. *Statistics in Medicine*, 8:785–794, 1989. [342]

[193] W. W. Hauck and A. Donner. Wald's test as applied to hypotheses in logit analysis. *Journal of the American Statistical Association*, 72:851–863, 1977. [190, 229]

[194] X. He and L. Shen. Linear regression after spline transformation. *Biometrika*, 84:474–481, 1997. [67]

[195] R. Henderson. Problems and prediction in survival-data analysis. *Statistics in Medicine*, 14:161–184, 1995. [410, 506, 507]

[196] J. E. Herndon and F. E. Harrell. The restricted cubic spline hazard model. *Communications in Statistics – Theory and Methods*, 19:639–663, 1990. [399, 400]

[197] J. E. Herndon and F. E. Harrell. The restricted cubic spline as baseline hazard in the proportional hazards model with step function time-dependent covariables. *Statistics in Medicine*, 14:2119–2129, 1995. [399, 489, 507]

[198] I. Hertz-Picciotto and B. Rockhill. Validity and efficiency of approximation methods for tied survival times in Cox regression. *Biometrics*, 53:1151–1156, 1997. [468]

[199] K. R. Hess. Assessing time-by-covariate interactions in proportional hazards regression models using cubic spline functions. *Statistics in Medicine*, 13:1045–1062, 1994. [489]

[200] K. R. Hess. Graphical methods for assessing violations of the proportional hazards assumption in Cox regression. *Statistics in Medicine*, 14:1707–1723, 1995. [506]

[201] S. L. Hillis. Residual plots for the censored data linear regression model. *Statistics in Medicine*, 14:2023–2036, 1995. [441]

[202] S. G. Hilsenbeck and G. M. Clark. Practical p-value adjustment for optimally selected cutpoints. *Statistics in Medicine*, 15:103–112, 1996. [8]

[203] W. Hoeffding. A non-parametric test of independence. *Annals of Mathematical Statistics*, 19:546–557, 1948. [67, 153]

[204] H. Hofmann. Simpson on board the Titanic? Interactive methods for dealing with multivariate categorical data. *Statistical Computing and Graphics Newsletter, ASA*, 9(2):16–19, 1999. Article may be obtained from cm.bell-labs.com/cm/ms/who/cocteau/newsletter/issues/v92/v92.pdf. [299]

[205] J. W. Hogan and N. M. Laird. Mixture models for the joint distribution of repeated measures and event times. *Statistics in Medicine*, 16:239–257, 1997. [410]

[206] J. W. Hogan and N. M. Laird. Model-based approaches to analysing incomplete longitudinal and failure time data. *Statistics in Medicine*, 16:259–272, 1997. [410]

[207] M. Hollander, I. W. McKeague, and J. Yang. Likelihood ratio-based confidence bands for survival functions. *Journal of the American Statistical Association*, 92:215–226, 1997. [410]

[208] D. W. Hosmer, T. Hosmer, S. le Cessie, and S. Lemeshow. A comparison of goodness-of-fit tests for the logistic regression model. *Statistics in Medicine*, 16:965–980, 1997. [231]

[209] D. W. Hosmer and S. Lemeshow. Goodness-of-fit tests for the multiple logistic regression model. *Communications in Statistics – Theory and Methods*, 9:1043–1069, 1980. [231]

[210] D. W. Hosmer and S. Lemeshow. *Applied Logistic Regression*. Wiley, New York, 1989. [245, 265]

[211] D. W. Hosmer and S. Lemeshow. Confidence interval estimates of an index of quality performance based on logistic regression models. *Statistics in Medicine*, 14:2161–2172, 1995. [265]

[212] P. Hougaard. Fundamentals of survival data. *Biometrics*, 55:13–22, 1999. [390, 410, 441]

[213] P. J. Huber. The behavior of maximum likelihood estimates under nonstandard conditions. In *Proceedings of the Fifth Berkeley Symposium in Mathematical Statistics*, Volume 1, pages 221–233. University of California Press, Berkeley, CA, 1967. [193]

[214] S. Hunsberger, D. Murray, C. Davis, and R. R. Fabsitz. Imputation strategies for missing data in a school-based multi-center study: the Pathways study. *Statistics in Medicine*, 20:305–316, 2001. [51]

[215] C. M. Hurvich and C. Tsai. Regression and time series model selection in small samples. *Biometrika*, 76:297–307, 1989. [202]

[216] C. M. Hurvich and C. Tsai. Model selection for extended quasi-likelihood models in small samples. *Biometrics*, 51:1077–1084, 1995. [202]

[217] C. M. Hurvich and C. L. Tsai. The impact of model selection on inference in linear regression. *American Statistician*, 44:214–217, 1990. [84]

[218] L. I. Iezzoni. Dimensions of risk. In L. I. Iezzoni, editor, *Risk Adjustment for Measuring Health Outcomes*, Chapter 2, pages 29–118. Foundation of the American College of Healthcare Executives, Ann Arbor, MI, 1994. [5]

[219] R. Ihaka and R. Gentleman. R: A language for data analysis and graphics. *Journal of Computational and Graphical Statistics*, 5:299–314, 1996. [106]

[220] J. E. Jackson. *A User's Guide to Principal Components*. Wiley, New York, 1991. [84]

[221] N. L. Johnson and S. Kotz. *Distributions in Statistics: Continuous Univariate Distributions*, Volume 1. Houghton-Mifflin, Boston, 1970. [398, 399]

[222] I. T. Jolliffe. *Principal Component Analysis*. Springer-Verlag, New York, 1986. [84, 161]

[223] M. P. Jones. Indicator and stratification methods for missing explanatory variables in multiple linear regression. *Journal of the American Statistical Association*, 91:222–230, 1996. [50]

[224] A. C. Justice, K. E. Covinsky, and J. A. Berlin. Assessing the generalizability of prognostic information. *Annals of Internal Medicine*, 130:515–524, 1999. [101]

[225] J. D. Kalbfleisch and R. L. Prentice. Marginal likelihood based on Cox's regression and life model. *Biometrika*, 60:267–278, 1973. [468]

[226] J. D. Kalbfleisch and R. L. Prentice. *The Statistical Analysis of Failure Time Data.* Wiley, New York, 1980. [401, 402, 404, 410, 426, 430, 472, 485, 506]

[227] G. Kalton and D. Kasprzyk. The treatment of missing survey data. *Survey Methodology*, 12:1–16, 1986. [50]

[228] E. L. Kaplan and P. Meier. Nonparametric estimation from incomplete observations. *Journal of the American Statistical Association*, 53:457–481, 1958. [400]

[229] T. Karrison. Restricted mean life with adjustment for covariates. *Journal of the American Statistical Association*, 82:1169–1176, 1987. [396, 500]

[230] T. G. Karrison. Use of Irwin's restricted mean as an index for comparing survival in different treatment groups—Interpretation and power considerations. *Controlled Clinical Trials*, 18:151–167, 1997. [396, 491]

[231] R. E. Kass and A. E. Raftery. Bayes factors. *Journal of the American Statistical Association*, 90:773–795, 1995. [59, 202, 211]

[232] M. H. Katz. *Multivariable Analysis: A Practical Guide for Clinicians.* Cambridge University Press, 1999. [viii]

[233] R. Kay. Treatment effects in competing-risks analysis of prostate cancer data. *Biometrics*, 42:203–211, 1986. [269, 404, 483]

[234] R. Kay and S. Little. Assessing the fit of the logistic model: A case study of children with the haemolytic uraemic syndrome. *Applied Statistics*, 35:16–30, 1986. [265]

[235] P. J. Kelly and L. L. Lim. Survival analysis for recurrent event data: An application to childhood infectious diseases. *Statistics in Medicine*, 19:13–33, 2000. [411]

[236] J. T. Kent and J. O'Quigley. Measures of dependence for censored survival data. *Biometrika*, 75:525–534, 1988. [493]

[237] V. Kipnis. Relevancy criterion for discriminating among alternative model specifications. In K. Berk and L. Malone, editors, *Proceedings of the 21st Symposium on the Interface between Computer Science and Statistics*, pages 376–381, Alexandria, VA, 1989. American Statistical Association. [102]

[238] J. P. Klein, N. Keiding, and E. A. Copelan. Plotting summary predictions in multistate survival models: Probabilities of relapse and death in remission for bone marrow transplantation patients. *Statistics in Medicine*, 12:2314–2332, 1993. [405]

[239] J. P. Klein and M. L. Moeschberger. *Survival Analysis: Techniques for Censored and Truncated Data*. Springer, New York, 1997. [410, 506]

[240] W. A. Knaus, F. E. Harrell, C. J. Fisher, D. P. Wagner, S. M. Opan, J. C. Sadoff, E. A. Draper, C. A. Walawander, K. Conboy, and T. H. Grasela. The clinical evaluation of new drugs for sepsis: A prospective study design based on survival analysis. *Journal of the American Medical Association*, 270:1233–1241, 1993. [4]

[241] W. A. Knaus, F. E. Harrell, J. Lynn, L. Goldman, R. S. Phillips, A. F. Connors, N. V. Dawson, W. J. Fulkerson, R. M. Califf, N. Desbiens, P. Layde, R. K. Oye, P. E. Bellamy, R. B. Hakim, and D. P. Wagner. The SUPPORT prognostic model: Objective estimates of survival for seriously ill hospitalized adults. *Annals of Internal Medicine*, 122:191–203, 1995. [51, 70, 71, 443]

[242] G. G. Koch, I. A. Amara, and J. M. Singer. A two-stage procedure for the analysis of ordinal categorical data. In P. K. Sen, editor, *BIOSTATISTICS: Statistics in Biomedical, Public Health and Environmental Sciences*. Elsevier Science Publishers B. V. (North-Holland), Amsterdam, 1985. [342]

[243] C. Kooperberg and D. B. Clarkson. Hazard regression with interval-censored data. *Biometrics*, 53:1485–1494, 1997. [410, 441]

[244] C. Kooperberg, C. J. Stone, and Y. K. Truong. Hazard regression. *Journal of the American Statistical Association*, 90:78–94, 1995. [176, 410, 412, 441, 464, 506]

[245] E. L. Korn and F. J. Dorey. Applications of crude incidence curves. *Statistics in Medicine*, 11:813–829, 1992. [406]

[246] E. L. Korn and B. I. Graubard. Analysis of large health surveys: Accounting for the sampling design. *Journal of the Royal Statistical Society A*, 158:263–295, 1995. [206]

[247] E. L. Korn and B. I. Graubard. Examples of differing weighted and unweighted estimates from a sample survey. *American Statistician*, 49:291–295, 1995. [206]

[248] E. L. Korn and R. Simon. Measures of explained variation for survival data. *Statistics in Medicine*, 9:487–503, 1990. [204, 211, 492, 507]

[249] E. L. Korn and R. Simon. Explained residual variation, explained risk, and goodness of fit. *American Statistician*, 45:201–206, 1991. [204, 211, 265]

[250] A. Krause and M. Olson. *The Basics of S and S-PLUS*. Springer-Verlag, New York, second edition, 2000. [x]

[251] D. Kronborg and P. Aaby. Piecewise comparison of survival functions in stratified proportional hazards models. *Biometrics*, 46:375–380, 1990. [491]

[252] W. F. Kuhfeld. The PRINQUAL procedure. In *SAS/STAT User's Guide*, Volume 2, Chapter 34, pages 1265–1323. SAS Institute, Inc., Cary NC, fourth edition, 1990. [67, 68]

[253] J. M. Lachin and M. A. Foulkes. Evaluation of sample size and power for analyses of survival with allowance for nonuniform patient entry, losses to follow-up, noncompliance, and stratification. *Biometrics*, 42:507–519, 1986. [499]

[254] L. Lamport. *LaTeX: A Document Preparation System*. Addison-Wesley, Reading, MA, second edition, 1994. [524]

[255] R. Lancar, Λ. Kramar, and C. Haie-Meder. Non-parametric methods for analysing recurrent complications of varying severity. *Statistics in Medicine*, 14:2701–2712, 1995. [411]

[256] J. M. Landwehr, D. Pregibon, and A. C. Shoemaker. Graphical methods for assessing logistic regression models (with discussion). *Journal of the American Statistical Association*, 79:61–83, 1984. [265, 334]

[257] T. P. Lane and W. H. DuMouchel. Simultaneous confidence intervals in multiple regression. *American Statistician*, 48:315–321, 1994. [195]

[258] M. G. Larson and G. E. Dinse. A mixture model for the regression analysis of competing risks data. *Applied Statistics*, 34:201–211, 1985. [269, 404]

[259] P. W. Laud and J. G. Ibrahim. Predictive model selection. *Journal of the Royal Statistical Society B*, 57:247–262, 1995. [211]

[260] A. Laupacis, N. Sekar, and I. G. Stiell. Clinical prediction rules: A review and suggested modifications of methodological standards. *Journal of the American Medical Association*, 277:488–494, 1997. [4]

[261] B. Lausen and M. Schumacher. Evaluating the effect of optimized cutoff values in the assessment of prognostic factors. *Computational Statistics and Data Analysis*, 1996. [8]

[262] P. W. Lavori, R. Dawson, and T. B. Mueller. Causal estimation of time-varying treatment effects in observational studies: Application to depressive disorder. *Statistics in Medicine*, 13:1089–1100, 1994. [227]

[263] P. W. Lavori, R. Dawson, and D. Shera. A multiple imputation strategy for clinical trials with truncation of patient data. *Statistics in Medicine*, 14:1913–1925, 1995. [43]

[264] J. F. Lawless. *Statistical Models and Methods for Lifetime Data*. Wiley, New York, 1982. [410, 441, 474, 506]

[265] J. F. Lawless. The analysis of recurrent events for multiple subjects. *Applied Statistics*, 44:487–498, 1995. [411]

[266] J. F. Lawless and C. Nadeau. Some simple robust methods for the analysis of recurrent events. *Technometrics*, 37:158–168, 1995. [410, 411]

[267] J. F. Lawless and K. Singhal. Efficient screening of nonnormal regression models. *Biometrics*, 34:318–327, 1978. [58, 114]

[268] S. le Cessie and J. C. van Houwelingen. A goodness-of-fit test for binary regression models, based on smoothing methods. *Biometrics*, 47:1267–1282, 1991. [231]

[269] S. le Cessie and J. C. van Houwelingen. Ridge estimators in logistic regression. *Applied Statistics*, 41:191–201, 1992. [64, 207]

[270] M. LeBlanc and J. Crowley. Survival trees by goodness of fit. *Journal of the American Statistical Association*, 88:457–467, 1993. [37]

[271] M. LeBlanc and R. Tibshirani. Adaptive principal surfaces. *Journal of the American Statistical Association*, 89:53–64, 1994. [84]

[272] A. Leclerc, D. Luce, F. Lert, J. F. Chastang, and P. Logeay. Correspondance analysis and logistic modelling: Complementary use in the analysis of a health survey among nurses. *Statistics in Medicine*, 7:983–995, 1988. [67]

[273] E. T. Lee. *Statistical Methods for Survival Data Analysis*. Lifetime Learning Publications, Belmont CA, second edition, 1980. [410]

[274] E. W. Lee, L. J. Wei, and D. A. Amato. Cox-type regression analysis for large numbers of small groups of correlated failure time observations. In J. P. Klein and P. K. Goel, editors, *Survival Analysis: State of the Art*, NATO ASI, pages 237–247. Kluwer Academic, Boston, 1992. [193, 194]

[275] J. J. Lee, K. R. Hess, and J. A. Dubin. Extensions and applications of event charts. *American Statistician*, 54:63–70, 2000. [408, 410]

[276] K. L. Lee, D. B. Pryor, F. E. Harrell, R. M. Califf, V. S. Behar, W. L. Floyd, J. J. Morris, R. A. Waugh, R. E. Whalen, and R. A. Rosati. Predicting outcome in coronary disease: Statistical models versus expert clinicians. *American Journal of Medicine*, 80:553–560, 1986. [203]

[277] E. L. Lehmann. Model specification: The views of Fisher and Neyman and later developments. *Statistical Science*, 5:160–168, 1990. [6, 7]

[278] K. Li, J. Wang, and C. Chen. Dimension reduction for censored regression data. *Annals of Statistics*, 27:1–23, 1999. [84]

[279] K. C. Li. Sliced inverse regression for dimension reduction. *Journal of the American Statistical Association*, 86:316–327, 1991. [84]

[280] D. Y. Lin. Cox regression analysis of multivariate failure time data: The marginal approach. *Statistics in Medicine*, 13:2233–2247, 1994. [193, 194, 211, 407, 408]

[281] D. Y. Lin. Non-parametric inference for cumulative incidence functions in competing risks studies. *Statistics in Medicine*, 16:901–910, 1997. [405]

[282] D. Y. Lin. On fitting Cox's proportional hazards models to survey data. *Biometrika*, 87:37–47, 2000. [211]

[283] D. Y. Lin and L. J. Wei. The robust inference for the Cox proportional hazards model. *Journal of the American Statistical Association*, 84:1074–1078, 1989. [194, 211, 476]

[284] D. Y. Lin, L. J. Wei, and Z. Ying. Checking the Cox model with cumulative sums of martingale-based residuals. *Biometrika*, 80:557–572, 1993. [506]

[285] J. C. Lindsey and L. M. Ryan. Tutorial in biostatistics: Methods for interval-censored data. *Statistics in Medicine*, 17:219–238, 1998. [410]

[286] J. K. Lindsey and B. Jones. Choosing among generalized linear models applied to medical data. *Statistics in Medicine*, 17:59–68, 1998. [9]

[287] K. Linnet. Assessing diagnostic tests by a strictly proper scoring rule. *Statistics in Medicine*, 8:609–618, 1989. [94, 102, 247, 249]

[288] S. R. Lipsitz, L. P. Zhao, and G. Molenberghs. A semiparametric method of multiple imputation. *Journal of the Royal Statistical Society B*, 60:127–144, 1998. [48]

[289] R. J. Little. Missing data. In *Encyclopedia of Biostatistics*, pages 2622–2635. Wiley, New York, 1998. [50]

[290] R. J. A. Little. Missing-data adjustments in large surveys. *Journal of Business and Economic Statistics*, 6:287–296, 1988. [46]

[291] R. J. A. Little. Regression with missing X's: A review. *Journal of the American Statistical Association*, 87:1227–1237, 1992. [45, 47, 48]

[292] R. J. A. Little and D. B. Rubin. *Statistical Analysis with Missing Data*. Wiley, New York, 1987. [50]

[293] K. Liu and A. R. Dyer. A rank statistic for assessing the amount of variation explained by risk factors in epidemiologic studies. *American Journal of Epidemiology*, 109:597–606, 1979. [204, 247]

[294] J. S. Long and L. H. Ervin. Using heteroscedasticity consistent standard errors in the linear regression model. *American Statistician*, 54:217–224, 2000. [211]

[295] J. Lubsen, J. Pool, and E. van der Does. A practical device for the application of a diagnostic or prognostic function. *Methods of Information in Medicine*, 17:127–129, 1978. [98]

[296] M. Lunn and D. McNeil. Applying Cox regression to competing risks. *Biometrics*, 51:524–532, 1995. [410]

[297] G. S. Maddala. *Limited-Dependent and Qualitative Variables in Econometrics*. Cambridge University Press, Cambridge, UK, 1983. [205, 493]

[298] L. Magee. R^2 measures based on Wald and likelihood ratio joint significance tests. *American Statistician*, 44:250–253, 1990. [204, 493]

[299] L. Magee. Nonlocal behavior in polynomial regressions. *American Statistician*, 52:20–22, 1998. [18]

[300] C. Mallows. The zeroth problem. *American Statistician*, 52:1–9, 1998. [8]

[301] N. Mantel. Why stepdown procedures in variable selection. *Technometrics*, 12:621–625, 1970. [58]

[302] N. Mantel and D. P. Byar. Evaluation of response-time data involving transient states: An illustration using heart-transplant data. *Journal of the American Statistical Association*, 69:81–86, 1974. [392, 410]

[303] P. Margolis, E. K. Mulholland, F. E. Harrell, S. Gove, and the WHO Young Infants Study Group. Clinical prediction of serious bacterial infections in young infants in developing countries. *Pediatric Infectious Disease Journal*, 18S:S23–S31, 1999. [345]

[304] D. B. Mark, M. A. Hlatky, F. E. Harrell, K. L. Lee, R. M. Califf, and D. B. Pryor. Exercise treadmill score for predicting prognosis in coronary artery disease. *Annals of Internal Medicine*, 106:793–800, 1987. [498]

[305] G. Marshall, F. L. Grover, W. G. Henderson, and K. E. Hammermeister. Assessment of predictive models for binary outcomes: An empirical approach using operative death from cardiac surgery. *Statistics in Medicine*, 13:1501–1511, 1994. [85]

[306] E. Marubini and M. G. Valsecchi. *Analyzing Survival Data from Clinical Trials and Observational Studies*. Wiley, West Sussex, 1995. [210, 211, 405, 410, 489, 506]

[307] MathSoft. *S-PLUS 2000 Guide to Statistics*, Volume 1. MathSoft Data Analysis Products Division, Seattle, WA, 1999. [378]

[308] MathSoft. S-Plus *2000 User's Guide*. Data Analysis Products Division of MathSoft, Inc., Seattle, WA, 1999. [x, 105, 260]

[309] P. McCullagh. Regression models for ordinal data. *Journal of the Royal Statistical Society B*, 42:109–142, 1980. [333, 342]

[310] D. R. McNeil, J. Trussell, and J. C. Turner. Spline interpolation of demographic data. *Demography*, 14:245–252, 1977. [36]

[311] W. Q. Meeker and L. A. Escobar. Teaching about approximate confidence regions based on maximum likelihood estimation. *American Statistician*, 49:48–53, 1995. [211]

[312] S. Menard. Coefficients of determination for multiple logistic regression analysis. *American Statistician*, 54:17–24, 2000. [211, 265]

[313] X. Meng. Multiple-imputation inferences with uncongenial sources of input. *Statistical Science*, 9:538–558, 1994. [48]

[314] G. Michailidis and J. de Leeuw. The Gifi system of descriptive multivariate analysis. *Statistical Science*, 13:307–336, 1998. [67]

[315] M. E. Miller, S. L. Hui, and W. M. Tierney. Validation techniques for logistic regression models. *Statistics in Medicine*, 10:1213–1226, 1991. [249]

[316] R. G. Miller. What price Kaplan–Meier? *Biometrics*, 39:1077–1081, 1983. [403]

[317] S. Minkin. Profile-likelihood-based confidence intervals. *Applied Statistics*, 39:125–126, 1990. [211]

[318] M. Mittlböck and M. Schemper. Explained variation for logistic regression. *Statistics in Medicine*, 15:1987–1997, 1996. [211, 265]

[319] G. S. Mudholkar, D. K. Srivastava, and G. D. Kollia. A generalization of the Weibull distribution with application to the analysis of survival data. *Journal of the American Statistical Association*, 91:1575–1583, 1996. [410]

[320] L. R. Muenz. Comparing survival distributions: A review for nonstatisticians. II. *Cancer Investigation*, 1:537–545, 1983. [483, 490]

[321] R. H. Myers. *Classical and Modern Regression with Applications*. PWS-Kent, Boston, 1990. [65]

[322] N. J. D. Nagelkerke. A note on a general definition of the coefficient of determination. *Biometrika*, 78:691–692, 1991. [205, 247, 493]

[323] W. B. Nelson. Theory and applications of hazard plotting for censored failure data. *Technometrics*, 14:945–965, 1972. [403]

[324] N. H. Ng'andu. An empirical comparison of statistical tests for assessing the proportional hazards assumption of Cox's model. *Statistics in Medicine*, 16:611–626, 1997. [506]

[325] T. G. Nick and J. M. Hardin. Regression modeling strategies: An illustrative case study from medical rehabilitation outcomes research. *American Journal of Occupational Therapy*, 53:459–470, 1999. [viii, 84]

[326] P. C. O'Brien. Comparing two samples: Extensions of the *t*, rank-sum, and log-rank test. *Journal of the American Statistical Association*, 83:52–61, 1988. [227]

[327] M. K. B. Parmar and D. Machin. *Survival Analysis: A Practical Approach*. Wiley, Chichester, 1995. [410]

[328] P. Peduzzi, J. Concato, A. R. Feinstein, and T. R. Holford. Importance of events per independent variable in proportional hazards regression analysis. II. Accuracy and precision of regression estimates. *Journal of Clinical Epidemiology*, 48:1503–1510, 1995. [84]

[329] P. Peduzzi, J. Concato, E. Kemper, T. R. Holford, and A. R. Feinstein. A simulation study of the number of events per variable in logistic regression analysis. *Journal of Clinical Epidemiology*, 49:1373–1379, 1996. [61, 84]

[330] M. S. Pepe. Inference for events with dependent risks in multiple endpoint studies. *Journal of the American Statistical Association*, 86:770–778, 1991. [405]

[331] M. S. Pepe and J. Cai. Some graphical displays and marginal regression analyses for recurrent failure times and time dependent covariates. *Journal of the American Statistical Association*, 88:811–820, 1993. [407]

[332] M. S. Pepe, G. Longton, and M. Thornquist. A qualifier Q for the survival function to describe the prevalence of a transient condition. *Statistics in Medicine*, 10:413–421, 1991. [405]

[333] M. S. Pepe and M. Mori. Kaplan–Meier, marginal or conditional probability curves in summarizing competing risks failure time data? *Statistics in Medicine*, 12:737–751, 1993. [405]

[334] B. Peterson and S. L. George. Sample size requirements and length of study for testing interaction in a $1 \times k$ factorial design when time-to-failure is the outcome. *Controlled Clinical Trials*, 14:511–522, 1993. [499]

[335] B. Peterson and F. E. Harrell. Partial proportional odds models for ordinal response variables. *Applied Statistics*, 39:205–217, 1990. [335, 339, 342]

[336] A. N. Pettitt and I. Bin Daud. Investigating time dependence in Cox's proportional hazards model. *Applied Statistics*, 39:313–329, 1990. [486, 506]

[337] A. N. Phillips, S. G. Thompson, and S. J. Pocock. Prognostic scores for detecting a high risk group: Estimating the sensitivity when applied to new data. *Statistics in Medicine*, 9:1189–1198, 1990. [84]

[338] R. R. Picard and K. N. Berk. Data splitting. *American Statistician*, 44:140–147, 1990. [101]

[339] R. R. Picard and R. D. Cook. Cross-validation of regression models. *Journal of the American Statistical Association*, 79:575–583, 1984. [102]

[340] L. W. Pickle. Maximum likelihood estimation in the new computing environment. *Statistical Computing and Graphics Newsletter, ASA*, 2(2):6 15, November 1991. [210]

[341] M. C. Pike. A method of analysis of certain class of experiments in carcinogenesis. *Biometrics*, 22:142–161, 1966. [430, 432, 469]

[342] D. Pregibon. Logistic regression diagnostics. *Annals of Statistics*, 9:705–724, 1981. [245]

[343] D. Pregibon. Resistant fits for some commonly used logistic models with medical applications. *Biometrics*, 38:485–498, 1982. [264, 265]

[344] R. L. Prentice, J. D. Kalbfleisch, A. V. Peterson, N. Flournoy, V. T. Farewell, and N. E. Breslow. The analysis of failure times in the presence of competing risks. *Biometrics*, 34:541–554, 1978. [404]

[345] S. J. Press and S. Wilson. Choosing between logistic regression and discriminant analysis. *Journal of the American Statistical Association*, 73:699–705, 1978. [217]

[346] D. B. Pryor, F. E. Harrell, K. L. Lee, R. M. Califf, and R. A. Rosati. Estimating the likelihood of significant coronary artery disease. *American Journal of Medicine*, 75:771–780, 1983. [265]

[347] D. B. Pryor, F. E. Harrell, J. S. Rankin, K. L. Lee, L. H. Muhlbaier, H. N. Oldham, M. A. Hlatky, D. B. Mark, J. G. Reves, and R. M. Califf. The changing survival benefits of coronary revascularization over time. *Circulation (Supplement V)*, 76:13–21, 1987. [497]

[348] C. Quantin, T. Moreau, B. Asselain, J. Maccaria, and J. Lellouch. A regression survival model for testing the proportional hazards assumption. *Biometrics*, 52:874–885, 1996. [506]

[349] D. R. Ragland. Dichotomizing continuous outcome variables: Dependence of the magnitude of association and statistical power on the cutpoint. *Epidemiology*, 3:434–440, 1992. [8]

[350] M. Reilly and M. Pepe. The relationship between hot-deck multiple imputation and weighted likelihood. *Statistics in Medicine*, 16:5–19, 1997. [51]

[351] B. D. Ripley and P. J. Solomon. Statistical models for prevalent cohort data. *Biometrics*, 51:373–374, 1995. [410]

[352] J. S. Roberts and G. M. Capalbo. A SAS macro for estimating missing values in multivariate data. In *Proceedings of the Twelfth Annual SAS Users Group International Conference*, pages 939–941, Cary NC, 1987. SAS Institute, Inc. [47]

[353] J. M. Robins, S. D. Mark, and W. K. Newey. Estimating exposure effects by modeling the expectation of exposure conditional on confounders. *Biometrics*, 48:479–495, 1992. [227]

[354] L. D. Robinson and N. P. Jewell. Some surprising results about covariate adjustment in logistic regression models. *International Statistical Review*, 59:227–240, 1991. [227]

[355] E. B. Roecker. Prediction error and its estimation for subset-selected models. *Technometrics*, 33:459–468, 1991. [84, 92]

[356] W. H. Rogers. Regression standard errors in clustered samples. *Stata Technical Bulletin*, STB-13:19–23, May 1993. [193]

[357] P. R. Rosenbaum and D. Rubin. The central role of the propensity score in observational studies for causal effects. *Biometrika*, 70:41–55, 1983. [3, 227]

[358] P. R. Rosenbaum and D. B. Rubin. Assessing sensitivity to an unobserved binary covariate in an observational study with binary outcome. *Journal of the Royal Statistical Society B*, 45:212–218, 1983. [227]

[359] P. Royston and S. G. Thompson. Comparing non-nested regression models. *Biometrics*, 51:114–127, 1995. [211]

[360] D. Rubin and N. Schenker. Multiple imputation in health-care data bases: An overview and some applications. *Statistics in Medicine*, 10:585–598, 1991. [42, 46, 51]

[361] D. B. Rubin. *Multiple Imputation for Nonresponse in Surveys*. Wiley, New York, 1987. [48, 50]

[362] W. S. Sarle. The VARCLUS procedure. In *SAS/STAT User's Guide*, Volume 2, Chapter 43, pages 1641–1659. SAS Institute, Inc., Cary NC, fourth edition, 1990. [65, 66, 85]

[363] SAS Institute, Inc. *SAS/STAT User's Guide*, Volume 2. SAS Institute, Inc., Cary NC, fourth edition, 1990. [335]

[364] W. Sauerbrei and M. Schumacher. A bootstrap resampling procedure for model building: Application to the Cox regression model. *Statistics in Medicine*, 11:2093–2109, 1992. [59, 93, 175]

[365] R. M. Scammon, A. V. McGillivray, and R. Cook, editors. *America Votes 20: A Handbook of Contemporary American Election Statistics*. Congressional Quarterly, Washington, DC, 1992. [121]

[366] M. Schemper. Analyses of associations with censored data by generalized Mantel and Breslow tests and generalized Kendall correlation. *Biometrical Journal*, 26:309–318, 1984. [507]

[367] M. Schemper. Non-parametric analysis of treatment-covariate interaction in the presence of censoring. *Statistics in Medicine*, 7:1257–1266, 1988. [37]

[368] M. Schemper. The explained variation in proportional hazards regression (correction in 81:631, 1994). *Biometrika*, 77:216–218, 1990. [492, 493, 495]

[369] M. Schemper. Cox analysis of survival data with non-proportional hazard functions. *The Statistician*, 41:445–455, 1992. [506]

[370] M. Schemper. Further results on the explained variation in proportional hazards regression. *Biometrika*, 79:202–204, 1992. [493]

[371] M. Schemper. The relative importance of prognostic factors in studies of survival. *Statistics in Medicine*, 12:2377–2382, 1993. [211, 493]

[372] M. Schemper and G. Heinze. Probability imputation revisited for prognostic factor studies. *Statistics in Medicine*, 16:73–80, 1997. [47, 176]

[373] M. Schemper and R. Henderson. Predictive accuracy and explained variation in Cox regression. *Biometrics*, 56:249–255, 2000. [507]

552   References

[374] M. Schemper and T. L. Smith. Efficient evaluation of treatment effects in the presence of missing covariate values. *Statistics in Medicine*, 9:777–784, 1990. [47]

[375] M. Schemper and J. Stare. Explained variation in survival analysis. *Statistics in Medicine*, 15:1999–2012, 1996. [211, 507]

[376] C. Schmoor, K. Ulm, and M. Schumacher. Comparison of the Cox model and the regression tree procedure in analysing a randomized clinical trial. *Statistics in Medicine*, 12:2351–2366, 1993. [37]

[377] D. Schoenfeld. Partial residuals for the proportional hazards regression model. *Biometrika*, 69:239–241, 1982. [334, 486, 487, 504]

[378] D. A. Schoenfeld. Sample size formulae for the proportional hazards regression model. *Biometrics*, 39:499–503, 1983. [499]

[379] G. Schwarz. Estimating the dimension of a model. *Annals of Statistics*, 6:461–464, 1978. [202]

[380] S. C. Scott, M. S. Goldberg, and N. E. Mayo. Statistical assessment of ordinal outcomes in comparative studies. *Journal of Clinical Epidemiology*, 50:45–55, 1997. [342]

[381] M. R. Segal. Regression trees for censored data. *Biometrics*, 44:35–47, 1988. [37]

[382] J. Shao. Linear model selection by cross-validation. *Journal of the American Statistical Association*, 88:486–494, 1993. [84, 93, 101]

[383] J. Shao and R. R. Sitter. Bootstrap for imputed survey data. *Journal of the American Statistical Association*, 91:1278–1288, 1996. [48]

[384] Y. Shen and P. F. Thall. Parametric likelihoods for multiple non-fatal competing risks and death. *Statistics in Medicine*, 17:999–1015, 1998. [411]

[385] R. Simon and R. W. Makuch. A non-parametric graphical representation of the relationship between survival and the occurrence of an event: Application to responder versus non-responder bias. *Statistics in Medicine*, 3:35–44, 1984. [392, 410]

[386] J. S. Simonoff. The "unusual episode" and a second statistics course. *Journal of Statistics Education*, 5(1), 1997. Online journal at www.amstat.org/-publications/jse/v5n1/simonoff.html. [299]

[387] J. C. Sinclair and M. B. Bracken. Clinically useful measures of effect in binary analyses of randomized trials. *Journal of Clinical Epidemiology*, 47:881–889, 1994. [264]

[388] J. D. Singer and J. B. Willett. Modeling the days of our lives: Using survival analysis when designing and analyzing longitudinal studies of duration and the timing of events. *Psychological Bulletin*, 110:268–290, 1991. [410]

[389] L. A. Sleeper and D. P. Harrington. Regression splines in the Cox model with application to covariate effects in liver disease. *Journal of the American Statistical Association*, 85:941–949, 1990. [20, 36]

[390] A. F. M. Smith and D. J. Spiegelhalter. Bayes factors and choice criteria for linear models. *Journal of the Royal Statistical Society B*, 42:213–220, 1980. [211]

[391] L. R. Smith, F. E. Harrell, and L. H. Muhlbaier. Problems and potentials in modeling survival. In M. L. Grady and H. A. Schwartz, editors, *Medical Effectiveness Research Data Methods (Summary Report), AHCPR Pub. No. 92-0056*, pages 151–159. US Dept. of Health and Human Services, Agency for Health Care Policy and Research, Rockville, MD, 1992. [61]

[392] P. L. Smith. Splines as a useful and convenient statistical tool. *American Statistician*, 33:57–62, 1979. [36]

[393] R. H. Somers. A new asymmetric measure of association for ordinal variables. *American Sociological Review*, 27:799–811, 1962. [70, 247, 493]

[394] A. Spanos, F. E. Harrell, and D. T. Durack. Differential diagnosis of acute meningitis: An analysis of the predictive value of initial observations. *Journal of the American Medical Association*, 262:2700–2707, 1989. [255, 256, 258]

[395] P. Spector. *An Introduction to S and S-Plus*. Duxbury Press, Belmont, CA, 1994. [x, 105]

[396] I. Spence and R. F. Garrison. A remarkable scatterplot. *American Statistician*, 47:12–19, 1993. [76]

[397] D. J. Spiegelhalter. Probabilistic prediction in patient management and clinical trials. *Statistics in Medicine*, 5:421–433, 1986. [81, 84, 95, 96, 511]

[398] D. M. Stablein, W. H. Carter, and J. W. Novak. Analysis of survival data with nonproportional hazard functions. *Controlled Clinical Trials*, 2:149–159, 1981. [489]

[399] E. W. Steyerberg, M. J. C. Eijkemans, F. E. Harrell, and J. D. F. Habbema. Prognostic modelling with logistic regression analysis: A comparison of selection and estimation methods in small data sets. *Statistics in Medicine*, 19:1059–1079, 2000. [58, 84]

[400] E. W. Steyerberg, M. J. C. Eijkemans, F. E. Harrell, and J. D. F. Habbema. Prognostic modeling with logistic regression analysis: In search of a sensible strategy in small data sets. *Medical Decision Making*, 21:45–56, 2001. [84, 264]

[401] C. J. Stone. Comment: Generalized additive models. *Statistical Science*, 1:312–314, 1986. [23]

[402] C. J. Stone, M. H. Hansen, C. Kooperberg, and Y. K. Truong. Polynomial splines and their tensor products in extended linear modeling (with discussion). *Annals of Statistics*, 25:1371–1470, 1997. [410, 441]

[403] C. J. Stone and C. Y. Koo. Additive splines in statistics. In *Proceedings of the Statistical Computing Section ASA*, pages 45–48, Washington, DC, 1985. [20, 23, 36]

[404] D. Strauss and R. Shavelle. An extended Kaplan–Meier estimator and its applications. *Statistics in Medicine*, 17:971–982, 1998. [406]

[405] S. Suissa and L. Blais. Binary regression with continuous outcomes. *Statistics in Medicine*, 14:247–255, 1995. [8]

[406] G. Sun, T. L. Shook, and G. L. Kay. Inappropriate use of bivariable analysis to screen risk factors for use in multivariable analysis. *Journal of Clinical Epidemiology*, 49:907–916, 1996. [60]

[407] B. Tai, D. Machin, I. White, and V. Gebski. Competing risks analysis of patients with osteosarcoma: a comparison of four different approaches. *Statistics in Medicine*, 20:661–684, 2001. [410]

[408] J. M. G. Taylor, A. L. Siqueira, and R. E. Weiss. The cost of adding parameters to a model. *Journal of the Royal Statistical Society B*, 58:593–607, 1996. [84]

[409] H. T. Thaler. Nonparametric estimation of the hazard ratio. *Journal of the American Statistical Association*, 79:290–293, 1984. [506]

[410] P. F. Thall and J. M. Lachin. Assessment of stratum-covariate interactions in Cox's proportional hazards regression model. *Statistics in Medicine*, 5:73–83, 1986. [471]

[411] T. Therneau and P. Grambsch. *Modeling Survival Data: Extending the Cox Model*. Springer-Verlag, New York, 2000. [410, 506]

[412] T. M. Therneau, P. M. Grambsch, and T. R. Fleming. Martingale-based residuals for survival models. *Biometrika*, 77:216–218, 1990. [194, 404, 476, 480, 482, 492]

[413] T. M. Therneau and S. A. Hamilton. rhDNase as an example of recurrent event analysis. *Statistics in Medicine*, 16:2029–2047, 1997. [410, 411]

[414] R. Tibshirani. Estimating transformations for regression via additivity and variance stabilization. *Journal of the American Statistical Association*, 83:394–405, 1988. [377]

[415] R. Tibshirani. Regression shrinkage and selection via the lasso. *Journal of the Royal Statistical Society B*, 58:267–288, 1996. [59, 212, 371]

[416] R. Tibshirani. The lasso method for variable selection in the Cox model. *Statistics in Medicine*, 16:385–395, 1997. [59, 371]

[417] R. Tibshirani and K. Knight. Model search and inference by bootstrap "bumping". Technical report, Department of Statistics, University of Toronto, http://www-stat.stanford.edu/~tibs/, 1997. Presented at the Joint Statistical Meetings, Chicago, August 1996. [196]

[418] R. Tibshirani and K. Knight. The covariance inflation criterion for adaptive model selection. *Journal of the Royal Statistical Society B*, 61:529–546, 1999. [9, 102]

[419] N. H. Timm. The estimation of variance-covariance and correlation matrices from incomplete data. *Psychometrika*, 35:417–437, 1970. [47]

[420] W. Y. Tsai, N. P. Jewell, and M. C. Wang. A note on the product limit estimator under right censoring and left truncation. *Biometrika*, 74:883–886, 1987. [410]

[421] A. A. Tsiatis. A large sample study of Cox's regression model. *Annals of Statistics*, 9:93–108, 1981. [474]

[422] B. W. Turnbull. Nonparametric estimation of a survivorship function with doubly censored data. *Journal of the American Statistical Association*, 69:169–173, 1974. [410]

[423] Ü. Uzunoğullari and J.-L. Wang. A comparison of hazard rate estimators for left truncated and right censored data. *Biometrika*, 79:297–310, 1992. [410]

[424] W. Vach. *Logistic Regression with Missing Values in the Covariates*, Volume 86 of *Lecture Notes in Statistics*. Springer-Verlag, New York, 1994. [50]

[425] W. Vach. Some issues in estimating the effect of prognostic factors from incomplete covariate data. *Statistics in Medicine*, 16:57–72, 1997. [47, 50]

[426] W. Vach and M. Blettner. Logistic regression with incompletely observed categorical covariates—Investigating the sensitivity against violation of the missing at random assumption. *Statistics in Medicine*, 14:1915–1929, 1995. [50]

[427] W. Vach and M. Blettner. Missing data in epidemiologic studies. In *Encyclopedia of Biostatistics*, pages 2641–2654. Wiley, New York, 1998. [47, 50]

[428] W. Vach and M. Schumacher. Logistic regression with incompletely observed categorical covariates: A comparison of three approaches. *Biometrika*, 80:353–362, 1993. [50]

[429] M. G. Valsecchi, D. Silvestri, and P. Sasieni. Evaluation of long-term survival: Use of diagnostics and robust estimators with Cox's proportional hazards model. *Statistics in Medicine*, 15:2763–2780, 1996. [506, 507]

[430] S. van Buuren, H. C. Boshuizen, and D. L. Knook. Multiple imputation of missing blood pressure covariates in survival analysis. *Statistics in Medicine*, 18:681–694, 1999. [50]

[431] H. C. van Houwelingen and J. Thorogood. Construction, validation and updating of a prognostic model for kidney graft survival. *Statistics in Medicine*, 14:1999–2008, 1995. [84, 102, 212]

[432] J. C. van Houwelingen and S. le Cessie. Logistic regression, a review. *Statistica Neerlandica*, 42:215–232, 1988. [264]

[433] J. C. van Houwelingen and S. le Cessie. Predictive value of statistical models. *Statistics in Medicine*, 8:1303–1325, 1990. [63, 64, 84, 93, 95, 102, 103, 202, 211, 248, 249, 265, 495, 496, 507]

[434] W. N. Venables and B. D. Ripley. *Modern Applied Statistics with S-Plus*. Springer-Verlag, New York, third edition, 1999. [x, 85, 105, 107]

[435] D. J. Venzon and S. H. Moolgavkar. A method for computing profile-likelihood-based confidence intervals. *Applied Statistics*, 37:87–94, 1988. [211]

[436] P. Verweij and H. C. van Houwelingen. Penalized likelihood in Cox regression. *Statistics in Medicine*, 13:2427–2436, 1994. [64, 207, 208, 209, 212]

[437] P. J. M. Verweij and H. C. V. Houwelingen. Cross-validation in survival analysis. *Statistics in Medicine*, 12:2305–2314, 1993. [84, 102, 205, 212, 496, 507]

[438] P. J. M. Verweij and H. C. van Houwelingen. Time-dependent effects of fixed co-variates in Cox regression. *Biometrics*, 51:1550–1556, 1995. [207, 209, 489]

[439] S. K. Vines. Simple principal components. *Applied Statistics*, 49:441–451, 2000. [85]

[440] S. H. Walker and D. B. Duncan. Estimation of the probability of an event as a function of several independent variables. *Biometrika*, 54:167–178, 1967. [12, 216, 331, 333]

[441] A. R. Walter, A. R. Feinstein, and C. K. Wells. Coding ordinal independent variables in multiple regression analyses. *American Journal of Epidemiology*, 125:319–323, 1987. [34]

[442] M. Wang and S. Chang. Nonparametric estimation of a recurrent survival function. *Journal of the American Statistical Association*, 94:146–153, 1999. [411]

[443] R. Wang, J. Sedransk, and J. H. Jinn. Secondary data analysis when there are missing observations. *Journal of the American Statistical Association*, 87:952–961, 1992. [47]

[444] Y. Wang and J. M. G. Taylor. Inference for smooth curves in longitudinal data with application to an AIDS clinical trial. *Statistics in Medicine*, 14:1205–1218, 1995. [212]

[445] Y. Wang, G. Wahba, C. Gu, R. Klein, and B. Klein. Using smoothing spline ANOVA to examine the relation of risk factors to the incidence and progression of diabetic retinopathy. *Statistics in Medicine*, 16:1357–1376, 1997. [37]

[446] Y. Wax. Collinearity diagnosis for a relative risk regression analysis: An application to assessment of diet-cancer relationship in epidemiological studies. *Statistics in Medicine*, 11:1273–1287, 1992. [65, 116, 244]

[447] L. J. Wei, D. Y. Lin, and L. Weissfeld. Regression analysis of multivariate incomplete failure time data by modeling marginal distributions. *Journal of the American Statistical Association*, 84:1065–1073, 1989. [407]

[448] R. E. Weiss. The influence of variable selection: A Bayesian diagnostic perspective. *Journal of the American Statistical Association*, 90:619–625, 1995. [84]

[449] S. Wellek. A log-rank test for equivalence of two survivor functions. *Biometrics*, 49:877–881, 1993. [441]

[450] T. L. Wenger, F. E. Harrell, K. K. Brown, S. Lederman, and H. C. Strauss. Ventricular fibrillation following canine coronary reperfusion: Different outcomes with pentobarbital and α-chloralose. *Canadian Journal of Physiology and Pharmacology*, 62:224–228, 1984. [256]

[451] H. White. A heteroskedasticity-consistent covariance matrix estimator and a direct test for heteroskedasticity. *Econometrica*, 48:817–838, 1980. [193]

[452] J. Whitehead. Sample size calculations for ordered categorical data. *Statistics in Medicine*, 12:2257 2271, 1993. [2, 61, 333, 342]

[453] J. Whittaker. Model interpretation from the additive elements of the likelihood function. *Applied Statistics*, 33:52–64, 1984. [203, 206]

[454] A. S. Whittemore and J. B. Keller. Survival estimation using splines. *Biometrics*, 42:495–506, 1986. [410]

[455] A. R. Willan, W. Ross, and T. A. MacKenzie. Comparing in-patient classification systems: A problem of non-nested regression models. *Statistics in Medicine*, 11:1321 1331, 1992. [203, 211]

[456] J. P. Willems, J. T. Saunders, D. E. Hunt, and J. B. Schorling. Prevalence of coronary heart disease risk factors among rural blacks: A community-based study. *Southern Medical Journal*, 90:814–820, 1997. [379]

[457] C. F. J. Wu. Jackknife, bootstrap and other resampling methods in regression analysis. *Annals of Statistics*, 14(4).1261–1350, 1986. [93]

[458] J. Ye. On measuring and correcting the effects of data mining and model selection. *Journal of the American Statistical Association*, 93:120–131, 1998. [8]

[459] T. W. Yee and C. J. Wild. Vector generalized additive models. *Journal of the Royal Statistical Society B*, 58:481–493, 1996. [342]

[460] F. W. Young, Y. Takane, and J. de Leeuw. The principal components of mixed measurement level multivariate data: An alternating least squares method with optimal scaling features. *Psychometrika*, 43:279–281, 1978. [67]

[461] H. Zhang. Classification trees for multiple binary responses. *Journal of the American Statistical Association*, 93:180–193, 1998. [37]

[462] H. Zhang, T. Holford, and M. B. Bracken. A tree-based method of analysis for prospective studies. *Statistics in Medicine*, 15:37–49, 1996. [37]

[463] B. Zheng and A. Agresti. Summarizing the predictive power of a generalized linear model. *Statistics in Medicine*, 19:1771–1781, 2000. [211, 265]

[464] X. Zheng and W. Loh. Consistent variable selection in linear models. *Journal of the American Statistical Association*, 90:151–156, 1995. [211]

[465] X. Zhou. Effect of verification bias on positive and negative predictive values. *Statistics in Medicine*, 13:1737–1745, 1994. [346]

[466] D. M. Zucker. The efficiency of a weighted log-rank test under a percent error misspecification model for the log hazard ratio. *Biometrics*, 48:893–899, 1992. [506]

Index

Entries in `this font` are names of software components. Page numbers in **bold** denote the most comprehensive treatment of the topic.

Springer Series in Statistics   *(continued from p. ii)*

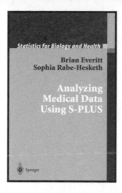
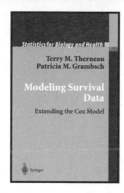
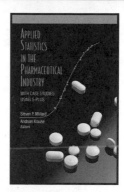
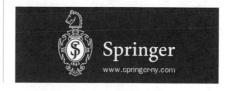